D1303439

Advanced Practice
NURSING

EMPHASIZING
COMMON ROLES

Edition 3

Advanced Practice
NURSING

EMPHASIZING
COMMON ROLES

Joan M. Stanley,
PhD, RN, CRNP, FAAN
Senior Director of Education Policy
American Association of Colleges of Nursing
Washington, DC

F.A. Davis Company • Philadelphia

F. A. Davis Company
1915 Arch Street
Philadelphia, PA 19103
www.fadavis.com

Copyright © 2011 by F. A. Davis Company

All rights reserved. This book is protected by copyright. No part of it may be reproduced, stored in a retrieval system, or transmitted in any form or by any means, electronic, mechanical, photocopying, recording, or otherwise, without written permission from the publisher.

Printed in the United States of America

Last digit indicates print number: 10 9 8 7 6 5 4 3 2 1

Publisher, Nursing: Joanne Patzek DaCunha, RN, MSN
Developmental Editor: Barbara Tchabovsky
Director of Content Development: Darlene D. Pedersen
Project Editor: Tyler R. Baber
Manager of Art and Design: Carolyn O'Brien

As new scientific information becomes available through basic and clinical research, recommended treatments and drug therapies undergo changes. The author(s) and publisher have done everything possible to make this book accurate, up to date, and in accord with accepted standards at the time of publication. The author(s), editors, and publisher are not responsible for errors or omissions or for consequences from application of the book, and make no warranty, expressed or implied, in regard to the contents of the book. Any practice described in this book should be applied by the reader in accordance with professional standards of care used in regard to the unique circumstances that may apply in each situation. The reader is advised always to check product information (package inserts) for changes and new information regarding dose and contraindications before administering any drug. Caution is especially urged when using new or infrequently ordered drugs.

Library of Congress Cataloging-in-Publication Data

Advanced practice nursing : emphasizing common roles / [edited by] Joan M. Stanley. — Ed. 3.
p. ; cm.
Includes bibliographical references and index.
ISBN 978-0-8036-2207-4 (pbk. : alk. paper)
1. Nurse practitioners—United States. 2. Midwives—United States. 3. Nurse anesthetists—United States
I. Stanley, Joan M. (Joan Marlene), 1949-
[DNLM: 1. Advanced Practice Nursing. WY 128 A2445 2011]
RT82.8.A37 2011
610.7306'92—dc22   2010013948

Authorization to photocopy items for internal or personal use, or the internal or personal use of specific clients, is granted by F. A. Davis Company for users registered with the Copyright Clearance Center (CCC) Transactional Reporting Service, provided that the fee of $.25 per copy is paid directly to CCC, 222 Rosewood Drive, Danvers, MA 01923. For those organizations that have been granted a photocopy license by CCC, a separate system of payment has been arranged. The fee code for users of the Transactional Reporting Service is: 8036-2207/11 0 + $.25.

This book is dedicated to all of the APRNs who have worked tirelessly for the past five decades to bring us to where we are today!

The current healthcare reform debate in Congress and across the nation raises the possibility of major changes in the emphasis and structure of our healthcare system. Regardless of the immediate outcome, concerns about cost, quality, access, effectiveness of interventions, prioritizing prevention, and workforce inadequacy are likely to persist and provoke transformations far beyond the legislative horizon. Once Pandora's Box is open, it is impossible to shut again. In this context, the contribution of nursing to the quality of care and patient outcomes—and especially the contribution of advanced practice registered nurses (APRNs)—is attaining growing recognition. APRNs are seen increasingly as a promising, long-overlooked source of solutions to the shortage of primary care physicians and the inadequate management of chronic diseases. The potential for nurse practitioners and other APRNs to influence the form and substance of healthcare delivery has never been so manifest. New models of care and new practice structures are being proposed that harness the knowledge and skills of APRNs.

This book, now in its third edition, provides an in-depth understanding of the past, present, and future of advanced practice nursing and why APRNs are poised to lead the reconceptualization of health care and assume greater prominence in its delivery. The authors ably describe current issues and trends faced by APRNs, their historical antecedents, and the major policy implications of practice, education, and regulatory developments. Although each of the four APRN roles—certified nurse-midwife, certified registered nurse anesthetist, clinical nurse specialist, certified nurse practitioner—has evolved along a different path, collectively they have changed nursing education and the way care is delivered. APRNs continue to lead changes in practice and in the healthcare system.

The chapters in this book cover a wide range of topics, from microsystems thinking, practice inquiry, intra- and interprofessional education, and ethics to credentialing, reimbursement, and marketing. The implications of pay for performance and retail clinics are detailed, as are issues related to scope of practice. The description of recent education/practice developments, such as the Doctor of Nursing Practice degree and the *Consensus Model for APRN Regulation*, documents the evolution of APRNs and provides a vision for the future of advanced practice nursing.

Each chapter presents perspectives on issues relevant to current APRN practice, education, certification, and licensure. A valuable part of each chapter is the suggested exercises. Thinking through the questions will give APRNs and others a chance to explore issues from a perspective they may not have considered. In addition, new to this third edition is a complementary instructor online resource that provides suggestions for teaching the content, a selection of PowerPoint slides for classroom use, and additional learning exercises for faculty to help them integrate this content into the APRN curriculum and learning experiences. Also, provided online for students are additional learning exercises and useful Web links.

This book will be a valuable resource for students, faculty, practicing APRNs, health systems that employ APRNs, policy makers, and certifying organizations.

Janet D. Allan, PhD, RN, NP, FAAN
Dean and Professor
The University of Maryland School of Nursing

ACKNOWLEDGMENTS

As an APRN for the past 37 years, I have made many lasting and cherished friends among the APRN community. Heartfelt thanks go out to all on whom I called and who allowed me to cajole them into contributing to this project. Their collegiality continues to be demonstrated over and over.

Special thanks go to my editor, Joanne DaCunha, and her staff for their patience and support through the many stages of writing and production.

Finally, loving thanks go to my husband, Jack, and my two sons, Jon and Jeff, for their understanding, love, and support. And to my sister, June, an FNP, who has always been there for me when I needed a listening ear or a laugh: Thank you!

Janet D. Allan, PhD, RN, NP, FAAN
Dean and Professor
The University of Maryland School
of Nursing
Baltimore, Maryland

Geraldine "Polly" Bednash, PhD, RN, FAAN
Chief Executive Officer
American Association of Colleges of
Nursing
Washington, DC

Linda A. Bernhard, PhD, RN
Associate Professor of Nursing and Women's
Studies
Ohio State University
Columbus, Ohio

Margaret T. Bowers, MSN, RN, FNP-BC
Assistant Clinical Professor
Duke University School of Nursing
Nurse Practitioner in the Duke Heart Failure
Disease Management Program
Durham, North Carolina

Christine E. Burke, PhD, CNM
Clinical Practice
The Denver Health Authority
Denver, Colorado

Linda Callahan, PhD, CRNA
Professor, Department of Nursing
California State University
Long Beach, California

Katherine Crabtree, DNSC, APRN-BC, FAAN
Professor of Nursing
Oregon Health and Science University
Portland, Oregon

Linda Lindsey Davis,
PhD, RN, ANP, DP-NAP, FAAN
Professor, Duke University School of Nursing
Senior Fellow, Duke Center for Aging and
Human Development
Durham, North Carolina

Mary Anne Dumas,
PhD, RN, FNP-BC, FAANP
Professor, School of Nursing
Stony Brook University
Stony Brook, New York

Marilyn Winterton Edmunds,
PhD, ANP-BC/GNP-BC
Editor of the *Journal for Nurse Practitioners*

Margaret Faut-Callahan, PhD, CRNA, FAAN
Dean, Marquette University School of
Nursing
Milwaukee, Wisconsin

Francis R. Gerbasi, PhD, CRNA
Executive Director
Council on Accreditation of Nurse
Anesthesia Educational Programs
Chicago, Illinois

Elaine Germano, DrPH, CNM, FACNM
Education Projects Manager
American College of Nurse-Midwives
Silver Spring, Maryland

Catherine L. Gilliss, DNSC, RN, FAAN
Dean and Professor
Duke University School of Nursing
Vice Chancellor of Nursing Affairs at Duke
Medicine
Durham, North Carolina

Kelly A. Goudreau, DSN, RN, ACNS-BC
Designated Learning/Education Officer
Portland VA Medical Center
Portland, Oregon

Gene Harkless, DNSC, FNP-C, CNL
Associate Professor and Graduate Program
Coordinator
University of New Hampshire
Durham, New Hampshire
Visiting Professor
Sor Trondelag University College of Nursing
Trondheim, Norway

Anita Hunter, PhD, CPNP, FAAN
Professor
University of San Diego
San Diego, California

Jean Johnson, PhD, RN, FAAN
Senior Associate Dean for Health Sciences
Professor, Department of Nursing
George Washington University
Washington, DC

M. Christina Johnson, MS, CNM
Director of Professional Practice and Health
  Policy
American College of Nurse-Midwives
Silver Spring, Maryland

Mary Knudtson, DNSC, NP, FAAN
Executive Director of Student Health
  Services
University of California in Santa Cruz
Professor of Nursing
University of California, Irvine
Irvine, California

Michael J. Kremer, PhD, CRNA, FAAN
Associate Professor and Director of
  the Nurse Anesthesia Program
Rush University College of Nursing
Chicago, Illinois

Leo A. Le Bel, M.Ed, JD, APRN, CRNA
Certified Registered Nurse Anesthetist,
  Practicing in Connecticut
Co-owner of a Connecticut healthcare
  consulting company
Huntington, Connecticut

Mary Jeanette Mannino, JD, CRNA
Director, Anesthesia and Ambulatory
  Surgery
The Mannino Group
Washington, DC

Margaret McAllister, PhD, RN, CNS, FNP
Clinical Associate Professor and
  Coordinator of the Family Nurse
  Practitioner Program
University of Massachusetts Boston College
  of Nursing and Health Sciences
Boston, Massachusetts

Eileen T. O'Grady, PhD, RN, NP
Visiting Professor
Pace University Leinhard School of Nursing
New York City, New York

Julie A. Stanik-Hutt,
  PhD, ACNP-BC, CCNS, FAAN
Associate Professor and Director of the
  Master's Program
Johns Hopkins University, School of
  Nursing
Baltimore, Maryland

Joan M. Stanley, PhD, RN, CRNP, FAAN
Senior Director of Education Policy
American Association of Colleges of
  Nursing
Washington, DC

Deirdre K. Thornlow, PhD, RN, CPHQ
Assistant Professor
Duke University School of Nursing
Durham, North Carolina

Jan Towers,
  PhD, NP-C, CRNP, FAANP, FAAN
Director of Health Policy
American Academy of Nurse Practitioners
Washington, DC

Michelle Walsh, PhD, RN, CPNP
Pediatric Nurse Practitioner
Nationwide Children's Hospital
Columbus, Ohio

Tammy L. Austin-Ketch,
   PhD(c), APRN, BC, FNP
Clinical Assistant Professor
University at Buffalo
State University of New York
Buffalo, New York

Susan A. Bruce, PhD(c), ANP
Clinical Associate Professor
University at Buffalo
Buffalo, New York

Linda L. Lindeke, PhD, RN, CNP
Associate Professor, Director of Graduate
   Studies
University of Minnesota
Minneapolis, Minnesota

Joanne Farley Serembus,
   EdD, RN, CCRN, CNE
Director, MSN and RN-BSN Programs
Drexel University
College of Nursing and Health Professions
Philadelphia, Pennsylvania

Mary L. Shea, PhD(c)
Assistant Professor
Colby-Sawyer College
New London, New Hampshire

Sharon J. Thompson, PhD, RN, MPH
Assistant Professor and Graduate Nursing
   Program Director
Gannon University
Villa Maria School of Nursing
Erie, Pennsylvania

L. Diane Weed, PhD, FNP
Associate Professor
Troy University School of Nursing
Troy, Alabama

CONSULTANTS

Lynne M. Dunphy, PhD, FNP, CS
Associate Professor
Florida Atlantic University
Boca Raton, Florida

Laurie Kennedy-Malone,
   PhD, RN, APRN-BC, GNP
Associate Professor
Director of the Adult/Gerontological Nurse
   Practitioner Program
School of Nursing
University of North Carolina at Greensboro
Greensboro, North Carolina

CONTENTS

CHAPTER 9   **Advanced Practice Nursing: Inquiry and Evaluation**   **247**

Deirdre K. Thornlow, PhD, RN, CPHQ

CHAPTER 10   **Publishing in Nursing Journals**   **279**

Marilyn Winterton Edmunds, PhD, ANP-BC/GNP-BC

CHAPTER 11   **Legal and Ethical Aspects of Advanced Nursing Practice**   **293**

Linda Callahan, PhD, CRNA

Mary Jeanette Mannino, JD, CRNA

CHAPTER 12   **Global Health and International Opportunities**

Anita Hunter, PhD, CPNP, FAAN

Katherine Crabtree, DNSC, APRN-BC, FAAN

CHAPTER 13   Advanced Practice Nursing and Health Policy   351

Eileen T. O'Grady, PhD, RN, NP

CHAPTER 14   The Advanced Practice Registered Nurse as Educator   379

Margaret McAllister, PhD, RN, CNS, FNP

CHAPTER 15   Clinical Microsystem Thinking and Resources for Advanced Practice Nursing   401

Gene Harkless, DNSC, FNP-C, CNL

CHAPTER 16   The Future of APRN Practice and the Impact of Current Healthcare Trends   417

Jean Johnson, PhD, RN, FAAN
Joan Stanley, PhD, RN, CRNP, FAAN

INTRODUCTION

Joan M. Stanley, PhD, RN, CRNP, FAAN

One commonality that undergirds all four advanced practice registered nursing (APRN) roles—certified registered nurse anesthetist (CRNA), clinical nurse specialist (CNS), certified nurse-midwife (CNM), and nurse practitioner (NP)—is the discipline of nursing. At the same time, it is the unique combination of advanced nursing knowledge, science, and practice that differentiates each of the APRN roles from one another and from other health professional roles and practice. Now is an exciting time for APRNs. After many decades, the cost-effectiveness and beneficial outcomes of advanced nursing practice are being widely recognized by policy makers, other health professionals, and the public. Despite of or because of the increased recognition of APRNs and of the advances made, APRNs face many recurrent issues, including attempts to limit their scope of practice, rising costs of malpractice insurance premiums, establishing parity with other health professions, maintaining ongoing competence, and obtaining standardized recognition for reimbursement, primary care status, and practice privileges.

Two sentinel events in the past 5 years stand to shape the future of advanced practice nursing more than any other events have throughout history:

- Completion and endorsement of the *Consensus Model for APRN Regulation*
- Transition of Advanced Practice Nursing education to the Doctor of Nursing Practice (DNP) degree.

Increasingly over the past 10 years, leaders in the APRN community recognized the need for and benefit of collaborating in addressing common concerns surrounding licensure, accreditation, certification, education, and practice. The culmination of these collaborative efforts resulted in the *Consensus Model for APRN Regulation: Licensure, Accreditation, Certification, and Education.*[1] Now endorsed by 45 national nursing organizations, this bellwether document creates not only a standardized model for regulation of all APRNs but also a unified platform from which APRNs are poised to assume a leadership role in today's healthcare system.

Also over the past 10 to 15 years, the healthcare needs of the United States have changed dramatically. Increasing numbers of older adults, rapid increases in chronic conditions, new technologies, and genetics are just a few of the massive changes that are affecting the healthcare system. A number of landmark reports, including the Institute of Medicine (IOM) reports *To Err Is Human: Building a Safer Health System*[2] and *Crossing the Quality Chasm: A New Health System for the 21st Century*[3] have determined that healthcare professionals cannot continue to practice as usual. In a follow-up report, *Health Professions Education: A Bridge to Quality,*[4] the IOM charged all health professions to change the ways providers are educated and to include new required competencies. Nursing is not the only profession that has examined the way practitioners are educated. Medicine, physical therapy, occupational therapy, and pharmacy have all re-examined their educational programs and have made major recommendations regarding how future practitioners will be educated.

These massive changes in health care and the mandates to the healthcare community to change the way healthcare professionals are educated and practice have provided the impetus for the movement to the DNP for all advanced nursing practice education. The APRN community also recognized that the massive changes in the health arena had already resulted in increased credit requirements and length of educational programs over the past decade. Therefore, after many years of investigation and dialogue within and outside the nursing profession, the American Association of Colleges of Nursing (AACN) membership in 2004 approved the position that advanced practice nursing education evolve to the DNP level by 2015.[5] This position was reinforced by the National Research Council of the National Academy of Science in a subsequent report, which stated that "the need for doctorally prepared practitioners and clinical faculty would be met if nursing could develop a new non-research clinical doctorate, similar to the MD and PharmD in medicine and pharmacy."[6(p 74)] Other APRN organizations, including the National Organization of Nurse Practitioner Faculties (NONPF), have endorsed the transition to the DNP for entry into advanced nursing practice. The DNP programs will focus on practice, preparing clinicians with the expertise needed to function at the highest level in an area of advanced or specialty nursing practice.

Critical issues facing APRNs are changing constantly. Just since beginning work on this text, changes in economic policies, health policies, funding sources, and even organizational policies have significantly affected, both positively and negatively, APRN practice and education. An overall and ongoing awareness of these issues, and of others not yet evident, is imperative if each APRN is to navigate the current and future healthcare environment successfully.

Four nursing leaders, each recognized for leadership and expertise in one of the APRN roles, were asked to identify and briefly discuss the critical issues facing their specific APRN role now and in the near future. These perspectives represent the individual's opinion and personal thoughts and are presented here as a basis for reflection and discussion.

The Certified Registered Nurse Anesthetist: Key Issues Today and Tomorrow

Francis R. Gerbasi, PhD, CRNA
Executive Director
Council on Accreditation of Nurse Anesthesia Educational Programs (COA)

Nurses were first asked to provide anesthesia in the middle of the 18th century. The first nurse anesthetists were trained by surgeons to meet anesthesia workforce needs, which resulted from the discovery of ether by dentist William Morton in 1846. Agatha Hodgins, an anesthetist and teacher, was the instructor for an early anesthesia school, the Lake Side Hospital School of Anesthesia, in Cleveland, Ohio, begun between 1912 and 1915. She was also the driving force for starting a national organization for nurse anesthetists. In 1931 the National Association of Nurse Anesthetists, later renamed the American Association of Nurse Anesthetists, was formed by 40 founding members. They identified the need to establish standards for educational programs. A formal accreditation process for nurse anesthesia educational programs was approved in 1950 and recognized by the U.S. Department of Education in 1955. In the late 1970s separate councils for accreditation, certification, and recertification, as well as for public interest, were established as autonomous decision-making bodies. During the next 30 years, the nurse anesthesia profession continued to grow, and the requirements for educational programs evolved.

Today there are approximately 40,000 CRNAs providing anesthesia in all 50 states and in U.S. protectorates. Nurse anesthetists provide anesthesia in a wide variety of practice settings for patients of all ages. In fact, CRNAs provide more than 85% of the anesthesia in rural hospitals.

The educational programs for CRNAs are using technology, including simulation and distance education, to enhance educational offerings and are initiating the move to offer professional doctoral degrees for entry into practice. On July 7, 2008, the *Consensus Model for APRN Regulation: Licensure, Accreditation, Certification & Education* (LACE) was completed, and nursing organizations were requested to endorse the document. As of

July 2009, 45 organizations endorsed the *Consensus Model,* including, in January 2009, the AANA, and in April 2009, the COA. The target date in the *Consensus Model* for full implementation of the concepts of LACE is 2015.

As the nurse anesthesia profession looks further into the 21st century, there will be challenges as well as opportunities in the areas of education, practice, certification, and recertification. This brief introduction identifies some key issues currently facing CRNAs and some potential issues they may face in the future. For more information regarding these issues, refer to the AANA Web site (http://www.aana.com), or contact the AANA national office at 847-692-7050.

Accreditation and Education

Accreditation and education are critical components of the foundation upon which the nurse anesthesia profession is built. The standards for educational programs have helped advance the nurse anesthesia profession by expanding the knowledge and clinical skills of program graduates. The COA is recognized by many regulatory agencies as the "gold standard" for the accreditation of CRNAs. To maintain this recognition, the organization must address key issues facing nurse anesthesia accreditation and education. These issues include:

- Continuing to ensure high-quality educational programs while meeting ever-growing workforce demands
- Maintaining an adequate number of qualified faculty members
- Moving to the professional doctorate degree
- Using new technology (e.g., distance education and simulation)
- Facing the strain of economic instability and uncertainty

In addition, the implementation of the *Consensus Model* will affect nurse anesthesia accreditation and education as it relates to requirements for establishing separate courses in advanced physiology/pathophysiology, health assessment, and pharmacology, and for providing content on the use and prescription of pharmacological interventions in the curriculum.

While these issues and requirements may present challenges, they also represent opportunities to enhance the knowledge and skills of graduate CRNAs. The incorporation of topics such as health informatics and evidence-based practice in doctoral curricula will help ensure CRNAs possess the knowledge and skills needed to provide high-quality anesthesia care in the future healthcare environment.

Practice

Anesthesia is fifty times safer today than it was 20 years ago. One reason for this is the highly skilled and knowledgeable CRNAs who provide anesthesia services. However, there are still several key practice-related issues facing the nurse anesthesia profession. These include:

- Continually incorporating evidence-based practice into the rapidly changing realm of clinical care delivery, research, administration, and education
- Ongoing development and updating of the standards of nurse anesthesia practice
- Increasing the focus on error reduction in anesthesia as well as in health care in general
- Developing performance-based measures linked to the assessment and delivery of quality care. For example, several healthcare organizations are exploring the implementation of Lean Six Sigma methods, business management and quality improvement strategies, and simulation into the healthcare setting

In addition, the implementation of the *Consensus Model* may affect nurse anesthesia practice for new graduates in some states by not allowing them to be granted a temporary license to practice and by not allowing new graduates to practice prior to receiving certification.

Certification and Recertification

The National Board on Certification and Recertification of Nurse Anesthetists (NBCRNA) consists of two councils—the Council on Certification of Nurse Anesthetists (CCNA) and the Council on Recertification of Nurse Anesthetists (COR); each council has autonomous authority to carry out its credentialing functions. The CCNA and the COR requirements are recognized in nurse practice acts in all states as well as by individual employers. This national recognition attests to the value of the CRNA credential and strengthens the nurse anesthesia profession. The NBCRNA credentialing programs are accredited by the National Commission for Certifying Agencies and the American Board of Nursing Specialties.

To ensure continued national recognition, several key issues facing the certification and recertification of CRNAs will need to be addressed. These will likely include:

- Devising and implementing methodologies to ensure continued competency
- Incorporating new technology in assessment methods (for example, simulation and online educational offerings)
- Changing trends in recertification, such as requiring re-examination via simulation or computerized testing

The implementation of the *Consensus Model* may also affect certification and recertification. For example, specialty certification in areas such as pediatrics, pain management, and obstetrics is not required at this time; however, specialty certification is considered highly desirable by some members of the CRNA profession. In the future, the CCNA may need to certify and the COR to recertify not only in the general CRNA role but also in specific specialties.

Clinical Nurse Specialists: What Does The Future Hold?

Kelly A. Goudreau, DSN, RN, ACNS-BC
Designated Learning/Education Officer, Portland VA Medical Center
Past President, National Association of Clinical Nurse Specialists

The role of the clinical nurse specialist (CNS) has undergone some significant changes over the last 50 years. The role, initially conceived in psychiatric nursing practice, has grown and expanded to include almost every area in which nursing is a key component of the healthcare system. The most rapid change has occurred during the past 15 years. In the 1990s, the cost-to-value ratio of the CNS was questioned, but more recently the CNS role has been recognized and affirmed for the intrinsic and versatile skills it brings in a time of needed change. The skills of a CNS include working within three spheres of influence: patient, nursing and healthcare worker, and systems.[7] These three areas of practice continue to have clear and broad application across healthcare settings. Some individuals would say that the skills of the CNS are needed more now than at any other time in the evolution of health care. As the IOM[2,3,8] and the Institute for Healthcare Improvement (IHI)[9,10] describe, there are gaps in the current healthcare system. The CNS is uniquely prepared to be the trans-professional collaborator, agent of change, integrator of evidence-based practice, and driver of patient/client outcomes that are needed, now more than ever before, to ensure the safety and quality of care for patients.

The release and subsequent implementation of the *Consensus Model for APRN Regulation: Licensure, Accreditation, Certification and Education*[1] will assist in recognizing the CNS and the role the CNS plays in health care. Additionally, the emphasis on healthcare reform by the Obama administration will provide further, as yet undefined, opportunities for the CNS and advanced practice skills.

Change in the CNS Role: Into the Future

The role of the CNS is seeing resurgence in the healthcare system. This can be attributed to numerous factors, but two that are clearly driving the increased demand are (1) the desire to attain Magnet designation by hospital facilities and (2) the recognition that the CNS role is ideally suited to lead patient safety and quality-of-care initiatives.

Under the American Nurses Credentialing Center (ANCC) Magnet Designation process, a program to recognize healthcare organizations that exemplify nursing excellence, CNSs are recognized as the advanced practice role that provides primary support to the nursing staff.[11] NPs, CRNAs, and CNMs are also advanced practice nurses, but when they work within an acute care setting, their focus is, appropriately, on the care of their patients. Their focus is not primarily on the provision of support for the nursing staff caring for complex patients nor on systems-level issues that may prevent nurses from providing the best possible care. Facilities that have embraced the CNS role and the IHI and IOM initiatives identified above are realizing clearly improved outcomes as the CNS assumes a leadership role in addressing these initiatives. The CNS is educated to be a leader in the healthcare system and to manage the changes associated with improving outcomes of care for patients at all levels in the system. Therefore, the CNS is the natural choice to lead change initiatives that will ultimately improve patient care.

The increasing demand for CNSs in the clinical environment means that there needs to be a thorough reassessment of the processes used in each of the four elements of licensure, accreditation, certification, and education.

Implications for the CNS in Implementing the Consensus Model

The *Consensus Model* was crafted through a long process of dialogue among a large number of stakeholder nursing organizations. After 4 years of discussion, the document was released, and it continues to be endorsed by nursing organizations. The document outlines the areas of consensus regarding regulation of the four current advanced practice roles. Specifically discussed throughout this process were the four pillars of regulation (LACE) as defined by Margaretta Styles, former president of the American Nurses Association (ANA) and Chair of the International Council of Nurses. The *Consensus Model* defines these four elements as they pertain specifically to the regulation of APRNs.

The implications of this document for CNSs are multiple and extend far into the future. The *Consensus Model* outlines several key points for consideration and definitive change within current CNS regulation.

- The CNS will receive a second license to practice as a CNS; this license will be based on the role and population within which the CNS was educated and certified and in which the CNS practices. Other APRNs will also be required to have a second license.

- The accreditation of CNS education programs must be consistent with education standards set by the professional organization(s).

- The CNS must be certified in order to demonstrate entry-level competency in the role and population in which educated.

- CNS educational programs must prepare the CNS with a broad foundation in three separate graduate-level courses: pathophysiology, pharmacology, and health assessment/physical assessment. These courses for all APRNS are commonly known as the 3Ps.

As for the first issue, the National Association of Clinical Nurse Specialists (NACNS) has long stated that the educational preparation of the CNS should be validation enough that they are capable and able to practice in their role as an advanced practice nurse.[7] The requirement for a second license has both positive and negative implications for CNSs. The positive is that the CNS title will be protected and that only those who have been educationally prepared as a CNS will be able to use the title. The negative is that by requiring a second license there is a perceived devaluing of the education already received as it must now be validated through testing for a second license.

The second issue is, again, both positive and negative. The positive aspect is that CNS programs will need to use standardized educational criteria developed through a consensus process, and the programs will need to be preaccredited or preapproved prior to enrolling students. The negative aspect is that this is a process that is not currently being used, so it may potentially be perceived as a barrier to the creation of new programs at a time when many more such programs are needed.

The third issue is related to certification, and it may also prove to be both positive and negative for CNS programs and their graduates. There are a number of CNS programs whose graduates do not currently have a certification examination available to them upon completion of the degree. This has proved problematic for graduates of programs located in states where certification examinations are already being used as a proxy for licensure examinations. One limiting factor is that, in many instances of CNS practice, there are insufficient numbers of test takers to sustain the psychometric soundness and legal defensibility of a test in a specific specialty area of practice. States in which the board of nursing has already ruled that a certification examination is the basis for licensure have essentially eliminated a number of specialty areas of CNS practice, including women's health, forensics, and genetics. The NACNS is working collaboratively with the ANCC to establish and maintain a core certification examination that will test the APRN core requirements (pathophysiology, pharmacology, and physical/health assessment), the core role competencies for the CNS, and the population-focused competencies of the individual across the life span. This proposed ANCC core examination will not test specialty content but will instead provide an option for licensure under the *Consensus Model* where no other certification examination exists for that particular area of practice. Under this certification process, in addition to the core examination, the CNS will need to demonstrate expertise in a specialty area of practice through another assessment process, such as an examination or a portfolio. Oncology and orthopedics are examples of specialty practice areas that currently have specialty examinations, and genetics is an example of a specialty area of practice that now uses a portfolio process to validate knowledge of the specialty content. This additional layer of competency measurement will allow specialty certification to continue to be a mark of excellence for CNS practice, rather than a test of minimal competency to enter into practice or a proxy for licensure.

The fourth issue concerns CNS education. CNS education has consistently been of high quality but, to date, the CNS curriculum has varied, depending on the school, on the beliefs of the faculty, and on how the CNS role is implemented and understood in each geographic area. For example, some CNS education programs teach the 3Ps, but others do not. This has created a broad tapestry of differences in CNS education.

The *Consensus Model* provides an opportunity for the CNS community to do some "spring cleaning" over the next few years as the model is fully implemented. Requiring CNSs to be educated with the 3Ps as a foundation will bring change and consistency to the curricula. Additional in-depth knowledge and content in these three areas must be customized to meet the needs of the various populations and specialized areas of practice.

Summary

Although the CNS role has seen times of strength and times of weakness, it is now poised on the brink of an emerging future. Many changes over the years have led to this point, a point at which the CNS role is again valued and needed in a healthcare system that is in need of reform. The CNS role also is in need of reform and rethinking about how it can best be ready to address the challenges of the future. Through active participation on a variety of fronts, nursing is now ready to license and protect the title of CNS; acknowledge the educational standards that CNS programs meet; recognize certification not only as a mark of entry-level competency but also as a mark of excellence; and provide consistent education for CNSs across the nation so that individual CNSs and their employers fully understand what skills CNSs bring that can assist in the attainment of excellent patient outcomes.

Midwifery: The Future Is in Our Hands

M. Christina Johnson, MS, CNM
Director of Professional Practice and Health Policy
American College of Nurse-Midwives

Elaine Germano, CNM, DrPH, FACNM
Education Projects Manager
American College of Nurse-Midwives

As the nation's leadership grapples with the need to make sweeping reforms in the delivery of health care, certified nurse-midwives (CNMs) and certified midwives (CMs) stand ready to provide solutions to some of the complex problems plaguing the healthcare system. CNMs and CMs, primary care providers focusing on pregnancy, birth, gynecology, and the health needs of women throughout the life span, are working to raise awareness of the need for change. Escalating healthcare costs, workforce shortages, and an increasing number of individuals without adequate health insurance have combined to create real economic and public health challenges. Yet rising healthcare spending has not improved outcomes in maternity care. In order to best serve women and families, the American College of Nurse-Midwives (ACNM), the professional organization representing CNMs and CMs, has provided guidance in the form of the following seven key principles of healthcare reform:

- Provide universal coverage
- Eliminate health disparities
- Focus healthcare resources on wellness, disease prevention, and primary care
- Improve care integration and coordination
- Align payment systems with evidence-based practice and optimal outcomes rather than on maximizing billable interventions
- Improve women's access to high-quality care
- Significantly improve maternal and infant health

In order to turn these principles into practice realities, many more midwives will need to be integrated into the healthcare system. While there is overwhelming evidence supporting the quality, safety, and value of midwifery care, most American women are not offered the opportunity to benefit from it. ACNM is focusing its current activities on strategic organizational goals designed to increase public awareness of the high value of midwifery care, to eliminate barriers to midwifery practice, and to produce the midwifery workforce required to effect change.

History and Education

Nurse-midwives have been practice in the United States since the 1920s, when Mary Breckinridge began the Frontier Nursing Service in eastern Kentucky with American public health nurses who were trained as nurse-midwives in Great Britain. The first midwifery education program was established in 1932. The profession grew slowly but steadily throughout the 20th century, and there are currently 38 education programs, with several more in development. Nurse-midwives now attend 11% of all vaginal births and provide primary health care to women throughout the country, with 24% of CNMs practicing in rural areas.

Incorporated in 1955 in New Mexico, ACNM now represents more than 11,500 CNMs and CMs nationwide. The mission of the ACNM is "to promote the health and well-being of women and infants within their families and communities through the development and support of the profession of midwifery as practiced by certified nurse-midwifes and certified midwives." Certification in midwifery is granted by the American Midwifery Certification Board (AMCB), which is responsible for developing and administering the national certification examination. AMCB is a member of the National Organization for Certifying Agencies and is accredited by the National Commission for Certifying Agencies. Candidates for certification must sit for the national examintion after completion of a midwifery education program accredited by the Accreditation Commission for Midwifery Education (ACME) in order to be eligible for state licensure. Standards for education and certification in midwifery are identical for CNMs and CMs. The difference between the two credentials reflects the background of the individual prior to entering the profession of midwifery: the CNM is also a registered nurse, the CM is not. ACME assesses the quality and content of midwifery education programs and has been recognized as an accrediting agency by the United States Department of Education since 1982.

ACNM maintains a commitment to competency-based education, yet it values graduate-degree preparation in midwifery, nursing, and public health. The majority of the midwifery workforce is prepared at the graduate level, and education programs have evolved to include many options for advanced degrees. Most recently, the Doctor of Nursing Practice (DNP) degree is being widely promulgated as an entry-level requirement for advanced clinical practice in nursing. CNMs have a higher proportion of doctoral preparation than other APRN groups[12]; however, ACNM does not currently support a requirement for doctoral preparation for entry-level midwifery practice. In light of the evidence that graduates from ACME-accredited midwifery education programs provide safe and cost-effective care, ACNM is concerned that the requirement of a doctoral degree will result in a substantive increase in time and expense for students and educational institutions.

Increasing the numbers of practicing midwives is critical to the ACNM strategy for future growth. By 2015, ACNM plans to graduate 1,000 new midwives annually. In order to accomplish this goal, the number of available education programs, clinical sites, and qualified faculty must be substantially increased. Hospital administrators often turn away midwifery students, opting to utilize seasoned staff midwives for the education and training of physician residents. The healthcare system must assign equal value to the education of midwifery students, who are often trained alongside resident physicians. Institutions need to be reimbursed for the training of midwives at the same rate as they are for the training of physicians, and nurse-midwives need to be reimbursed for training medical students and residents as well as midwifery students.

Scope of Practice

In addition to their roles as attendants to women during childbirth, nurse-midwives provide a full range of primary care services to women throughout the life span. These services include providing contraceptive and gynecological services, addressing adolescent and menopausal needs, and caring for many common primary care concerns of women. The focus of all care is on wellness, prevention, and client education. CNMs have prescription writing authority in all states, are considered independent practitioners in all but six states, and receive mandated Medicaid reimbursement for nurse-midwifery practice in all states.

Despite these facts, the inability to practice to the full extent of one's licensure is perhaps the most serious threat to midwifery, healthcare reform, and the advanced practice nursing community in general. ACNM is striving to achieve full autonomy in practice and equitable reimbursement for midwives by 2015. Midwives face barriers to practice, including but not limited to inequitable and outright denial of reimbursement for services, exorbitant professional liability rates, lack of collaborative employment opportunities, and restrictive institutional privileging and state regulations. While quality, high-value care involves the recruitment of more qualified providers, the insidious practice inequities that exist for midwives and other APRNs are a daily reality and discourage the growth of the professions. Ongoing, co-ordinated efforts at the local, state, and national levels to address a wide range of deeply in-grained problems within the healthcare system publicly are critical.

According to the most recent National Center for Health Statistics data, the number of CNM-/CM-attended births has increased by 33% since 1996, reaching a record high of 317,168 in 2006. In order to continue to promote the growth of the profession, ACNM is highlighting the opportunities that exist to advance maternal and infant health outcomes through midwifery care. An active campaign providing guidance to national and state leaders and lawmakers is currently under way. ACNM utilizes social media technologies, print and Internet publications, and television and film opportunities for messages regarding the value of midwifery. Educational outreach programs target women, families, youth, government officials, community leaders, institutional administrators, and other key stakeholders. Collaborative coalitions among the obstetric, nursing, advanced practice, and greater healthcare leadership focus on common goals and the dissemination of important health information.

Longstanding Commitment to Research

ACNM continues its long-standing commitment to a vigorous research agenda and is recognized for its internationally acclaimed, peer-reviewed *Journal of Midwifery and Women's Health*. The body of independent evidence supporting the quality, safety, and cost-effectiveness of midwifery care also continues to grow, as demonstrated by publications such as the *2008 Report: Evidence-Based Maternity Care: What It Is and What It Can Achieve* by Childbirth Connection, the Reforming States Group, and the Milbank Memorial Fund.[13] The recent Cochrane Review, "Midwife-Led Versus Other Models of Care for Childbearing Women,"[14] recommends that in order to achieve optimal outcomes, all pregnant women should be offered midwife-led models of care.

The ancient practice of midwifery has evolved into an innovative, respected, and well-studied profession that is alive, flourishing, and charting the course for women's health care in the 21st century. CNMs and CMs, along with other APRNs, provide a viable solution to the nation's need for high-value primary care. As ACNM President Melissa Avery proclaimed during the 2009 ACNM annual meeting and exhibit in Seattle, Washington, "I am a midwife. The future is in my hands."

Nurse Practitioners: Providing Access to Health Care in 2009 and Beyond

Mary Anne Dumas, PhD, RN, FNP-BC, FAANP
Professor, School of Nursing, Stony Brook University
Immediate Past President, National Organization of Nurse Practitioner Faculties

Health care and the provision of care have evolved over time. The role of the nurse practitioner (NP) also continues to evolve to meet the healthcare needs of the nation. As APRNs, NPs provide cost-effective, high-quality care, achieving outcomes similar to those of physicians.[15] Factors that have increased the demands on clinical practice include increasing numbers of older adults, particularly the frail elderly; multisystem, complex medical problems; higher patient acuity levels; limited number of primary care providers (PCPs); and an increased number of uninsured individuals and families.

The Obama Administration is seeking to reform the healthcare system to enable all individuals to have access to health care. More than 46 million individuals in the United States are uninsured. A more effective healthcare system and an adequate number of healthcare providers are needed to meet the healthcare needs of all Americans.

A constant decline in the number of medical school graduates choosing primary care specialties—internal medicine, family practice, primary care pediatrics—has been well documented in workforce data and is a major concern in meeting national healthcare needs. Although the numbers "stabilized" in 2009, with a minimal decline in residency applicants for primary care specialties, many residency positions in these specialty areas are unfilled. The decreased number of physicians choosing primary care as a practice choice adds to the growing dilemma of having adequate numbers of PCPs to meet the growing needs of the population and a reformed healthcare system. This growing need for primary care and other healthcare services has strengthened the need and urgency to prepare NPs in both primary and acute care to meet these burgeoning healthcare needs across all populations.

NP Education

NP educators will be challenged to identify opportunities and innovative methods for teaching and preparing the next generation of NPs. NP education has evolved from the traditional classroom only to the virtual classroom, normally referred to as distance education. Distance education has enabled nurses who do not have or are unable to access graduate education to advance their education and career using electronic technology to facilitate their education in the geographical location in which they work and live. Regardless of the method of delivery, NP educators must continue to provide the highest quality education, implement curricula redesign, and develop new evaluation methods that adhere to national regulations and guidelines.

In 2008, two important documents were published. The first document, the *APRN Consensus Model,* was developed through the collaboration of national APRN organizations and the National Council of State Boards of Nursing. It addresses the licensing, accreditation, certification, and education of all APRNs. The *Consensus Model* has been endorsed by 45 nursing organizations, including the NONPF and all NP certification organizations. All faculty must transition the NP curriculum to meet the program criteria delineated in the *Consensus Model.* These criteria include three courses for the 3Ps and preparation in the NP role across the health-wellness-illness continuum in at least one of the six population foci: family/individual across the life span, adult-gerontology, neonatal, pediatrics, women's health–gender-related, and psychiatric–mental health. Graduates must be prepared with the national consensus-based competencies recognized for the population they are to care for (e.g., pediatric, adult-gerontology, or neonatal). Preparation in a specialty area of practice (e.g., oncology or diabetes) will not be regulated but will require *additional* knowledge and expertise in a more discrete area of clinical practice. The ability of an APRN to become licensed and practice in the future will depend on educational preparation and certification that conform to the *Consensus Model.*

The second document, which is specific to NP education, is the *Criteria for Evaluation of Nurse Practitioner Programs,* 3rd Edition,[16] produced by the National Taskforce on Quality Nurse Practitioner Education. This document, which reflects the changes required by the *Consensus Model,* has been updated from earlier editions and provides clarification and guidelines for accreditation of NP programs. New criteria include education and practice standards for NP program faculty and post-master's program criteria.

Both of the above documents are sentinel to the education of NPs. The NP profession has responded over the years to the healthcare needs of the population by evolving from a focus on primary care to a focus that includes, in addition to primary care, acute care, psychiatric–mental health, and neonatal care. In addition, blending of the NP role and population foci with specialties, such as oncology, diabetes, cardiology, and palliative care, (e.g., a pediatric NP specializing in diabetes care) have evolved and will continue to address the growing and diverse healthcare needs of the population.

The growing complexity of the healthcare system and the expanding role of NPs require knowledge and competence in addition to those of the role, population foci, and/or specialty. Leadership and fiscal management, as well as technology-, policy-, and systems-related skills are required of all NPs to meet future challenges and expectations.

In 2008 the NONPF Board of Directors approved the position that entry into NP practice evolve to the doctoral level.[17] NPs prepared with this expanded knowledge and competence in a DNP program have the potential to make significant contributions and achieve even greater influence in the evolving healthcare system. The DNP graduate is prepared with advanced skill sets to meet the NONPF DNP role competencies[18] and the AACN's *Essentials of Doctoral Education for Specialty Nursing Practice.*[19] NP education in the future should also reflect an interprofessional sharing of knowledge and clinical experiences. Collaborative education across the professions can serve to promote teamwork in practice, improve patient care outcomes, and identify patient-centered care as a common goal among all health professionals.

Research Needed

Ongoing research that evaluates and documents the outcomes of NP practice is greatly needed. NPs need to document their clinical practice outcomes (e.g., diabetics with normal hemoglobin A_1C levels, smoking cessation rates) to validate the quality and cost effectiveness of NP practice. Implementation of the electronic health record (EHR) provides NPs with the opportunity to collect data, evaluate adherence to standardized guidelines, and document patient outcomes. Although NPs use evidence-based guidelines in their clinical practices, the EHR also provides opportunities for NPs to develop clinical guidelines and publish quality improvements and care outcomes. Many more outcome and comparative studies are needed to secure the NP profession a sound footing as independent healthcare providers and a place at the health-policy table.

References

1. APRN Joint Dialogue Group. (2008). *The Consensus Model for Advanced Practice Registered Nurses (APRN): Licensure, Accreditation, Certification and Education.* Accessed May 27, 2010 at http://www.aacn.nche.edu/Education/pdf/APRNReport.pdf

2. Institute of Medicine. (1999). *To Err Is Human: Building a Safer Health System.* National Academy Press, Washington, DC.

3. Institute of Medicine Committee on the Quality of Health Care in America. (2001). *Crossing the Quality Chasm: A New Health System for the 21st Century.* National Academy Press, Washington, DC.

4. Institute of Medicine. (2003). *Health Professions Education: A Bridge to Quality.* National Academy Press, Washington, DC.

5. American Association of Colleges of Nursing. (2004). *Position Statement on the Practice Doctorate in Nursing.* Accessed at http://www.aacn.nche.edu/DNP/DNPPositionStatement.htm.

6. National Research Council of the National Academies. (2005). *Advancing the Nation's Health Needs: NIH Research Training Programs.* Washington, DC: National Academies Press.

7. National Association of Clinical Nurse Specialists. (2004). *Statement on Clinical Nurse Specialist Practice and Education,* 2nd ed. Harrisburg, PA: Author.

8. Institute of Medicine. (2004). *Quality Chasm Series: Patient Safety—Achieving a New Standard for Care.* National Academy Press, Washington, DC.

9. Institute for Healthcare Improvement. (2004). *Transforming Care at the Bedside.* Cambridge, MA: Author.

10. Institute for Healthcare Improvement. (2006). *A Framework for Spread: From Local Improvements to System-Wide Change.* Cambridge, MA: Author.

11. Goudreau, K.A., Baldwin, K., Clark, A., et al. (2007). *A Vision of the Future for Clinical Nurse Specialists.* Clinical Nurse Specialist, 21(6), 310-320.

12. Sipe T.A., Fullerton J.T., Schuiling K.D. (2009). *Demographic profiles of certified nurse-midwives, certified nurse anesthetists, and nurse practitioners: Reflections on implications for uniform education and regulation.* Journal of Professional Nursing, 25(3), 178-185.

13. Sakala, C., Corry, M.P. (October 2008). *Evidence-Based Maternity Care: What It Is and What It Can Achieve.* Copublished by Childbirth Connection, the Reforming States Group, and the Milbank Memorial Fund. Available at http://www.milbank.org/reports/0809MaternityCare/0809MaternityCare.html

14. Hatem M., Sandall J., Devane D., et al. (2008). *Midwife-Led Versus Other Models of Care for Childbearing Women.* Cochrane Database of Systematic Reviews 2008, Issue 4. Art. No.: CD004667. DOI: 10.1002/14651858.CD004667.pub2.

15. Mundinger, M.O., Kane, R.L., Lenz, E.R., et al. (2000). *Primary care outcomes in patients treated by nurse practitioners or physicians: A randomized trial.* Journal of the American Medical Association, 283(1)59-68.

16. National Task Force on Quality Nurse Practitioner Education. (2008). *Criteria for Evaluation of Nurse Practitioner Programs.* Accessed at http://www.nonpf.com/displaycommon.cfm?an=1&subarticlenbr=15

17. National Organization of Nurse Practitioner Faculties. (2008, August 28). *White Paper: Eligibility for NP Certification for Nurse Practitioner Students in Doctor of Nursing Practice Programs.* Message posted to the NONPF electronic membership mailing list, archived at http://www.nonpf.org

18. National Organization of Nurse Practitioner Faculties. (2006). *Practice Doctorate Nurse Practitioner Entry-Level Competencies.* Accessed at http://www.nonpf.com/displaycommon.cfm?an=1&subarticlenbr=14

19. American Association of Colleges of Nursing. (2006). *Essentials of Doctoral Education for Specialty Nursing Practice.* Accessed at http://www.aacn.nche.edu/DNP/pdf/Essentials.pdf

Advanced Practice
NURSING

EMPHASIZING
COMMON ROLES

Jan Towers is the Director of Health Policy for the American Academy of Nurse Practitioners. She received her BSN from Duke University in Durham, North Carolina; her MS from the University of North Carolina at Chapel Hill; her FNP postmaster's certification from Pennsylvania State University; and her PhD from the University of Pennsylvania in Philadelphia.

She has held positions in the School of Medicine, Pennsylvania State University, Department of Family and Community Medicine and on the faculty of the nurse practitioner program at Pennsylvania State University. She has also served as the director of the nurse practitioner program at Georgetown University and Widener University.

Clinically Dr. Towers has been a family nurse practitioner at Health Care for the Homeless in Frederick, Maryland. In addition, she has held clinical nurse practitioner positions in the Department of Family and Community Medicine, Pennsylvania State University, Hershey, Pennsylvania; Dickinson College Health Program, Carlisle, Pennsylvania; and the Adams County Migrant Clinic, Gettysburg, Pennsylvania.

Dr. Towers has been active in the area of health policy at the national and state levels for more than 25 years, working on behalf of nurse practitioners and their patients to facilitate appropriate regulation, use, and support for nurse practitioner practice during that time. She has served as a health policy consultant for multiple government and private programs and agencies, including the national advisory committee for the primary care initiatives grants sponsored by the Robert Wood Johnson Foundation and the Joint Commission on Accreditation of Healthcare Organizations. The author of numerous publications related to nurse practitioner practice, Dr. Towers is also founding editor of the *Journal of the American Academy of Nurse Practitioners*. She is a fellow of the American Academy of Nurse Practitioners and the American Academy of Nursing.

Dr. Towers would like to recognize the contribution of Pauline Komnenich, PhD, RN, author of the chapter "Evolution of Advanced Practice in Nursing" in the second edition of *Advanced Practice Nursing: Emphasizing Common Roles*.

CHAPTER 1

The Evolution of Advanced Practice in Nursing

Jan Towers, PhD, NP-C, CRNP, FAANP, FAAN

CHAPTER OUTLINE

CERTIFIED NURSE-MIDWIVES
  Early history
  Sociopolitical context
  Influence of government agencies
  Influence of professional associations
  Influence of private foundations, colleges, and universities
  Forces influential in marketing and effective use

CERTIFIED REGISTERED NURSE ANESTHETISTS
  Early history
  Sociopolitical context
  Influence of government agencies

CLINICAL NURSE SPECIALISTS
  Historical context
  Sociopolitical context
  *Influence of government agencies, a private foundation,
    and professional associations*

NURSE PRACTITIONERS
  Historical and sociopolitical context
  Influence of government agencies
  Influence of private foundations, colleges, and universities
  Forces influential in marketing and effective use

INTERFACE AMONG CERTIFIED NURSE-MIDWIVES, CERTIFIED
  REGISTERED NURSE ANESTHETISTS, CLINICAL NURSE
  SPECIALISTS, AND NURSE PRACTITIONERS
  Consensus on advanced practice registered nurse education
  *Similarities and differences among different advanced
    practice registered nurses*
  Trends and the future for advanced practice registered nurses

SUGGESTED LEARNING EXERCISES

CHAPTER OJECTIVES

*After completing this chapter, the reader
will be able to:*

1. Understand the evolution of advanced
   practice nursing within the historical
   context of each of the four roles—
   nurse-midwives, nurse anesthetists,
   clinical nurse specialists, and nurse
   practitioners.
2. Identify and discuss the sociopolitical
   forces that stimulated the expanded
   role for nurses in each of these practice
   domains.
3. Evaluate critical trends in the
   educational preparation of nurses
   and the implications of those trends in
   preparing nurses for advanced practice
   roles.
4. Synthesize common or shared role
   parameters and concerns of advanced
   practice nurses from a historical
   perspective.

3

Loretta Ford,[1] an influential leader in the nurse practitioner movement, pointed out that myths and fallacies surround any movement. This chapter describes the evolution of each advanced practice role from the perspective of history and sociopolitics, identifies key events, and discusses common role parameters. It concludes with a discussion of the common themes and distinguishing characteristics of each role and some thoughts on the future.

Certified Nurse-Midwives

According to Dickerson,[2] as of 2008, there were 45 accredited nurse-midwifery education programs in the United States. These programs include 41 master's education programs and four certificate programs. In addition to these nurse-midwifery programs, there are two accredited midwifery programs that prepare individuals who are not nurses as certified midwives (CMs).

The development of these programs in the United States has a history dating back to the early 1900s. During the period from 1900 to 1935, attention focused on the extension of the education of midwives, and from 1935 to the present, the focus has been on the growth of nurse-midwifery programs. This development of nurse-midwifery educational programs has occurred with the placement of nurse-midwifery education in post-nursing or post-baccalaureate programs within institutions of higher education.[3] The overall purposes of nurse-midwifery education, as stated in the Carnegie Foundation for the Advancement of Teaching report,[4] are the provision of better health care for mothers and babies, infants, and the promotion of midwifery as "a quality profession, requiring emphasis on caring, competence, and public education" (p. 29).

Early History

Although the established date for the inception of modern nursing is 1873, there are records of midwifery practice in the North American colonies dating back to 1630 and of attempts to educate midwives dating back to early 1762.[5,6] In these early times, the provision of obstetrical care was outside the purview of medical practice and remained in the exclusive domain of midwives. According to Roberts,[3] efforts to establish formal midwifery schools, such as the effort of William Shippen, Jr., in Philadelphia in 1762, were unsuccessful. Throughout the 1800s, the midwife was "self or apprenticeship-taught and was isolated from medicine, nursing, or the hospital"[3] (p. 123). Although interest in promoting education for midwifery practice renewed with the immigration of European midwives and physicians to the United States in the latter part of the 19th century, it was not sustained.

Historians consider many factors as contributing to the demise of midwifery's occupational identity. The medical specialty of obstetrics[7,8] arose against the backdrop of the lack of formal midwifery education[5] and the relatively inexact training requirements for midwives. Other social and economic events contributed to the decline of the native midwife.[9] Between 1900 and 1935, midwife deliveries decreased from 50% to 10% as the flow of immigration decreased and the emigrated midwife's clients became integrated into the dominant society, as home deliveries were replaced with hospital deliveries, and as physicians became increasingly critical of midwives.

An exception to this pattern of declining midwifery use in the United States existed among the Mormon pioneer midwives. During the late 1800s and early 1900s, the Mormons relied on midwives trained initially in their native countries and further educated in the medical-obstetrical arena available in the United States at that time.[3] In 1874, women who were able to travel to study at the Women's Medical College in Philadelphia returned to Utah and established midwifery courses. Licensure for practice was required in Utah from 1894 to 1932, during which time 208 midwives were licensed in Salt Lake City.

According to Roberts,[3] medical care in the early 20th century was no better than midwifery care. A 1912 survey, carried out by J. Whitridge Williams, a professor of obstetrics at

Johns Hopkins University in Baltimore, found that the lack of preparation of obstetricians rendered their practices as harmful as those of midwives, if not more so, and noted that more deaths occurred from improper operations by physicians than from infections at the hands of midwives. A 1914 report by Carolyn van Blarcom, RN, to the New York Committee for the Prevention of Blindness acknowledged that women may have been better cared for by less educated midwives than by the physicians who were responsible for the puerperal septicemia and infant eye infections that were occurring at that time.

Although major reform in medical education began to occur after the Flexner Report of 1910 (a sentinel report from the Carnegie Foundation on medical education in the United States and Canada), no similar efforts to improve the education or preparation of midwives occurred. Roberts[3,10] perceived that the lack of education and opportunity for training further led to diminished opportunities for midwives. Because midwives perceived childbirth as a "normal" phenomenon and within the female domain of competence, few of them sought formal education. The predominantly male physicians' attitudes toward midwifery were that midwives were unsafe and that no "true" woman would want to learn the knowledge and skills needed for midwifery.[3]

Van Blarcom, instrumental in developing the Bellevue School for Midwives, became known as the first nurse in the United States to be licensed as a midwife.[11] She advocated the training, licensure, and control of midwives, whereas Williams recommended the abolishment of midwives and better education of physicians. Although this controversy led to a decline in midwifery deliveries, Roberts[3] noted that "the negative indicators surrounding childbirth actually rose with the decline of midwives" (p. 128). Lower maternal and infant mortality rates existed only where midwives were retained, notably in Newark, New Jersey,[12] and in New York City.[13] If one considers that midwives were attending to poor, higher risk women, these findings were even more impressive. Some poorer birth outcomes attributed to medicine were thought to be due to physicians' lack of training and experience with childbirth and to the techniques they used to hurry labor.

Positive midwifery outcomes in Germany and England were noted by some American nurses who, according to Roberts,[3,10] believed that midwives should play a role in maternity care. This view led to the integration of the roles of the midwife and public health nurse into the preparation of the nurse-midwife. American nursing leaders in the early 1900s did not consider midwifery to be a part of nursing preparation or practice. In 1901, Dock,[14] in a report on nursing education, pointed out: "The nurse never takes up midwifery work and in private practice or district nursing goes only to obstetric cases where a doctor is in atten-dance" (p. 485).

Because so many births were being carried out in the community, nurses involved in the supervision of midwives worked predominantly in public health and community nursing. During this time, nurses concerned with maternal-child health care tended to be actively involved in social and health reforms, including Lillian Wald, the founder of the New York Henry Street Settlement. One result of these reform efforts was the formation of a federal Children's Bureau. Established between 1909 and 1912, the Children's Bureau, according to Roberts,[3] was a "major force in health reforms and subsequent midwifery practice" (p. 130).

Sociopolitical Context

During World War I, the limited fitness of men for military service resulted in legislative initiatives that were instrumental in leading to social and health-care reform and, eventually, to changes in maternity care.[15] The poor physical condition of potential recruits also captured the attention of physicians and public health officials, who noted that if one-half of these men were properly cared for during childhood, they would have qualified for military service. Tom[15] noted that the investment of state and federal funds into public health programs was not stimulated by high maternal and infant mortality rates, but rather by the concern for a fit fighting force to ensure the nation's security. According to Tom,[15] "For the first time, children were recognized as future members of the military and thus deserving of federal funds" (pp. 4–13). Childbearing women were considered to be producers of future fighting men, so their health became a national resource.

NEED FOR BETTER-EDUCATED MIDWIVES

The need for better maternity services in the context of opposition to midwives by physicians contributed to the controversy in nursing about the role of nurses in the practice of obstetrics. In 1909, the American Society of Superintendents of Training Schools for Nurses (ASSTSN) acknowledged that nurses' training in obstetrics should be included in the program, and in 1911, a resolution was passed to support that position. The association directed that the training be limited, however, to emergency preparation, observing symptoms, and reporting problems to a more general practice. In 1911, the ASSTSN passed another resolution to provide training for registration, licensure, and training in the practice of midwifery.

Around the same time, the Bellevue School for Midwives in New York City initiated a program to educate midwives. This occurred largely through the efforts of van Blarcom, who, as noted earlier, was a strong advocate for midwifery. Clara Noyes, Superintendent of Training Schools, Bellevue and Allied Hospitals, including the School for Midwives, also supported the education of nurses as midwives. The training program for midwives at Bellevue was supported by public monies from 1911 until 1935, when the diminishing need for midwives made it difficult to justify its existence.[3] The movement of maternity care into the hospitals excluded midwifery. The joint proposal of the Maternity Center Association (MCA) in New York and the Bellevue School of Midwifery to educate nurse-midwives was opposed by medical and nursing leaders. Although the need for better maternal-child health services and midwifery practice continued, such opposition inhibited nurses from engaging in the practice of midwifery. The continuing need eventually led to the advanced preparation of public health nurses who could supervise midwifery practice and prepare nurse-midwives.

In 1921, the controversial Sheppard-Towner Act was enacted to provide money to states to train public health nurses in midwifery.[3] There was a major political effort to prohibit passage of the bill, but, according to Roberts,[3] the joint efforts of women represented "one of the most effective expressions of women's political influence" (p. 131). In 1929, major opposition by the American Medical Association (AMA) resulted in the lapse of the bill, however. Roberts[3] attributed the bill's demise to the desire of the AMA to "establish a 'single standard' of obstetrical care" (p. 131) and to its concern that governmental regulation of midwifery would lead to regulation of medical practice.

FIRST MIDWIFERY SCHOOLS

According to Shoemaker,[16] despite the opposition to midwifery in nursing, the first school for nurse-midwifery was established in the United States in 1928. Started by Mary Richardson, a public health nursing instructor who had taken a midwifery course in England, the Manhattan Midwifery School was, however, short-lived. Two of the graduates from the Manhattan Midwifery School were identified as joining the Frontier Nursing Service in 1928.[3] Earlier, in 1925, Mary Breckenridge had brought nurse-midwives from England to help establish the Frontier Nursing Service. The Frontier Nursing Service in Kentucky (1925) and the MCA (education) in New York City (1932) were two public health–oriented agencies that characterized the midwifery practice area for public health nurses prepared in nurse-midwifery. According to nurse-historian Elizabeth Baer,[17] the Lobenstine Midwifery Clinic was established in 1931 to prepare public health nurses to be midwives. In contrast to the Manhattan School, considered the first "unofficial" school of midwifery[3] (p. 133), the Lobenstine Clinic was the first recognized nurse-midwifery school.

After the opening of the Lobenstine Midwifery Clinic, the School of the Association for the Promotion and Standardization of Midwifery was established in 1932. Priority for attendance in the school was given to nurses from states that had high infant mortality rates and many lay midwives. The intent was for the graduates to return to their home states to establish public health department programs for training and supervising "granny midwives."[3] In 1934, the school merged with the Lobenstine Clinic under the MCA and was known thereafter as the Clinic.

A key figure in the education of nurse-midwives was Hattie Hemschemeyer, a public health nurse educator and graduate of the Clinic's first nurse-midwifery class. She was later appointed director of the Clinic, where the emphasis was on the provision of care to women during pregnancy and childbirth in neighborhood settings staffed by public health nurses and physicians. The MCA, a prototype of this type of service, developed about 30 centers in New York City in 1918.[3] Nurse-midwives began to provide services in these centers around 1931, and the role of the public health nurse as a nurse-midwife emerged. At the same time, the role of the nurse in maternity care was evolving, but seemed to be quite different from midwifery and medical practice.

In 1937, according to Roberts,[3] the National League for Nursing Education (NLNE) described the role of the midwife in obstetrics as involving the "overall promotion of the health and comfort of the mother and baby" (p. 135). The obstetric nurse, in contrast, was described as a "bedside assistant" and "teacher of health."[18] Although preparation of the nurse in obstetrics was relatively poor in the early part of the 20th century, development of programs in nurse-midwifery during the 1940s showed progress in the education for the role. According to Diers, as cited by Roberts,[3] nurse-midwives have been described as

> the oldest of the specialized practice roles for nurses, providing...an unusually good example of the issues nurses face in addressing public policy considerations of manpower, economics, costs of care, quality and access to care, and interprofessional politics (p. 136).

Positive publicity for nurse-midwives was enhanced further by the results of a study of Frontier Nursing Service outcomes that Mary Breckenridge asked Metropolitan Life statistician Louis Dublin to complete. The report found that the Frontier Nursing Service protected the life of the mother and baby, saving 10,000 lives a year in the United States, preventing 30,000 stillbirths, and ensuring that there would be 30,000 more children alive at the end of the first month of life.[19] According to Roberts,[3]

> There is an irony in the notion that an insurance company would serve to stimulate the expansion of nurse-midwifery services (p. 141).

World War II had a significant impact on the development of nurse-midwives. As a consequence of the war, there was a diminished supply of nurse-midwives. This situation led to the establishment of another nurse-midwife education program, the second in the United States. It was initiated as part of the Frontier Nursing Service in Kentucky and was assisted by the MCA in New York.

CONTINUED EXPANSION OF EDUCATIONAL PROGRAMS

The formalization of nurse-midwifery as an extension of public health nursing continued after World War II. With increasing professionalization in nursing and healthcare services, the progress of nurse-midwifery education went hand-in-hand with the development of public health education, which was considered to be essential for nurse-midwifery practice. With the advocacy of clinical nursing specialization within universities, the nurse-midwife or advanced maternity nurse became more qualified to work with physicians within a professional framework.

Influence of Government Agencies

In the 1970s and 1980s, efforts of government and professional associations continued to advance the development of nurse-midwifery. The Children's Bureau (later known as the Maternal Child Health Bureau), and the Division of Nursing, Bureau of Health Professions Education, were instrumental in facilitating the nurse-midwifery movement by providing training grants.[10,17] According to Baer,[17] Senator Daniel K. Inouye of Hawaii assisted with lobbying efforts on Capitol Hill and with the development of contacts between nursing and other key people. During the same time, Senator Daniel Patrick Moynihan of New York sponsored the Civilian Health and Medical Program for the Uniformed Services (CHAMPUS) in the Omnibus Reconciliation Act of the Defense Appropriations Bill. These activities on the part of both Senators had a positive impact on legislation that influenced education and advanced practice initiatives for nurses, nurse practitioners, and nurse-midwives.

The medical malpractice crisis, a key sociopolitical event that occurred in 1985, slowed the growth of nurse-midwifery. Insurance carriers, fearing financial drains associated with litigation, dropped malpractice coverage for nurse-midwives. This situation created a difficult challenge for the American Nurses Association (ANA), the American College of Nurse-Midwives (ACNM), and the Nurse Association of the American College of Obstetrics and Gynecology, all of which stepped in and worked to assist in getting the Risk Retention Act passed. Passage of this law allowed independent carriers to provide malpractice insurance to individuals on a state-by-state basis.

Influence of Professional Associations

During the mid-1940s, the National Organization of Public Health Nurses (NOPHN) created a section for nurse-midwives. The NOPHN was dissolved in 1952 and subsequently was subsumed into the ANA and the National League for Nursing (NLN). A separate entity for nurse-midwives with the ANA and NLN was not created. Nurse-midwives were included in the Maternal and Child Health–NLN Interdivisional Council, which included obstetrics, pediatrics, orthopedics, crippled children, and school nursing. The general concern of the membership was that this Council was too diverse to represent nurse-midwifery; however, nurse-midwives assumed much of the leadership of the council. In 1954 at the ANA Convention, the Committee on Organization was formed to explore the possibility of creating a separate organization for nurse-midwifery. After long deliberation and consideration of four options, the Committee on Organization voted unanimously to form the American College of Nurse-Midwifery (ACNM).[20]*

The ACNM was officially incorporated in 1955 as an outgrowth of the recommendations of the Committee on Organization.[20] Hattie Hemschemeyer was elected the first president of the ACNM. Her tenure occurred during a time when there were no provisions for nurse-midwives in federal programs. Consistent leadership was needed to maintain intense lobbying efforts for midwives concerning key legislation that influenced programs such as Medicare, Medicaid, and CHAMPUS. These lobbying efforts opened the door for more autonomous nursing practice, the potential for third-party reimbursement, and greater recognition of the certified nurse-midwife (CNM) as a healthcare provider.

Further movement toward professional development occurred during 1987 to 1989, when ACNM developed a Division of Research.[17] A time of marked growth in the number and quality of educational programs for nurse-midwives followed. Participation in the International Confederation of Nurse-Midwives (ICNM)[21] led to involvement in the international development of midwifery. During this time, a formal liaison developed between the ICNM and the Royal College of Midwives in London, England.

Among international organizations, the Agency for International Development (AID) and the World Health Organization (WHO) were probably most influential in promoting midwifery in developing countries. The ICNM,[21] founded in Europe in 1919, also worked to advance education in midwifery, with the aim of improving the standard of care provided to

---

*In 1969, the American College of Nurse-Midwifery merged with the American Association of Nurse-Midwives to form the American College of Nurse-Midwives.

mothers, babies, and their families throughout the countries of the world. The Confederation is the only international midwifery organization that has official relations with the United Nations and works closely with WHO and the United Nations International Children's Emergency Fund (UNICEF) to achieve common goals in maternal and child care.

Although its activities were interrupted during World War II, the first World Congress of Midwives began a new era and the start of a series of triennial meetings. These meetings brought together midwives from all over the world to share ideas and experiences and to improve knowledge in the field. The first triennial meeting, hosted by the United States, was held in 1972 in Washington, D.C.,[17] during the presidency of Lucille Woodville. Currently, nine other organizations work with the confederation, including the International Council of Nurses and the International Federation of Gynecology and Obstetrics.[21]

Influence of Private Foundations, Colleges, and Universities

The Carnegie Foundation served as a definite stimulus for the nurse-midwifery movement. Ernest Boyer, president of the Carnegie Foundation until his death in 1995 and whose wife was a nurse-midwife, strongly supported nurse-midwifery programs. At an exploratory meeting convened by the Carnegie Foundation in July 1989, Boyer posed a critical and continuing question, however, regarding the issue of accreditation of a program designed for individuals who were not first educated as nurses. The ACNM responded by saying that accreditation of a program for non-nurse-midwives would require identification of all the relevant knowledge, skills, and competencies that nurses bring to nurse-midwifery education and would require that those essential competencies be acquired by completion of the midwifery education program.

A key principle underlying the ACNM, Division of Accreditation (DOA) program, was that

> [T]he ultimate competencies attained in an ACNM accredited midwifery program for non-nurses would be the same as those required of graduates of DOA-accredited nurse-midwifery programs (p. 1).

The ACNM articulated this principle by stating that ACNM standards for nurse-midwifery education and practice would "have to be maintained and upheld by every accredited program"[12] (p. 1). The ACNM Certification Council, now separately incorporated and known as the ACNM Certification Board (AMCB) further required that individuals sitting for the ACNM Certification Council (ACC) examination be registered nurses (RNs), who on passing the examination were certified as certified nurse-midwives (CNMs).

In 1998, the AMCB began to offer certification to professionally educated midwives who were not nurses. They were called certified midwives (CMs). Although some concern has been expressed regarding this issue, the AMCB points out that only individuals graduating with a minimum of a baccalaureate degree from an ACNM-accredited midwifery program would be eligible to take the CM certification examination. As of 2009, there are two direct-entry programs, one a certificate and one a master's degree program. Both programs require applicants to hold a baccalaureate degree—but not necessarily in nursing—before admission.[2]

Nurse-midwifery programs have received notable and growing support from many major colleges and universities throughout the United States. Support for doctoral education for nurse-midwives who hold positions within university-based programs and for the preparation of leaders with the skills of scientific inquiry, health-policy formulation, educational administration, and research also has become increasingly important.

Forces Influential in Marketing and Effective Use

According to Baer,[17] professional association and legislative support have encouraged the use of nurse-midwives by consumers. Although nurse-midwives have been involved in health maintenance organizations (HMOs) since 1980, consumer support was probably the most influential in the marketing and effective use of their services. When the recipients of health care became aware of what nurse-midwives could do, earlier misconceptions about midwifery were dispelled. The benefits of midwifery practice, especially among the underserved populations, were appreciated and disseminated.

Certified Registered Nurse Anesthetists

Although midwifery as a vocation dates back to the 1600s, nurse anesthesia predates nurse-midwifery as a specialty area of nursing in the United States. From the perspective of world history, the history of women attending other women in labor can be documented in pre-Christian times. Nurses attending patients in surgery to administer anesthesia is more recent. Today, certified registered nurse anesthetists (CRNAs) practice in all 50 states and administer more than 32 million anesthetics a year. This section considers their history in its sociopolitical context, its evolving educational programs and certification requirements, and its ongoing battle for autonomy.

Early History

Anesthesia in the United States reportedly dates back to the mid-19th century, with rival claimants to its discovery. Allegedly, William T. G. Morton successfully demonstrated anesthesia in surgery on October 16, 1846, at a centennial event held at Massachusetts General Hospital. This demonstration was followed by numerous reported studies, all of which failed to mention any involvement of nurse anesthetists. In response to this apparent oversight, Thatcher[22] emphasized the role of the nurse specialist in her book, *History of Anesthesia, with Emphasis on the Nurse Specialist*. In the preface to the book, she stated,

> If the place of the nurse as an anesthetist receives special emphasis in this history, it is because she has been derogated or ignored (p. 15).

Bankert[23] also described the difficulty associated with identifying the first nurse anesthetist and the limited recognition of the prominence of nurses in anesthesia.

According to Thatcher,[22] church records of 1877 identify Sister Mary Bernard as being called on to function as an anesthetist within a year of enrolling in St. Vincent's Hospital, in Erie, Pennsylvania. As a result of this recording, Sister Bernard has been recognized as the first nurse anesthetist to practice in the United States. The further contribution of members of the religious orders to the development of the field of anesthesia was illustrated by many others, including Sister Aldonza Eltrich (1860–1920) and certain religious nursing orders.

According to Bankert,[23] the Hospital Sisters of the Third Order of St. Francis managed five hospitals that served employees of the Missouri Pacific Railroad between 1884 and 1888. During this period, nuns from the order served as anesthetists for the five settings. In 1912, Mother Superior Magdalene Wiedlocher, an anesthetist, developed a course in anesthesia for sisters who were graduate nurses. In 1924, this course was made available to secular nurses. Based on Thatcher's research, Bankert detailed the contributions of Catholic and Protestant nursing orders whose members served as nurse anesthetists since the 1850s, providing poignant narratives of these committed women. Included in this group are Alice Magaw, known as the "Mother of Anesthesia," and Sister Secundina Mindrup (1868–1951).

The emergence of nurse anesthesia in the United States cannot be considered outside the context of the development of nursing itself. In 1873, nurses' training schools were established in New York, New Haven, and Boston. These American schools were referred to as "Nightingale Schools" and were credited with bringing the art of nursing into a more reputable view. At that time, there was some controversy over the philanthropic desire to make nurses' training attractive to the middle-class American woman. Some physicians supported the idea, but many did not. As quoted by Bankert,[23] one physician (Starr) voiced his concern that "educated nurses would not do as they were told," a remarkable comment on the status anxieties of 19th-century physicians" (p. 20).

Women reformers paid little attention to these remarks and, similar to Florence Nightingale, moved forward. The schools were established to attract respectable women and were modeled after the Saint Thomas Hospital Training School for Nurses founded in London in 1860 by Nightingale.

Eventually, physicians were forced to accept nurses who were trained to carry out the more complex work that hospitals were assuming. Bankert[23] includes a quotation that vividly described this change in attitude toward nurses:

> *All of this related to the public opinion of medical service in general, since the nurses came into more continuous contact with the patient than did any other figure in the whole range of medical personnel. Good nursing was invaluable from a technical point of view. It might make all the difference in the outcome of the individual case, and patients sometimes realized this. Better nursing was an essential feature in the gradual improvement of hospitals, and this in turn modified the earlier popular attitude toward these institutions....The whole spirit of hospitals changed (p. 21).*

Nursing historian Ellen Baer, as quoted by Bankert,[23] made yet a stronger statement when she asserted that "nursing made medicine look good" (p. 21). She continued to illustrate this point:

> *Medicine's ultimate success, technological advances, and subsequent impressive social power were achieved through hospitals, and nurses made those hospitals work. Nurses made them reasonable choices for sick-care, providing the environment in which patients felt safe enough to permit medical instrumentation to occur. The development of medical practice, education, therapeutics, etc. proceeded from that point. Happily, one prominent physician understood that and reminded his contemporaries in 1910: "Now one must have some understanding of the value of the profession of nursing in modern medicine....It has changed the face of modern medicine: it is revolutionary in its influence upon the progress of modern medicine (p. 21).*

Sociopolitical Context

The advent of anesthetics occurred simultaneously with the acceptance and promotion of asepsis and the emergence of nursing in hospital care; the elements "were in place for a removal of the remaining obstacle in the path of the advancement of surgery"[24] (p. 22). Discussion concerning problems associated with anesthesia delivery began at the time of Morton's first successful induction and continued without resolution for some 40 years. Most anesthesia was given by novice interns who were more interested in the surgery than in the safe administration of anesthesia. Bankert[23] provides a quote illustrating the nonchalant attitude toward anesthesia characteristic of the times:

> *Unfortunately, in most hospitals one of the younger interns is, as a rule, selected to administer the anaesthetic. The operator accustomed to having a novice give chloroform or ether for him is kept on the qui vive while performing the operation and watching the administration of the anaesthetic. Such a condition of affairs is not conducive to the best work of the surgeon (p. 23).*

EARLY NURSE ANESTHETISTS

One of the hospitals established by the Sisters of St. Francis played a particularly noteworthy role in the development of anesthesia care. Established in 1889 as St. Mary's Hospital, it later became known as the Mayo Clinic. During the early years at the Mayo Clinic, no interns were available to assist in surgery. The clinic relied on nurse anesthetists, initially as a matter of necessity and later as a matter of choice.

The Mayo Clinic's first nurse anesthetists were Dinah and Edith Graham, sisters who had graduated from the school of nursing at the Women's Hospital in Chicago. To train the Graham sisters while continuing to support the work of the clinic, five staff nurses took over the patient care and housekeeping duties, while the Grahams administered anesthesia and did general office and secretarial work. According to Bankert,[23] Dinah's career as a nurse anesthetist at the clinic was brief, but her sister Edith continued there until she married William W. Mayo in 1893. Edith was succeeded by Alice Magaw (1860–1928), reported to be brilliant not only as an anesthetist, but also as a scholar and researcher.

Bankert[23] noted that although Magaw "won more widespread notice than that of any other member of the Rochester group apart from the [Mayo] brothers" (p. 30), she was not given membership in the medical society because she was a nurse. According to Garde,[25] Magaw administered anesthesia, was a meticulous data collector, and wrote articles. One of her studies was included in the Collected Papers by the Staff of St. Mary's Hospital, Mayo Clinic, Rochester, Minnesota, 1905–1909. A 1941 catalogue revealed that her first comprehensive paper, reporting more than 3000 cases, was titled "Observations in Anesthesia," and was published in *Northwestern Lancet* in 1899.[24] A year later, the *St. Paul Medical Journal* published Magaw's update of the year's work, and in 1906, Magaw published another review of more than 14,000 successful anesthesia cases.

According to Bankert, Magaw made numerous recommendations that shaped contemporary anesthesia practice. She stressed individual attention for all patients and identified the experience of the anesthetist as a critical element in quickly responding to the patient. Magaw's success also was attributed to her attention to the psychological dimension of the anesthetic experience. In her words, she believed that "suggestion" was a great help "in producing a comfortable narcosis"[23] (p. 32).

The model of nurse anesthesia at the Mayo Clinic drew the attention of medical people from all over the United States and the world. The Mayo Clinic's reputation gave credibility to the movement, and Magaw's efforts provided a particular advantage to careful documentation and publication. As Garde[25] noted:

> We lose so many opportunities in clinical areas because people do not take the time to write articles that could be major contributions to the literature. [By her writing], Alice Magaw really made a name for the nurse anesthetists.

In 1936, Crile,[26] who was hailed as one of the greatest surgeons in the United States, praised the nurse anesthetist movement. In these nursing professionals, he found a special quality of "finesse" for administration of anesthesia not present in medical interns. His choice for the prototype nurse anesthetist was Agatha Cobourg Hodgins, a native of Canada. According to Bankert, she "proved herself to be not only a brilliant anesthetist, but a woman of vision" (p. 39)[23] in her dedication to the development of professional nursing and the establishment of a national nurse anesthesiology association.

A graduate of the Boston City Hospital Training School for Nurses at age 21, Hodgins went to Cleveland to work as a head nurse at Lakeside Hospital. There she was selected by Crile to administer anesthesia. She avidly read all she could about anesthesia and "walked the wards" at night listening to sleeping patients' breathing to detect subtle differences. According to Crile, as quoted by Bankert,[23] "Miss Hodgins made an outstanding anesthetist for she had to a marked degree both the intelligence and the gift" (p. 41).

EARLY CENTERS FOR TEACHING ANESTHESIA TO NURSES

Crile and Hodgins inaugurated the Lakeside School of Anesthesia, which immediately was recognized as an organized center for teaching anesthesiology, contributing to the education of nurse anesthetists, and furthering the work of the graduates.[23]

World Wars I and II, the Korean conflict, and the Vietnam War all had a significant impact on the development of anesthesia. Crile and Hodgins were part of the Lakeside Unit at the

American Ambulance at Neuilly in 1914. After 2 months, Crile returned to the United States to present a plan to the U.S. Surgeon General for the creation of hospital units composed of doctors, nurses, and anesthetists for service internationally. Hodgins stayed on in Neuilly to teach nurses, dentists, and physicians how to administer anesthesia. She later returned to Cleveland to resume her work at the Lakeside School of Anesthesia. The first graduating class consisted of 6 physicians, 2 dentists, and 11 nurses. After the formal declaration of war by the United States on April 6, 1917, the Lakeside Hospital Unit, Base Hospital No. 4, was mobilized. Hodgins did not accompany the unit at the time, instead remaining as director of the school and training nurse anesthetists for military service.

In addition to training at the Mayo Clinic, preparation of nurse anesthetists was also occurring in other parts of the United States. Sophie Gran Winton (1887–1989), a graduate of Swedish Hospital in Minneapolis, had trained as an anesthetist. After garnering 5 years of anesthesia experience and having established a record of more than 10,000 cases without a fatality, she joined the Army Nurse Corps. Winton and other nurses from the Minneapolis Hospital Unit No. 26 were assigned to Mobile Hospital No. 1 in the Chateau-Thierry area of France. Working with the physician anesthetist James T. Gwathmey, the unit succeeded in pioneering anesthesia in mobile hospital units.

As suggested, a repeated theme in the nurse anesthetist movement has been that of an acknowledgment of the intelligence and dedication of women, while pointing out, with some bias, that the gender differences made anesthesia a natural place for women to display their intelligence and feminine attributes. Bankert[23] described the following expectations as characteristic of persons administering anesthesia in 1896. She noted that these qualities were found in women who were recruited into a field shunned by physicians. According to Bankert, women of that period, as perceived by physicians such as Dr. Frederic Hewitt, should

- have been satisfied with the subordinate role that the work required,
- not have made anesthesia their one absorbing interest,
- not have looked on the situation of anesthetist as one that put them in a position to watch and learn from the surgeon's technique,
- have accepted comparatively low pay, and
- have had the natural aptitude and intelligence to develop a high level of skill in providing the smooth anesthesia and relaxation that the surgeon demanded (p. 50).[23]

As Bankert suggested, this "glorified handmaiden" image was part of the expectation of the surgeon and was one that came to be associated with nursing.

The first battle between nurse anesthetists and medicine was waged in the 1920s. At that time, Francis Hoeffer McMechan, a third-generation Cincinnati physician, began to promote the organization of physician anesthetists. Before nurse anesthetists could assume McMechan's challenge to "cease and desist" practice, they first had to win a battle of acceptance within the profession of nursing. Hodgins led the movement to integrate nurse anesthetists into mainstream nursing through the ANA.

RESISTANCE FROM ORGANIZED NURSING

For years, the nurse anesthetist movement had met resistance from organized nursing. In 1909, nurse anesthetists were stunned when Florence Henderson, a successor of Magaw's, was invited to present a paper at the ANA with the unmet expectation of an invitation to join the association. In 1931, Hodgins initiated a formal effort for nurse anesthesia to become a section within the ANA. (See Bankert,[23] p. 65, for a comprehensive account of this effort.) According to notes in Bankert, Hodgins mobilized the Lakeside alumni and other nurse anesthetists around the United States to "attend a meeting for the purpose of considering the organization of [a] nurse anesthetist group" (p. 67).[23] She was committed to separating nurse anesthetists from hospital service, but retaining nurse anesthesia within the ANA framework.

The ANA eventually rejected this proposal, accepting nurse anesthetists only into the Medical-Surgical Nursing section. According to Bankert, when the ANA rejected the affiliation of nurse anesthetists, Hodgins made a profound statement that led to an alliance with the American Hospital Association (AHA). The following words, excerpted from Bankert,[23] are part of the speech Hodgins made to nurse anesthetists:

> It seems to us that anesthesia, being in no sense nursing, could not be absorbed into a strictly nursing group such as the ANA, as we hope to include in our sustaining membership surgeons, hospital superintendents, and others interested in advancing the cause (p. 73).

The nonacceptance by organized nursing stimulated nurse anesthetists to form the International Association of Nurse Anesthetists (later changed to the National Association of Nurse Anesthetists [NANA] in an effort to merge with the ANA). By 1938, the NANA had changed its name to the American Association of Nurse Anesthetists (AANA) and had moved to a new one-room office at the offices of the AHA in Chicago. The affiliation with the AHA provided a home that fostered the profession of nurse anesthesia.

INCREASED EFFORTS FOR EDUCATION AND CERTIFICATION

The recognition by the AHA and the subsequent onset of World War II, bringing a need for an increased number of military nurses trained in anesthesia, stimulated further development of the nurse anesthetist movement and later prompted other efforts to standardize nurse anesthetist education and to establish a national certification examination.[27] According to Bankert,[23] leading nurse anesthetist Gertrude Fife addressed the first national convention of the NANA in 1933, calling for a committee to

> investigate nurse anesthesia schools for the purpose of accreditation and for a national board examination for nurse anesthetists (p. 96).

Fife's stand on the direction for nurse anesthetist education was different from that of Hodgins and ultimately was opposed by Hodgins. Although Fife had the support of prominent physicians and the help of Dr. Howard Karsner, professor of pathology at Western Reserve University, in the development of national accreditation and procedures, opposition by Hodgins was based on the perception that under Fife's plan, the nurse anesthetist would not have a separate legal status.

Despite being ill and semiretired, Hodgins continued to influence the progress of the professional movement of nurse anesthetists. It was Fife who carried the ball, however. Others involved joined Fife in her efforts, and together they produced a nurse anesthesia program and moved forward to achieve the following objectives:

- advance the science and art of anesthesiology;
- develop educational standards and techniques in the administration of anesthetic drugs;
- facilitate efficient cooperation between nurse anesthetists and the medical profession, hospitals, and other agencies interested in anesthesiology; and
- promulgate an educational program to help the public understand the importance of the proper administration of anesthetics (pp. 67–77).[27]

Although Hodgins died before the first qualifying examination for membership in the AANA was held on June 4, 1945, and before the first Institute for Instructors of Anesthesiology was convened in Chicago later that same year, her efforts, along with those of other leaders, came to fruition in peacetime after World War II. Education became the primary goal of the association, and an increased effort was made to form standards and to develop a standardized curriculum to teach nurses to be nurse anesthetists.

The move toward accreditation of schools of anesthesia was approved in September 1950 with the encouragement of the AHA Council on Professional Practice and under nurse anesthetist Helen Lamb's leadership as chair of the Advisory Committee of the AANA.[23] The AANA accreditation program for schools of nurse anesthesia became effective on January 19, 1952. Although the program allowed for an interim period during which schools in existence could meet the accreditation criteria, new schools were required to meet accreditation requirements from the outset.

The rift between organized nursing and nurse anesthesia continued as deans of nursing schools and colleges resisted the inclusion of nurse anesthetist academic programs into their curricula. According to Garde,[25] this dilemma of nonacceptance led to the development of many anesthetist programs in colleges of allied health and education. Although allied health was most receptive to nurse anesthesia, the profession wanted and needed more than a certificate program.

NEW EDUCATIONAL PROGRAMS

The 1970s witnessed pivotal and profound changes in society: the nation's economic recession, the energy crisis, inflation, involvement in Vietnam, and President Nixon's articulation of a healthcare crisis, to name a few. The general direction of nursing education preparation was changing as well. As the educational requirement in nursing moved from a diploma to a baccalaureate degree, the requirement for nurse anesthesia moved from certification to a baccalaureate and master's framework. A major breakthrough in nurse anesthesia preparation occurred when Rush University decided to offer a master's of science in nursing for anesthesia through its Graduate School. Another major move to higher education for nurse anesthetists was the establishment of the first master's program in nurse anesthesia through the Department of Nursing at California State University,[25] an effort promoted through the leadership of Joyce Kelly, a nurse anesthetist affiliated with Kaiser Permanente.

CERTIFIED REGISTERED NURSE ANESTHETIST AS AN ADVANCED PRACTICE REGISTERED NURSE AND INCREASED AUTONOMY

Currently, nurse anesthesia is considered to be an advanced clinical nursing practice and CRNAs are one of four advanced practice registered nurse (APRN) roles. Requirements for admission to a nurse anesthesia program are

- a bachelor's of science in nursing or another appropriate baccalaureate degree,
- a license as a registered nurse, and
- a minimum of 1 year of acute care nursing experience (determined by the individual program).

After completion of and graduation from an accredited nurse anesthesia education program, the nurse must pass a national certification examination to become a CRNA. All nurse anesthesia education programs now offer a master's degree, which can be in nursing, allied health, or the biological and clinical sciences.[27]

In the 1970s, the AANA experienced a change in leadership and a continued controversy with organized medicine. Although Florence A. McQuillen ("Mac") had single-handedly held the organization together since 1948, the time had come for a new approach, marking the end of an era for the Association. The conflict between the American Society of Anesthesiologists (ASA) and the AANA centering on issues of control and autonomy has not yet been fully resolved.

Influence of Government Agencies

The various state boards of nursing, who worked closely on licensing issues with the National Council of State Boards of Nursing (NCSBN) and the U.S. Department of Health, were most influential in supporting nurse anesthesia. Controversy over the authority and licensing of nurse anesthetists continues to the present day. The consensus was that state boards of nursing should regulate nursing, including advanced practice nursing. According to Garde,[25] the AANA monitored very closely the recommendations of the Pew Commission as they pertained to advanced practice. The association viewed the report as a way of collapsing barriers and opening doors to allow nurse anesthetists to practice unencumbered.

Currently, CRNAs are "qualified and permitted by state law or regulations to practice in every state of the nation"[27] (p. 3). A CRNA can practice solo, in groups, and collaboratively. In addition, CRNAs have the legal authority to practice anesthesia without anesthesiologist supervision in all 50 states, typically in every setting where anesthesia is administered. Some states have placed restrictions and supervisory requirements in some settings, however.[28] CRNAs may have independent contracts with physicians or hospitals. They are the sole anesthesia providers in more than two-thirds of rural hospitals in the United States.

In 2001, at the end of the Clinton Administration, a Medicare regulation was signed that would have removed the federal physician supervision requirement for nurse anesthetists. The AHA and the National Rural Health Association (NRHA) supported Medicare's ruling. When the Bush Administration took over later that month, however, a freeze was placed on the enactment of all regulations signed at the end of the Clinton Administration. Subsequently, in November 2001, a Medicare Rule was enacted that allowed state governors to opt out of the supervision requirement by sending a written letter to the Centers for Medicare and Medicaid Services (CMS). Before sending the letter, the governor must consult with the state boards of medicine and nursing, determine that removal of the supervision requirement is in the best interests of the citizens of that state, and determine that opting out of the requirement is consistent with state law.[24] As of April 2009, 29 states have opted out of the Medicare supervision requirement.

Clinical Nurse Specialists

According to Hamric and Spross,[29] the concept of nurse specialties is not new in the profession of nursing. Minarik[30] referred to DeWitt's article in the *American Journal of Nursing* (see Bibliography), in which DeWitt attributed the development of nursing specialties to present civilization and modern science (p. 14). According to Sparacino and colleagues,[31] DeWitt's view of specialty nursing follows the medical model, basically practicing within a limited domain with certain types of conditions or "working for a specialty physician" (p. 4).

Historical Context

During the first half of the 20th century, the term "specialist" implied

> *a nurse with extensive experience in a particular area of nursing, a nurse who completed a hospital-based "postgraduate" course, or a nurse who performed with technical expertise* (p. 3).[26]

Although, at that time, such nurses were recognized for their expert knowledge regarding nursing practice in a specific area, most postgraduate nursing courses before World War II were limited to functional courses that prepared a nurse administrator or nurse educator. Although there is some controversy about when the title "clinical nurse specialist" (CNS) was first used, there is clear agreement that, in 1943, Frances Reiter, RN, coined the term "nurse clinician" and promoted the idea.[29,30,32] According to Hamric and Spross,[29] her perception of the nurse clinician was one of

> *a nurse with advanced knowledge and clinical competence committed to providing the highest quality of nursing care* (p. 3).

Reiter did not believe that a master's degree was the distinctive qualification to be a nurse clinician, but she did recognize that graduate education was the most efficient means of preparing such practitioners.

Norris[33] dated the inception of the CNS to 1944 and the NLNE Committee to Study Postgraduate Clinical Nursing Courses. Smoyak[34] credited a national conference of directors of graduate programs, sponsored by the University of Minnesota in 1949, for the genesis of the clinical nurse specialty. Even though the NLNE had recommended a plan to develop nurse specialists and urged qualified universities to undertake the experiment, one major difficulty with advancing the concept of the CNS was that the predominant level of education for nurses at the time was the diploma. Another difficulty was that in the 1950s many nurses in baccalaureate and master's level courses shared the same classroom. Eventually, psychiatric nursing was credited with being the first specialty to develop graduate level clinical experiences.

Sociopolitical Context

Several factors inhibited the growth of specialization in nursing. After World War II, there was an increased demand for nurse generalists and an increased demand for advanced education of such nurses with many veteran nurses being eligible for educational benefits under the GI bill. These factors, as well as the focus of preparation of the early graduate leaders in nursing at Teachers' College, Columbia University, and the post–World War II increase in hospital care, resulted in nursing shifting from a private-duty model to a supervisory model within a hospital bureaucracy. In response, the National Mental Health Act was passed; it provided research and training funds for advanced study in core mental health disciplines. Because psychiatric nursing was identified as a core discipline, undergraduate and graduate education in this specialty were eligible for funding. Peplau,[35] a psychiatric nurse leader, educator, and clinician, developed the first master's program focused on advanced practice in psychiatric nursing.

Oncological nursing was another area that early on developed graduate education for specialization. These efforts were spearheaded by the American Cancer Society and the National Cancer Institute. According to Hamric and Spross,[29] the American Cancer Society continued its interest in the development of CNSs in oncology into the 1990s. The Oncology Nursing Society is credited with establishing cancer nursing as a specialty and with contributing to the development of the oncology CNS role and refining the advanced practice role in oncology.

STIMULUS FOR CLINICAL NURSE SPECIALIST EDUCATION

The Professional Nurse Traineeship Program of 1963 was a major force that stimulated education in the development of the CNS movement. This expansion, along with the increasing numbers of baccalaureate-prepared nurses and the profession's increasing interest in graduate education, led to the establishment of education for clinical specialization within graduate programs.[26]

The shortage of physicians in the 1960s helped to create a milieu for expanding clinical specialization in nursing. It also provided opportunities within the healthcare environment for more competent professionals prepared for advanced practice.

By the 1970s, there were master's level programs to prepare CNSs for a variety of practice settings and specialty areas. Without a clear mandate for entry-level preparation, however, confusion remained over the use of multiple-role titles, such as nurse clinician, nursing specialist, expert clinician, clinical nurse scientist, and CNS. Also during this time, questions regarding the purpose, preparation, function, responsibility, and practice setting for the CNS continued.

CLARIFICATION OF THE ROLE OF THE CLINICAL NURSE SPECIALIST

According to Minarik,[30] role confusion began to resolve with the publication of the ANA social policy statement, which defined specialization in nursing. Clarification of the various issues provided a public declaration of criteria for the title of CNS. Other groups embraced the definition and supported the characteristics, but without a doubt, the strongest support came from the ANA in 1980.[36] Specialty organizations and state nurses' associations reinforced this definition by formally describing the requisites and competencies of nurses assuming the CNS role (e.g., American Association of Critical Care Nurses' [AACN] position statements [1987],[37] the ANA paper [1986],[38] and the California Nurses' Association statement [1984][39]). According to Sparacino and colleagues,[31] further validation of acceptance of the CNS role within the ANA became a reality with the publication of a study undertaken by the Council of Clinical Nurse Specialists reporting that 19,000 RNs functioned as CNSs. A clear definition of the CNS role appeared in the ANA publication *The Role of the Clinical Nurse Specialist,* published in 1986 when Sparacino was chair of the CNS Council.[40]

Funding for advanced nursing education occurred through federal government agencies, such as the National Institute of Mental Health and the Bureau of Health Professions (BHPr), Division of Nursing. Private foundations, such as the Robert Wood Johnson Foundation, also provided funding.

Minarik's[30] perception of the evolution of the CNS role was that it grew out of needs recognized by nurse educators and clinicians. Before the development of the CNS role, there were no rewards or opportunities for advanced study and practice in clinical nursing; a graduate student had two role selections: educator or administrator.

The social forces noted by Minarik[30] that had a significant impact on the CNS movement included growing specialization; growing use of technology; growing acuity of care; and, in a phrase coined by Cooper,[41] a growing need for "attendance" in nursing. The CNS was similar to the attending nurse who, by virtue of confidence and skills gained through years of direct clinical contact with patients, was a refined expert in providing care and guidance to others. In contrast to the generalist nurse, the CNS had to be more than just a safe practitioner. As the ANA Social Policy Statement[36] emphasized, the CNS was expected to have attained competence in a clinical specialty over time. In addition, the role reflected the additional components of educator, consultant, and researcher.

In early conversations with Minarik[30] and Riddle,[32] one gains a view of the CNS as a special kind of nurse who is able to view the patient from a well-developed knowledge base in a specialized area of nursing. According to Riddle,[32] who is not a CNS but a master teacher and clinician in the nursing of children, the CNS could be viewed as a pioneer. These clinicians learned how to present themselves in a professional manner and to work with nursing service in innovative and creative ways. The CNS programs helped nursing students learn to upgrade the quality of the care that they delivered. The CNS has a broader set of responsibilities than the non-CNS in the service setting and needs a broader educational experience.

According to Minarik's personal experience,[30] inherent and invaluable in the CNS educational experiences are collegial relationships that can be sustained over time. Minarik[30] described her experience as follows:

> *The beautiful thing that happened to me was being at the University of California at San Francisco because of the colleague relationship....There were strong clinicians, strong thinkers. This resulted in my colleagues being editors for each other's work. We struggled through the thinking involved, it was a wonderful, exciting process of co-mentorship, editing and learning together.*

These comments by Minarik[30] reflect the collegiality, collaboration, and creativity that developed as these clinicians worked together to provide expert patient care in teams of nurses and physicians. Emerging from these collegial, creative, and collaborative relationships was a need to communicate through writing what occurred with patients. The shared experience resulted in innovative nursing care in which individuals learned from one another and shared that knowledge with others.

Boyle[42] attributed CNS continuity to a history rich in problem-solving and other skills responsive to change in the practice settings. She perceived the persistent involvement of the CNS with patients across the continuum of care as providing a special view of needs, concerns, and omissions that aids in providing for continuity of care. Shifting of care from the acute hospital setting to outpatient and home care provides an ideal milieu in which the CNS can translate the need for nursing care in a more contemporary context.

In 1998, the National Association of Clinical Nurse Specialists (NACNS) Legislative and Regulatory Committee completed a critical analysis of state statutes and developed a model of statutory and regulatory language governing CNS practice. The model was driven by the need to define qualifications for practice and scope of practice for the CNS. The model recognizes the CNS scope of practice as encompassing three spheres of influence identified in the NACNS statement on CNS Practice and Education (1998)—direct patient care, advancing the practice of nursing through nursing personnel, and system interventions to improve patient care cost-effectively.[43]

Influence of Government Agencies, a Private Foundation, and Professional Associations

In the 1970s and 1980s, the Robert Wood Johnson Foundation and the Division of Nursing of the BHPr were major funding agencies for CNS education. A particular influence in the marketing of the role has been the students themselves.[30,32] CNSs have generated numerous publications in which they have described patient care within their specialties and have attempted to clarify areas of responsibility, specialization, and multiplicity of the roles. According to Minarik,[30] however, because they did not write specifically about their roles as CNSs and the impact on patient care outcomes, they remained invisible as CNSs. The ANA remained a strong marketing force, working hard to increase the visibility of the CNS. The Oncology Nursing Society and the American Association of Critical-Care Nurses also focused on clinical practice problems and efforts.

The more recent history of the CNS role depicts a shift in the role from its traditional focus to a broader scope of practice as local and national health institutions change. The environment of the late 1980s and early 1990s created new challenges and the need for definition and conformity with the APRN model. Downsizing of hospitals and budget constraints, coupled with increasing role ambiguity, led to a need for a clearer definition of the CNS.[44] Around 2000, a CNS was defined as a registered professional nurse with a graduate degree or post-master's certificate from an accredited CNS program and nationally certified in a CNS specialty. In addition, the CNS must meet all board of nursing requirements to practice as a CNS.

Nurse Practitioners

The nurse practitioner (NP) movement—the most modern of the four advanced practice roles—arose against the backdrop of the 1960s and in response to changes needed in the healthcare environment and the education of graduate nurses.

Historical and Sociopolitical Context

The time of transition from the post–World War II generation to the baby boomers' developmental years was one of social activism and scientific advancement. The assassination of President John F. Kennedy created a sense of deep national commitment to public service among young people. According to Ford,[45] a national leader in the NP movement whose contributions and vision of advanced practice for nurses have improved the quality of health care, there was, at that time, a true concern for the "haves and have nots." While the war in Vietnam was accelerating, President Lyndon Johnson declared the war on poverty. As the increase in technology was driving the need for knowledge, information systems began to emerge, and the pace of life began to accelerate.

During this time, society exhibited a sincere concern about the maldistribution of health resources, especially physicians. The increasing concerns relating to health care and the emerging emphasis on health promotion made it a good time for change in the nursing profession. Ford[45] described the time as one in which nurses were able to try new things. Although there was some uncertainty and resistance to change, mainly within the profession, the window of opportunity was clearly open.

BIRTH OF THE NURSE PRACTITIONER MOVEMENT

In a candid interview reported in the *Journal of the New York State Nurses Association,* Ford[1] described the NP movement as an

> *outgrowth (a) of the Western Interstate Commission on Higher Education for Nursing (WICHEN) Clinical Content study on Master's preparation in Community Health Nursing in which I was involved from 1963 to 1967 and (b) an experience that pediatrician Henry K. Silver had at a Child Health Nursing Conference which was organized in the mid-1960s by the public health nurses and the Colorado State Health Department* (p. 12).

Although there had been earlier attempts to expand the role of nurses, the WICHEN project provided a stimulus for the change needed in the healthcare environment and the education of graduate nurses. Dr. Silver's involvement provided the mechanism for that change. At that time, Ford and Silver designed a program for pediatric nurses that would assist in meeting the unmet healthcare needs of children from low-income families.[46]

FACTORS THAT HAVE INFLUENCED THE NURSE PRACTITIONER MOVEMENT

Ford[1] identified several factors or "myths" that have influenced the NP movement (and that continue to do so today). The first myth is that the development of the NP role was solely in response to a proclaimed physician shortage existing at the time. The reality is that the rationale for the development of the NP role came from nursing leaders who were committed to preparation of graduate nurses for clinical specialization. Four groups of faculty representing Western states[46] had worked together to identify the clinical content for a master's degree in nursing. Stimulated by social and professional developments and aided by the maldistribution of medical personnel, an "opportunistic" environment for changes in well-child care in ambulatory settings was created.[1,46] The aim of the clinical content model was not only to prepare graduate students for clinical specialization, but also, according to Levy,[12] to "reclaim a role that public health nurses had historically held" (p. 12).

To reclaim that role, nurses needed to be able to work in an autonomous and collegial way with physicians. The experience with Silver provided an opportunity for Ford and Silver to promote an experiment that would allow nurses to reclaim the role. Dr. Silver, who had been introduced to Ford by a fellow pediatrician, had not been enthusiastic about the idea of NPs. He returned from his attendance at the Child Health Nursing Conference with a new and enthusiastic view of nurses, however. Thus, the liaison began.[1,45]

This association between Ford and Silver led to a collegial relationship in which the role of nursing in well-child care was tested to determine if nurses could competently care for well children in community-based settings. That model was fashioned after the nursing profession's criteria for clinical practice, set forth by the ANA. The emphasis was on professional, direct client/patient care, health and wellness, collegiality with physicians, and prevention-oriented care, including consumer education.

The initial NP program at the University of Colorado began as part of a demonstration project in which a post-master's student worked in an expanded role for nursing. Ford[45] dated the inception of the practitioner program to the admission of the first student to the University of Colorado's program in the fall of 1965. The demonstration project tested the scope of practice by building on what had existed as part of community health nursing and doing it more thoroughly. A survey of health needs identified major problems commonly encountered by nurses in the community. More than just collecting data, the survey also focused on data interpretation and management of the well child. Results of the demonstration project helped to extend the focus of practice toward

> *testing a nursing role in well-child care to determine whether nurses could competently deliver care to well children in community-based settings.*[46]

Included in the project were efforts to increase the sensory input of nurses and to increase the nurse's ability to share that input with parents, assisting the parents in making decisions for themselves that were based on an informed consideration of options and consequences.[46] As a result, the observations of the nurse and her decision-making abilities were sharpened.

The intent of the project was not only to teach nurses how to provide care competently and confidently, but also to establish an advanced nursing practice grounded in, and held to, a post-baccalaureate academic standard. The program was successful and led to the establishment of nine accredited programs, with the standard for entry being a baccalaureate in nursing. Initially, the first programs awarded certificates given jointly by the American Academy of Pediatrics and the ANA. By 1973, the number of master's degree programs began to increase and soon outnumbered the certificate programs.[47] The early nurse practitioner programs attracted nurses with international experience, including those who had completed mission work or had broad community experience or both.

The second myth that influenced the NP movement was the suggestion that the NP movement was a medical model with nurses performing as junior physicians. According to Ford,[1,45] the model was anything but medical: It was based on well-child care, health promotion, and disease prevention, and it afforded the nurse an opportunity to assess autonomously, innovate, and work collaboratively with physicians and families in providing care. Although the myths about the program may have been negative, the outcomes were very positive. Ford also considered the statement from the National League of Nursing[48] that the early programs

> *have been considered a means of controlling costs by introducing lower-paid health care providers....as an answer to distribution problems in geographic areas short of physicians.* (p. 2)

Ford[1] believed that the distribution problems provided an opportunity to test the expanded role of nurses.

The third myth focused on the educational pattern followed to prepare NPs, suggesting that "short-term continuing education courses were the educational pattern used to prepare nurse practitioners from any nursing background"[1] (p. 12). To counter this myth, Ford[1] clarified that the first pediatric NP program, which was at the University of Colorado and was funded through the Medical Research Fund at the University of Colorado, required a baccalaureate degree in nursing and qualifications to meet graduate school admission requirements. Findings from the first pediatric experimental program, which first admitted students in 1965, were to be incorporated into collegiate nursing programs at the appropriate degree level.[48] This initial interest in an expanded role for nurses was not shared by much of the professional nursing community, however, resulting in programs being developed outside the academic framework that was originally intended by Ford and Silver. As a result, for a period, "certificate programs" through continuing education venues were developed in a variety of settings, including hospitals and medical schools.

The recommendations of the National Advisory Commission on Health Manpower and the Committee to Study Extended Roles for Nursing stimulated the interest of the government in expanding the role of nurses to meet health promotion, disease prevention, and primary care needs of patients. With this interest came funding for nurse practitioner programs. It was probably an increase of federal support in the 1970s that accelerated the development of CNS (educator-oriented role) and NP (practice-oriented role) programs.[49]

The fourth myth, according to Ford,[1] is that the "innovations in expanded roles came from professionals other than nurses" (p. 12). The fifth myth addresses the issue of laws governing practice. Ford emphasized that the model was within the practice of nurses and did not necessitate changing nurse practice acts. The sixth myth, according to Ford,[1] is that "physician supervision was necessary for nurse practitioners" (p. 12). Ford pointed out that the University of Colorado program was collegial; it was only when academic standards were compromised that the NP role became confused with the physician assistant role (which does require physician supervision) and control by the medical profession became an issue.

The seventh myth surrounds the acceptance or lack of acceptance of the NP by physicians and patients. According to Ford,[45] when collegiality was experienced, problems between or among groups diminished, resulting in the mutual acceptance of roles.

Influence of Government Agencies

Federal support came late to the movement, mainly for political reasons. Without the strong support of the professional organizations, it was difficult to promote the developing programs. The first attempt to gain federal support for the demonstration project at the University of Colorado was through the Children's Bureau. This approach was unsuccessful, however, because the perception was that the project did not fit the mold or mission of the Children's Bureau. According to Ford,[45,49] the bureau's rejection turned out to be fortunate because it motivated a search for other funding sources that proved to be very productive. The other source of federal funding was through the Division of Nursing of the BHPr. Following the initiation of the Colorado program in 1965, the 1970s opened up a significant increase in master's programs for NPs. By 1977, there were 84 master's programs, and 20% had support of the then Department of Health, Education, and Welfare (DHEW). There were also 131 certificate programs at that time. Length of time for completion of the programs ranged from 9 to 18 months and required 270 to 1440 hours of experience under the supervision of a preceptor.[50]

In 2008, 323 schools offered one or more master's NP programs.[53] The mean length of these master's programs was 21.5 months, and they required a mean of 485 didactic hours and 650 clinical practice hours.[54]

Influence of Private Foundations, Colleges, and Universities

Despite the lack of support and the resistance of professional associations, the NP movement made continued progress through the support of private foundations and specialty organizations. The Robert Wood Johnson Foundation and the Commonwealth Fund were very supportive of the NP role. Through their efforts, including moral and financial support, the program, according to Ford, was "put on the map."[45] University nursing faculty were slow to do more than challenge the ideas; it seemed that faculty were more interested in preparing the CNS than the NP. In addition, the few faculty who were in practice feared medical control.

Because the ANA and the schools did not support the early NP effort, the NP movement went to the American Academy of Pediatrics for sponsorship and certification. From 1970 and into the 1980s, NPs persisted in their attempts to be recognized by nursing organizations and academies, making repeated demands of the traditional organizations. In the 1990s, according to Ford[1]:

> *The goals of the first nurse practitioner educational programs—to be integrated and institutionalized in collegiate nursing programs—are coming to fruition* (p. 13).

The NP is clinically competent, well accepted by patients and healthcare professionals, cost-effective, and professionally credentialed.[45,46] The NP has continued to expand into new settings and new specialty areas as needs, demands, and opportunities have increased. The NP has also been influential in academic settings, introducing the concept of faculty practice and influencing graduate and undergraduate curricula.[49] The breadth of the role has expanded from a 9- to 12-month formal preparation beyond the basic nursing program to a master's level and now to doctoral preparation in family health, pediatrics, gerontology, adult health, women's health, neonatal care, acute care, and psychiatric/mental health.

Forces Influential in Marketing and Effective Use

From Ford's perspective,[45] the use of pilot projects, spurred by the academic credentials and success of Ford and Silver, helped to keep programs afloat. The Colorado Health Department and private pediatricians helped to study the process and to identify outcomes by following students into the practice arena. Ford served on the State Board of Nursing in Colorado and, as president, helped to keep the health community informed. She made visits to the medical and nursing boards and described what NPs were doing, reassuring the boards that the nurses were not changing the nature of nursing practice, but remaining within its scope.

The students themselves were probably most influential in marketing and communicating the effective use of NPs.[45] Articles, published books, personal testimonies, and invitations to visitors for direct observation at practice sites contributed to highlighting the progress and distributing the message of the NP. As healthcare issues assumed a larger part of the public agenda, newspapers begin to pick up on the trend.

Interface Among Certified Nurse-Midwives, Certified Registered Nurse Anesthetists, Clinical Nurse Specialists, and Nurse Practitioners

Coordination and continuity of care are important considerations for all APRNs. So, too, is recognition of the specific education each APRN has and the similarities and differences among the different APRN roles.

Consensus on Advanced Practice Registered Nurse Education

In July 2008,[52] a coalition comprising members of the Alliance for Advanced Practice Credentialing and the NCSBN published a document entitled the *Consensus Model for APRN Regulation: Licensure, Accreditation, Certification, and Education.* The document was the culmination of 4 years of work by representatives from the Alliance and the NCSBN to make recommendations for the standardization of APRN education, accreditation, certification, and licensure throughout the United States. The two groups comprised NPs, CNMs, CRNAs, and CNSs.

The document creates a framework for APRNs that includes the definition, educational expectations, titling, and recommendations and regulatory framework for all APRNs. This document has been endorsed by more than 45 national nursing organizations and is the basis for the APRN Model Act/Rules developed and approved by the NCSBN House of Delegates in August 2008. The documents recognize APRNs as licensed independent practitioners, regulated by boards of nursing with standardized educational requirements preparing all APRNs at the graduate level. Within this document, all APRNs will be

> educationally *prepared* to assume responsibility and accountability for health promotion and/or maintenance as well as assessment, diagnosis and management of patient problems, which includes the use and prescription of pharmacologic and nonpharmacologic interventions and has "clinical experience of sufficient depth and breadth to reflect the intended license" (p. 7).

The clarification and implementation of the guidelines in this document are anticipated to standardize and move forward the roles of the four advanced practice nursing groups[52] discussed in this book.

Similarities and Differences Among Different Advanced Practice Registered Nurses

Within the historical and sociopolitical contexts of the evolution of the four advanced practice roles of CNM, CRNA, CNS, and CNP, certain similarities and differences are evident. From the educational perspective, the most common theme—a similarity among all four groups—is that all four roles were influenced by the early development of nursing, which, through the Nightingale Schools, stimulated better education and professional development for nurses. As each practice area has evolved, education has been a significant force in enabling greater autonomy in practice.

Trends in educational preparation have gradually moved toward post-baccalaureate preparation and now are focused on doctoral preparation as the entry level. As has been stated, the professional organizations have made great strides in identifying competencies and educational and regulatory requirements for advanced practice nursing. Although each role retains a distinctive definition, the standardization of educational requirements has clarified the preparation and functions of each of the roles with the APRN framework.

In each of the four practice areas, there is also a recognized movement toward autonomy in decision making and professionalism. For CNMs, CRNAs, and NPs, acceptance of the autonomous nature of their roles by the healthcare community helped connect responsibility and accountability to authority in independent decision making in areas of assessment and care normally requiring medical management under the purview of the physician.

The CNS, in contrast, needs similar autonomy, but is not so closely aligned to medical management as are the other three advanced practice roles. Responsibilities of the CNS are broader within the specialty and focused more on nursing management of illness in acute care, consultation, education, and research.

In all four roles, support from medicine, more specifically from individual practicing physicians; from state and federal legislatures; and, most importantly, from the consumer has been of significant importance. The primary source of consumer support for nurse-midwives came from the underserved populations who benefited from their attendance at home deliveries. Nurse anesthetists gained recognition through physicians and patients, especially because of their impeccable records with survival rates through surgery. Similarly, but in different practice arenas, CNSs and NPs have been their own best advocates. Consumer satisfaction and physician advocacy have proved to be powerful stimuli for both of these movements. In contrast to the NP and CRNA movement, the CNS movement had the benefit of support from the ANA from its inception. All four groups were actively involved in scholarly and lay publications as their specialties developed, keeping professionals and the public informed.

Other significant influences included public and private initiatives. The Children's Bureau was significant in the nurse-midwifery movement. The National Council of State Boards was important for maintaining standards for the CRNA, and Robert Wood Johnson, Pew, and the BHPr Division of Nursing helped to support educational programs that moved the CNS and NP movements forward. While the ANA initially focused its support on the CNS movement, the Commonwealth Fund was a particularly helpful source of support for the NP movement. In addition, advancing technology and growing acuity in care gave further impetus to the need for clinical specialization, assisting the CNS movement. In contrast, the current emphasis on primary care and community-based illness, prevention and health promotion have created greater opportunities for the NP.

Each of the roles has experienced its own struggle in establishing credibility and acceptance by the profession and public. Educational preparation, certification, licensure, and accreditation are overriding concerns for all four roles. Increasing competition in the healthcare market in the 1970s and 1980s was a concern to people practicing in each of the areas, but especially to the emerging NP, who is particularly susceptible to the issues of equitable economic reimbursement for services, hospital privileges, and prescriptive authority. Collaboration, interdisciplinary emphasis, and mutual support are emerging as key common elements in a changing healthcare environment.

The distinctive feature of the nurse-midwifery practitioner is the focus on the health and comfort of mothers and babies during the birthing experience in the home and in the hospital. CRNAs and CNMs have engaged in systematic data collection to demonstrate competency. Probably the most distinctive feature of the CNS role is coordination, evaluation, and planning for the individual within the broader context of acute and, to some extent, community-based health care. According to Sparacino and colleagues,[31] the CNS role incorporates theory, clinical practice content, and research in a particular specialty area, promoting the "integration of education, consultation, and leadership with the clinical practice component" (p. 7). The early hallmarks of the NP role were an emphasis on primary care and health promotion that occur in an independent or collegial setting and the fact that the NP role provides an excellent opportunity for independence and innovation in practice. Table 1-1 provides a comparison of the four APRN roles.

Table 1-1 Comparison of Four Advanced Practice Registered Nurse Roles

Characteristics	Certified Nurse-Midwife	Certified Registered Nurse Anesthetist	Clinical Nurse Specialist	Certified Nurse Practitioner
Mechanisms that helped operationalize role	Autonomy Professional development War Medical support Access to consultation Legislative support Consumer support (dealing with underserved populations) Publications	Autonomy Professional development War Medical support Access to consultation Publications	Autonomy Professional development War Medical support Access to consultation Legislative support (primarily ANA lobby) Publications Managing illness in acute care Growing specialization Increased use of technology in acute care created need for an attending nurse	Autonomy Professional development War Medical support Access to consultation Legislative support Consumer support Publications Academic support of Ford and Silver Communication with state board (Colorado) Pilot projects
Forces that influenced marketing and effective use	Wars Focus on improving education Federal initiatives (Frontier Nursing Service) Development of American College of Nurse-Midwives Malpractice crisis in 1985 Consumer support	Wars Focus on improving education Certification Department of Health National Council of State Boards Private foundations Pew HCFA	Federal initiatives Private foundations (Robert Wood Johnson) Students Consumer support Support of nursing service administration	Federal initiatives (not initially but later) Private foundations (The Commonwealth Fund and the Robert Wood Johnson Foundation) Students Consumer support

Continued

Table 1-1 **Comparison of Four Advanced Practice Registered Nurse Roles—cont'd**				
Characteristics	Certified Nurse-Midwife	Certified Registered Nurse Anesthetist	Clinical Nurse Specialist	Certified Nurse Practitioner
Distinguishing characteristics	Health and comfort of mothers and babies Distinctive medical support Development of core competencies in 1978 Well grounded in childbirth Community-based and hospital-based	Medical focus nature of distinctive medical support Systematic and orderly data collection Hospital-based	Direct care broad within specialty Filled gap for the need for attending nurse to coordinate care within specialty in acute care setting Depth and breadth of clinical knowledge in one specialty Fully developed specialty	Good public relations Health and wellness focus within community-based primary care context Systematic and orderly data collection with feedback Consumer advocacy within independent role
Interaction with other specialties	National Organization for Specialty Nurses Frontier Nursing Service	National Organization for Specialty Nurses	National Organization for Specialty Nurses	National Organization for Specialty Nurses
Commonalities among roles	Autonomy in practice Interdisciplinary emphasis and sharing of each other's skills Joint effort to practice without artificial barriers Recognition of each other's areas of expertise Practice in acute-care and community-based settings Now graduate preparation	Autonomy in practice Interdisciplinary emphasis and sharing of each other's skills Joint effort to practice without artificial barriers Recognition of each other's areas of expertise Shared role in selling services in managed care Practice in diverse settings Now graduate preparation	Autonomy in practice Interdisciplinary emphasis and sharing of each other's skills Joint effort to practice without artificial barriers Recognition of each other's areas of practice Movement to community-based care, potential for overlap with NP role Graduate preparation	Autonomy in practice Interdisciplinary emphasis and sharing of each other's skills Joint effort to practice without artificial barriers Recognition of each other's areas of practice Movement to acute care, potential for overlap with CNS role Now graduate preparation

ANA = American Nurses Association, HCFA = Health Care Financing Administration.

Trends and the Future for Advanced Practice Registered Nurses

Trends indicate that the future of advanced practice nursing will continue to expand, including the emphasis on community-based primary care. For the NP and the CNM, this increased focus on primary care and the need for expanded clinical prevention and chronic disease management services will increase the potential for new growth. The CRNA has been, and will continue to be, affected by the healthcare changes, with more emphasis on 1-day outpatient surgery. The implications of this type of surgical experience in a changing environment will create a need for continuity and better communication among providers. The focus on quality improvement and patient safety with attention to the system at all levels provides the CNS with significant opportunities as well. Finally, the debate surrounding improved access to healthcare services provides opportunities for all APRNs.

Although many NPs originally foresaw the CNS role eventually being absorbed into the NP role, Minarik[30] and Riddle[32] put forth a different view of the future of the NP and CNS roles. Minarik and Riddle questioned who "will provide direct care in the acute care setting" and express concern that the "broad responsibility and creative nursing care of the CNS" may be lost in the transition.

The nursing shortage and changes in the United States and the world have created a new focus for health care providers. In recent years, nursing and the nation have faced some major crises. The increased concerns regarding bioterrorism and pandemic illnesses, the current need for healthcare reform, and the current state of the economy make it clear that all APRNs have a major role to play in providing the resources to meet the demands of the nation. As APRN roles continue to evolve, the public's expectations for nurses, particularly APRNs, to join forces and provide leadership for maintaining the welfare of individuals and communities will provide new opportunities and challenges.

The current state of uncertainty surrounding healthcare reform presents the greatest window of opportunity for APRNs to unite and be seen as a vital force or answer in addressing health and illness. A response to the rapid changes in medical technologies, the concerns over healthcare resources, and the ethical considerations inherent in the pressure to deliver high-quality, cost-effective health care requires collective strength that demands a joining of forces of these four autonomous APRN roles. It is important for the profession to remain true to its essence while continuing to develop. With our predecessors as prototypes, the secure and successful future of nursing in the emerging model of health care can best be accomplished by collaboration and cooperation and by drawing on the intellect, integrity, and vigor that have marked the best of nursing's past.

SUGGESTED LEARNING EXERCISES

1. Briefly trace the historical development of the four APRN roles discussed in this chapter. From a historical perspective, identify the forces that have influenced the development of each of these roles. From your perspective, which of these forces do you view as having the most significant impact and why?

2. Identify a key player for each of the APRN roles and discuss his or her major contributions to the advanced practice nursing movement.

3. Describe the role of the federal government and private foundations in the advanced practice nursing movement. Compare and contrast the similarities and differences of these organizations in moving advanced practice forward in each of the four roles.

4. After reading this chapter and thinking about the four APRN roles and your personal experience, where do you perceive the greatest need for collaboration, and what mechanisms or strategies would you identify as critical in enabling advanced practice nursing to move forward in a unified way?

5. Create a scenario in which representatives from each of these roles have been called forward to testify at a congressional hearing to convince members of Congress to continue to support advanced practice nursing. What points would you identify that each representative could make unique to each role and collective for all four roles that would support continued funding?

6. Consider yourself a consumer advocate for each of the four roles. Describe what you consider the strengths of each role and how it contributes to improving health care of the U.S. population.

References

1. Ford, LC. (1995). Nurse practitioners: myths and misconceptions. *J NYS Nurses Association* 26:12.

2. Dickerson, N. (2003). Personal communication, June 2003.

3. Roberts, J. (1995). The role of graduate education in midwifery in the USA. In Murphy-Black, T. (ed). *Issues in Midwifery*. Churchill Livingstone, Tokyo.

4. American College of Nurse-Midwives. (1993). Background on the AENM/MAWA Interorganization workgroup on midwifery education (IWG). *Quickening* 24:29.

5. Hiestad, WC. (1978). The development of nurse-midwifery education in the United States. In Fitzpatrick, ML. (ed). *Historical Studies in Nursing. Teachers' College Press*. Columbia University, New York.

6. Chaney, JA. (1980). Birthing in early America. *J Nurse-midwifery* 25:5.

7. Litoff, JB. (1978). *American Midwives: 1860 to the Present*. Greenwood Press, Westport, CT.

8. Litoff, JB. (1982). The midwife throughout history. *J Nurse-midwifery* 27:3.

9. Stern, CA. (1972). Midwives, male-midwives, and nurse-midwives. *Obstet Gynecol* 39:308.

10. Roberts, J. (1996). Personal communication, March 1996.

11. Hawkins, JW. (1987). Annual Report of the ANA Council on Maternal-Child Nursing. American Nurses Association, Kansas City, June 1987.

12. Levy, J. (1968). The maternal and infant mortality in midwifery practice in Newark, NJ. *Am J Obstet Gynecol* 77:42.

13. Baker, J. (1913). The function of the midwife. *Woman's Medical Journal* 23:196.

14. Dock, LL. (1901). In Robb, IA, Dock, LL, and Banfield, M. (eds). *The Transactions of the Third International Congress of Nurses with the Reports of the International Council of Nurses*. JB Savage, Cleveland, OH.

15. Tom, SA. (1982). The evolution of nurse-midwifery 1900–1960. *J Nurse-midwifery* 27:4.

16. Shoemaker, MT. (1947). *History of Nurse-Midwifery in the United States*. Dissertation. The Catholic University of America Press, Washington, DC.

17. Baer, B. (1996). Personal communication, February 1996.

18. Hall, CM. (1927). Training the obstetrical nurse. *Am J Nursing* 27:373.

19. Willeford, MB. (1933). The frontier nursing service. *Public Health Nurs* 25:9.

20. The History of the American College of Nurse-Midwives. Adapted from Varney's *Midwifery*, 3rd ed. http://www.midwife.org/about/history.cfm. Accessed January 4, 2010.

21. International Confederation of Midwives. Fact sheet. nd.

22. Thatcher, VS. (1953). *History of Anesthesia, with Emphasis on the Nurse Specialist*. JB Lippincott, Philadelphia.

23. Bankert, M. (1989). *Watchful Care: A History of America's Nurse Anesthetists*. Continuum, New York.

24. American Association of Nurse Anesthetists. Capitol corner. http://www.aana.com/capcorner /finalrule_111301.asp. Accessed June 6, 2003.

25. Garde, J. (1996) Personal communication, February 1996.

26. Crile, GW. (ed). (1947). *George Crile: An Autobiography*. JB Lippincott, Philadelphia, PA.

27. Questions and Answers: A Career in Nurse Anesthesia. http://aana.com/crna/careerqna.asp.

28. Tobin, M. (2003). Personal communication, June 2003.

29. Hamric, AB, and Spross, JA. (1989). *The Clinical Nurse Specialist in Theory and Practice,* 2nd ed. WB Saunders, Philadelphia.

30. Minarik, PA. (1996). Personal communication, March 1996.

31. Sparacino, PA, Cooper, DM, and Minarik, PA. (1990). *The Clinical Specialist Implementation and Impact.* Appleton & Lange, Stamford, CT.

32. Riddle, I. (1996). Personal communication, February 1996.

33. Norris, CM. (1977). One perspective on the nurse practitioner movement. In Jacox, A, and Norris, C. (eds). *Organizing for Independent Nursing Practice.* New York, Appleton-Century-Crofts.

34. Smoyak, SA. (1976). Specialization in nursing: From then to now. *Nurs Outlook* 24:676.

35. Peplau, HE. (1965). Specialization in professional nursing. *Nursing Science* 3:268.

36. American Nurses' Association. (1980). *Nursing: A Social Policy Statement.* American Nurses' Association, Kansas City, MO.

37. American Association of Critical Care Nurses. (1986). *AACN Position Statement: The Critical Care Clinical Nurse Specialist.*

38. American Nurses' Association. (1986). *Clinical Nurse Specialists: Distribution and Utilization.* American Nurses' Association, Kansas City, MO.

39. California Nurses' Association. (1984). *Position Statement on Specialization in Nursing Practice.* California Nurses' Association, San Francisco, CA.

40. Sparacino, P. (1986). The clinical nurse specialist. *Nursing Practice* 1:215.

41. Cooper, DM. (1983). A refined expert: The clinical nurse specialist after five years. *Momentum* 1:1.

42. Boyle, C. (1997). Lesson learned from clinical nurse specialist longevity. *J Advance Nursing* 26:168.

43. Lyons, BL. (2003) NACNS Model Statutory and Regulatory Language Governing CNS Practice. http//www.nacns.org/legis.

44. Quaal, SJ. (1999). Clinical nurse specialist: Role restructuring to advanced practice registered nurse. *Crit Care Nurs Q* 21:37.

45. Ford, LC. (1996). Personal communication, February 1996.

46. Ford, LC, Cobb, M, and Taylor, M. (1967). *Defining Clinical Contact Graduate Nursing Programs: Community Health Nursing.* Western Interstate Commission for Higher Education, Boulder, CO.

47. Bullough, B. (1995). Professionalization of nurse practitioners. *Annu Rev Nurs Res* 13:239.

48. National League of Nursing. (1979). *Position Statement on the Education of Nurse Practitioners.* National League of Nursing, New York, publication 11-1808.

49. Ford, LC. (1982). The contribution of nurse practitioners to American health care. In Aiken, LH. (ed). *Nursing in the 1980's: Crises, Opportunities, Challenges.* JB Lippincott, Philadelphia.

50. Malasanos, L. (1981). Health assessment skills in nursing: From conception to practice in a single decade. In McCloskey, JC, and Grace, HK. (eds). *Current Issues in Nursing.* Blackwell Scientific Solutions.

51. Snyder, M, and Yen, M. (1995). Characteristics of the advanced practice nurse. In Snyder, M, and Mirr, M. (eds). *Advanced Practice Nursing: A Guide to Professional Development.* Springer Publishing Company, New York.

52. Consensus Model for APRN Regulation: Licensure, Accreditation, Certification and Education, 2008.

53. Fang, D, Tracy, C, and Bednash, GD. (2009). *2008-2009 Enrollment and Graduations in Baccalaureate and Graduate Programs in Nursing*. American Association of Colleges of Nursing, Washington DC.

54. Berlin, L, Harper, D, Werner, K, and Stennett, J. (2002). *Master's-Level Nurse Practitioner Education Programs*. Washington, DC, American Association of Colleges of Nursing and National Organization of Nurse Practitioner Faculties.

Julie Stanik-Hutt is an Associate Professor and Director of the Master's Program at Johns Hopkins University, School of Nursing. Dr. Stanik-Hutt completed master's preparation for practice as an adult critical care clinical nurse specialist and is nationally certified as an adult medical surgical and an adult critical care clinical nurse specialist. She also completed post-master's preparation and is certified as an adult acute care nurse practitioner. She has practiced as a clinical nurse specialist (CNS) and a nurse practitioner (NP) and has taught in master's programs for both roles since 1992. She continues to maintain a practice as an adult acute care nurse practitioner.

Dr. Stanik-Hutt is past president of the American College of Nurse Practitioners (ACNP). She has served as the co-chairperson of the ACNP Task Force for the American Association of Critical Care Nurses, as a member of the Content Expert Panel for the American Nurses Credentialing Center ACNP Certification Examination, and as a member of the NP Peer Review and Advisory Committee of the Maryland Board of Nursing. She is a co-investigator for the Tri-Council for Nursing–funded systematic review of research regarding APRNs, *An Assessment of the Safety, Quality, and Effectiveness of Care Provided by Advanced Practice Nurses.*

Dr. Stanik-Hutt would like to recognize the contribution and work of Lucille Joel, EdD, RN, FAAN, to the development of this chapter in the first two editions of this text. Lucille Joel is a Professor at Rutgers–the State University of New Jersey College of Nursing.

CHAPTER 2

Advanced Practice Nursing in the Current Sociopolitical Environment

Julie A. Stanik-Hutt, PhD, ACNP-BC, CCNS, FAAN

CHAPTER OJECTIVES

After completing this chapter, the reader will be able to:

1. Estimate the qualities of advanced practice registered nurses (APRNs) most valued by the public.
2. Articulate current issues related to advanced nursing practice that may become formidable obstacles as the healthcare delivery system evolves.
3. Formulate a strategy for facilitating the practice of APRNs.
4. Critique the sociopolitical tactics used by organized nursing to promote the advanced practice nursing agenda.

What advanced practice nursing is and what it will become largely depend on the choices that the people in the United States make about their health care. Ideally, public opinion is a major force in determining governmental policy and consequently the form and function of the healthcare delivery system. With the election of President Obama in 2008, immediate reforms in the U.S. healthcare system were proposed. The recent dramatic shift in the U.S. economy has become the domestic priority, however.

During the Clinton administration, many people thought that the time was ripe for significant healthcare reform. Commissions were formed, congressional committees were convened, and the electronic and paper media reported constantly on the public's demand for healthcare reform. Then in 1994, control of Congress went to the Republicans, and balancing the budget became the priority. Health care ceased to be a concern except to the extent that social welfare and public entitlement programs represented a large target for budget cuts. Between 2000 and 2008, passage of Medicare Part D providing older adults with prescription drug coverage was the only successful major health-related policy initiative.

The public's desire for significant government-initiated health-care reform may be difficult to sustain unless it is linked to economic recovery. The need for healthcare reform is tied to economic factors and to the need for improved safety, quality, and effectiveness of care. In 2005, U.S. healthcare expenditures accounted for more than 2 trillion dollars, or 16% of the gross domestic product.[1] Employer healthcare premiums have increased by 87% since 2000, significantly threatening the financial survival of large and small businesses.[2] At the same time, an estimated 46 million people in the U.S. are uninsured.[3] Even with health insurance, 50% of personal bankruptcies and many mortgage foreclosures are reported to be associated with medical expenses.[4,5]

The U.S. healthcare system boasts the most up-to-date technology, but when compared with similar developed nations, it scores poorly on basic measures of quality, such as infant mortality.[6] The current system provides primarily illness care rather than health care. Management of chronic diseases consumes 75% of healthcare spending, with hospitalization alone accounting for 30% of the expenditures.[7] During hospitalizations, it is estimated that 98,000 patients die, and hundreds of thousands are injured because of preventable errors.[8] In addition, it is reported that patients receive the correct diagnosis and treatment only 55% of the time.[9,10] A great deal of money is being spent for a very dysfunctional system.

The sequence of events by which the sociopolitical environment forges public policies is familiar. These policies or their absence shape the healthcare industry, including the role of advanced practice registered nurses (APRNs) as participants in the industry. That being the case, society must move deliberately to ensure a future for advanced nursing practice. An understanding of the preferences of consumers, their familiarity with APRNs, and their attitudes toward health services, combined with an appreciation of the economic and political forces that influence the form and function of the emerging healthcare delivery system can enable APRNs to decide how and if they fit into the system.

People and Their Health

A healthcare system is the product of political, sociological, economic, cultural, and demographic trends of the time. Change in every aspect of life is the norm, but never has change been as quick and penetrating as in recent years. Given this reality, it is amazing that the healthcare industry has not undergone comparable change. It is impossible to identify all of the factors that have conspired to maintain the status quo and equally challenging to define all of the reasons that have compelled recent changes. Political, sociological, and economic perspectives provide the backdrop for this chapter. Demographics are presented here to illustrate current population trends because any discussion of healthcare services must begin with an appreciation of the people they serve.

Aging Society

The U.S. population is aging rapidly. In 2011, 80 million "baby boomers," born between 1946 and 1965, will begin reaching their 65th birthdays. These individuals constitute more than 27% of the population. The growth among the old-old, individuals older than 85 years, is predicted to be the greatest. In 1994, this segment of older people numbered 3 million; it is expected to increase to 19 million by 2050.[11,12] At least 84% of older adults have at least one chronic illness compared with 38% of young adults.[13] More than 18% of people older than 85 years live in nursing and convalescent homes. Such facilities are caring for nearly 1 out of every 20 people older than 65.[14] Although the current boomers hope to remain independent, perhaps with help in their own homes, it is likely that the number needing residential care will increase significantly. Challenges presented because of the growth in the number and health needs of older individuals are compounded by the growing shortage of all types of healthcare providers.[15]

Ethnic Makeup

The United States is also experiencing a dramatic shift in ethnic and racial diversity. Immigration is at an all-time high, rivaling the numbers of people who entered the United States around the turn of the 20th century. In contrast to the great European migrations of earlier times, the new immigrants are primarily of Hispanic and Asian origins. Between 1990 and 2000, about 33 million people were added to the U.S. population. Hispanics were the fastest-growing racial/ethnic group, adding almost 13 million people to the population. Hispanic Americans tend to be relatively young, with half being younger than 26 years of age. For the first time in history, most immigrants speak one language—Spanish. Many of the newest immigrant groups tend to live in ethnic enclaves or neighborhoods, where they sometimes are insulated from assimilation. This insulation creates a population that is more a "mosaic" than a "melting pot." These observations provide insights essential for the design and location of healthcare services and for the education and recruitment of providers.

Families

The new millennium has been a period of restabilization for the U.S. family, which shrunk to its smallest size ever, 2.62 people, in 1992 and rebounded to 3.14 people in the 2000 census. Of the 70.8 million children younger than 18, 69% live in households with two parents, and 27% live with one parent. Where children live with one parent, 38% of those parents are divorced, and 35% were never married. In two-parent families, it continues to be common for both parents to work outside the home, and the single-parent family is usually headed by a working woman. The number of families headed by single mothers has increased 25% since 1990 to more than 7.5 million households. For most of the first decade of the 21st century, about one-third of all babies were born to unmarried women; this compares with 3.8% in 1940.[11,12]

Economic Issues

The last 50 years have been an economic roller coaster in the United States, with more highs than lows. There have been fewer poor people, and median family income has been higher since 1995. A dramatic recession occurred in 2008, however, leading to an unemployment rate greater than 7.2% (13 million people), nearly a 3% increase.[15] The greatest job losses were among people with a high school education or less. An additional 8 million people are underemployed, working one or more part-time jobs. Because most Americans rely on employer-provided health insurance, loss of employment is likely to affect their healthcare decisions and increase the costs of uncompensated and governmental healthcare programs.

About half of poor people in the United States are either younger than 18 years or older than 65 years. The last census found about 12 million children (16.1%) living in poverty.

By race and ethnicity, 34% of these children are black, 28% are Hispanic, 12% are Asian and Pacific Islanders, and 13% are white.[16] Poor children are twice as likely as non-poor children to experience stunted growth or lead poisoning and to be kept back in school. One-third of children of divorced mothers and more than half of children of never-married women were poor in 2000, whereas only 9% of children in married families were poor.[17,18]

About 3.4 million elderly adults (10.2%) were below the poverty level in 2000. Another 2.2 million, or 6.7%, of elderly adults were classified as "near-poor" (income between the poverty level and 125% of this level). One of every 12 (8.9%) elderly whites was poor in 2000 compared with 22.3% of elderly African Americans and 18.8% of elderly Hispanics. Older women had a higher poverty rate (12.2%) than older men (7.5%) in 2000.[16] Although the middle class previously had a great deal of sympathy for these needy people, sympathy has turned into backlash, with financial pressures, crime, unemployment, and international hostilities all testing their patience.

Health Disparities

Poor health is associated with poverty and membership in a racial/ethnic minority group.[19] Members of minority groups are also more likely to be uninsured. Uninsured individuals are less likely to have a usual source of care or to receive preventive health services. When ill, they postpone seeking care and are subsequently sicker when they do present for care. Poor health can affect earning power and ultimately results in higher rates of disability and mortality.[20] These health disparities (or inequalities) challenge the healthcare system to provide both payment systems and providers to reverse these trends.

Future Selves

To anticipate the future of our healthcare delivery system from socioeconomic and sociopolitical perspectives, it is important to remember that each generation is a product of its times. Today's "thirty-something" adults are the subject of much commentary. Many were raised by surrogates while their baby boomer parents were caught up in the perceived need for dual incomes and the all-too-common eventuality of divorce and the "supermom" phenomenon. At least half of these 51 million "generation Xers" are college-educated, value independence and work-life balance, and are not afraid to change jobs to attain these attributes. They resent paying the price for the uncontrolled spending and environmental indiscretions of their parents. Also labeled "13ers" because they are the 13th generation in U.S. history, they have strengthened the family and long-term commitments to marriage, looked suspiciously on public assistance, supported conservative public policy, and favored the needs of the young over the old, who, ironically, are their boomer parents. They have supported volunteerism and have a no-nonsense attitude about social welfare programs.[21,22]

The rising millennial generation, also called "generation Y," is another factor in the intergenerational equation, bringing with it values and attitudes that are more aligned with the baby boomers than with generation X. The generation Xers are disillusioned and pessimistic, whereas members of generation Y seem to embody the optimism and idealism that baby boomers hold dear. Generation Y is of particular interest because by 2020, this group will compose 32% (70 million) of the population. Generation Y is ethnically diverse; with minorities constituting 34% of its total. It is intensely computer driven and skeptical of government and the media, although well aware of societal issues and problems.[23]

Each generation has characteristics that affect their employer/employee and client/provider relationships. How these two generations will influence health and health care in the United States is yet to be revealed, but one thing that can be expected is that "generational changes in values, perceptions, and expectations will have a significant impact"[24] (p. 59).

Health and Lifestyle

In the midst of all this turbulence, some things remain constant. Heart disease, cancer, stroke, chronic obstructive pulmonary disease (COPD), diabetes mellitus, pneumonia, and accidents continue to claim the most lives. Minority distinctions in morbidity and mortality continue to be notable in all areas and have become an ethical issue. Although the statistics are confusing, some general statements can be made. People in the United States have shared in life expectancy gains, although life expectancy for blacks is 73.8 years in contrast to 78.3 years for whites.[25] In 2005, death rates from hypertension, diabetes, kidney disease, septicemia, stroke, and heart disease were 30% to 250% more prevalent in minority populations.[26] The largest discrepancies in health outcomes for minorities were related to hypertension, renal disease, diabetes, and septicemia. Minority citizens are more likely to have problems gaining access to care and to have a poor experience of care when they do obtain care. These factors are evident in higher frequency of emergency department visits, higher likelihood of leaving the emergency department without being seen, and higher numbers of reports of communications problems with healthcare providers such as physicians and nurses. Perhaps partly because of problems with access, minorities are less likely to receive preventive care, such as colon cancer screening, influenza and pneumococcal vaccinations; to receive recommended diabetes care (e.g., glycosylated hemoglobin assessment, eye and foot examinations); and to have their blood pressures controlled to recommended levels.[27] Similar ethnicity-based differences are evident in maternal-child health statistics, such as the high incidence of low-birth-weight babies born to African-American mothers.[27]

Factors contributing most significantly to death and disability in the United States are associated with lifestyle and include smoking, diet, lack of exercise and activity, substance abuse, stress, firearms, risky sexual behavior, vehicular accidents, and environmental pollution. Appreciating the wisdom of investing in health, in 1991 the U.S. Department of Health and Human Services (DHHS) initiated the *Healthy People 2000* project.[28] The aim of the project was to increase the years of health and to decrease the disparities in health among people. The project involved periodic monitoring of quality-of-life indicators. By the middle of the decade, decreases were noted in cigarette smoking and alcohol-related vehicular accidents and deaths. People were noted to be consuming less fat and salt and using more supplementary vitamins and minerals. At the same time, industrial accidents, homicides, and teenage pregnancies had increased, and people were more overweight than ever before. Deaths from heart disease, cancer, and stroke were slightly decreased, but deaths from COPD and AIDS had increased. By 1993, almost 11% of the U.S. population was disabled by chronic disease, a direct result of the sophisticated medicine practiced and lifestyles.[29]

The new phase of *Healthy People* began in January 2000. With *Healthy People 2010*, the emphasis has been on health status; quality years, not just longevity; and the elimination of health disparities.[30] A broadened perspective has come from the development of the science of prevention, improved data systems and surveillance activities, consumer demand for health promotion, and a renewed appreciation of the public health. *Healthy People 2000* put a participatory and decentralized process into operation, and *Healthy People 2010* aimed to capitalize on those dynamics. The agenda continues to be a variation on the theme of increasing quality and years of healthy life and eliminating health disparities. The national dialogue is already under way to identify health objectives for the United States for 2020.

Sociopolitical Attitudes Regarding Health Care

Values that spurred the creation of the United States more than 200 years ago underlie our unique American healthcare system. These values include preference for personal freedom and rugged individualism; disdain for governmental interference; innovation and entrepreneurship; capitalism and the opportunity to "get ahead"; and compassion for the less fortunate. The healthcare system inspired by these values incorporates private-sector and public-sector resources, personal choice, a taste for specialization, and state-of-the-art technology. At the same time, consumers' expectations of unfettered choice and access to the newest and best in health care have created serious problems with regard to access, cost, and quality. Constitutional provisions supporting states' rights interfere with efforts to standardize processes and systems to improve cost-effectiveness and contributes to significant differences in contiguous jurisdictions.

The public recognizes that the healthcare system is flawed and needs to be reformed. People are simultaneously highly satisfied with their own health care but critical of the U.S. healthcare system.[31] For the most part, the voting public has access to health care and does not want to risk losing it. Because of the prevalence of employer-based health insurance, many people feel trapped in their jobs, afraid to seek more challenging or satisfying work because of preexisting conditions that jeopardize insurance coverage and because of fear that an illness would threaten their financial security.

Many consumers believe that the major problems are greed and waste and point to insurance company and pharmaceutical industry profits and to physicians' income as evidence. There is general suspicion about many of our traditional leaders, including politicians, lawyers, and clergy. In contrast, nurses are repeatedly reported to be the most honest and trusted professional. Most people feel powerless when they enter the healthcare delivery system. They rely on nurses to keep them safe, tell them the truth in language they can understand, help them maintain their autonomy, and help them to learn how to help themselves.

Despite apparent discontent with the system, when confronted with the possibility of change, many Americans seem to prefer inaction. President Clinton's Health Security Act of 1993 provided the vehicle for broad change. After much debate, this legislation failed in September 1994. As the United States now refocuses on healthcare reform, there are lessons to be learned from the experience. To begin with, Americans are not willing to jeopardize the domestic economy. According to Joel,[32] Americans want:

- Incremental reform—proceeding with caution, building on successes, allowing one change to be assimilated before requiring that another change be accommodated

- Freedom of choice in health care, even though most do not realize that their healthcare choices have already been limited

- Options, but they also want the safe haven associated with relinquishing some of those options (p. 7).

The U.S. passion for freedom of choice in health care is closely associated with a distaste for the heavy hand of government. The Clinton plan seemed to guarantee a bloated bureaucracy and federal mandates that would have preempted states' rights. It appeared to create a mushrooming social-welfare state, funded by heavier taxation on the middle-class majority. The government's response was to propose reduced funding for entitlement programs, notably Medicare and Medicaid. An intuitive public recognized that the private sector would ultimately be required to subsidize the funding deficit created in these programs.

In 2003, the 107th Congress attempted to reinstate some of the deep financial cuts made to Medicare and Medicaid, and block grants were created to fund healthcare insurance for near-poverty children. Democrats and Republicans voiced sympathy regarding the need to introduce some type of prescription drug program for elderly adults. Further talk of health care or cost containment was upstaged, however, by international affairs, the threat to American security, and partisan politics. It was not until 2005 that Congress was able to reach agreement to establish a prescription drug benefit under Medicare. This legislation was the most significant healthcare reform of the Bush administration.

Healthcare reform was prominent in the 2008 election. After passing a $787 trillion economic stimulus package, the Obama administration and Congressional leaders turned to healthcare reform. The White House hosted meetings with business and community leaders in Washington and across the United States. Congress scheduled hearings to begin examining various proposals for reform. Yet nurses, the largest single group of healthcare professionals, did not provide a significant voice early in the discussion. Physicians are typically, but not totally, the most prominent healthcare providers called on to discuss healthcare issues. Although at least 10 physicians attended the White House Health Care Summit, only one nurse, the president of the American Nurses Association (ANA), was invited. Although a few other nurses were later invited, along with many more physicians, to "second-tier" regional meetings addressing healthcare reform, the imbalance in physician to registered nurse or APRN representation influences the impression produced, leaving the dominant imprint of a medical, rather than a health-based, perspective.

The outcomes and changes generated by the Patient Protection and Affordable Care Act signed in to law March 2010 remain to be seen. Meaningful change will require considerable public support, support that in previous years has proved to be difficult to sustain. Advanced practice nurses have a special responsibility to become visible and provide leadership to these ongoing discussions and decisions.

Healthcare Delivery System

Enactment of Titles 18 and 19 of the Social Security Act created Medicare and Medicaid more than 45 years ago. After only a few years of experience operating the programs, the federal government began to anticipate a serious financial crisis. Hoping to find some solution that would contain the rapidly accelerating costs, the government supported a variety of demonstration projects. By 1982, the Medicare prospective payment system, using diagnostic related groups (DRGs), became the model for healthcare payment. Targeted at hospitals, the most costly offenders in the system, use of this model began an era of technical game-playing to reduce cost while the issue of quality care became secondary.

Early Attempts to Control Costs

Although the financial pressure on hospitals was first applied by Medicare, other public and private sector insurers quickly adopted similar reimbursement strategies. The healthcare industry responded with a rapid migration to community-based services. The variety of clinical situations managed in ambulatory care and the supportive technology in those settings grew rapidly. Many office-based practices began to resemble mini-hospitals, although largely unregulated. Concentrating their practices in these settings allowed physicians to circumvent the use constraints and oversight imposed on hospitals.

The all-inclusive DRG rate for hospitalization also prompted hospital administrators to begin monitoring physician care processes. Attempts to standardize and streamline care of inpatients included the development of care maps and critical pathways. Physicians who remained insensitive to the length-of-stay limitations and who ordered expensive diagnostic tests and therapeutic regimens, when less expensive options were available and appropriate, were considered a liability and pressured to rethink their practice patterns. Given their virtually exclusive ability to admit patients—which is essential to hospital survival—physicians retained their unquestioned influence in hospitals.

Observing the escalating cost of Part B of Medicare, the Health Care Financing Administration, now known as the Centers for Medicare and Medicaid Services (CMS), began the search for algorithms (similar to DRGs) that would place reimbursement limits on the activities of providers. Common procedural technology codes and the resource-based relative value scale (RVS) were developed for this purpose. So far, these algorithms have been unsuccessful; they do not seem to control costs but rather fuel discontent in the medical community. They have created counterproductive incentives for physicians to use therapeutic options that offer higher reimbursement rates. These payment systems may actually be driving physicians out of primary care and into specialty practices.

Managed Care

Still lagging in its ability to control cost, government looked to private-sector models, notably managed care. Although fee-for-service (payment for each activity or service) and episode-of-illness (DRG) models continued, further economies from these models were deemed unachievable. The success of managed care in the private sector piqued the interest of government and politicians.

Although managed care comes in many structural forms and financial arrangements, the goals are to control costs through use of a primary care gatekeeper, to limit the use of less cost-effective diagnostic and treatment options, and to encourage the use of integrated care systems to improve continuity of care and streamline transitions across settings. Some managed care plans are capitated, which means that instead of being paid a fee for each individual service or episode of care, providers are paid a maximum, preset, contracted fee per patient per year. A transition to managed care was a major part of the Clinton Administration's Health Security Act.

Managed care plans strive to guarantee the consumer a sound relationship with a primary care provider (PCP), but these relationships can often be strained by managed care policies. The emphasis on appropriate, but not unlimited, care can cause patient-provider conflict. Attempts to incorporate data regarding clinical utility and even medical futility into clinical discussions are branded as rationing. Payer policies that reward providers who use fewer tests and specialists (control costs) create financial conflicts of interest for PCPs, threatening the patient-provider relationship. Patient satisfaction is important to payers, however, because adequate enrollment in a plan is a prerequisite to their fiscal stability. To resolve these patient-provider-payer conflicts, managed care plans offer patients the opportunity to "buy out at the point of service." This policy ensures that patients have access to out-of-network healthcare services and provider choices for an additional out-of-pocket cost. In a managed care environment, multiple levels of care come together in a vertically integrated system. Primary and specialty care; acute, subacute, and long-term care; home care; and rehabilitation services are combined into what is intended to be a seamless continuum of services. This essential characteristic creates the need for alliances and prompted an industry merger-and-acquisition frenzy to build a full range of services.

Physician reactions to managed care have not been universally positive. Unwilling to accept any scrutiny of their practice, many physicians reject managed care arrangements. They also strenuously object to payer interference with individual professional judgments through imposition of clinical guidelines, which physicians call "cookbook medicine."

Despite these negative physician responses, managed care plans continue as an option that promises a more cost-efficient future. Medicaid, in particular, has contributed to a growing managed care market. In 2004, 61% of Medicaid recipients were in managed care plans, whereas only 21% of people with private-sector health plans and only 11% of Medicare recipients were in managed care.[33] Although not all managed care plans are capitated, this form seems to promise the best dollar value. Whether quality is sacrificed in managed care remains an unanswered question. Medicaid managed care specifically does not seem to be meeting quality expectations. Children cared for in Medicaid managed care plans received lower-quality care (fewer immunizations; fewer well-child visits; increased need for ear, nose, and throat surgeries) than children in commercial managed care plans.[34] Ratings for provision of preventive health services, screenings, prenatal and postnatal care, and chronic disease management were poor in Medicaid managed care.[35]

Primary care is the backbone of high-quality health care regardless of its form. The PCP is the linchpin in any care system, filling the roles of direct care provider, first contact at point of entry into the system, and coordinator of continuing care. The PCP is expected to shape the health behavior of patients. Often gaining access to patients through the management of minor acute illness and chronic conditions, the PCP seizes the opportunity to prevent disease and develops consumers' attitudes and skills for healthy living. Although this philosophy may be inconsistent with the medical model, it is totally consistent with the orientation of nursing.

In addition, contemporary practice should include the intense use of information systems for decision support and patient healthcare records, active patient participation, appreciation of limited resources relative to the concept of value (the relationship of quality to cost), and an interdependence among a variety of providers. Providers should be as concerned with populations as with individuals, promising a renewed commitment to public health.

Medical Home

The medical home, first described by pediatricians in 1967 as a way to emphasize care integration and quality, has been proposed to support the value of primary care.[36] For several years, it has been promoted by medical societies as a strategy to improve outcomes from and preserve physician participation in primary care. According to these groups, a medical home (also referred to as a patient-centered medical home or a primary care medical home) is a physician PCP–led practice that complies with the following principles:

- Whole-person orientation
- Care that is coordinated and integrated across all care settings
- Emphasis on quality and safety
- Strategies to enhance patient access to information, care, and providers[37]

A medical home also sets expectations for additional payments to the practice to recognize the added value provided by care coordination, adoption and use of health information technology, telephone or electronic physician-to-patient consultation, direct face-to-face physician visits, improved performance on quality measures, and sharing of cost savings achieved with the model. A medical home demonstration project was included in the Tax Relief and Health Care Act of 2006. Although that demonstration is just now being implemented, the medical home strategy is already being widely adopted by many state and private insurer projects. Most of these projects follow the exclusively physician–led model, which excludes APRNs from participation as PCPs. These studies also fail to document whether nurses of any type are present in the practice or have any role in the care.

There is significant concern that if the medical home model is adopted as an exclusively physician PCP–led model, APRN practice and reimbursement, especially for NPs, would be dramatically restricted. National NP and nursing organizations have worked to ensure that the authority of NPs to participate as PCPs is not restricted in these medical home projects. These efforts have met with some success, most notably in the revised American College of Physicians policy position regarding nurse practitioners. That document acknowledges "the important role that nurse practitioners play in meeting the current and growing demand for primary care, especially in underserved areas." It goes on to suggest that the effectiveness of NP-led medical homes be evaluated along with physician-led medical homes.[38]

The Accountable Care Organization (ACO), another demonstration program authorized under the Patient Protection and Affordable Care Act (2010), rewards practices that take responsibility for costs and quality of care received by their patient panel over a period of time. Healthcare providers include physician groups, hospitals, NPs, PAs and others. ACOs that meet quality of care targets and reduced costs of their patients relative to benchmarks would be rewarded with a share of the Medicare savings achieved.[98]

The APRN and the Healthcare Delivery System

APRNs include certified registered nurse anesthetists (CRNAs), certified nurse-midwives (CNMs), clinical nurse specialists (CNSs), and NPs. The foundations of nurse anesthesia go back to the mid-to-late 1800s when nurses first administered anesthetic agents during surgical procedures.[39] The specialty of nurse midwifery was established soon after, in the 1920s.[40] Thirty years later, Peplau created the role of CNS in 1954 and used it to enhance nurses' expertise in psychiatric care.[41] Finally in 1965, Silver and colleagues[42] began to prepare experienced nurses to provide expanded practice services to children as pediatric NPs.

Today, APRN practice is based on advanced knowledge, skills, and practice expertise attained through graduate study in nursing. In the past, preparation for APRN roles could be completed through certificate programs. Some APRNs educated in those early certificate programs continue to practice today, but they are quickly reaching retirement age. These nurses overcame enormous barriers to secure legal authority for advanced practice and established the strong record of practice excellence that forms the sociopolitical foundation for advanced nursing practice in the 21st century. They should be commended for their leadership contributions to the advanced practice movement.

Now, all CNS and NP educational programs award at least the master's degree; however, the number of schools offering the practice doctorate is growing. Although the trend is toward the master's degree for nurse midwifery practice, two post-licensure certificate programs that do not award a master's degree are still recognized. At the same time, a clinical doctorate in the CNM role can be earned at 11 schools.[43] Of the 108 accredited nurse anesthesia educational programs nationwide, all offer a master's degree, and at least 5 offer clinical nursing doctorate options for CRNAs.[44]

Underpinnings of APRN Practice

All 50 states and the District of Columbia address advanced practice in public policy. For the most part, state boards of nursing (BONs) hold the authority to license and regulate APRNs, and nearly all of them require nationally recognized certification in the specialty.[45] By this arrangement, many state BONs have deferred to the profession's right to recognize its specialists through certification and to develop and promulgate the standards of practice on which certification is based. In the past, certification standards were seen as vague and lacked precise competency statements on which to build rigorous and reliable certification examinations. At its annual meeting in the summer of 1995, the National Council of State Boards of Nursing (NCSBN), an association of state and territorial BONs, postponed plans to develop a certification or licensing examination for NPs and CNSs under the aegis of the state BON.

All the APRN groups have created documents that describe expectations for their respective educational programs and practitioner knowledge, skills, and abilities. Standards and policies for accreditation of nurse anesthesia programs have existed since 1952 and have been used by the Council on the Accreditation of Nurse Anesthesia Educational Programs to monitor the quality of CRNA education for nearly 20 years.[46,47] The *Standards for Nurse Anesthesia Practice* were first published in 1974; it has subsequently been revised seven times, and the eighth edition was published in 2007.

The American College of Nurse-Midwives published performance standards, *Core Competencies for Basic Nurse-Midwifery Practice*, in 1978.[48] These competencies have also been subsequently revised five times, most recently in 2007. In addition, educational programs preparing CNMs have met requirements of the Accreditation Commission for Midwifery Education since 1982.

The American Association of Colleges of Nursing (AACN)[49,50] and the National Organization of Nurse Practitioner Faculties (NONPF)[51] have developed educational standards for advanced nursing practice and entry-level core competencies for NPs. In October 2002, the AACN and NONPF completed work on primary care NP competencies in the specialty areas of adult, family, gerontological, pediatric, and women's health.[52] Competencies for psychiatric and for acute care NPs were similarly developed in 2003 and 2004.[53,54] Additionally, in 2001 and again in 2008, the NONPF and AACN convened a national task force to create *Criteria for Evaluation of Nurse Practitioner Programs*.[55] This landmark work, completed collaboratively by NP organizations with an interest in NP education, certification and accreditation established standards for NP programs.

From the logic of developing all these scope-of-practice and standards documents and educational program criteria, it follows that nursing educational accreditation boards should incorporate these competencies in their program evaluation and that certification boards should design their examinations based on these competencies. This is not merely an option but a necessary step for the profession to maintain any control over advanced practice. Application of the same standard by the accrediting and the certifying agencies provides the best assurance of competence for the consumer. The fact that these competency statements originated with practitioners and are nationally recognized by the profession means they exhibit professional unity and provide enhanced credibility.

Medicine has ensured the credibility of its specialists (advanced practitioners) by the creation of an oversight board, the American Board of Medical Specialties (ABMS). The ABMS recognizes specialty boards based on their adherence to specific standards defined by their specialties, on the processes and testing instruments used to ensure the competency of their diplomats, and on the quality of their residencies, among other program aspects. In 1992, nursing established the American Board of Nursing Specialties (ABNS) for the purpose of assuming a similar leadership role in certification. As the *Consensus Model for APRN Regulation*[56] is implemented, the ABNS could provide a vital link between internal and external regulation of the roles and professional regulation of the specialties.

APRN Roles and Public Policy

APRNs are licensed in such a variety of ways across the United States that their regulations, authorizations, and limitations most closely resemble a crazy quilt. Most CNSs practice nursing, at the highest level of expertise, under the authority of their registered nurse license. Some states (e.g., Connecticut, Minnesota, Ohio, Texas) have separate designation or secondary licensure for CNSs using the title "advance practice registered nurse." A few use this title for CNSs and NPs. In 33 states, the BONs retain sole authority over NP practice, but in 17 states the state boards of medicine are involved to some extent. Depending on interpretation of state law, NPs are authorized to practice completely independently in 11 to 23 states, but they are required to submit to some form of collaboration with physicians in up to 28 states.[45,57] Supervision language is used in 11 states.

The regulatory process for CNMs and CRNAs sometimes give the appearance of being more straightforward. This appearance could be due in part to the fact that the CNM is commonly recognized in the law through amendments to medical practice acts, which legally require CNMs, and frequently CRNAs as well, to practice collaboratively with a physician. The CRNA has a long history of credibility, and CRNAs were the first APRNs to assume leadership in focusing on practice changes to ensure patient safety. Despite this record, CRNAs continue to defend against medicine's attempts to require anesthesiologist supervision of their practice.

Some regulatory proposals have called for a one-on-one supervisory relationship between a CRNA and anesthesiologist. An alternative tactic has been to insert language in facility licensing regulations requiring oversight of CRNA practice. This amount of dependency would make the use of CRNAs inefficient and at the very least would result in increased cost to the consumer and, more ominously, place severe limitations on the availability of anesthesia services, especially in rural areas. It could also lead to the loss of anesthesia practice to nurses.

In the 1980s, the ANA began to link the NP with the CNS in public policy language, using the term "advanced practice nurse (APN)" to refer to both. Legislators already understood the NP role and its benefit to the public. This appreciation was based largely on the ability of the NP to substitute for the physician in many settings, offering many of the same services at a lower cost. The unintended consequence of this comingling of the CNS with the NP for policy advancement has been some confusion regarding the roles of these two unique and equally valuable roles. In the early 1990s, use of the term APN was expanded to include the CRNA and CNM. The purpose of this language was political and directed largely toward the reimbursement agenda; it is not intended to imply that the four roles are comparable.

Although there is agreement that the CNS and NP are APRNs, there has been less support among nurses for the use of a single generic title. Citing a 1990 curriculum study that reported similarities in CNS and NP education, some schools of nursing blurred the distinctions between these two roles.[58] Subsequent role delineation studies have shown clear distinctions in practice activities of these two APRN roles, however, with a few areas of overlap.[59-63] Additionally, practicing CNSs and NPs assert that significant role crossover is impossible without additional education and would dilute the benefits attributed to each role. Debate continues over the body of knowledge and skills common to both roles. Meanwhile, the job market for NPs has created a demand for post-master's and second master's degree programs to prepare CNSs for NP practice. Academic program accreditation criteria, certification examination eligibility requirements, and some state laws now require that the graduate transcripts specify the type of role and patient population preparation the APRN has completed. Consequently, role crossover is no longer left to the discretion of the educator or individual practitioner. In contrast, CRNA and CNM roles and practice boundaries have always been more clearly circumscribed. It is important, however, that nurse educators and advanced nursing practitioners form advisory relationships and work together with government agencies to create appropriate legislation and regulations related to APRNs.

The form of tomorrow's healthcare system is uncertain. All the participants have not yet been identified, and statements of philosophy and policy positions are often contradictory. The system is still evolving, and part of that process requires public education about advanced nursing practice. The value of health promotion, disease prevention, and self-sufficiency is gaining momentum. Consumers are demanding more control over their healthcare decisions, even if the freedom of choice in providers is limited to individuals who have the financial ability to seek and purchase care outside of a provider's plan.

NPs, CRNAs, and CNMs, who provide healthcare services directly to patients, have clearly established roles. In contrast, the CNS, whose primary role is to improve healthcare delivery indirectly through provider and systems improvements, is often in a more tenuous position. It is a role that has frequently been undervalued, even by nurses themselves, and it is too often considered expendable when money gets tight in healthcare institutions. The fact that CNSs are not a luxury, but a necessity, must continue to be shown through research and evaluation.

Strategic Roles for APRNs

For many, access to the system is through a PCP who continues to coordinate services and manage problems that can be resolved at the level of competence of the PCP. In the ideal situation, the PCP is both a skilled clinical generalist and a developer of people.

Counseling and teaching must be a strength, and consumer satisfaction is a requisite outcome. NPs are well suited to the PCP role, given their clinical competence, emphasis on health promotion, nursing expertise in care coordination and patient education, and commitment to the goal of increasing the independence of their clients. Physicians historically have been more interested in disease management than in health promotion and disease prevention and in specialization and subspecialization rather than in generalist practice. APRNs—more specifically NPs, CNMs, and some CNSs—are the natural competitors with physicians for the PCP role. Although only a handful of medical school graduates select primary care practice, many groups propose the government create greater incentives for them to pursue this option.[64] There are almost 150,000 nurses who could potentially assume the PCP role. Payment incentives, the current physician supply, and emphasis of preparation of most

APRNs in primary care practice must be considered in any strategy to increase the presence and prominence of APNs in any future healthcare reform.

The policies of health plans should also be carefully monitored to determine where APRN services can be incorporated. It is common to allow female health plan subscribers to have a relationship with two PCPs, one for women's health and a second for general health concerns. This policy has strategic implications and should cause NPs and CNMs to emphasize their respective educational preparation to fill these roles. Women's health is an attractive clinical focus and, if broadly prepared for practice as PCPs in women's health, CNMs would be logical choices, as would women's health NPs.

The placement of NPs within provider panels is another area to be examined. After fighting for years to have NPs included in provider panels, some health plans have added NPs but have categorized them as "specialists" on their provider lists. Although patients are able to find NPs, they may be required to pay higher co-pays or to obtain a referral or preapproval to receive care from an NP.

The acceptance of primary care as a valued component of an evolving healthcare system is significant, but it should not cause APRNs to ignore traditional markets for nursing services. CNMs continue to offer family-centered birthing as well as women's health care. They also lend their expertise to improve hospital maternity and newborn services and systems. The skills of CRNAs, although still concentrated in the perioperative area, have been applied to improve care of individuals with acute and chronic pain. The increased complexity of patients at every level of care creates the need for APRNs in various direct and indirect roles in acute and critical care, rehabilitation, and long-term care settings.

CNSs are well prepared to assume indirect care roles in case management, care coordination, quality improvement, and development of the practice of staff nurses. Success in these roles requires a "mental set" that integrates clinical and financial information. Much of the frustration facing individuals who practice in the CNS role derives, however, from the fact that it is a highly mediated role. Positive patient outcomes are frequently accomplished by other nurses, but only because the CNS has addressed systems' problems and helped to develop the nurses' capacity for more sophisticated practice. Because patient outcomes cannot be attributed directly to CNSs, they must become masters of inference to document their invaluable contributions. Information systems that can be used to quantify the impact of CNSs on patient populations and the system would support the important role they play and preserve their positions while justifying their salaries.

Two growth areas for APRNs are direct care of acutely and critically ill adults and children and all types of care for elderly adults. The first acute care NPs were neonatal NPs. Adult acute care NPs became established in the 1990s when hospitals were challenged by managed care to streamline care while maintaining continuity across settings. Soon after, NPs began to practice in subspecialties such as cardiac surgery, trauma, solid organ transplant, and oncology. Pediatric NPs specialize in the care of acutely and critically ill children.

The market for NPs in acute care has increased dramatically as they have shown the ability to deliver high-quality care. At the same time, graduate medical education work hours decreased the availability of physician house staff. Many of the resulting provider gaps were filled by acute care NPs. The impending retirement of baby boomers and resultant increase in demand for health and long-term care services provide untold opportunities for NPs and CNSs.

There is a critical shortage of direct care providers (NPs and physicians) with expertise in the care of older adults. Although there is a growing body of evidence that NPs can improve the health and quality of life of older adults, NP programs in the specialty are in jeopardy because of low enrollments. APRNs directly and indirectly affect the health of residents in nursing homes, providing education and leadership to nursing staff and monitoring and improving the quality of care. Both types of APRN providers are needed to provide direct patient care management services and to develop new methods and models of care for this large population of patients, which carries a heavy burden of chronic disease. In response to these challenges, the nursing profession is taking steps to increase the competencies of current and future APRNs to meet the unique needs of this growing population.

Continuing Issues for Advanced Nursing Practice

Most external obstacles to advanced practice have, in one way or another, been associated with public policy. Although doors open slowly, APRNs have achieved positive legislative and regulatory gains. The goal has been for the APRN to secure direct access to the public. In this fragmented, litigious, and medicalized system, nurse practice acts and credentialing systems attest to competency of APRNs and their authority to practice. The safety and efficacy of nurses in advanced practice has been proved many times over.[65-73] Despite this, efforts to ensure appropriate prescriptive authority, clinical privileges, direct reimbursement, and enrollment on managed care provider panels have been frustrated by the resistance of other health professionals, particularly organized medicine, to expanding the scope of practice of APRNs. Availability of adequate professional liability insurance has also hindered full APRN practice.

APRN Licensure, Accreditation, Certification, and Education

As APRN practice has evolved, state BONs have struggled to determine appropriate regulatory standards. Most BONs are composed of a variety of types of nurses: licensed practical nurses (LPNs), registered nurses (RNs), academic nurse educators, nurse administrators, and community members. Some BONs have an APRN member or receive consultation from an APRN advisory committee. The NCSBN provides a national forum for boards to discuss common concerns and develop recommendations regarding regulatory issues.

In February 2006, the NCSBN APRN Advisory Group (now designated the APRN Advisory Committee) released a draft document, *Vision Paper: The Future Regulation of Advanced Practice Nursing,* and requested comments.[74] The *Vision Paper* contained three controversial items:

- The development of a core generalist licensure examination for all NPs
- The exclusion of CNSs from the definition of advanced practice, which would mean that only NPs, CNMs, and CRNAs would be licensed for advanced practice
- The addition of a residency before full APRN licensure

The Committee's position regarding the need for APRN licensure for CNSs was based on its assessment that the practice of CNSs was within the RN scope of practice and did not require additional regulation by BONs or separate licensure to practice.

Over the 2 years that followed the release of the *Vision Paper,* an APRN Joint Dialogue Group, comprising representatives from national APRN organizations and the NCSBN, continued to work on development of a consensus-based model for APRN regulation (commonly called the Consensus Model). In 2008, the model, which addresses APRN education, accreditation of educational programs, certification, and licensure, was disseminated.[56] This Consensus Model is intended to create an integration of APRN preparation with credentialing for practice and a uniform approach to recognition of APRNs. The members of the APRN Joint Dialogue Group hoped to create a model that would minimize state-by-state differences in APRN regulation and allow APRNs to move from one jurisdiction to another without encountering new and divergent licensing requirements.

The Consensus Model recommends second licensure using the title APRN and title protection for each of the APRN roles—CNS, CNM, CRNA, and CNP. It defines an APRN as an RN with substantial "specialized knowledge and skills acquired through graduate level education"[56] (p. 5), whose practice focus is primarily on direct patient care in a scope of practice that extends beyond that of an RN and requires additional regulatory oversight by a BON.[56] To be included within the APRN definition, the CNS role was reconceptualized to have a significant component of direct patient care and to encompass skills of diagnosis and management, including prescriptive authority. If adopted into state regulations, this means that in the future, a nurse who did not complete required educational preparation to provide direct patient care with prescriptive authority, including graduate courses in physiology/pathophysiology, pharmacology, advanced health assessment, and is not nationally certified as a CNS would not hold second licensure as an APRN and would not be able to use the title CNS. Although this Consensus Model has been endorsed by the NCSBN and 45 national APRN and other nursing organizations, its full implementation will require many changes, including changes to nurse practice acts in a majority of states.

Prescriptive Authority

Almost everyone entering the healthcare system receives a prescription for drug therapy. Historically, the right to prescribe medications was the exclusive domain of the physician. As NPs become more widely established, many continue to manage illness, including the prescription of medication, in a joint practice or collaborative relationship (sometimes a euphemism for supervision) with a physician. The reasoning for this requirement is inconsistent. NPs are proposed as a physician substitute because they represent at least equal outcomes at lower cost. This rationale loses its credibility when medical management cannot proceed without physicians' approval. If APRNs are to be PCPs, they must have full prescriptive authority on their own signature, including that for controlled substances.

The authority to prescribe independent of any physician involvement exists for one or more categories of APRNs in 13 states (the District of Columbia is treated as a state for this analysis); 38 others maintain a requirement for some formal physician involvement.[57] Although NPs have prescriptive authority in all 50 states and the District of Columbia, they may prescribe independently in only 11, and physician collaboration is required to perform this activity in the remaining 40 states.[45] Prescriptive authority of NPs includes controlled substances in 48 states. CNSs may also prescribe in a few states (e.g., Illinois, Ohio, Minnesota, Texas).

Prescriptive authority for APRNs is often controlled in various ways. The range of drugs permitted to be prescribed by APRNs is sometimes limited to a formulary developed jointly by state BON, medicine, and pharmacy. Prescriptive authority may also be limited to drugs common to a specialty area. CRNAs are frequently allowed to select and administer, but not to prescribe, medications. CNMs are often prevented writing for legend drugs–medications for which a prescription is required but does not include controlled substances–to manage conditions such as hypertension, dyslipidemia, and seizure disorders, but are allowed to prescribe medications traditionally seen as related to women's health, such as prenatal vitamins, hormone replacement therapy, and birth control. The variety of constraints is creative and often obviously self-serving. The medical community seems to be determined to maintain as much control as possible over access to drug therapy. In the interim, prescriptive authority contingent on collaboration can be workable. Joint practice arrangements between APRNs and physicians or medical directors in community practice settings or with a service chief in inpatient settings can be used until this involvement is unnecessary.

With characteristic patience and tenacity, APRNs will continue to make progress related to prescriptive authority and independence. Other non-nursing professional groups are making inroads, which could establish further precedents. Physician assistants are authorized to prescribe in all 50 states.[75] Psychologists and pharmacists have successfully argued that they are qualified to prescribe, prompting many states to allow them some degree of prescriptive authority. The goal and expectation for unencumbered APRN independent prescriptive authority will likely take years and considerable sociopolitical will. Similar to all other efforts to remove unnecessary barriers to practice, achievement of this goal will be contingent on public demand for APRNs to provide these services and APRN involvement in the political process, including the election of supportive legislative representatives. As APRNs become more involved in this process, state authorizations are improving; the best source of up-to-date detail on state-to-state variations in prescriptive authority for NPs in particular can be found each year in the *Pearson Report*, published in the *American Journal for Nurse Practitioners*, and in the *Annual Legislative Update*, published in the January issue of *The Nurse Practitioner*.[57,76]

Professional Staff Privileges

The educational and experiential background of an APRN should result in peer status within the multidisciplinary healthcare environment. Criteria for the approval and accreditation of healthcare programs and facilities have been fairly consistent in adopting an expanded definition of the term "professional staff." This expanded definition awards professional staff privileges to various providers. Healthcare systems often impose more specific restrictions, however, for the express purpose of denying privileges to emerging or nontraditional providers, such as APRNs, podiatrists, chiropractors, and dentists. Over the past decade, the question has been raised whether the withholding of privileges is an act of discrimination or of restraint of trade[77] (p. 326).

Professional staff privileges recognize the right to admit, discharge, treat, visit, or consult on the clinical management of patients. Withholding privileges denies patient access to the excluded providers when patients are admitted to a particular system. Providers with the authority to admit patients to a system hold stature (influence) in the system through their ability to contribute to its financial stability.

The Joint Commission requires that healthcare facilities credential any licensed independent provider with privileges to order tests or treatments.[78] This requirement applies to physicians and other healthcare providers whom the Joint Commission categorizes as licensed independent providers (LIPs). APRNs may be credentialed as members of the professional (medical) staff organization as LIPs and given privileges based on their state-authorized scope of practice. Many NPs, CRNAs, and CNMs have inpatient management privileges based on this credentialing. Up to 40% of NPs have admitting privileges, although this is primarily in rural and underserved areas.[79] In some situations, privileges are associated with the imposition of the requirement for joint or collaborative practice with a physician. Other limitations may require APRNs to restrict their activities to a specialty scope of practice (e.g., psychiatric–mental health CNS, women's health NP). The ability to obtain professional privileges is more important if payers refuse to empanel providers who do not have admitting privileges and for APRNs who are providers in rural and medically underserved areas.

The creation of a nursing staff organization has been proposed by some as the counterpart of the medical staff organization (also called the professional staff organization) as a method to offer privileges to APRNs. Such arrangements do not carry the same recognition, however, and could be confused with nursing staff who organize for purposes of negotiating conditions of employment. This is an unacceptable solution for many reasons. One reason is parity and a need for appropriate recognition within a multidisciplinary environment. A second concerns a technicality of labor law in which an organized effort such as forming a nursing staff organization could be misconstrued and used later to challenge the right of staff nurses to choose a collective bargaining agent or unionize. Other dynamics and dilemmas are contingent on whether the APRN with privileges is an employee of or an independent contractor in the institution. To the extent that an APRN is viewed by an institution as a "mere employee," the power of the admitting privileges could be limited.

CNMs are a contrasting story of success. Just 25 years ago, few states permitted nurse midwives to practice. Between 1975 and 1991, the number of hospital births attended by CNMs increased sevenfold. Mandatory access of CNMs to Medicaid recipients ensures practice viability in every state and territory. The preferred practice setting for CNMs has become the hospital, perhaps owing to the legal requirement to maintain a collaborative arrangement with an obstetrician. In addition, dramatic increases in malpractice premiums for this specialty often prevent CNMs from attending births, sometimes limiting them to labor coaching and other women's health and maternity service activities.

CRNAs have the legal authority to practice anesthesia without anesthesiologist supervision in all 50 states, typically in every setting where anesthesia is administered. The most restrictive proposals concerning CRNA practice in recent years have tended to occur in the context of laws, rules, guidelines, or position statements regarding physician office and outpatient surgery center practice, but many of the proposed restrictions have been rejected.[80] These observations support the prevalence of hospital practice privileges among CNMs and CRNAs.

Reimbursement

Achieving reimbursement for APRN services has been a tortuous and costly agenda. Progress has been slow but steady. All categories of APRNs are reimbursable in the Federal Employees Health Benefits (FEHB) program. Similar provisions are included in TRICARE (previously known as the Civilian Health and Medical Program for the Uniformed Services [CHAMPUS]), the government's health benefits program for military active duty and retired personnel and their family members. TRICARE includes options for standard and managed care plans. It shares the costs of inpatient and outpatient medical care from civilian hospitals and physicians when care is unavailable through a military hospital or clinic. NPs, psychiatric CNSs, CNMs, and CRNAs are authorized to provide TRICARE services and are directly reimbursed.[81]

There is a federal mandate for the reimbursement of pediatric and family NPs and CNMs through Medicaid (at 70% to 100% of the physician rate), but state discretion prevails for other NPs and for CRNAs and CNSs. "Mandatory" in terms of federal legislation means that a provider must be reimbursed through Medicaid (or other federal programs as specified) for services within the provider's scope of practice as recognized within that state, but some states bar APRNs from Medicaid reimbursement. None of the federal reimbursement laws supersede the states' responsibility for health and safety.

Medicare was opened to direct reimbursement of APRNs with the provisions of the Balanced Budget Act of 1997, although only at 85% of the fee received by physicians. Before the Balanced Budget Act, NPs and CNSs were limited to serving Medicare recipients in rural and medically underserved areas. CNMs and CRNAs were already recognized under Medicare. CMS rules regarding NP authority and reimbursement for long-term care, acute inpatient care, and home and hospice services are convoluted, although evolving. Physicians are still the designated provider of care for Medicare recipients in nursing homes; they must perform the initial comprehensive visit and sign the certificate of necessity. NPs may do alternating and medically necessary visits, and, if not an employee or contractor of the facility, they may sometimes sign certifications of necessity as well.[82] CMS rules also allow a primary care or hospital-based NP to perform a patient's admission history and physical examination before surgery. If the salary support of the NP is unbundled from the Medicare cost report, hospital-employed NPs may bill for the services they provide. Although they cannot initially order home care and hospice, NPs may provide ongoing evaluation and management of care of these patients and be designated as the "attending physician" for hospice patients.[83]

On March 9, 2000, CMS announced that removal of the federal requirement that CRNAs be supervised by physicians when administering anesthesia to Medicare patients was forthcoming. Delays continued until July 5, 2001, when CMS published a proposed rule that would maintain the existing supervision requirement but allow a state's governor the right to petition CMS requesting exemption from this requirement when the governor had consulted with the state's boards of medicine and nursing, determined that opting out of the requirement was consistent with state law, and decided that it is in the best interests of the state's citizens. By 2009, 15 states had opted out of the federal physician supervision requirement—Iowa,

Nebraska, Idaho, Minnesota, New Hampshire, New Mexico, Kansas, North Dakota, Washington, Alaska, Oregon, Montana, South Dakota, Wisconsin and California.[46] Although CMS directed the Agency for Health Research Quality to conduct a study comparing anesthesia outcomes in the states that selected to "opt out" of the CRNA supervision requirement with outcomes in the states that did not, results of that investigation are not yet available.

Indemnity and commercial insurance is governed by state laws, and these laws recognize advanced practice nursing to a varying extent. The picture is confusing, however. APRNs report reimbursement in 37 states,[57] and many APRNs report billing "incident to" the practice of a physician in federal and state programs and in many private sector plans. In this situation, the physician or practice is paid a fee equal to what a physician would have received for the same services, but the nurse must meet strict physician-NP practice conditions. If the APRN bills independently, the fee is 65% to 85% of the physician's reimbursement amount. This continues to be a controversial issue.

Reimbursement is honeycombed with social bias and self-serving behavior. A particularly blatant example can be seen in the work of the Physician's Payment Review Commission (PPRC). Charged with proposing a rate structure for Part B of Medicare, the PPRC based its fee-setting techniques on the service to the patient, as opposed to the identity of the provider. The commission justified this move by alleging the need to increase the attractiveness of primary care to physicians by reducing the financial differential between generalists and specialists. When it came time to apply the same standard to non-physician providers, the PPRC recanted and proposed that the extent of the provider's education should be built into the reimbursement formula for this group.

A surge in the NP job market has been associated with growth in community-based services and primary care. The fact that NPs are comfortable in the employee role and excel in their ability to work within systems has not been lost on employers. NPs are seen as low-cost physician substitutes. In some settings—such as emergency department non-urgent care fast-track areas—their ability to practice independently or under collaborative agreements has been seen as an advantage over physician assistants, who must be supervised.

Disease prevention, health promotion, and self-care services now hold higher value than in some earlier paradigms. Reimbursement may become a nonissue with managed care or other prepaid forms of care delivery, but APRNs must continue to work with legislators and regulators to remove idiosyncrasies in insurance laws that are barriers to plan participation. Payers must be convinced to include APRNs within care networks and as members of approved primary care and specialty care provider panels. The goal is to attain reimbursement options that are on par with those of other healthcare professionals, such as physicians, who provide the same services.

Professional Liability Insurance

A liability insurance crisis occurred in 1985, when CNMs sustained an increase in their premiums so great that it could not be absorbed by their incomes. CNMs were assumed to represent a liability risk equal to that of obstetricians, who have the highest claims experience in the medical field. Nurse midwives, with their long-standing mandatory relationship with physicians to ensure backup in the event of intrapartum complications, had been tainted by physicians' malpractice experience. The solution to the crisis was a self-insured arrangement involving the American College of Nurse-Midwives and a consortium of insurance companies. Liability issues again surfaced between 2002 and 2004, prompting significant premium increases and the layoff of some CNMs from private practices, along with the closure of some community-based CNM birthing centers. CRNAs, who have the greatest experience related to malpractice claims, organized their own self-insurance system through the American Association of Nurse Anesthetists.[84]

Although NPs and CNSs in some specialties have experienced malpractice increases, these increases have not been so large as to surpass earning capacity or salary. Their claims experience is still relatively low, and coverage is still universally available, although at significantly higher rates than those for staff nurses.

The National Practitioners Data Bank (NPDB), which collects reports of medical malpractice claims against all providers, provides hard evidence about APRN claims experience. First, the NPDB holds 36 reports regarding physician malpractice for every 1 report regarding malpractice of a nurse and 93.7 physician reports for every 1 APRN report.[84] Second, two-thirds of the malpractice payments against nurses were made on behalf of RNs rather than APRNs. When adverse event reports (e.g., employment events, licensure actions) are added to the data, the rate of malpractice claims and adverse actions for NPs and physicians are 1 in 173 and 1 in 4.[85] NPDB results and a study of NP closed claims reveal that NPs are most often accused of errors related to diagnosis, treatment, or medication management, whereas errors by CRNAs are predominantly related to anesthesia and surgery, and errors of CNMs are related to obstetrical care.[84,86]

Of the 2384 NPDB reported payments for APRN malpractice during the period September 1990 through December 2004, CRNAs were the most frequently sued, accounting for 49.5% ($n = 1181$) of the reported payments. CNM and NP payments were 25% ($n = 596$) and 24.5% ($n = 594$) of the total. The NPDB began collecting CNS data in 2002, and so far CNS payments account for only 0.5% ($n = 13$) of the payments. In 2004, the number of payments for all nurses was 645 with a mean value per claim of $277,431. Although the number of nurse-related payments has increased from 364 in 2000, the inflation-adjusted mean and median payments for claims for nurse malpractice have not increased markedly.[86]

Although it is likely that malpractice attorneys have discovered that authority of APRNs and their accountability for errors more closely resemble those of a physician than a nurse, APRNs do not yet suffer as severely with respect to malpractice claims. Many choose to believe that this is because of the safe, effective, and satisfying service provided by APRNs. Instead of interpreting their low claims experience as an indication of quality, however, critics prefer to assert that a litigant will target providers with assets ("deep pockets") in hope of greater financial recovery. APRNs so far are not seen as providers with these deep pockets. Regardless, each malpractice crisis brings calls for tort reform that would establish new standards for financial recovery. APRNs have joined forces with physicians to try to change related statutes, but so far legislative efforts to change malpractice laws significantly have been unsuccessful.

Emerging Issues for Advanced Nursing Practice

Although some issues, such as prescriptive authority, staff privileges, and reimbursement, have concerned APRNs for many years—and continue to do so—new issues are emerging, including the invisibility of APRNs, scope of practice issues, and educational innovations.

Invisibility

As APRN roles and responsibilities grow, their invisibility becomes a more significant problem. It used to be said, "What is important is that the patient gets the care, not who gets the credit." If APRNs are to survive and continue to offer patients the added value of their services, however, they must become visible.

Visibility is achieved in many ways. Identity is the first way. Much of the public is still unaware that APRNs exist or of the services they provide. To obtain public support, APRNs need to publicize their product. This includes the ability of all APRNs to describe briefly who they are and what they do, or, in other words, to deliver the proverbial "elevator speech." It also requires concerted efforts to showcase APRN providers and practices in the mass media at every opportunity through letters to the editor, clips on evening news programs, blogs, and Web sites.

In addition, APRNs must step out from under the shadow of nursing and clearly differentiate the value that advanced practice brings to health care and to the profession as a whole.

Although APRNs should embrace what they have in common with all nurses, they must articulate their own perspectives, issues, and needs. Whenever nursing groups assemble, APRN representatives need to have their own seats at the table to ensure their unique voice is heard. In public, APRNs should speak for APRNs rather than relying on other nurses to do so. Control over APRN education and certification and practice through active participation in associations and regulatory bodies is also the responsibility of APRNs.

Visibility is also built through numbers. Although there are more than 250,000 nurses prepared as APRNs, most fail to maintain membership in their respective professional associations.[87,88] Inadequate participation limits the influence these organizations command in the public domain. Lack of participation and membership also limits the ability of professional associations to keep APRNs updated on issues and to mobilize grassroots activities to support much needed legislative change. It also threatens the financial well-being of the respective organizations. Membership is a professional obligation for APRNs.

Data also support visibility. Legislators and regulators want to know how many people will be affected and how much it will cost before they make decisions. APRNs in general, and NPs and CNSs in particular, are poorly represented in national databases. Because all CRNAs are certified by a single professional organization and all CNMs are certifed by a single professional organization, data regarding these two types of APRNs are available from those organizations. The same is not true of NPs, however, who can be certified by any one of at least five different organizations. Fewer than half of CNSs are certified at all, and if they are, it may be through several organizations.[88]

Federal databases collect, at best, incomplete data on APRNs. Although they are included in the National Sample Survey of Registered Nurses, it is impossible to determine where and how APRNs are practicing and to whom they provide services.[88] In 2008, after repeated requests from APRN organizations, the Office of Management and Budget added new categories to the Standard Occupational Classifications to differentiate NPs, CNMs, and CRNAs from RNs, although they failed to create a unique classification for CNSs. The addition of the three new classifications will allow federal agencies to describe these components of the labor workforce more accurately in the future.

The National Ambulatory Medical Care Survey (NAMCS), the Center Studying Health Systems Change (HSC), and the Area Resource File (ARF), which is the basis for determining health professional shortage areas, do not collect any data regarding APRNs and their practices.[87] The result is that there are no good data regarding the number, specialties, practice settings, populations served, or distributions for APRNs. This means that APRNs and their contributions are invisible to analysts and policy makers. To influence policy, APNs must be counted and included in analyses.

Transparency regarding the identity of the care provider also increases visibility. Many APRNs are "ghost providers." Similar to "ghost writers," APRNs do the work, and someone else, commonly physicians, take the credit. This happens most frequently through convoluted billing in which the APRN sees the patient and provides the service and then, usually to obtain higher reimbursement, bills under the physician's name. Although this practice may be legal, it undermines the credibility, contributions, and visibility of APRNs. To be visible, APRNs must consistently bill under their own unique identifier numbers. This practice allows payers to discriminate among provider types in databases and clearly see contributions of APRNs. These data can also be used to show the amount and type of care APRNs are providing and to analyze differences among providers.

APRNs need to push for legislative authority to sign their own orders for home health care, hospice services, and any other therapy or document that currently requires a physician's signature. Many state organizations have successfully improved APRN visibility by passing so-called signature bills, which authorize APRNs to sign commonly used forms, ranging from handicapped parking tags to death and birth certificates. The days are over of passing these forms on for a signature from a physician who does not even know the patient. It is bad practice and needs to be stopped.

"Work-arounds," used to overcome unnecessary day-to-day practice barriers, are also dangerous for patients and create subtle threats to visibility. This practice occurs most commonly when APRNs are restricted from ordering prescriptions or authorizing laboratory or diagnostic tests. In states where prescriptive authority of APRNs is limited, it is common for the APRN to see the patient, determine the therapy, and then provide the patient with a prescription that has been signed by another provider, typically a physician. This practice is dangerous because it can cause delays when a pharmacist needs to discuss the prescription with the provider who actually knows the patient and the condition or when refills are needed. Some pharmacists contribute to this problem when a physician's name, rather than the name of the prescribing APRN, is used on the medication container given to the patient. When this type of name switching occurs on laboratory or diagnostic test requisitions, it jeopardizes patient safety by interfering with timely communication to the provider who knows the patient. APRNs need to refuse to use these "work-arounds" and change any statutes or policies that contribute to them.

Most of the general public believes that physicians are the ultimate experts on everything related to health care. APRNs need to communicate clearly to their patients, the public, and, most importantly, government officials about what they do. They need to inform the patient that it is the APRN who is performing the service, analyzing the results, making the decision, prescribing the care, and monitoring the outcomes.

The American Medical Association and Scope of Practice Partnership

"Scope of practice can be defined as the range of healthcare-related activities and services which a healthcare professional is educated and certified or licensed to provide."[89] Because physicians were the first healthcare professionals to develop licensing processes, they defined the scope of practice of medicine to be all-inclusive.[90] They refer to "general undifferentiated medical practice" as their domain. Over time, health care has improved as its scientific foundations and the educational preparation and abilities of all providers have increased. It is logical that many disciplines have expanded their scopes of practice and sought more rights and responsibilities.[91] Today, the scope of practice of one profession frequently overlaps with the scope of practice of another.

The role of government bodies in regulating professions is to protect the public health and welfare. Some groups of healthcare providers believe the government's role is to protect their traditional professional privileges. In reality, the only relevant criteria to use in determining who should be authorized to perform a service is who is qualified to perform the activity safely and effectively.[91]

The safety and efficacy of nurses in advanced practice has been proven many times.[65-73] Despite this significant body of evidence, many unnecessary barriers to full use of APRNs continue to exist. When legislators or regulators consider removing these barriers, physicians object, perpetrating "unsubstantiated concerns for public safety."[92] Many organized medical groups direct considerable energy and money toward foiling the attempts of APRNs to expand their practice into what they consider the exclusive domain of medicine. In 2004, the American Medical Association (AMA) declared that it would join other specialty medical societies to fund investigations of the educational preparation of nonphysician providers, monitor systematically and oppose policy changes that would expand the scope of practice of nonphysician providers, and take legal action to overturn policy changes.[93] This partnership, called the Scope of Practice Partnership (SOPP), began with six state and six specialty medical societies and has grown to include state medical societies from all 50 states and 25 national specialty medical organizations. SOPP has committed full-time staff, legal resources, and hundreds of thousands of dollars to this divisive effort.

SOPP has proposed positions to restrict or control the practice of most other health professions. Initiatives have been introduced in several states to eliminate profession-specific regulatory boards and replace them with a single "super board" under the control of physicians. They have filed state and federal bills to undermine other practitioners and restrict their practice—for example, limit the number of NPs with whom a physician may collaborate or impose higher standards for facilities, resources, and care processes for convenient care clinics than exist for physician offices and other ambulatory care settings. They have even tried to lay claim to ownership of the words "doctor" and "resident."

SOPP has used the AMA Litigation Center to support actions against individual practitioners and regulatory boards and even state legislatures to interfere with the free practice of other professions.[93,94] The Missouri State Medical Association sued the State of Missouri attempting to overturn a law allowing CNMs to practice independently. In Louisiana, SOPP successfully sued the State Board of Nursing over a rule allowing CRNAs to perform interventional pain management procedures. In Texas, SOPP sued the State Board of Examiners of Marriage and Family Therapists over regulations allowing marriage and family therapists to diagnose patients. SOPP also triggered a Federal Trade Commission (FTC) hearing in 2008 to examine the quality of care provided in convenient care clinics. Ironically, the role of the FTC is to prevent antitrust activities, and some people believe that SOPP activities constitute restraint of trade, which falls under the control of the FTC.

In response to these divisive efforts to limit patient access to healthcare services and choice of provider and to wrench control of all health-care practice from the respective professions, 37 national healthcare organizations representing more than 10 healthcare professions formed the Coalition for Patient's Rights.[89] This organization is dedicated to preserving patients' unrestricted access to the full range of high-quality healthcare services and providers. These diverse professionals are working in collaboration to promote the value of all the respective healthcare disciplines and providers and to highlight the additive and distinct services that these practitioners provide. National organizations representing all four APRN roles are prominent leaders in this organization. APRNs need to remain active in these kinds of activities to ensure that patients will continue to be able to access the services they provide.

Educational Innovation

Schools of nursing continue to create innovative educational programs to attract new young people to the profession and prepare students for practice in a rapidly changing healthcare system. These programs include direct enrollment into an APRN graduate program and new paths to doctoral education.

DIRECT ENROLLMENT IN AN APRN PROGRAM

Many schools offer applicants with a baccalaureate degree in another field direct enrollment into APRN graduate programs. These students complete basic preparation for RN licensure, and move directly into APRN training without any or only minimal postlicensure practice experience. These graduates enter the nursing workforce for the first time as APRNs. Most are successful on national certification boards and generally have no difficulty finding employment, especially in primary care settings. They tend to be happy with their educational preparation, but they may lack confidence that comes from independent practice as a nurse. Practicing APRNs express concerns regarding the integration of these novice providers into the profession.

Practicing APRNs cite concerns that the newly minted APRNs may have deficits in knowledge or skills because of their lack of basic nursing experience. They question if patient outcomes will be comparable to those of nurses entering APRN practice with experience in basic nursing. They also ask if it is possible to internalize the nursing philosophy and create a strong professional identity as a nurse without independent practice experience as an RN, especially because most APRNs practice in settings with few RNs or few RN role models but with many physicians: Will the lack of a strong professional identity as a nurse undermine the nursing perspective that is the basis of APRN practice? Will the novice APRN use the nursing model for care when surrounded by physicians using the medical model of care? Perhaps most important, how will these novice APRNs affect the public's perception of APRNs?

NEW PATHS TO DOCTORAL EDUCATION

Schools of nursing are creating new paths to doctoral education as well. Although the first PhD program for nurses was created in 1932, most universities did not offer doctoral degrees until the last 20 years.[95] In the 1970s, in an effort to expand the availability of doctoral education for nurses, universities introduced practice doctoral degrees, the Doctor of Nursing (ND), Doctor of Nursing Science (DNS), and Doctor of Science in Nursing (DSN). Most of these doctoral degrees except for the ND quickly evolved into research degrees, comparable to the Doctor of Philosophy (PhD) degree, and most universities now award a PhD degree on completion. Graduates of these programs conduct research to expand the scientific and theoretical basis for practice, and many teach in academic settings.

In 2004, the AACN membership approved the recommendation that by 2015, a new practice doctoral degree—the Doctor of Nursing Practice (DNP)—replace the master's degree as the educational preparation for all advanced nursing practice specialties, including the four APRN roles. DNP graduates would be prepared not only for advanced practice roles, but also would be prepared to address many of the issues in a changing, complex healthcare system.[96] This recommendation was based partly on the increasing complexity of the healthcare system and associated demands on healthcare providers. It also addresses calls from a variety of health policy groups for reform of education of health professionals.[97] The called-for reforms would design new curricula and learning experiences to improve transdisciplinary communication and care coordination, increase translation of evidence to practice, enhance care safety and quality, increase knowledge of healthcare finance and economics, and expand leadership to transform the healthcare system. Several other health professions, such as pharmacy, audiology, and physical and occupational therapy, have made changes to their discipline's educational preparation and award practice doctorates (e.g., PharmD, DPT, DOT).[97] Transitioning APRN education in the same manner to a DNP would maintain parity of educational preparation among peer providers. Graduates of these programs would focus on transforming practice, although, similar to their PhD colleagues, they may also teach in academic settings.

Currently, most DNP programs admit APRNs after completion of a master's degree and require 18 to 24 months of study. A few schools admit experienced baccalaureate-prepared nurses who would complete their APRN education en route to the DNP. Practicing APRNs, although they do not expect to be required to return to school to complete this additional degree, have expressed concerns that their master's degree educational preparation will be considered inadequate in the future. National certification bodies and the NCSBN have indicated their intent to continue to recognize currently practicing master's-prepared APRNs.

Detractors say that these programs, which increase the training time to become an APRN, would slow down or decrease the production of sorely needed providers. They point out that financing 3 to 4 years rather than 2 to 3 years of graduate education increases the cost of education and adds to graduates' debt. The harshest critics call the DNP an example of "degree creep." Concern has been expressed that most post-master's DNP curricula emphasize content related to health systems (e.g., evidence-based practice, health policy, health information technology, economics and finance, organizational ethics) rather than traditional clinical topics (e.g., pharmacology, therapeutics, pathology, clinical decision making). Advocates point out, however, that these post-master's graduates have previously completed their preparation for direct clinical practice and need to expand their skills to transform their practice and address the issues that confront the healthcare system. It remains to be seen whether the 2015 recommendation will be met or if it, similar to the recommendation for BSN entry to the profession, will require much longer to be accomplished.

Summary

For more than 100 years, nurses in APRN roles have provided high-quality health care. CRNAs are the sole anesthesia providers in most rural hospitals, but they have been less dominant in areas with more physicians. CNMs, whose roots are in working with the poor and underserved, have gained popularity with women of moderate and substantial means. CNSs are the unsung heroes quietly working behind the scenes to improve the safety and quality of healthcare systems. NPs have achieved the greatest autonomy working in rural areas and with underserved populations. All of these APRNs provide crucial healthcare services to meet the needs of society. The difficulty is that many people still do not know about APRNs or the services they provide although this is changing with the increased focus on reforming the healthcare system. What advanced practice nursing will become largely depends on the choices that people make about their health care individually and through their government representatives. The actions of APRNs will influence those choices.

APRNs are limited by the "crazy quilt" of convoluted regulations that impose unnecessary barriers to their autonomous practice. To meet their full potential, APRNs must create a more coherent system. The decision for APRNs is whether to walk away from the challenge or to overcome their invisibility and communicate their value to society. To be successful, APRNs must mobilize their own members and their patients. The consumers of health care, from urban and middle class areas and rural and underserved areas, and their acceptance and demand for APRNs will establish their credibility. APRNs must continue to resist organized medicine's opposition to patient choice of provider, nurse-managed centers, convenient care clinics, and birthing centers—all ideal settings in which to prove and promote APRN services and excellence.

The future of APRNs is closely associated with the concept of value: the value of caring in its own right, the added value derived from care provided by an APRN in partnership with a patient, the economic value of APRNs as physician substitutes, and the inherent value of primary care and the exceptional suitability of many APRNs for the PCP role. Given the urgency implicit in today's healthcare debate, APRNs must be open to a broad range of interpretations of value. The safety and efficacy of nurses in advanced practice has been proved many times over.[65-73]

Although nursing should continue to support research that verifies the credibility and value of APRNs in care processes and patient outcomes and APRN-led models of care, efforts should not end there. The research focus should shift to the value of caring in its own right and, more specifically, to the value of nursing in the PCP role. Educated risk taking, a commitment to excellence, dogged pursuit of visibility, and the courage of one's convictions must become watchwords as APRNs shape a future that is good for nursing.

SUGGESTED LEARNING EXERCISES

1. Design a strategic plan to ensure the competency of APRNs to the public. Include the roles of professional and government entities in the plan.

2. Develop a multipronged strategy to improve public recognition of APRN services and the added value and benefits derived from APRN care.

3. Identify the reimbursement and prescriptive authority rights of the four APRN roles in your state and all contiguous states.

4. Identify restrictions placed on APRN practice that set up barriers to access to care. Outline the next stage in policy development to overcome these barriers and increase patient access to APRNs.

5. Describe anticipated opportunities for APRNs in the emerging healthcare delivery system and the areas of resistance that APRNs will encounter.

6. Propose a plan to mobilize larger numbers of APRNs to influence better federal and state legislative and regulatory agencies to remove unnecessary barriers to APRN practice.

7. Write a 30-second "elevator speech" that describes your role as an APRN and the associated benefits to care for consumers. Practice delivering this message to a colleague. Critique the colleague's speech.

References

1. Catlin, A, Cowan, C, Hartman, M, and Heffler, S. (2008). National health spending in 2006: A year of change for prescription drugs. *Health Affairs* 27:14–29.

2. Taylor, A. (2007). Behind Ford's scary $12.7 billion loss. *Fortune*. http://money.cnn.com/2007/01/26/news/companies/pluggedin_taylor_ford.fortune/index.htm?postversion=2007012611. Accessed January 23, 2009.

3. Wilson, K. (2005). Health Care Costs 101. *California Health Care Foundation*. http://www.chcf.org/topics/healthinsurance/index.cfm?itemID=109369. Accessed January 23, 2009.

4. Himmelstein, D, Warren, E, Thorne, D, and Woolhander, S. (2005). Illness and injury as contributors to bankruptcy. *Health Affairs Web Exclusive* W5-63. http://content.healthaffairs.org/cgi/content/full/hlthaff.w5.63/DC1. Accessed January 23, 2009.

5. Robertson, C, Egelhof, R, and Hoke, M. (2008). Get sick, get out: the medical causes of home mortgage foreclosures. *Health Matrix* 18:65–105.

6. CIA World Fact Book. (2009). Rank order—infant mortality rate. https://www.cia.gov/library/publications/the-world-factbook/rankorder/2091rank.html. Accessed January 23, 2009.

7. Centers for Disease Control and Prevention. (2008). Chronic disease overview. http://www.cdc.gov/nccdphp/overview.htm. Accessed January 23, 2009.

8. Institute of Medicine. (2000). *To Err Is Human: Building a Safer Health System*. National Academies Press, Washington, DC.

9. McGlynn, E, Asch, S, Adams, J, Keesey, J, Hicks, J, DeCristofaro, A, and Kerr, E. (2003). The quality of health care delivered to adults in the United States. *N Engl J Med* 348:2635–2645.

10. Schuster, M, McGlynn, E, and Brook, RL. (2005). How good is quality of healthcare in the United States. *Milbank Q* 83:843–895.

11. United States Aging Demographics. (2006). UNC Institute on Aging. http://www.aging.unc.edu/infocenter/slides/usaging.ppt. Accessed April 3, 2009.

12. U.S. Census Bureau. (2006). Newsroom. http://www.census.gov/Press-Release/www/releases/archives/facts_for_features_special_editions/006105.html. Accessed April 10, 2009.

13. Center for Health Workforce Studies. (2005). *The Impact of the Aging Population on the Health Workforce in the United States*. SUNY School of Public Health, Albany, Rensselaer, NY.

14. U.S. Census Bureau. (2001). The 65 and older population: 2000. Census 2000 Brief. http://www.census.gov/prod/2001pubs/c2kbr01-10.pdf. Accessed April 3, 2009.

15. Bureau of Labor Statistics. (2009). The employment situation: December 2008. U.S. Department of Labor. http://www.bls.gov/news.release/pdf/empsit.pdf. Accessed January 23, 2009.

16. U.S. Census Bureau. (2006). Annual estimates of the population by sex, race and Hispanic or Latino origin for the United States: April 1, 2000 to July 1, 2005 (NC-EST2005-03). Population Division. http://www.census.gov/popest/national/asrh/NC-EST2005-srh.html. Accessed April 19, 2009.

17. Rector, R, Johnson, K, and Fagan, P. (2002). The effect of marriage on child poverty. Center for Data Analysis Report #02-04. The Heritage Foundation. http://www.heritage.org/research/Family/CDA02-04.cfm#pgfId=1002049. Accessed April 8, 2009.

18. Lichter, D, Qian, Z, and Crowley, M. (2005). Child poverty among racial minorities and immigrants: Explaining trends and differentials. *Soc Sci Quart* 86(Suppl):1037–1059.

19. Agency for Healthcare Research and Quality. (2008). 2007 National Health Care Disparities Report. AHRQ Publication No. 08-0041. U.S. Department of Health and Human Services, Rockville, MD. http://www.ahrq.gov/qual/qrdr07.htm. Accessed January 23, 2009.

20. Hadley, J. (June 2003). Sicker and poorer—the consequences of being uninsured: A review of the research on the relationship between health insurance, medical care use, health, work, and income. *Med Care Res Rev* 60:2.

21. Quinn, JB. (1994). The luck of the Xers. *Newsweek,* June, p 66.

22. Lankard BA. (1995). Career development in generation X: Myths and realities. Clearinghouse on Adult, Career, and Vocational Education. http://listserv.aera.net/scripts/wa.exe?A2=ind9611&L=aera-j&D=0&F=P&T=0&P=1220.

23. Gibson, S. (2009). Enhancing intergenerational communication in the classroom. *Nurs Educ Perspectives* 30:37–39.

24. Academy of Academic Health Centers. (2008). *Out of Order Out of Time: The State of the Nations Health Workforce.* Academy of Academic Health Centers, Washington, DC.

25. Centers for Disease Control and Prevention. (2008). Table 26. Life expectation at birth, at 65 years of age and at 75 years of age by race and sex, United States: 1900–2005. http://www.cdc.gov/nchs/data/hus/hus08.pdf#026. Accessed April 9, 2009.

26. Kung, H, Hoyert, D, Xu, J, and Murphy, S. (2008). Deaths: Final data for 2005. *National Vital Statistics Report* 56:1–124. http://www.cdc.gov/nchs/data/nvsr/nvsr56/nvsr56_10.pdf. Accessed April 9, 2009.

27. Agency for Healthcare Research and Quality. (2006). *National Healthcare Disparities Report.* AHRQ Pub. No. 07-0012. U.S. Department of Health and Human Services, Agency for Healthcare Research and Quality, Rockville, MD.

28. Institute of Medicine. (1990). *Healthy People 2000: Citizens Chart the Course.* National Academy Press, Washington, DC.

29. McGinnis, JM, & Lee, PR. (1995). Healthy People 2000 at mid-decade. *JAMA* 273:1123.

30. U.S. Department of Health and Human Services. (2000). *Healthy People 2010: Understanding and Improving Health,* 2nd ed. U.S. Government Printing Office, Washington, DC. http://www.healthypeople.gov/Document/pdf/uih/2010uih.pdf. Accessed April 19, 2009.

31. Blendon, R, Brodie, M, Benson, J, Altman, D, and Buhr, T. (2006). Americans' views of health care costs, access, and quality. *Milbank Q* 84:623–657.

32. Joel, L. (1995). Health care reform: Getting it right this time. *Am J Nurs* 95:6–7.

33. Kaiser Family Foundation. (2005). Trends and indicators in the changing health care marketplace, section 2: Trends in health insurance enrollment. http://www.kff.org/insurance/7031/index.cfm. Accessed April 9, 2009.

34. Thompson, J, Ryan, K, Pinidiya, S, & Bost, J. (2003). Quality of care of children in commercial and Medicaid managed care. *JAMA* 290:1486–1493.

35. Landon, B, Schneider, E, Normand, S, Scholle, S, Pawlson, L, and Epstein, A. (2007). Quality of care in Medicaid managed care and commercial health plans. *JAMA* 298:1674–1681.

36. American College of Physicians. (2006). The impending collapse of primary care medicine and its implications for the state of the nation's health care. http://www.txpeds.org/u/documents/statehc06_1.pdf. Accessed April 3, 2009.

37. American Academy of Family Physicians, American Academy of Pediatrics, American College of Physicians, and American Osteopathic Association. (2007). Joint principles of the patient-centered medical home. http://www.medicalhomeinfo.org/joint%20statement.pdf. Accessed January 23, 2009.

38. Ginsburg, J, Taylor, T, and Barr, M. (2009). Nurse practitioners in primary care. American College of Physicians. http://www.acponline.org/advocacy/where_we_stand/policy/np_pc.pdf. Accessed April 3, 2009.

39. Gunn, I. (1991). The history of nurse anesthesia education: Highlights and influences. *AANA J* 59:53–61.

40. Thompson, J. (1986). Nurse midwifery care: 1924–1984. *Ann Rev Nurs Res* 4:153–173.

41. Rust, J. (2004). Dr. Hildegard Peplau. *Clinical Nurse Specialist* 18:262–263.

42. Silver, H, Ford, L, and Steady, S. (1967). A program to increase health care for children: The pediatric nurse practitioner program. *Pediatrics* 39:756–760.

43. American College of Nurse Midwives. http://www.acnm.org/index.cfm. Accessed January 23, 2009.

44. American Association of Nurse Anesthetists. http://www.aana.com/. Accessed January 23, 2009.

45. Christian, S, Dower, C, and O'Neil, O. (2007). Overview of nurse practitioner scopes of practice in the United States—chart and discussion. Center for the Health Professions, University of California, San Francisco. http://www.futurehealth.ucsf.edu/pdf_files/Chart%20of%20NP%20Scopes%20 Fall%202007.pdf. Accessed April 5, 2009.

46. American Association of Nurse Anesthetists. http://www.aana.com/Advocacy.aspx?ucNavMenu_ TSMenuTargetID=49&ucNavMenu_TSMenuTargetType=4&ucNavMenu_TSMenuID=6&id=2573. Accessed May 15, 2010.

47. AANA. (2007). Scope and standards for nurse anesthesia practice. http://www.aana.com/ uploadedFiles/Resources/Practice_Documents/scopestds_nap07 2007.pdf. Accessed April 3, 2009.

48. American College of Nurse Midwives. (2007). Core competencies for basic midwifery practice. http://acnm.org/core_competencies.cfm. Accessed April 3, 2009.

49. American Association of Colleges of Nursing. (1996). *The Essentials of Master's Education for Advanced Practice Nursing.* American Association of Colleges of Nursing, Washington, D.C.

50. American Association of Colleges of Nursing. (2006). *The Essentials of Doctoral Education for Advanced Nursing Practice.* American Association of Colleges of Nursing, Washington, DC. http://www.aacn.nche.edu/. Accessed April 5, 2009.

51. National Organization of Nurse Practitioner Faculties. (2002). *Core Competencies for Nurse Practitioners.* National Organization of Nurse Practitioner Faculties, Washington, DC.

52. National Organization of Nurse Practitioner Faculties and American Association of Colleges of Nursing. (2002). *Nurse Practitioner Primary Care Competencies in Specialty Areas: Adult, Family, Gerontological, Pediatric, and Women's Health.* U.S. Department of Health and Human Services Health Resources and Services Administration Bureau of Health Professions Division of Nursing, Rockville, MD.

53. National Panel for Psychiatric-Mental Health NP Competencies. (2003). *Psychiatric-Mental Health Nurse Practitioner Competencies.* National Organization of Nurse Practitioner Faculties, Washington, DC.

54. National Panel for Acute Care Nurse Practitioner Competencies. (2004). *Acute Care Nurse Practitioner Competencies.* National Organization of Nurse Practitioner Faculties, Washington, DC.

55. National Task Force on Quality Nurse Practitioner Education. (2008). *Criteria for Evaluation of Nurse Practitioner Programs.* National Task Force on Quality Nurse Practitioner Education, Washington, DC. http://www.aacn.nche.edu/.

56. APRN Joint Dialogue Group. (2008). *Consensus Model for APRN Regulation: Licensure, Accreditation, Certification and Education.* www.aacn.nche.edu/education/pdf/APRNReport.PDF. Accessed January 23, 2009.

57. Pearson, L. (2008).The Pearson Report. *Am J Nurse Practitioner* 12:7–80.

58. Forbes, K, Rafson, J, Spross, J, and Koslowski, D. (1990). Clinical nurse specialist and nurse practitioner core curricula survey results. *Nurse Practitioner* 15:43, 46–48.

59. American Association of Critical-Care Nurses. (2004). *Standards of Clinical Practice and Scope of Practice for Acute Care Nurse Practitioner.* Aliso Viejo, CA, American Association of Critical Care Nurses.

60. American Association of Critical Care Nurses. (2002). *Scope of Practice and Standards of Professional Performance for the Acute and Critical Care Clinical Nurse Specialist.* Aliso Viejo, CA, American Association of Critical Care Nurses.

61. Kleinpell-Nowell, R. (2001). Longitudinal survey of acute care nurse practitioner practice: Year 2. *AACN Clinical Issues* 12:447–452.

62. Williams, CA, and Valdiviesco, GC. (1994). Advanced practice models: A comparison of clinical nurse specialist and nurse practitioner activities. *Clinical Nurse Specialist* 8:311–318.

63. Mick, DJ, and Ackerman, MH. (2000). Advanced practice nursing role delineation in acute and critical care: Application of the Strong Model of Advanced Practice. *Heart Lung* 29:210–221.

64. Residency match results demonstrate need to address national primary care workforce goals. www.ACPonline.org/pressroom/09_match.htm?hp. Accessed April 3, 2009.

65. Sox, H. (1979). Quality of patient care by nurse practitioners and physician's assistants: A ten-year perspective. *Ann Intern Med* 91:459–468.

66. U.S. Congress Office of Technology Assessment. (1981). *The Costs and Effectiveness of Nurse Practitioners.* U.S. Government Printing Office, Washington, DC.

67. U.S. Congress Office of Technology Assessment. (1986). *Nurse Practitioners, Physician Assistants, and Certified Nurse-Midwives: A Policy Analysis.* U.S. Government Printing Office, Washington, DC.

68. Ventura, M, Feldman, M, and Crosby, F. (1991). An information synthesis to evaluate nurse practitioner effectiveness. *Milit Med* 156:286–291.

69. Brown, S, and Grimes, D. (1995). A meta-analysis of nurse practitioners and nurse midwives in primary care. *Nurs Res* 44:332–339.

70. Horrocks, S, Anderson, E, and Salisbury, C. (2002). Systematic review of whether nurse practitioner working in primary care can provide equivalent care to doctors. *BMJ* 324:819–823.

71. Laurant, M, Reeves, D, Hermens, R, Braspenning, J, Grol, R, and Sibbald, B. (2005). Substitution of doctors by nurses in primary care. *The Cochrane Library,* Issue 4.

72. Hatem, M, Sandall, J, Devance, D, Soltani, H, and Gates, S. (2008). Midwife-led versus other models of care for childbearing women. *Cochrane Database Syst Rev* (4):CD004667.

73. Newhouse, R, Stanik-Hutt, J, White, K, Johantgen, M, Zangaro, G, Heindel, L, Steinwachs, D, Weiner, J, Bass, E, Wilson, R, and Fountain, L. (2009). *An Assessment of the Safety, Quality, and Effectiveness of Care Provided by Advanced Practice Nurses.* TriCouncil for Nursing, Washington, DC.

74. National Council of State Boards of Nursing. (2007). NCSBN "Vision Paper" ignites controversy. *Am J Nurs* 106:25–26.

75. American Academy of Physician Assistants. (2009). Facts at a glance. http://www.aapa.org/glance.html. Accessed January 24, 2009.

76. Twentieth Annual Legislative Update. (2008). *Nurse Practitioner* 33:14–34.

77. Kelly, L, and Joel, L. (1999). *Dimensions of Professional Nursing,* 8th ed. McGraw-Hill, New York.

78. Joint Commission on Accreditation of Healthcare Organizations. (2004). *The Medical Staff Handbook: A Guide to Joint Commission Standards,* 2nd ed. Joint Commission on Accreditation of Healthcare Organizations, Oakbrook Terrace, IL.

79. Towers, J. (2005). After forty years. *J Am Acad Nurse Practitioners* 17:9–13.

80. Bruton-Maree, N, and Rupp, R. (2001). Federal healthcare policy: How AANA advocates for the profession. In Foster, SD, and Faut-Callahan, M. (eds). *A Professional Study and Resource Guide for the CRNA.* AANA Publishing, Park Ridge, IL, pp 357–379.

81. Mittelstadt, P. (1993). Federal reimbursement of advanced practice nurses' services empowers the profession. *Nurse Practitioner* 18:43–49.

82. Sollins, H. (2006). Medicare developments and explanations affecting nurse practitioners. *Geriatric Nurs* 27:149–150.

83. Sollins, H. (2006). New Medicare guidance for nurse practitioners providing services in a home care or hospice setting. *Geriatric Nursing* 27:271–272.

84. Health Resource and Services Administration. (2006). *National Practitioner Data Bank Annual Report.* U.S. Department of Health and Human Services Bureau of Health Professions, Washington, DC. http://www.npdb-hipdb.com. Accessed April 19, 2009.

85. Pearson, L. (2009). The Pearson report. *Am J Nurse Practitioner* 13:8–82.

86. Miller, K. (2007). Feeling the heat: Nurse practitioners and malpractice liability. *J Nurs Pract* 3:24-26

87. O'Grady, E. (2008). Advanced practice registered nurses: The impact on patient safety and quality. In Hughes, R. (ed). *Patient Safety and Quality: An Evidence-Based Handbook for Nurses.* Vol 2. AHRQ Publication No. 08-0043. Agency for Healthcare Research and Quality, Rockville, MD, pp 601–620. http://www.ahrq.gov/qual/nurseshdbk/.

88. Health Resource and Services Administration. (2004). *The Registered Nurse Population: National Sample Survey of Registered Nurses.* U.S. Department of Health and Human Services Bureau of Health Professions, Washington, DC. http://bhpr.hrsa.gov/healthworkforce/rnsurvey04/. Accessed April 19, 2009.

89. Coalition for Patient's Rights. (2009). Giving patients a choice of providers. http://www. patientsrightscoalition.org/. Accessed April 10, 2009.

90. Safriet, B. (2009). Regulation and scope of practice issues for APRNs. Presentation at 35th Annual Meeting National Organization of Nurse Practitioner Faculties, April 17, 2009.

91. DeAngelis, D, Hatherill, W, Safriet, B, Robin, L, Grace, P, Apple, K, and Gatizone, C. (2006). Changes in healthcare professions' scope of practice: Legislative considerations. https://www.ncsbn.org/ScopeofPractice.pdf. Accessed January 23, 2009.

92. Henderson T, and Chovan, T. (1994). *Removing Practice Barriers of Non-Physician Providers: Efforts by States to Improve Access to Primary Care.* Intergovernmental Health Policy Project, George Washington University, Washington, DC.

93. Sorrel, A. (2008). AMA meeting: Physicians demand greater oversight of doctors of nursing. *American Medical News* (amednews.com). http://www.ama-assn.org/amednews/2008/07/07/prsd0707.html. Accessed April 10, 2009.

94. Sorrel, A. (2009). Scope of practice expansions fuel legal battles. *American Medical News* (amednews.com). http://www.ama-assn.org/amednews/2009/03/09/prl20309.htm. Accessed April 10, 2009.

95. Cherry, B, and Jacob, S. (2005). *Contemporary Nursing Issues, Trends and Management.* Elsevier, St. Louis, MO.

96. American Association of Colleges of Nursing. (2004). *Position Statement on the Practice Doctorate in Nursing.* http://www.aacn.nche.edu/DNP/pdf/DNP.pdf. Accessed April 9, 2009.

97. Greiner, A, and Knebel, E. (eds). *Health Professions Education: A Bridge to Quality.* National Academies Press, Washington, DC.

98. The SCAN Foundation. (2010). A summary of the patient protection and affordable care act (P.LO.111-148) and modifications by the health care and education reconciliation act of 2010 (H.R.4872). Policy Brief No. 2, March 2010.

Mary Knudtson is the executive director of student health services at the University of California in Santa Cruz and also a professor of nursing at the University of California, Irvine. Prepared as both a family and a pediatric nurse practitioner, Dr. Knudtson has completed a Robert Wood Johnson Executive Nurse Fellowship and a Department of Health and Human Services (DHHS) Primary Health Care Policy Fellowship. She has practiced in a variety of settings for more than 18 years as an advanced practice registered nurse. Currently, she is involved in clinical practice in student health. Dr. Knudtson is a past president of the American College of Nurse Practitioners and is a fellow of the American Academy of Nursing.

CHAPTER 3

The American Healthcare System: Implications for Advanced Practice Registered Nursing

Mary Knudtson, DNSC, NP, FAAN

CHAPTER OUTLINE

CHAPTER OBJECTIVES

After completing this chapter, the reader will be able to:

1. Analyze the influence of economics on the restructuring of the healthcare delivery system in the United States.

2. Compare and contrast various challenges facing both publicly and privately financed health care.

3. Synthesize information regarding cost-containment efforts as they affect advanced practice nursing.

4. Compare and contrast various models proposed for the delivery and financing of health care.

5. Debate the advantages and disadvantages of different reimbursement strategies as they might apply to the advanced practice registered nurse (APRN) in a capitated care environment.

6. Delineate strategies that can be used by APRNs to gain entry into healthcare markets.

In Dr. Jan Tower's retrospective of the evolution of advanced practice registered nursing (see Chapter 1), the past echoes with several themes for today's APRNs[1]:

- Times of change create opportunities for APRNs to define and shape themselves.
- Forces outside the profession of nursing—often economic—have been the stimulus for this development.
- At the same time, the professional establishment—both within nursing and within medicine—has at times erected barriers to independent advanced nursing practice.

Today's healthcare revolution is a similar time of change for APRNs. To position themselves as leaders in the reform movement, APRNs must become sensitive to the various forces that have stimulated the movement toward healthcare restructuring. Healthcare reform is not only about who is going to pay for coverage—businesses, individuals, and families as taxpayers—but also about who is going to manage the plan—private companies, the government, and/or consumers themselves. To compete, APRNs must better understand factors related to payment and reimbursement mechanisms and the aggregate resources necessary for this new order.

This chapter provides a brief history of the evolution of healthcare financing and describes the current state of the American healthcare system. It also delineates strategies that APRNs can use to gain entry into healthcare markets.

The American Healthcare Revolution

It is likely that the 1990s will be remembered as the decade in which the nation acknowledged, albeit grudgingly, that the demand for medical services is apparently unlimited—but that the capacity of the society to pay for such services is not.[2] Three factors characterized health care in the 1990s: excess and deprivation, the development of managed care, and the public's changing view of the U.S. healthcare system. All three factors combined to create the system as it exists today and to generate the overriding feeling among healthcare professionals, consumers of health care, the government, and private companies/organizations that the system needs to be fixed.

Excess and Deprivation

A paradox of excess and deprivation characterized the 1990s in that people with comprehensive health insurance could receive unnecessary and inappropriate health services while those without insurance, or with inadequate insurance, could be deprived of needed care.[3] Some patients receive too little care because they are uninsured, or inadequately insured, while others receive too little care because they have Medicaid or Medicare coverage, which some healthcare providers will not accept. The United States spent $2.3 trillion on health care in 2007, yet 45.7 million Americans lacked basic health coverage.[4] For most of the past 20 years, the number of people without health insurance has been on the rise. Many of the uninsured are victims of the changing economy, which has shifted from a manufacturing economy based on highly paid, full-time jobs with good fringe benefits toward a service economy with lower-paid jobs that are often part-time and have no paid benefits. Two-thirds of the uninsured are in families with an employed adult. The number of uninsured declined in 2007 for the first time since 2000. However, that number is expected to rise again because of a weakened economy and layoffs at many companies. Currently, some 45.7 million Americans lack health coverage, down from 47 million in 2006; this number includes 8 million children.[4]

Underinsurance is also an important issue. Medicare covers only 43% of the healthcare costs of the elderly.[3] Since Congress established the program, the benefits covered by Medicare have remained largely unchanged, with the exception of a few added preventive services. Coverage for prescription drugs was added in 2006; that coverage requires a monthly premium and a yearly deductible. A major problem for many patients is that private health plans as well as Medicare and Medicaid do not cover all healthcare needs, requiring patients to pay out-of-pocket for uncovered services. For people with low or moderate incomes, insurance deductibles and co-payments may represent a substantial financial burden.

While some people cannot access the care they need, others receive too much care that is costly and may be unnecessary or harmful. Most studies that have looked for overuse have discovered that the percentage is at least in the double digits. Brooke, in extrapolating from the available literature, found one-fourth of hospital days, one-fourth of procedures, and two-fifths of medications could be omitted.[5] Fisher in 2003 found that elderly patients in certain areas of the country receive 60% more services—hospital days, specialty consultations, and medical procedures—than similar patients in other areas. However, surprisingly, the patients receiving fewer services had the same mortality rates, quality of care, access to care, and patient satisfaction as those receiving more service.[6]

Managed Care

In the 1990s, the U.S. healthcare system experienced a paradigm shift. Managed care became the overarching concept describing and influencing the system. It revolutionized the system and pervades all aspects of healthcare financing and organization, forging a new relationship among the purchasers, insurers, and providers of care in the United States. In the past, healthcare providers were able to make most healthcare decisions and determine their compensation with minimal intrusion. With managed care, providers have had to share or give up decision making to insurers and purchasers and accept financial risk. Medical practices that had been in business for decades went bankrupt.

Health maintenance organizations (HMOs) are one type of managed care. HMOs cover approximately 80 million people in the United States. They increasingly use capitation, a system in which a medical provider is paid a set fee per patient per month regardless of how many times the patient is seen during that time period. Capitation was expected to slow rising costs, reduce unnecessary medical services, and correct the imbalance between specialty and primary care. However, by the 21st century, the organizing principle of managed care had begun to falter. Patients and healthcare providers expressed a growing concern over a conflict between the HMO's desire to increase profits and their responsibility to provide necessary care.[7]

The Public's View of the System

The healthcare system is now evolving. For people with private or public insurance who have access to healthcare services, the melding of high-quality primary care and preventive services with the appropriate specialty care can produce the best medical care in the world. Unfortunately, health care in the United States encompasses a wide spectrum, ranging from the highest-quality, cutting-edge technology and most compassionate treatment of the ill to the turning away of the very ill because of their lack of ability to pay; from well-designed practice guidelines for the prevention or treatment of disease to inappropriate or unnecessary surgical procedures performed on uninformed patients. Despite the upheaval in the healthcare system over the past 15 years, the United States still has the least universal, most costly system in the industrialized world.[8] In 2001, only 18% of the U.S. population felt that the healthcare system worked well. Almost 79% felt that the system needed fundamental changes or a complete overhaul. About 21% of Americans had difficulty paying medical bills during the previous year compared with 7% of Canadians and 3% of Britains.9

Financing Health Care

The U.S. healthcare system is unique among nations in that it is the most expensive, outstripping by over half again the healthcare expenditures of any other country. The problem of soaring costs is not a new one. From 1970 to 1990, health expenditures in the United States increased at a yearly rate of 12%.[7] Americans spent $42 billion on health care in 1965, representing 6% of the gross national product (GNP) for that year. In 1981, that figure rose to $287 billion, or 9.8% of GNP. In 2000, the figure rose to 1.310 trillion, or 13.3% of GNP. In 2007, costs jumped to $2.3 trillion, or 16% of GNP.[10] Per capita healthcare spending was $4631 in 2000 in the United States, an increase of 6.3% over 1999. In 2007, healthcare spending averaged about $7600 per person.[10] These expenditures far exceeded the overall inflation rates prevalent in the American economy at the time. Two of the fastest-growing expenditures were prescription drugs and physician services. Prescription drug spending—which made up $200.7 billion of total health spending—continued to grow faster than all other areas.

In the past decade, there has been a decrease in hospital spending. Hospital spending continued a gradual deceleration from an 8.2% growth rate in 2002 to a 7.0% growth rate in 2006, or $648.2 billion. This trend was partially driven by a lower utilization of hospital services, especially within Medicare, as fee-for-service inpatient hospital admissions declined. Critics of the current system have stated that the overall spending increases are proof that once-touted HMOs are losing their ability to control costs. In 2007, health insurance premiums grew 6.1%, two times the rate of inflation, while workers contributed 10% more in premiums than they did in 2006.[10]

The system for financing healthcare services is a key factor in shaping the delivery of health care in the United States. Unlike many European systems, which are largely publicly financed, the American system, as it has evolved during the past 40 years, involves a complex blend of private and public responsibilities. To better understand the U.S. healthcare system and its financing, APRNs and the public should look at what the healthcare dollar buys, where the dollar comes from, and how it is paid out. Finally, we should look at the need for change in the system.

What the Healthcare Dollar Buys

To better understand healthcare financing, one first must understand what is being accomplished with the ever-increasing expenditures for health care. As measured by the federal Center for Medicare and Medicaid Services (CMS), national health expenditures are grouped into two categories: research and medical facilities construction and payments for health services and supplies.

Five types of personal healthcare expenditures (PCHEs) accounted for more than 84% of the 2005 total spending on health care. Ranked in order of spending, the five are:

- Hospital care
- "Physician" services
- Drugs and other medical nondurables
- Nursing home care
- Dental services

Not included in the CMS figures were medical education costs, except insofar as they are inseparable from hospital expenditures and biomedical research. The five types of PHCEs constituted the bulk of the national healthcare "bill"—more than $1726.7 billion in 2006.[10] As noted, the United States spends more on health per capita than any other country, and U.S. health spending continues to increase, although the rate of increase has slowed for the third consecutive year, due to the increased intensity and cost of services and a higher volume of services needed to treat an aging population.[11]

Where the Healthcare Dollar Comes From

In the early part of this century, people paid for medical care "out of their own pockets," much as they would purchase any other service. Costs and utilization were kept at a minimum because there was little in the way of medical care that physicians or hosptials could offer and that money could buy. In the 1930s, with the introduction of ether as an anesthetic, and with the advent of other advances in surgical technology, physicians and hospitals had more to sell. Consequently, resource utilization increased and the price of medical care climbed. In response to this increased demand and escalated cost for medical services, the first health insurance plan, Blue Cross, was jointly developed and offered by a group of hospitals and surgeons. Although the plan limited coverage to inpatient care, with physician services and medications remaining available only to those who could afford to pay for them, the third-party reimbursement system, with its attendant insensitivity to economics, was established.[12]

Although some say that healthcare monies come from different sources, what they really mean is that dollars take different routes on their way from consumers to providers. The current tax-financed share of health spending is far higher than most people think: 59.8%.[13] Ultimately, the American people pay all healthcare costs, indirectly or directly, regardless of whether payment occurs via government, private insurance companies, or independent plans. Moreover, third-party costs are paid in addition to the out-of-pocket payments. Out-of-pocket spending for health care consists of direct spending by consumers for all healthcare goods and services. Included in this estimate is the amount paid out-of-pocket for services not covered by insurance and the amount of coinsurance and deductibles required by private health insurance and by public programs such as Medicare and Medicaid (and not paid by some other third party).

Total public funding (which paid for 46% of all health care) continued to accelerate in 2005, increasing 7.7%, and exceeded private funding growth by 1.4 percentage points. In 2006, total Medicare spending grew to $401.3 billion. The introduction of the Part D benefit, which provided beneficiaries with coverage for prescription drugs, accelerated total Medicare spending; it grew 18.7% in 2006 compared to 9.3% in 2005. Medicaid, the state–federal health insurance program for the poor, grew to $308.6 billion in 2006. However, total Medicaid spending declined for the first time since the program's inception, falling 0.9%. The introduction of Part D, which shifted drug coverage for people eligible for both Medicaid and Medicare into Medicare contributed to this decline in Medicaid spending. Other reasons for the decline included continued cost-containment efforts by states and slower enrollment growth due to more restrictive eligibility criteria.[14]

Private health insurance premiums grew 5.5% in 2006 to $723.4 billion. This is the slowest rate of growth since 1997. This slowdown reflects a decline in private health insurance spending for prescription drugs, as well as a slowdown in underlying benefits. Benefit payment growth slowed, from 6.9% in 2005 to 6.0% in 2006, reaching $634.6 billion. Consumer out-of-pocket spending grew 3.8% to $256.5 billion, a deceleration from 2005. This slowdown is attributable to the negative growth in out-of-pocket payments for prescription drugs, mainly due to the introduction of Medicare Part D benefit. Out-of-pocket spending accounted for 12% of national health spending in 2006; this share has steadily declined since 1998, when it accounted for 15% of health spending. Out-of-pocket spending relative to overall household spending, however, has remained fairly flat since 2003.[14]

Hospital spending continued a gradual deceleration (from 8.2% growth in 2002), growing 7.0% in 2006 to $648.2 billion. The 2006 trend was partially driven by a lower utilization of hospital services, especially within Medicare, as fee-for-service inpatient hospital admissions declined. Spending on physician and clinical services also slowed, growing 5.9% in 2006 to $447.6 billion; this is the slowest rate of growth since 1999. The slowdown was driven by a deceleration in price growth, fueled by a near freeze on Medicare physician payments. Prescription drug spending accelerated for the first time in 6 years, from a low of 5.8% in 2005 to 8.5% in 2006. Spending reached $216.7 billion.

Figures 3-1 and 3-2 are pie charts of the nation's healthcare spending for 2006 and show where the money came from and where it went.

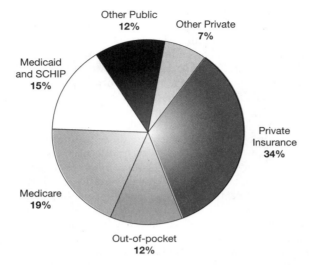

The statistics were taken from the Centers for Medicare & Medicaid Services, Office of the Actuary, National Health Statistics Group, 2008.

Other Public includes programs such as workers' compensation, public health activity, Department of Defense, Department of Veterans Affairs, Indian Health Service, state and local hospital subsidies, and school health. Other Private includes industrial in-plant, privately funded construction, and non-patient revenues, including philanthropy.

Figure 3-1: *The Nation's Health Dollar, Calendar Year 2006: Where It Came From.*

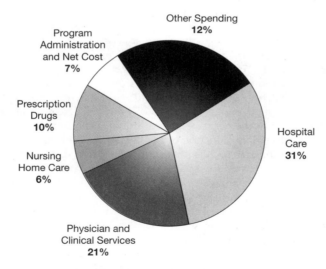

Note: Other Spending includes dentist services, other professional services, home health, durable medical products, over-the-counter medicines and sundries, public health, other personal health care, research, and structures and equipment.

Source: Centers for Medicare & Medicaid Services, Office of the Actuary, National Health Statistics Group, 2008.

Figure 3-2: *The Nation's Health Dollar, Calendar Year 2006: Where It Went.*

How the Money Is Paid Out

PUBLIC OUTLAYS

The significant rise in federal spending is accounted for by the Medicare, Medicaid, and SCHIP (State Children's Health Insurance Program) programs and by Titles XVIII and XIX of the Social Security Act (SSA).

Types of Public Outlays

Federal spending through the three main programs—Medicare, Medicaid, and SCHIP—targets different populations and is administered in different ways. Still other programs—for example, medical services for veterans—provide coverage for other sections of the population.

Medicare

Medicare is a federally funded health insurance program created by Title XVIII of the Social Security Act of 1965; it was originally designed to protect people 65 years of age and older from the high cost of health care. The program also covers permanently disabled workers eligible for old-age, survivors, and disability-insurance benefits and their dependents, as well as people with end-stage renal disease.

Implemented in 1966, when it enrolled 19 million persons, the program has increased the number served to 43.2 million. Expenditures for Medicare have risen faster than those for any other major federal program; it now insures one of every seven Americans. The program remains at the forefront of debate because of the aging of the baby-boom generation and the likelihood that expenditures will continue to increase. By 2031, the program is expected to serve 77 million people—more than one of every five Americans—and to account for about 4.4% of the gross domestic product (GDP).[15] The increase in life expectancy in the United States since 1965 is undoubtedly attributable in part to Medicare.

As currently structured, Medicare comprises four programs, each of which has its own trust fund[16]:

1. Part A, the hospital insurance program, is financed by payroll taxes collected under the Social Security system. It provides coverage for inpatient hospital services, post-hospitalization skilled nursing services, home healthcare services, and hospice care.

2. Part B, a voluntary supplemental medical insurance (SMI) program, pays certain costs for physicians' services, outpatient hospital services and therapy, and other health expenses. The SMI program is financed by monthly premiums collected from elderly enrollees and by general tax revenues.

3. Part C, Medicare Advantage plans was implemented by the passage of the Balanced Budget Act of 1997, which gave Medicare beneficiaries the option to receive their Medicare benefits through private health insurance plans, instead of through the original Medicare plan (Parts A and B). These programs were known as "Medicare+Choice" or "Part C" plans. The Medicare Prescription Drug, Improvement, and Modernization Act of 2003, changed the compensation and business practices of insurers that offer these plans, and "Medicare+Choice" plans became known as "Medicare Advantage" (MA) plans.

4. Medicare Part D, the prescription drug plans, went into effect on January 1, 2006, with the passage of the Medicare Prescription Drug, Improvement, and Modernization Act. Anyone with Part A or B is eligible for Part D. To receive this benefit, a person with Medicare must enroll in a stand-alone Prescription Drug Plan (PDP) or Medicare Advantage plan with prescription drug coverage (MA-PD). These plans are approved and regulated by the Medicare program, but they are actually designed and administered by private health insurance companies. Unlike original

Medicare (Parts A and B), Part D coverage is not standardized. Plans choose which drugs (or even classes of drugs) they wish to cover, at what level (or tier) they wish to cover them, and are free to choose not to cover some drugs at all.

Medicaid

Medicaid was established by the federal government in 1965 to provide health care to the poor. This program was designed to ensure healthcare services to the aged poor, the blind, the disabled, and families with dependent children if one parent is absent, unemployed, or unable to work. Persons become eligible for Medicaid on the basis of their financial status and by fitting into one of these federally defined categories. Medicaid, authorized by Title XIX of the SSA in 1965 as a joint federal/state entitlement program, pays for medical assistance to both "categorically" and "medically" eligible groups with limited resources. It provides health and mental health care coverage for children and families with low incomes, long-term healthcare services for seniors and people with disabilities, and provides gap funding for seniors who qualify for both Medicare and Medicaid.

Unlike Medicare, which is solely a federal program, the Medicaid program is jointly funded and administered by the federal and state governments. The name "Medicaid" is more or less a blanket label for 50 different state programs designed specifically to serve welfare recipients. Different states give their individual Medicaid programs different names. For example, in California, Medicaid is known as MediCal; in Arizona, the program is called Access; and in Tennessee, it is called TennCare. Medicaid provides federal funds to states on a cost-sharing basis according to each state's per capita income.

The Medicaid program represents a high degree of decentralization in that the federal government's requirements are only minimally restrictive. States exercise significant control over Medicaid eligibility and benefit packages within federal guidelines. For the most part, Medicaid is available only to very low income persons. The program also has categorical restrictions; that is, only families with children, pregnant women, and those who are aged, blind, or disabled can qualify.

The basic set of services mandated by the federal government for Medicaid programs includes:

- Inpatient and outpatient hospital care
- Other laboratory and x-ray services
- Physicians' services
- Nursing-facility care for persons older than 21 years
- Home health for those entitled to nursing-facility services
- Screening, diagnostic, and treatment services for persons younger than 21 years;
- Family planning

Although states must provide the basic set of services, they can set their own rates based on how much they are willing to spend on their percentage of the cost. Generally, the federal government will reimburse states between 50% and 83% of what they spend. Because each state can determine how much it will pay for services under the Medicaid program, much variability exists. For instance, in Massachusetts, a physician might be reimbursed about $1500 for delivering a baby, while in New Mexico, a physician might only receive about $900 for the identical service.

SCHIP

SCHIP is a federal government program that gives funds to states to provide health insurance to families with children. The program was designed to cover uninsured children in families with incomes that are modest but too high to qualify for Medicaid. At its creation in 1997, SCHIP was the largest expansion of health insurance coverage for children in the

United States since Medicaid began in the 1960s. States are given flexibility in designing their SCHIP eligibility requirements and policies within broad federal guidelines. SCHIP covered 7.8 million children during the federal fiscal year 2008, and every state has an approved plan.

Other Public Expenditures

Medicare and Medicaid account for more than 76% of public outlays for personal healthcare services. State and local government outlays represent the next largest expenditure category, but they only account for about 10% of the total amount. The remaining four major personal healthcare categories for which government monies are spent include:

1. Federal outlays for hospital and medical services for veterans
2. Department of Defense provision of care for the armed forces and military dependents
3. Workers' compensation medical benefits;
4. Other federal, state, and local expenditures for personal health care

Finally, public spending for research and facilities construction totaled approximately $58 billion in 2006. Of this amount, public outlays for research totaled $37.7 billion, with the federal government representing the primary source for most of the money spent.[14]

THE CURRENT CHALLENGE TO PUBLICLY FINANCED HEALTH CARE

Medicare has large deductibles, co-payments, and gaps in coverage. Two-thirds of Medicare beneficiaries carry supplemental private "Medigap" insurance, and 20% are enrolled in a Medicare HMO plan. Medicare now has a program to subsidize the costs of outpatient prescription medications. The average beneficiary pays more than $3000 out of pocket each year for health care, excluding long-term care.[15] Limitations on the amount of coverage exist as well. For example, hospital benefits cease after 90 days if the patient has exhausted the lifetime reserve pool of 60 additional hospital days, and extended-care facility benefits terminate after 100 days. Medicare payments represent approximately 65% of the total annual national expenditure on hospital services and 27% of physicians' services. Because Medicare clarified its conditions for nursing home payment in 1988 with the Catastrophic Coverage Act, it seems likely that Medicare will maintain its current share of total spending for nursing home care at 4% to 5%.[16]

As of 2006, approximately 60 million people received some type of Medicaid benefit, up from approximately 51 million in 2002, with approximately $316 billion of combined federal and state funds being spent for personal health care in 2006. As a result of its accelerated growth, Medicaid's share of the nation's public health PHCEs has increased significantly. In 2006, the Medicaid program financed health care and social services for more than one in every five Americans. In 2006, the federal government provided 57% of all Medicaid expenditures, totaling $190 billion dollars. Medicaid pays for more than one-third of all births. It is the nation's largest purchaser of long-term-care services, and it funds more than half of all nursing home expenditures. It is also the largest payer of medical care for persons with HIV infection or AIDS.

Medicaid also provides major support to hospitals that are "safety-net" providers. Medicaid's expenditures are largely institutional, with more than 40% of its budget spent on hospital care and approximately 35% spent on nursing home care annually. Medicaid continues to be the largest third-party payer of long-term-care expenditures, financing almost 50% of nursing home care annually.

Confronted with increasing numbers of recipients and recent legislative expansions to the Medicaid program in the face of limited revenues available to finance the program, states have been pressured to control their individual Medicaid costs. Strategies used or proposed by states include:

- Overall spending cuts
- Reallocation of available funds from high-cost services to lower-cost services

- Rationing of high-technology services to selected recipients to provide lower-cost services to a broader group of recipients
- Provider-specific taxes
- "Voluntary donations" from physicians and hospitals

PRIVATE OUTLAYS

Although the amount of public funding for health care is staggering, the predominant source of funding for the American healthcare system comes from private sources. The bulk is derived from individuals receiving treatment and from third-party insurers making payments on the behalf of individuals.

In 1929, private payment represented 88.4% of the total amount spent on PHCEs. In 1935, that figure dropped to 82.4%. In 1965, before the advent of Medicare and Medicaid, such private payments accounted for nearly 77% of the total. In 1998, private payment accounted for 56% of all PHCEs. By 2005, private health insurance paid for only 36% of PHCEs.[11] The decline in the private share of PHCEs is primarily due to the sharp drop in out-of-pocket payments associated with the increase in federal spending. In 1965, 53% "of PHCEs were paid for by the patient, and in 2005, 15%. Yet because of inflation and other factors, the per capita dollar amount paid directly by a patient has increased dramatically.[11]

Types of Private Outlays

Private outlays come from private third-party reimbursement, Blue Cross and Blue Shield indemnity plans, commercial insurance, self-insurance, nonindemnity insurance plans (HMOs), and preferred provider organizations (PPOs).

Private Third-Party Reimbursement

Most Americans receive their health insurance as a tax-free benefit through their employers.[11] This employer-based financing of health care was started during World War II and has grown steadily ever since. The system relies predominantly on private, employment-based, insurance-type financing schemes that, at least until recently, divorced financing from the delivery of services.

Private health insurance companies constitute one of the largest sectors of the health industry. The United States has more than 1000 for-profit, commercial health insurers and 85 not-for-profit Blue Cross and Blue Shield plans. These private insurance organizations, along with HMOs, PPOs, and other third-party payers, paid for 36% of the total healthcare expenditures in 2005.[11]

Employment is the foundation of the private health insurance system in the United States. In 2005, 81% of Americans under the age of 65 had some form of health insurance coverage; of these, 68% were covered by an employment-based plan.[17] Employment enables many workers to obtain health coverage. Six out of every 10 workers (60%) are offered health insurance by their own employers, and 8 out of 10 (82%) receive employment-based coverage through their jobs.[18] In 2006, employer-based insurance covered some 158 million people. This includes 18 million retirees who also have Medicare and use the employer-based health insurance as a supplement to Medicare. About an additional 22 million people purchased their own insurance; these people are usually self-employed or employed by an employer who does not offer health insurance as a benefit.

Overall, employer-based health insurance touches the lives of nearly two out of every three Americans. PPOs enroll the largest proportion of workers (57%), followed by HMOs (21%), and point-of-service (POS) plans (13%). PPO enrollment has grown substantially in recent years, while HMO enrollment has decreased. Enrollment in conventional insurance plans constitutes only 3% of workers, down from 27% in 1996. [18,19]

Blue Cross and Blue Shield and the Rise of Indemnity Insurance

The term "insurance" originally meant, and often still refers to, the contribution by individuals to a fund to provide protection against financial loss following relatively unlikely but damaging events. Thus, there is insurance against fire, theft, and death at an early age. All of those events occur within a group of people at a predictable rate, but they are rare occurrences for any one individual in a group.[20]

Medical insurance was introduced in the mid-1800s to defray costs associated with unexpected disabilities. Essentially, it consisted of cash payments by some carriers to individuals to offset income losses attributed to accident-related disabilities. Medical insurance continued in this tradition until the 1930s when, coincident with the rise in available medical services, a number of prepayment plans that offered care at various hospitals were organized in several cities. These hospital insurance plans soon became known as Blue Cross.[21] Shortly thereafter, Blue Shield was developed independently as an insurer for physicians' services. With the organization of Blue Cross and Blue Shield, a new policy for reimbursing general healthcare costs began.

The "Blues" were established as nonprofit membership plans that served state and regional areas and offered both individual and group membership. For many years, the Blues were committed to community rating.[22] In exchange for offering coverage to anyone in the community, the Blues were able to secure significant discounts in costs by way of negotiations and through regulations known as "most-favored-nation status," which ensured that they would have the lowest rates allowed to any payer.

In recent years, this community-rating approach has placed the Blues at a disadvantage when competing with commercial insurers adhering to a policy of experience rating. Experience rating has allowed commercial insurers to charge different individuals and groups different premiums, based on individual risk and on the use of services. Low-risk groups could secure benefits at lower premiums because of the "healthy worker effect," whereas high-risk groups were only able to receive commercial insurance coverage at prohibitively high premium rates. Consequently, the Blues have been left as the insurers of last resort for those individuals who might have chronic illnesses and/or are unable to obtain employer-based group insurance coverage.

Commercial Insurance

Like the Blues, commercial insurance plans offer comprehensive coverage for hospital and physicians' services; however, they differ in that they also sell medical and cash-payment policies. Regular medical coverage is a form of insurance that provides coverage of physicians' fees in cases that do not involve surgery. The medical care may be provided in the home, in a hospital, or in a physician's office. A regular medical policy may also cover diagnostic x-ray and other laboratory expenses. Major medical policies usually contain deductibles. After an insured has reached a specified hospital-medical expense level, the insurer will also pay, for example, 80% of all remaining expenses to a set maximum. In contrast, insurance companies that sell cash-payment policies provide a cash payment for each day that a patient receives care. If the costs exceed the limit set, the patient or the family is responsible for the extra costs.

The commercial portion of the industry has grown rapidly in this country, primarily because experience rating has allowed them to respond to consumer demand for reduced out-of-pocket costs for medical care and because of the "employer-based" model for financing health care that developed during World War II. Initially, commercial insurance companies were slow to enter a market dominated by the Blues. However, during and after World War II, tax laws changed to permit employers to offer tax-free health coverage as part of employee benefit packages, allowing commercial companies that previously had offered limited coverage to individuals to offer hospital insurance to groups. Since that time, commercial insurance companies have acquired more than half of the health insurance market from Blue Cross and

Blue Shield. Currently, there are more than 1000 private insurance companies providing individual and group health coverage in the United States.[17]

Self-Insurance

To avoid high tax premiums, administrative overhead, and marketing expenses, a majority of large corporations have become self-insured. Commercial insurance companies have found themselves to be little more than transaction processors for these corporations, providing claims payment services to the self-insured on a cost-plus basis. Consequently, these insurance companies are experiencing operating losses due to the shrinking of the fully insured market. To compete and survive, group insurance carriers have transformed themselves into managed care companies, thereby improving internal operating and marketing efficiencies. However, it is estimated that only 25 of the nearly 500 group health insurance carriers have the capability, financial support, management, and customer volume to accomplish this task.[23]

Health Maintenance Organizations and the Rise of Nonindemnity Insurance

As healthcare costs escalated in the 1970s, Congress passed legislation that encouraged the formation of HMOs, or systems that would integrate the delivery and financing of health care. These operate differently from traditional indemnity insurance plans that reimbursed on a fee-for-service basis. HMOs provide comprehensive health "maintenance" care (and restorative care when necessary) for its enrollees at a flat, prepaid fee. Although this "capitated" form of health insurance has been available for the past 30 years, it has more recently reshaped the way many Americans relate to the healthcare system.

Although several different types of prepaid plans are available, the basic notion of each is that an annual fixed payment is made by or for beneficiaries in exchange for the delivery of all necessary health care by a group of providers within the scope of their contracts. Distinctions among HMOs pertain to the ways in which fiscal agents or the financing organizations relate to groups of care providers. Most prepaid plans contract with providers for scheduled reimbursement, capitated payments, discounted charges, or per-episode payments. Currently, there are five distinct HMO models in operation in the United States (Table 3-1).

Regardless of the type of plan, a capitated annual insurance premium is paid in exchange for all necessary care, including preventive and routine services not generally covered under indemnity plans. Presumably, HMOs reduce healthcare costs (owing, for the most part, to lower rates of hospitalization) while providing coverage that has fewer co-payment features and fewer uncovered services. These plans have grown popular with employers who are

---

Table 3-1 **Health Maintenance Organization Models in the United States**

Model Description

Staff model: In this traditional HMO system, the fiscal agent engages individual physicians who are paid a salary to deliver services to the HMO's enrollees.

Group model: This model is similar to the staff model; however, it varies in that a single group of physicians contracts with the fiscal agent to deliver services.

Network model: Fiscal agents contract with multiple groups of physicians to deliver services to enrollees. Physicians in this model do not have exclusive contracts with fiscal agents and generally provide services to non-HMO enrollees.

Independent model: Fiscal agents contract with a range of independent physicians or multispecialty group practices to deliver care to its enrollees.

IPA model: As in the network model, physicians in the IPA model provide services to HMO enrollees as well as to patients with other forms of insurance. Usually, HMO enrollees represent a small percentage of IPA physicians' practices.

looking for ways to reduce healthcare benefits spending. Between 1984 and 1993, the proportion of employees enrolled in HMOs increased from 5% to 50%. By 1998, 85% of employees with health insurance coverage were in some form of managed care plan, whereas 15% were in fee-for-service indemnity plans.[24] Enrollment in managed care plans grew because managed care cost less than fee-for-service care. Managed care business practices, such as preauthorization of hospital and other services and restricted formularies for medications, reduced utilization and cost.[24]

In the late 1990s, more than 50% of HMOs lost money. The financial downturn in HMO performance coincided with growing public and physician disenchantment with managed care. In 2000, HMO enrollment dropped for the first time in history and has continued to drop. PPOs now insure more Americans than HMOs. HMOs—with slightly cheaper premiums and no deductibles—could become the health plans for low-income people, while PPOs would insure those with higher incomes.

The next trend in healthcare insurance is the defined contribution approach in which employers limit their exposure to rising healthcare costs by shifting cost increases onto their employees. Under the defined contribution approach, the employer contributes a fixed sum for each employee's health insurance with the employee paying the balance—less for a low-cost plan and more for a high-cost plan.

Preferred-Provider Organizations

The success of the HMO independent practice association (IPA) model increased experimentation with varying levels of consumer and physician choice, eventually leading to the introduction of PPOs. PPOs, like HMOs, offer the consumer a choice of full coverage for ambulatory and inpatient services provided by a selected panel of providers, combined with a limited range of coverage for consumers who choose a provider that is not part of the selected panel of providers, known as out-of-plan use. Frequently, PPOs are established by groups of physicians who are interested in maintaining patients and revenues in the face of competition from HMOs.

PPOs provide health care at a lower cost to those beneficiaries who use participating providers, who are paid on the basis of negotiated or discounted rates. Beneficiaries are usually given some type of incentive, such as lower insurance premiums or waivers of cost-sharing requirements, for selecting a preferred provider. PPOs are gaining popularity, especially in markets where there is significant competition among physicians and other healthcare providers.

In such competitive areas, providers can be persuaded more easily to offer discounted services in exchange for a larger share of the patient volume. The enhancement in consumer choice afforded by PPOs mimics the freedom of choice found in traditional fee-for-service medicine. Enrollment in PPO plans has been growing steadily since 1996, and PPOs now cover more than half of workers.[25]

Point-of-Service Plans

Point-of-service (POS) healthcare plans allow enrollees to choose whether to receive a specific service from a contracted preferred provider or a noncontracted provider. POS plans are a combination of either an HMO or PPO plan with a traditional indemnity plan. For the maximum level of benefits, the enrollee must consult the primary care physician prior to obtaining treatment or services. If the enrollee seeks care without authorization or out of network from a contracted provider, the enrollee will have a higher out-of-pocket cost.

THE CURRENT CHALLENGE TO PRIVATELY FINANCED HEALTH CARE

Although private health insurance coverage for Americans is extensive, it is far from complete. According to one report, more than 45 million Americans are uninsured and their numbers are growing as the economy weakens.[26] The problem of the uninsured is one of America's biggest health challenges. Too many families do not have access to affordable health insurance, and they live sicker and die younger as a result. And being uninsured is not primarily a problem for the unemployed. Nearly 70% of the uninsured come from families with at least one full-time worker. Nearly one in five Americans under the age of 65 were without health insurance in 2005, a number that has continued to increase. The demographics of the nearly 45 million uninsured are a mix of people living below the poverty line, adults between the ages of 19 and 54 (who make up 71% of the nonelderly uninsured), and 9 million children. About two-thirds of the nonelderly uninsured are from low-income families (income below 200% of the federal poverty line, or about $42,400 for a family of four in 2007). More than one in three people (35%) living in poverty are uninsured, compared with 1 in 20 people (5%) with family incomes at or above four times the poverty level.[26] These data support the notion that the proportion of the population that has insurance is directly related to income.

At the same time, employers are applying pressure on insurers to pare down premiums. Between the spring of 2006 and spring 2007, premiums increased an average of 6.1% for employer-sponsored health insurance, a slower rate than the 7.7% increase in 2006.[18] Premium increases affect all employees with health insurance coverage. Insurers, at the behest of employers, are also redesigning their benefit packages in ways that will have the greatest effect on workers who seek medical care. These packages generally feature fewer benefits, larger cost-sharing requirements at the point of service, or both, but also smaller premium increases than would have otherwise been the case. Structuring benefits in ways that subject patients to larger out-of-pocket expenditures is a reversal of a pattern that had been in place for decades, according to the Centers for Medicare and Medicaid Services. The agency estimates that approximately 15% of PHCEs were borne by consumers in the form of out-of-pocket costs in 2000, down from 20% in 1990 and 48% in 1960. In 2005, 34% of PHCEs were paid by the federal government and 11% by state and local government; private health insurance paid 36% and consumers paid 15% out of pocket.

Cost sharing by patients comes in a variety of forms: an annual deductible (an amount that a patient pays up front, before using healthcare services), a specific deductible for hospital admission, a co-payment (an amount that a patient pays per unit of service, such as an office visit or a hospital stay), and various cost-sharing features for generic and brand-name drugs, all of which can be "mixed and matched to achieve whichever premium price point is desired by the purchaser."[27]

One of the newest cost-containment methods being used by insurers differentiates prescription drugs, hospitals, and, in California, medical groups and physicians on the basis of cost. This approach was first used with prescription drugs. About three in four covered workers are in plans with three- or four-tier cost-sharing arrangements, and most face co-payments rather than coinsurance for the first three tiers.[18] Under such coverage, the lowest co-payment is required if a generic drug is prescribed, a higher co-payment is required for a preferred brand-name drug, and the highest co-payment is required for a nonpreferred brand-name drug. In 2007, among workers with three- or four-tier plans, the average co-payment was $11 for generic drugs, $25 for preferred drugs, and $43 for nonpreferred drugs. The most recent form of tiered benefits—different levels of co-payments for hospital care that are based on costs—is being offered by some of the nation's largest insurers on either a trial or a permanent basis. PacifiCare and Blue Shield of California are exploring ways to provide tiered benefits for physicians' services based on the fees the physicians charge and possibly on selected indicators of the quality of care they provide. Blue Shield of California will evaluate hospitals not only on the basis of their costs but also on the basis of data on patient satisfaction and the quality of care, compiled by two independent organizations.

The basic change that many employers are considering is to abandon the traditional approach of offering employees a defined set of insurance benefits and instead offer them a fixed amount of money to pay for coverage. Under the defined contribution approach, the employer contributes a fixed sum for each employee's health insurance with the employee paying the balance—less for a low-cost plan and more for a high-cost plan. Under this approach, the employee would pay for any costs that exceeded the employer's contribution, up to a maximum amount, beyond which insurance would cover the cost of a serious or catastrophic illness.

A health savings account (HSA) is a tax-advantaged medical savings account available to taxpayers in the United States who are enrolled in a high-deductible health plan (HDHP). The funds contributed to the account are not subject to federal income tax at the time of deposit. Unlike a flexible spending account, funds roll over and accumulate year to year if not spent. HSAs are owned by the individual, which differentiates them from the company-owned health reimbursement arrangement, which is an alternate tax-deductible source of funds paired with HDHPs. HSA funds may currently be used to pay for qualified medical expenses at any time without federal tax liability or penalty.

How the Money Is Paid Out

The predominant manner of payment to hospitals and providers has been the retrospective fee-for-service method. However, with the spiraling costs associated with Medicare and Medicaid, the federal government began to exercise its prerogative to scrutinize the value received for the healthcare reimbursements to hospitals and physicians. Commercial health insurance companies were quick to follow the government's lead by adopting similar payment policies.

With the proliferation of HMOs and PPOs and with increased fee regulation by public programs, physicians and hospitals are now less able to freely set prices for their services. At this time, there are several approaches that insurers may use to pay hospitals and physicians for their services:

- Fee-for-service, which means the physician is paid a set fee for a specific level of service.
- The preferred provider approach, which means physicians or hospitals that are listed as preferred by the insurance company have a higher level or percent reimbursement. Capitation, which can be for both the hospital component and the physician fee component.
- Point of service, a hybrid plan that is part HMO and part PPO; the HMO benefit pays a higher benefit than selecting a specialist on one's own.
- Pay for performance for both hospitals and physicians; for example, if the institution has fewer secondary infections, then Medicare pays a higher rate.
- Global fees for both hospital and physician services; for example, each group (physician/surgeon and hospital) is reimbursed for a knee replacement at a set fee for the procedure and hospitalization.

Although there are many permutations within these reimbursement categories, the two dominant approaches are retrospective payment and prospective payment. These two approaches are described next, along with the measures used to contain the costs of physician services.

FEDERAL COST CONTROL AND ITS EFFECT ON HOSPITAL REIMBURSEMENT

Beginning in the 1970s, the related issues of the cost and the quality of the care delivered under federal entitlement programs were addressed by the passage of legislative amendments. Professional standards review organizations (PSROs) were established in an effort to monitor the quality and quantity of institutional services delivered to Medicare and Medicaid recipients. Subsequent amendments attempted to limit the growth in healthcare expenditures by changing the manner in which the amount to be reimbursed hospitals and physicians was calculated.

In 1982, Congress passed the Tax Equity and Fiscal Responsibility Act (TEFRA). Designed to provide incentives for cost containment in institutions, it replaced the PSROs with a "utilization and quality-control peer review organization" (PRO). The TEFRA legislation introduced to hospitals the cost-per-case reimbursement system known as diagnosis-related groups (DRGs) and, simultaneously, placed limits on the rates of increase in hospital revenues. Additional legislation mandated that hospitals covered under Medicare's new case-based reimbursement system contract with a PRO by 1984.

Prospective Payment System

The 1983 amendments to the Social Security Act further refined the case payment system by establishing a prospective payment system. These amendments created a revolutionary method based on DRGs of reimbursing hospitals for inpatient care of Medicare patients. Under the prospective payment system, hospitals are paid a pre-fixed amount per case treated. Research exploring the impact of DRGs suggests that the utilization patterns of hospitals are changing as a result of the reimbursement system. Most notably, hospital admissions and length of hospital stays have significantly decreased, and post-hospital care, including the use of home health services and nursing homes, has sharply increased.

Retrospective Payment System

While prospective payment represents the most significant change in reimbursement methods in the past 20 years, it is not the exclusive means by which institutions are paid. Retrospective payment, or paying for services already provided, remains a mode by which some third-party payers reimburse hospitals. Most commercial insurers, such as Blue Cross, pay hospitals on the basis of submitted charges, or the prices set by hospitals for the care they provide. A more sophisticated retrospective repayment system is based on cost. In this system, third-party payers take a sum of total hospital costs and then, based on allowable items, reimburse hospitals on a per-patient-day basis.

FEDERAL COST CONTROL AND ITS EFFECT ON PHYSICIAN PAYMENT

Physician reimbursement mechanisms were changed as a result of federal legislation, primarily under provisions in the Omnibus Budget Reconciliation Acts (OBRAs), especially OBRA 1989 and OBRA 1993.[28–32] Before the enactment of OBRA 1989, physicians were permitted wide discretion in establishing their own prices for each type of service they delivered. Once care was received, patients or their insurers paid the set price. Since the OBRA legislation, new physician reimbursement mechanisms have been put into place—prevailing rates, resource-based value systems, discounted rates for PPOs, salaries for physicians, and payments based on performance.

Prevailing Rates

After OBRA 1989 was enacted, the amount that Medicare reimbursed physicians was equal to the "prevailing" fee (also known as "usual and customary rates") that physicians in the specific community charged for each type of physician service. Whether the patient is charged for any amount billed in excess of the prevailing rate depends on the specific plan. Many insurers have followed Medicare's approach by adopting a wide range of methods for establishing scales for covered services, limiting the ability of the physician to establish prices.

Resource-Based Relative Value System

The resource-based relative value system (RBRVS) went into effect in 1992 and represents another attempt by the federal government to control physician-related costs. With its introduction, Medicare substantially changed its approach to paying physicians. Based on a national fee schedule, the RBRVS assigns cash values to services based on the time, skill, and intensity required to provide the services. The relative values are then further adjusted for geographic variations in payment. The RBRVS attempts to correct the bias of physician payment that has historically paid for surgical and other procedures at a far higher rate than primary care and cognitive services. Unfortunately, evidence suggests that the RBRVS has not been as successful as expected.

PPOs and Discounted Payment Schedules

In the private arena, the approach to paying physicians used by PPOs offers a variation on the fee-for-service system. Using this approach, insurers pay physicians discounted amounts for care delivered to enrollees on a service-by-service basis. The discounted payment schedule is usually negotiated between the insurers and the physicians or by physician groups. With fee-for-service payments, physicians and other healthcare providers have an economic incentive to perform more services because more services bring in more revenue. With the discounted approach to paying physicians or physician groups, there is not the same incentive to perform more services as there is with the fee-for-service approach.

Salary and Capitation

Salary and capitation are the two other forms of provider reimbursement. The use of salary arrangements as a payment mechanism for health professionals is widespread and needs little explanation. Generally, this arrangement proves satisfactory to both employer and provider. In a salaried arrangement, employers can generally enjoy administrative simplicity, while providers are usually assured a more protected income compared to those being reimbursed through other arrangements.

Capitation is another form of physician reimbursement for healthcare services. The physician is paid a contracted rate for each member assigned, referred to as a "per-member-per-month" rate, regardless of the number or nature of services provided. The contractual rates are usually adjusted for age, gender, illness, and regional differences.

Pay for Performance

Pay for performance is part of a growing movement to better align financial incentives to increases in the quality of care and thereby reduce unnecessary costs. The concept is viewed as a way to narrow the well-documented gap between clinical practice and evidence-based guidelines.[33] The Institute of Medicine 2006 report supports pay for performance "as a stimulus to foster comprehensive and system-wide improvements in the quality of health care." This report also recommends that implementation of pay-for-performance programs should be carefully monitored to be sure that the stated goals are being achieved and that unintended consequences are recognized as early as possible.[34] Both private and public payers are increasingly developing new pay-for-performance initiatives. More than half of commercial HMOs in the United States currently use pay-for-performance incentives in their provider contracts.[35]

In 2003, the Centers for Medicare and Medicaid Services launched the Hospital Quality Improvement Demonstration project, the largest pay-for-performance pilot project to date in the United States.[36] The project tracks clinical quality and outcomes across five clinical conditions, including indicators for acute myocardial infarction, heart failure, pneumonia, coronary artery bypass surgery, and joint replacement. Pay-for-performance will affect both hospital and provider reimbursement. In the Medicare program, payment will be linked to quality measures, such that hospitals will receive differential payment according to their performance.

All major payers are piloting pay-for-performance systems measuring healthcare provider performance and offering financial incentives to those who meet quality targets. Primary care is a key target for these programs: 95% of the programs include primary care providers and 52% include specialists.[37] The programs use a variety of methods to reward healthcare providers financially for achieving targets. Fee differentials, which reflect a percentage increase in reimbursement when quality standards are met, and bonuses are the models of choice. Pay-for-performance programs focus on a range of performance measures, but clinical measures continue to be the primary focus. More than 80% of the measures used are Health Plan Employer Data and Information Set (HEDIS) measures from the National Committee for Quality Assurance.[37] Fifty percent of pay-for-performance programs include efficiency measures such as the number of inpatient admissions or the rate of prescribing generic drugs.[37] Use of information technologies, such as electronic medical records and electronic prescribing, are rewarded in 42% of programs.[37]

Another emerging model of payment reform is nonpayment for "never events." In this model, providers are not paid if they perform surgery on the wrong body part; nor are providers paid for patients with preventable inpatient complications, such as urinary tract infections and decubiti.

The Need for Change

All healthcare systems face the same challenges: improving health, controlling costs, prioritizing allocation of resources, enhancing the quality of care, and distributing services fairly.[3] Almost everyone agrees that the U.S. healthcare system is broken and needs to be fixed. Everyone also agrees that healthcare costs need to be controlled, but people disagree on the best methods of addressing the escalating costs for government, employers, employees, and the uninsured.

One of the most basic conflicts affecting health-care providers is the tension between caring for the individual patient and caring for the larger community or population.[3] Many of the most important decisions to be made in health policy—decisions such as allocating healthcare resources, addressing the social context of health and illness, and augmenting activities in prevention and public health—depend on broadening the practitioner's view to encompass the population health perspective. The challenge for physicians and other clinicians will be to make room for this broader perspective while preserving the ethical duty to care for the individual patients under their charge.[3]

According to advocates of managed care and others who have studied health-spending trends, patients and physicians had grown insensitive to the rising cost of health care in this country. Previously, insured patients were paying very little directly for every dollar spent for hospital care and physicians' services. Most of the expense was borne by either employers or the government. The expectation of patients to receive all potentially beneficial care and the unwillingness of these same individuals in their role as purchasers to spend unlimited amounts to finance health care creates a strain for all caregivers and systems of care. This trend is changing. Cost sharing has become the norm for all types of healthcare plans. Cost sharing refers to making patients pay directly out-of-pocket for some portion of their health care.

Because patients previously felt relatively little financial burden associated with their healthcare expenses, they exerted little pressure on providers to keep costs low. Similarly, providers generally had no real incentive to seek and use lower-cost medical services that would yield the same outcome as more expensive services. Rather, they were, and to a great extent continue to be, rewarded for delivering as many of the most expensive services as possible. Consequently, there has been little competition among providers to produce services efficiently and pass savings on to consumers. In light of these perceptions, most proposed healthcare reform initiatives, regardless of their origin, are directed toward restraining medical inflation by sensitizing consumers and providers to the high cost of health care.

Healthcare providers increasingly are being called upon to incorporate considerations of costs when making clinical decisions. Debate will continue about the best ways to encourage providers to be more accountable for the costs of care in a manner that is socially responsible and does not unduly intrude on the provider's ability to serve the individual patient. The healthcare system as a whole will continue to struggle over finding the proper balance between the provision of acute care services and preventive and chronic care services, as well as striking the right balance between the levels of tertiary and primary care.

Possible Solutions to Evolving Healthcare Concerns

Continuing concerns about the healthcare system in the United States, along with disappointment over HMOs and other proposed "fixes" for the system, have highlighted three major themes on the health policy agenda and have led to several proposals for new possible solutions. These three themes that have dominated the nation's health policy agenda in the past few decades are access, cost, and quality. Policies that influence access focus on providing services to the underserved, such as the elderly and the poor, and ensuring availability of commercial health insurance. Cost containment has been a primary focus of both public and private policy initiatives since the early 1970s. Fueled by technology and increases in longevity, the United States witnessed a 15-fold increase in healthcare spending in the years between 1960 and 2002.[39] More recently, public attention has focused on the quality of health services and patient safety as several reports have concentrated on health system inefficiencies, medical errors, and preventable deaths.

One proposed solution that the states, the federal government, and private insurers are experimenting with is promoting primary care through the use of patient-centered medical homes. Another proposed solution has been the proliferation of retail medical clinics. Lastly, the size, makeup, and efficiency of the healthcare workforce must be considered.

Medical Homes

The medical home is an emerging concept. The definitions vary, but the basic model is a bundling of medical practice characteristics that improve both individual patient outcomes and the health of populations.[39] Medical homes not only improve patient care but also make a positive contribution to health policy. They improve quality by ensuring that the right services are provided at the right times. They reduce costs by reducing avoidable hospitalizations for many chronic conditions. And they enhance access by increasing provider availability and using patient-centered scheduling.[39]

A medical home provides primary care that is accessible, continuous, comprehensive, compassionate, and culturally effective. The program provides financial incentives to primary care providers to take responsibility for all of a patient's healthcare needs and to arrange appropriate care with other healthcare providers. The primary care provider is expected to be the leader of the patient's healthcare team and ensure that all stages of care—preventive care, acute care, chronic care, and end-of-life care—are coordinated and/or integrated across all elements of the healthcare system. In the medical home model, the primary care provider is not the gatekeeper, but a care facilitator. The model encourages shared decision-making and feedback from patients about their experiences and the quality of care (Box 3-1).

Providers seeking designation as patient-centered medical home practices must evaluate their practices against nine different standards, each of which has numerous sub-elements and some of which are designated as "must pass." Three levels of accreditation are determined by a practice's cumulative score. A practice can earn up to 100 points; but the minimum requirement for the PCMH designation is 25 points, provided that certain must-pass elements are also fulfilled.[40] Those who commit to the patient-centered medical home model can receive better compensation. The proposed payment formula in the medical home model differs from the managed care or the current fee-for-service payment systems. Capitation encourages very little volume, and fee-for-service encourages lots of volume, but neither one encourages good results. The medical home payment model uses blended fees. The blended fee combines fee-for-service; a care management fee, which ideally will be risk-adjusted to account for the demands of a particular provider's patient population; and performance-based compensation, which could include a shared-savings model or more traditional pay for performance. This system of reimbursement for medical home payments introduces accountability and responsibility at the level of practice for satisfying quality, cost of care, and safety metrics.

BOX 3-1 | The Characteristics of a Medical Home

Accessible

- Practice is accessible by public transportation.
- Practice is open evening and weekend hours.
- Patients can speak to a provider about a medical problem 24/7.
- Practice has adopted open-access scheduling of appointments.

Patient-Centered

- Practice has adopted a whole-person orientation to care delivery.
- Practice provides clear, unbiased, and complete information about health and disease that is shared with patients.
- Patients have access to their medical records.
- Patients share responsibility in decision making.
- Practice provides patient support and enabling services, such as reminders for routine preventive care, patient education, translation, and transportation.

Continuous

- The same professionals are available to provide care over time.
- The practice participates in discharge planning when the patient is hospitalized.

Comprehensive

- Preventive care is provided.
- Preventive, primary, and tertiary care needs are addressed.
- Patients are supported in managing their chronic conditions.
- Practice provides or arranges for providing other health services, such as oral and behavioral health.
- Care provided by multiple providers is coordinated through the medical home.
- A central record containing all pertinent health information is maintained at the practice.

Culturally Effective

- The patient's cultural background (beliefs, rituals, and customs) is recognized, valued, and respected.
- All efforts are made to assure that the patient understands the results of the clinical encounter and the treatment plan.
- Translators and interpreters are available as needed.
- Written instructions are provided in the patient's primary language.

Retail Health Clinics

A critical need exists for increasing access to health care in the United States. This need is especially acute for individuals with common health problems who need timely attention but who do not have a convenient place to go or a familiar provider to see for this type of care.[41] Barriers to care include difficulty getting an appointment, lengthy travel distances to care settings, long and unpredictable waits, limited hours of service, high out-of-pocket costs, complex health plan rules, and eroding health insurance coverage. To meet this need for improved access to health care, health clinics staffed primarily by nurse practitioners (NPs) have opened in retail settings like pharmacies, grocery stores, and malls. The growth of these clinics has been explosive due to the market need for accessible, affordable, high-quality health care.

NPs' services in retail settings bring affordable and accessible care to patients in a familiar, community-based environment and answer the needs unmet by the current U.S. healthcare system.[41]

Workforce Issues

More than 20% of the population living in the United States today currently resides in federally designated health professional shortage areas.[42] Currently, the United States is facing critical shortages of nurses, physicians, and pharmacists. If the healthcare system's purpose is to provide quality care and appropriate access to care, a critical factor is having an adequate supply of well-educated providers.

One area coming under increasing focus has been the current and future size of the U.S. physician workforce. The Council on Graduate Medical Education (COGME) stated that the number of full-time-equivalent physicians is expected to increase from 781,200 in 2000 to 971,800 in 2020. At the same time, though, because of an expanding and aging population, the demand for physicians is expected to grow even faster. COGME forecasts a shortage of about 85,000 physicians in 2020.[43] The weight of evidence indicates a future physician shortage; this may be another opportunity for APRNs, particularly NPs.

In recent years, the proportion of medical students choosing careers in primary care has declined significantly in the United States. At the same time, the number of NPs entering the workforce has continued to increase, from 76,306 in 1999 to 137,178 in 2008, an 82% increase.[44] Demand for primary care services will only rise as the population ages and develops more complex healthcare needs, such as chronic conditions. NPs play a vital role in the delivery of primary care; as of 2004, it was estimated that 80% of NPs work in a primary care discipline.

NPs have been providing excellent primary care to patients for several decades. They are competent practitioners who help our nation improve healthcare outcomes and lower healthcare costs. To meet the needs of patients, NPs must continue to pursue the goal of increasing their legislatively sanctioned autonomy. They must remove all barriers that restrict their access to patients and patient access to NPs.

In many areas of the United States, there also exists a shortage of specialty physicians. This is creating an opportunity for NPs and other APRNs, including certified nurse-midwives and clinical nurse specialists, to enter into specialty areas of practice. [45,46]

Implications for Advanced Practice Registered Nursing

APRNs must prepare themselves for the substantial opportunities and considerable challenges that are evolving in the healthcare system. For the first time since the beginning of this century, both the delivery and receipt of health care are operating on a budget. In addition, the consumer—whether an elderly person selecting from among several health insurance plans to supplement Medicare coverage or a large corporation's employee benefits administrator deciding between a self-insured health plan or an HMO—is once again in a position to exercise control over what to buy and how much to pay. The shift to a value-driven consumer in a cost-conscious environment translates into an opportunity for APRNs to become the value-conscious healthcare provider. This is an opportunity that should not be squandered. As repeatedly stated by past and present APRN leaders, APRNs have in the past—and should today—commit to promoting themselves and their advanced practice skills as essential elements in healthcare reform.

Some of the concepts integral to managed care have permeated all of health care, and APRNs are knowledgeable in all of these areas. APRNs need to become familiar with using clinical practice guidelines, which can lead to improvements in healthcare delivery. The guidelines should be well designed, goal oriented, specific, evidence based, and adapted for local use with input from the providers who will employ them. Although utilization management has been portrayed as favoring cost containment at the expense of quality, its guiding principles are to minimize inappropriate variations in practice and promote cost-effective patient care, which should meet best-practice standards and simultaneously reduce costs. The goal is to enable health professionals to practice comfortably and effectively in a high-quality, cost-effective healthcare system.

APRNs are additionally challenged by a system that increasingly demands the prevention and management of chronic diseases. Management of chronic diseases takes a systems-based approach to improving patient outcomes to help achieve the best possible health outcomes through the use of evidence-based practice guidelines. Pressures on the U.S. healthcare system and greater focus on health promotion and prevention have opened up opportunities for APRNs, since a population-based approach to health care is being promoted as a solution to the spiraling costs. This is an approach taught and promoted at all levels of nursing education and one in which APRNs have strength and expertise.

Another area APRNs need to be cognizant of is the focus on measuring the quality of care delivered. As one measure of quality, patient satisfaction is now emphasized. This is an area where APRNs have traditionally excelled. It is imperative APRNs be knowledgeable and aware of how quality is measured at their institutions and by the insurers, which commonly takes the form of HEDIS measures as well as practice profiling.

APRNs must also be knowledgeable about the business aspects of health care. Health care in the United States is, unfortunately, a business. APRNs need to obtain their own provider identification numbers and directly bill for Medicare, Medicaid, and any private plans that permit it. Many plans will credential and reimburse APRNs directly; some will allow APRNs to be primary care providers (PCPs) for their patients. APRNs need to continually query insurers regarding their policy on credentialing and reimbursement, and they must petition plans to recognize them as providers.

As was made clear in Chapter 1, the APRNs who brought advanced practice nursing to where it is today did so largely by their own initiative and by a commitment to excellence. They made their mark and thus made a place for today's APRNs by collecting and disseminating data that promoted their value, by refusing to accede to organized nursing's and medicine's efforts to constrain their vision to some preconceived idea about what a nurse should be, and by actively seeking out and seizing opportunities for advancement presented by others outside the profession or occasioned by sociological, political, and/or economic events.

SUGGESTED LEARNING EXERCISES

1. As a result of the healthcare revolution in America, medical care is evolving. Develop a platform that illuminates the actual and potential effects or consequences of this transformation on advanced practice nursing.

2. Many opportunities exist for APRN entrepreneurs in today's competitive market. Create a business plan for the new healthcare environment that recharacterizes the APRN identity, redefines APRN role components, and relocates advanced nursing practice venues.

3. Organize a portfolio to be presented to prospective employment markets that supports the position that APRNs are well suited to assume a variety of positions in integrated healthcare systems.

4. Debate whether APRNs would be better advised to assume complementary (value-added) or substitution positions in managed care markets or prospective payment systems.

5. Design a master plan for an IPA that consists exclusively of APRNs. Identify potential consumer groups to be served as well as payers/insurers to be approached. Discuss strategies for reimbursement.

6. How would you "sell" or market the concept of an APRN IPA to selected consumers and prospective insurers? Develop a marketing plan to accomplish that goal.

References

1. McCarthy, MC, and Berman, JA. (1998). Corporate health and managed competition: Implications for advanced practice nursing in the new American health-care system. *Advanced Practice Nursing: Emphasizing Common Roles*. F.A. Davis, Philadelphia.

2. Fox, JC. (1993). The role of nursing. *J Psychosocial Nurs* 31:9.

3. Bodenheimer, TS, and Grumbach, K. (2005). *Understanding Health Policy: A Clinical Approach*. 4th ed. Lange, New York, 1–208.

4. Robert Wood Johnson Foundation. (2008). Covering the Uninsured. http://covertheuninsuredweek. org/. Accessed September 29, 2008.

5. Brooke, RH. (1989). Practice guidelines and practicing medicine. *JAMA* 262:3027.

6. Fisher, ES, et al. (2003). The implications of regional variations in Medicare spending part 1 and part 2. *Ann Intern Med* 138:273, 288.

7. Blendon, RJ, et al. (1998). Understanding the managed care backlash. *Health Affairs* 17(4):80.

8. Brown, L. (2008). The amazing noncollapsing US health care system. *NEJM* 358:4, 325.

9. Blendon, RJ, et al. (2002). Inequities in health care: A five country survey. *Health Affairs* 21(3):182.

10. National Coalition on Health Care. (2008). Health Care Costs Fact Sheet. http://www.nchc.org/facts/costs. Accessed September 29, 2008.

11. Center for Disease Control and Prevention. (2008). National Center for Health Statistics: Health United States 2007 with Chartbook Trends. http://www.cdc.gov/nchs/data/hus/hus07. Accessed September 29, 2008.

12. Baldor, RA. (1996). *Managed Care Made Simple*. Blackwell Science, Cambridge, MA.

13. Woolhandler, S, and Himmelstein, D. (2002). Paying for national health insurance—and not getting it. *Health Affairs* 21(4):88–98.

14. Center for Medicare and Medicaid Services, Office of the Actuary. (2008). *National Health Care Expenditure Projections*.

15. Moon, M. (2001). Health policy: 2001 Medicare. *N Engl J Med* 344 (12):928–931.

16. Center for Medicare and Medicaid Services website: http://www.cms.hhs.gov/.

17. Health Insurance Industry of America. (2003). *Employment Based Health Insurance Coverage.* Health Insurance Association of America, Washington, DC.

18. Kaiser Family Foundation. *Employer Health Benefits* 2007.

19. Blumenthal, D. (2006). Employee sponsored health insurance in the United States. *New Engl J Med* 355(1):82–88.

20. Jonas, S, and Kovner, A. (2008). *Health Care Delivery in the United States.* Springer, New York.

21. Blue Cross/Blue Shield Corporate Report. (May 1990). Blue Cross/Blue Shield of Massachusetts, Boston, MA.

22. Robert Wood Johnson Foundation Alpha Center. (1994). *State Initiatives in Health Care Reform: New York Adopts Pure Community Rating—Other States Take Incremental Approach.*

23. America's Health Insurance Plans. (2008). AHIP's Center for Policy and Research; www.ahipresearch.org.

24. Dudley, RA. (2001). Managed care in transition. *N Engl J Med* 344:1087.

25. Gabel, J, et al. (2002). Job based health benefits in 2002: Some important trends. *Health Affairs* 21:143.

26. Kaiser Family Foundation. (2008). *Covering the Uninsured: Options for Reform.*

27. Inglehart, J. (2002). Changing health insurance trends. *N Engl J Med* 347:956.

28. Omnibus Budget Reconciliation Act of 1989, Public Law No. 101–239.

29. Omnibus Budget Reconciliation Act of 1990, Public Law No. 101–508.

30. Omnibus Budget Reconciliation Act of 1987, Public Law No. 100–203.

31. Omnibus Budget Reconciliation Act of 1980, Public Law No. 96–499.

32. Omnibus Budget Reconciliation Act of 1986, Public Law No. 99–509.

33. Glickman, S, et al. (2008). Evidence based perspectives on pay for performance and quality of patient care and outcomes in emergency medicine. *Ann Emerg Med* 51(5):622–631.

34. Institute of Medicine. (2006). *Rewarding Provider Performance: Aligning Incentives in Medicine.* National Academy Press, Washington DC.

35. Rosenthal, M, et al. (2006). Pay for performance in commercial HMO's. *N Engl J Med* 355:1895–1902.

36. Center for Medicare and Medicaid Services Hospital Quality Initiatives. http://www.cms.hhs.gov/.

37. Endsley, S, et al. (2006, July–August). What family physicians need to know about pay for performance. *Family Pract Mngmt* 13(7):69–74.

38. Goldman, D, et al. (2005). *US Healthcare Facts about Cost, Access and Quality.* RAND Corp.

39. Robert Graham Center. (2007, November). *The Patient Centered Medical Home.* Robert Graham Center, Washington DC.

40. Rubinstein, HG. (2008, Jan/Feb). Medical homes: The prescription to save primary care? *AHIP Coverage* 49 (1):44–47.

41. Kirch, D, and Vernon, D. (2008). Confronting the complexity of the physician workforce equation. *JAMA* 299(22):2679.

42. Mitka, M. (2007). Looming shortage of physicians raises concerns about access to care. *JAMA* 297 (10):1045–1046.

43. Pearson, L. (2008). The Pearson report. *AJNP* 12(2).

44. Resneck, J, and Kimball, A. (2008). Who else is providing care in dermatology practices? Trends in the use of nonphysician clinicians. *J Am Acad Dermatol* 58(2):211.

45. Hooker, RS. (2008). The extension of rheumatology services with physician assistants and nurse practitioners. *Best Practices and Research in Clinical Rheumatology* 22(3):523–533.

46. Lugo, N, et al. (2006). *Nurse Practitioner Survives in Retail Locations.* White Paper, Nurse Practitioner Healthcare Foundation.

Michelle Walsh is a pediatric nurse practitioner certified by the Pediatric National Certification Board. She has provided primary care to children of all ages in busy pediatric practices in Columbus, Ohio, and she has also served as a clinical preceptor for pediatric nurse practitioner students. She currently practices at Nationwide Children's Hospital in Columbus. Before becoming a nurse practitioner, she taught pediatric nursing, research, and nursing leadership to baccalaureate and masters' students. She is coauthor of *Leadership: The Key to the Professionalization of Nursing*.

Linda A. Bernhard is an associate professor of nursing and women's studies at The Ohio State University in Columbus, Ohio. Her specialty is women's health. She has taught nursing leadership for many years and is coauthor of *Leadership: The Key to the Professionalization of Nursing*.

CHAPTER 4

Selected Theories and Models for Advanced Practice Nursing

Michelle Walsh, PhD, RN, CPNP, and Linda A. Bernhard, PhD, RN

CHAPTER OUTLINE

THEORIES OF LEADERSHIP
Theory X and theory Y
Consideration and initiating structure
Path-goal theory
Fiedler's contingency model and cognitive resource theory
Tridimensional leadership-effectiveness model
Newer models of leadership

THEORIES AND STRATEGIES OF CHANGE
The freezing model
Strategies for changing
Diffusion of innovation
Change in practice by the APRN

MODELS OF HEALTH PROMOTION
Health belief model
Health promotion model
The transtheoretical model
PRECEDE-PROCEED model
Theory of care-seeking behavior

MODELS OF ADVANCED PRACTICE NURSING
Novice to expert
Advanced nursing practice
Differentiated practice

COMPARISON OF ADVANCED PRACTICE MODELS
Collaborative practice

SUMMARY

SUGGESTED LEARNING EXERCISES

CHAPTER OBJECTIVES

After completing this chapter, the reader will be able to:

1. Select a theory of leadership appropriate to an area of advanced practice.
2. Explain the research utilization process in the context of evidence-based practice and planned change.
3. Apply theories of health promotion to all types of advanced practice nursing.
4. Summarize a variety of advanced nursing practices and other related nursing models.
5. Evaluate a conceptual model of collaborative nurse-physician interaction for usefulness in advanced practice nursing.

This chapter provides an introduction to a variety of theories and models that can be used in advanced practice nursing. Theories provide a framework and may lead to new ways of thinking about practice situations. Advanced practice registered nurses (APRNs) think more broadly and perform at a higher level and within a broader scope of practice than other nurses. APRNs will be more successful when they apply concepts from various leadership or change theories in the assessment and management of clients. The chapter presents theories of leadership as well as related theories and models of change, health promotion, and advanced practice nursing.

Theories of Leadership

Leadership theories have important implications for APRNs. Leadership is a process that is used to move a group toward goal setting and goal achievement.[1] The components of leadership are the leader and group, the theory of leadership, and the organization. Leadership can be used by any nurse but is especially important for APRNs, who use leadership skills to promote the health of clients and families. We present the leadership theories in an historical manner, demonstrating how the theories have built on one another.

Theory X and Theory Y

Assumptions about motivation are the basis for McGregor's theories of leadership.[2] Theory X reflects the traditional view of direction and control, whereas Theory Y includes an integration of individual and organizational goals. McGregor was careful to indicate that X and Y are not opposite, but rather are separate philosophies. Theory X is the basis of managerial theory; Theory Y is operationalized through a strategy commonly referred to as management by objectives.

In Theory X, the assumption is that people dislike work and avoid it whenever possible. Because of the dislike of work, people must be controlled and directed to engage in goal-directed activity. Further, according to McGregor, people wish to avoid responsibility and prefer direction to feel secure. A different view of people is proposed in Theory Y, which states that work is as natural as play. People are self-directed and engage freely in goal-directed activity so long as they are in agreement with the goals. It is the commitment to the goals, as well as goal attainment, that is fulfilling, making external direction unnecessary. Because all individuals have the potential to succeed, the creation of conditions that allow the individual to pursue goals is essential. By creating conditions that enable goal setting, the leader fosters participation and creative problem solving.

Consideration and Initiating Structure

The two constructs of consideration and initiating structure were identified through investigations to determine which behaviors used by a leader had a positive influence on group satisfaction and productivity.[3] Consideration encompasses those behaviors of the leader that emphasize concern for the individual or group. It includes trust, respect, warmth, and rapport and thus encourages communication.[4] Initiating structure includes the behaviors of the leader that focus on the task to be accomplished or on the organizational goals. It includes defining roles, assigning tasks, planning, and encouraging production.[4]

Researchers found that group productivity is more closely associated with initiating structure, whereas individual satisfaction is more dependent on consideration. However, individuals seem to be more secure when they know what is expected of them; thus, both behaviors are important for success at both individual and organizational levels. Moreover, group cohesiveness is fostered by both consideration and initiating structure.

While reviewers of leadership theory indicate that the most effective leaders use both consideration and initiating structure,[5] the measures and, consequently, the validity of the measurement of these two behaviors have been questioned.[6] Inconsistent findings among the studies have led to further investigation of missing variables that could explain effective leader behavior.

Path-Goal Theory

The path-goal theory was an attempt to identify the missing variables by specifying the conditions under which the leader's behavior affects member satisfaction.[7] The degree to which the leader exhibits consideration determines the members' perceptions of available rewards, whereas the degree to which the leader initiates structure determines the members' perceptions of the paths that will ultimately lead them to their goals.[5]

Using the path-goal theory, the leader initiates structure to demonstrate to members how their actions will result in goal attainment. The leader also exhibits consideration by helping to remove barriers, and so makes the path to the goal easier.[8] Both consideration and initiating structure enhance members' motivation and satisfaction to the extent that such leadership behaviors clarify the path to the goal.

Fiedler's Contingency Model and Cognitive Resource Theory

Using similar variables to develop a model of leadership effectiveness, Fiedler[9] created the contingency approach, or contingency theory. Fiedler's model measures leadership effectiveness by examining group productivity. According to Fiedler, leadership is an interpersonal relation in which power and influence are unevenly distributed so that one person is able to direct and control the actions and behaviors of others to a greater extent than they direct and control those of the leader. In this model the leader has the primary responsibility for completion of the group task.

Because leadership is a relationship based on power and influence, the leader must classify each situation based on the amount of power and influence that the group members allow the leader. In any given situation, the amount of power and influence depend on a combination of three variables that yield a favorable or unfavorable situation for the leader.

The first variable that determines a favorable situation for the leader is the relationship between the leader and group members. The notion that the leader-member relationship is the single most important variable determining the leader's power and influence is well supported in the literature.[10] The extent to which group members accept the leader determines whether leader-member relationships are classified as good or poor.

The second variable is task structure. Routine or predictable tasks are classified as structured, whereas tasks that require analysis of multiple possibilities are classified as unstructured.

Finally, the third variable, position power, refers to the leader's place within the organization and the amount of authority given to the leader by virtue of that position. Position power is not a personality characteristic; rather, it measures the leader's status in the organization. Position power is classified as strong or weak.

According to Fiedler, these three variables create eight different situations that can be ranked from "most favorable" to "least favorable." Each possible situation is numbered and termed a cell, with cell 1 characterized as the most favorable situation and cell 8 the least favorable. On the basis of his earliest research, Fiedler predicted that cells 1, 2, and 3 were the very favorable situations and that cell 8 was the least favorable situation. Thus, using a task-centered, controlling behavior would be most effective. Cells 4, 5, 6, and 7 were intermediate situations that included both structured and unstructured tasks and strong and weak power positions. In those situations, a more effective approach for the leader is a permissive, relationship-centered one (Table 4-1).

Table 4-1 **Fiedler's Contingency Table**				
Cell	Leader-Member Relationship	Task Structure	Position Power	Situation Rating	Preferred Behavior
1	Good	Structured	Strong	Very favorable	Controlling
2	Good	Structured	Weak	Very favorable	Controlling
3	Good	Unstructured	Strong	Very favorable	Controlling
4	Good	Unstructured	Weak	Intermediate favorableness	Permissive
5	Poor	Structured	Strong	Intermediate favorableness	Permissive
6	Poor	Structured	Weak	Intermediate favorableness	Permissive
7	Poor	Unstructured	Strong	Intermediate favorableness	Permissive
8	Poor	Unstructured	Weak	Very favorable	Controlling

From Fiedler, FE. *A Theory of Leadership Effectiveness.* McGraw-Hill, New York, 1967, p. 142, with permission.

Fiedler continued to predict that with cells 1, 2, 3, and 8, the leader should use a more controlling or task-oriented behavior. However, he eventually determined that only cells 4 and 5 represented situations of intermediate or moderate favorableness, requiring a permissive or relationship-oriented approach.[11] Cells 6 and 7 were defined as unfavorable to the leader, and Fiedler predicted that little difference would occur in outcome, whether permissive or controlling behavior was used.[11] Even though the model is predictive, only two conclusions are specified:

1. Task-oriented leaders will perform best in groups in which the situation is either very favorable or very unfavorable.

2. Relationship-oriented leaders will perform best in groups in which the situation is either of moderate or intermediate favorableness.

Considerable research supports the validity of the contingency model of a leader's effectiveness. Although only three variables are evaluated to determine the favorableness of a situation, these variables are the most significant in a given situation. Nonetheless, the model has been criticized because it fails to explain the underlying processes that result in a leader's effective performance.

Fiedler addressed the limitations of the contingency model by developing the cognitive resource theory.[12] Cognitive resources include the intellectual abilities, technological competencies, and job-relevant knowledge of a leader. These resources are acquired during formal education and through experience. Cognitive resource theory is depicted in Figure 4-1. The theory attends to task accomplishment and the role that the group members play in task accomplishment. Task accomplishment is often the outcome of the leader's effectiveness. The leader's behavior results from both the situation and the leader's personality, as measured by the Least Preferred Coworker Scale.[12]

The most important idea from cognitive resource theory is that the situation is the most important variable. Only under certain conditions do the leader's and the members' abilities contribute positively to group performance.[12]

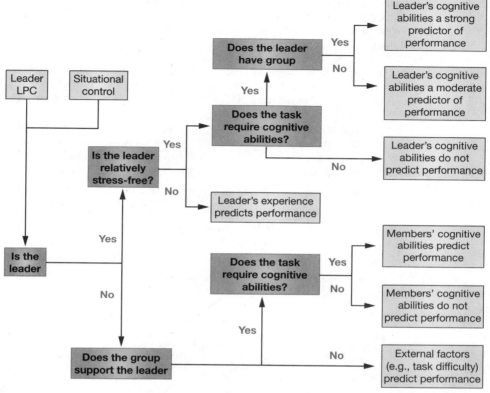

Figure 4-1: Fiedler's Cognitive Resource Theory. (From Fiedler, FE, and Garcia, JE., *New Approaches to Effective Leadership: Cognitive Resources and Performance.* John Wiley & Sons, New York, NY, 1987, p. 9, with permission.)

Tridimensional Leadership-Effectiveness Model

Hersey and Blanchard[13] used Fiedler's[9,11] early work and the consideration and initiating structure theories to propose another way of viewing leadership. They believed that no single leadership style or behavior could be effective in every situation. Combining the variables of task orientation and relationship orientation with effectiveness, Hersey and Blanchard created the tridimensional leadership-effectiveness model. In this model, the leader's behavior is integrated with situational dimensions. Leadership style is defined as the behavior pattern that a leader exhibits when attempting to influence the activities of others as perceived by those others.[13]

According to Hersey and Blanchard, task behaviors include organizing and defining roles of group members and directing activities. Task behaviors focus on production; relationship behaviors include facilitating, supporting, and maintaining personal relationships through open communication. The four basic leadership styles in the model are arranged in quadrant style, with high and low combinations of relationship and task behavior, that is, high relationship/low task, high task/high relationship, low relationship/low task, and high task/low relationship.

To the task and relationship behavioral dimensions, a third dimension, effectiveness, is added. Effectiveness depends on appropriateness to the situation and is conceptualized as a continuum from effective to ineffective. The four basic styles are effective or ineffective depending on their appropriateness for the situation as seen by the group members; hence the model has been expanded as the Situational Leadership® Model (Fig. 4-2).

Hersey and Blanchard[13] developed an instrument, the Leader Effectiveness and Adaptability Description (LEAD), to be used with their model. The LEAD instrument measures leadership style, style range or flexibility, and style adaptability or effectiveness. Style range and adaptability are particularly important, because the more flexible a leader can be, the more likely the leader is to be effective in any situation. There are two forms of the LEAD, one for leaders to evaluate themselves (LEAD-self) and a second for group members to rate their perceptions of the leader (LEAD-other).

Certain predictions are possible without using the LEAD instruments. An indication of group members' willingness or motivation in relation to a given task, in addition to their ability or competence, gives an indication of readiness (see Fig. 4-2). Four classifications of readiness can be determined[13]:

1. R4: Member is both willing and able to accept this responsibility.
2. R3: Member is able but a little insecure about accepting responsibility.
3. R2: Member is willing but unable to accept responsibility yet because he or she does not know what he or she does not know.
4. R1: Member is both unwilling or insecure and unable to accept this responsibility.

After determining which level of readiness members represent, the leader can select an appropriate style.

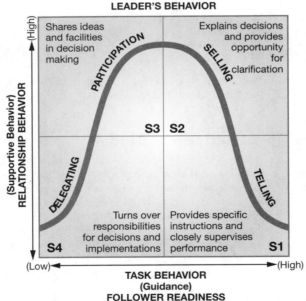

Figure 4-2: Situational Leadership Model. (From Hersey, P, and Blanchard, KH, *Management of Organization Behavior Utilizing Human Resources,* 5th ed. Prentice Hall, Englewood Cliffs, NJ, 1988, p. 171, with permission from Paul Hersey, Escondido, CA: The Center for Leadership Studies. All rights reserved.)

Research results demonstrate a curvilinear relationship within the quadrants.[13] The low-relationship, low-task quadrant style is called delegating; the high-relationship, low-task quadrant style is called participating; the high-task, high-relationship quadrant style is called selling; and the high-task, low-relationship quadrant style is called telling.[13] The relationships between style and readiness are depicted in Figure 4-2. The telling style is best used with group members who have the lowest level of readiness. Members with the second lowest level of readiness respond better to the selling style. For members in the third level of readiness, participating is the most effective style. Finally, delegating, or allowing a maximum amount of freedom, is most effective for members with the highest level of readiness.[13]

Another prediction that should help the leader become more effective is based on the readiness of the group as reflected in their actual performance.[13] The leader style should shift to the left on the curvilinear line (see Fig. 4-2) when performance in the group increases and should shift to the right when performance declines.

APRNs can use Situational Leadership theory by assessing their followers' readiness. Followers could be clients and families or other staff members. In the Situational Leadership theory, it is the followers who determine the appropriate leader behavior. Thus, it is the needs and characteristics of clients or others that dictate the leadership behavior that will be most effective. The APRN needs to be able to use a variety of leadership styles to fit each situation: persuading those who are willing while clarifying their abilities, guiding with specific clear instruction, empowering those with greater ability, and delegating.

Followers are not always in the same place on the continuum of readiness; thus the leader must use different strategies, as appropriate. When the follower/family caregiver is unable and insecure, the APRN gives information in small amounts, with step-by-step guidelines, helping to overcome insecurity by focusing on instructions and not overwhelming the caregiver with too much information at one time.

Healthcare colleagues usually may be perceived by the leader as competent, willing, and able, but they are not always. Sometimes followers are viewed as more ready, such as in an emergency, when one APRN takes the leadership and directs other staff in tasks needed in priority order. Thus, the APRN assesses their readiness and acts according to their readiness, moving from strategy to strategy as the situation changes.

Newer Models of Leadership

Newer models of and approaches to leadership have developed as society has changed and people use more systems than linear thinking. That is, leaders cannot predict the future, because no one knows what the future will bring, and even very small changes in the present will result in a different future. Chaos theory and complexity science are changing how leadership is theorized, studied, and practiced.

CHAOS THEORY AND COMPLEXITY SCIENCE

Chaos theory originated in mathematics. Chaotic systems are not random; in fact, they are deterministic, orderly, and sensitive to the initial situation. Chaos theory helps to identify the order that appears to be random. APRNs can use chaos theory to forecast service outcomes.[14] Complexity science grew out of chaos theory and new science. Because people in groups are complex adaptive systems, the use of complexity science can result in more natural, productive, enjoyable, and innovative outcomes than "old science."[15]

Complex adaptive systems have many parts that are interconnected and interdependent and that adapt dynamically to their constantly changing environment.[15] Principles of complex nonlinear systems include:

1. Small "inputs" can have very large consequences.
2. Very small differences in the initial situation produce very different outcomes.
3. The whole is greater than the sum of the parts.

4. These systems seek patterns, "learn" from experience, and adapt.

5. Most of these systems exhibit "attractors"; that is, there is an existing structure, but changes to the system may cause it to become an entirely different structure.[15]

What these principles mean for healthcare environments where APRNs are employed is that teams and collaboration are very important, small changes can lead to large effects, order will evolve but there is no certainty what that order will be (so detailed plans will not work), and diversity (e.g., age, gender, race, expertise) must be increased to enhance creativity. When members of a team work with one other and the environment to develop new skills and behaviors, something new and better can be achieved.[16]

TRANSFORMATIONAL LEADERSHIP THEORY

Transformational leadership theory is consistent with complexity science; it is nonlinear. Burns[17] conceptualized transforming leadership in contrast to transactional leadership. In transactional leadership, leaders merely exchange one thing for another with followers. That is, the leader only motivates workers with their salary, bonuses, and so on. These transactions are all about getting something done. The leader provides rewards to followers for meeting expectations. The leader also supervises closely and takes corrective actions on the basis of the results in the transactions between the leader and the followers.[18]

Transforming leadership still exploits followers, but the leader also seeks to satisfy some needs or personal motives of the followers. The result can be mutually stimulating and may convert followers into leaders.[17] Bass[19] built on Burns' work to describe transformational leadership. Transformational leadership begins with a vision for the future that the leader has and conveys to followers. The transformational leader creates a relationship with followers that is mutually beneficial and motivates followers to achieve. The four dimensions of transformational leadership are charisma or idealized influence, inspirational motivation, intellectual stimulation, and individualized consideration.[18] It is through the use of these dimensions or factors by the leader that followers work harder and are more satisfied.[19]

Theories and Strategies of Change

Change is inevitable both in nursing and in society. APRNs must be able to accept the changes they face, as well as function as change agents to foster change in individuals, groups, and systems. Integration of the theories and models of change into the knowledge base of APRNs will facilitate their relationship to change. The following sections discuss several theories/models of change.

The Freezing Model

According to the freezing model of change, planned change occurs in a three-step process[20]:

1. Unfreezing the present level of equilibrium

2. Moving to a new level of equilibrium

3. Refreezing the new level so that it is relatively permanent

The freezing theory derives from field theory, a method of analyzing causal relationships. In field theory, change is due to certain forces within the field. Forces are directional entities that work in opposition to each other to maintain a dynamic equilibrium. For every force, there is an opposite force. Positive, or driving, forces indicate the likelihood of moving a system toward a desired goal. Negative, or restraining, forces indicate obstacles that decrease the likelihood of a system moving toward a desired goal.

Three possible situations result from an analysis of the forces within a field:

1. A state of dynamic equilibrium exists when the sum of the driving forces is equal to the sum of the restraining forces.
2. Change occurs in the desired direction when the sum of the driving forces is greater than the sum of the restraining forces.
3. A change in the undesired direction, or away from the desired goal, occurs when the sum of the driving forces is less than the sum of the restraining forces (Fig. 4-3). Change occurs whenever the forces in a given field are unequal.

The three stages occur sequentially, with the moving phase dependent on the outcome of the unfreezing phase and with the refreezing phase dependent on the outcome of the moving phase.

UNFREEZING

During unfreezing, existing conditions are viewed as stable, or "frozen." Change begins with a felt need, or desire for change, because a desired goal has not been achieved. When one individual shares a felt need with another individual, unfreezing has begun. During the unfreezing phase, the current condition is critically analyzed.

The goal of the unfreezing phase is to clarify the present situation and make persons aware of the need for change by creating dissatisfaction with the existing situation. The target of change can be attitudes, knowledge, and/or behaviors. A change agent encourages group members to raise questions and explore their feelings and attitudes about present conditions. When group members acknowledge their dissatisfaction with the present situation, they begin to commit themselves to the change process. For change to occur, a plan that maximizes driving forces and minimizes restraining forces is made.

MOVING

The goal of the moving phase is to achieve the desired change. The moving phase is also known as the changing phase because it is during this phase that the change is implemented. The moving phase depends on the outcome of the unfreezing phase. If the equilibrium has been upset in a favorable fashion—driving forces exceed restraining forces—then the desired change can occur. The moving phase ends when the change has been fully implemented—that is, the desired change in knowledge, attitude, and/or behavior has occurred. When the target has been changed, refreezing can occur.

REFREEZING

The goal of the refreezing phase is stabilization of the change. The new knowledge, attitude, and/or behavior learned during the moving phase must continue to be practiced until the new knowledge and changed attitude and/or behavior becomes as familiar as the knowledge,

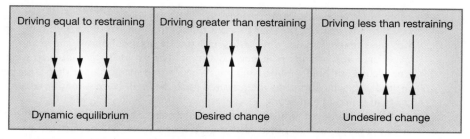

Figure 4-3: Driving and Restraining Forces. (From Bernhard, LA, and Walsh, M, *Leadership: The Key to the Professionalization of Nursing*, 3rd ed. Mosby St. Louis, MO, 1995, p. 169, with permission.)

attitudes, and/or behaviors that preceded the change. The change agent can help the group to refreeze by actions that help to legitimate the change, such as providing articles for the group to read about others who have made the same or a similar change.

Refreezing represents the end point in the change process and indicates that the change has been fully accepted and internalized. The change agent knows that refreezing has occurred when group members consistently demonstrate the new attitude or behavior and talk positively about it, their words and actions being congruent. Once it has been determined that refreezing has occurred, the group's performance should be evaluated periodically to confirm that the planned change is indeed refrozen.

Strategies for Changing

Chin and Benne[21] presented a model of strategies for changing. Strategies are approaches used by the change agent to influence a group to adopt a proposed change. Three strategies, which may be used individually or in combination, include:

1. Empirical-rational
2. Normative–re-educative
3. Power-coercive

The *empirical-rational strategy* is based on the closely related assumptions that human beings are rational and that they follow a pattern of self-interest. From these basic assumptions, it follows that people will change when they understand that a proposed change is rationally justified and is beneficial to them.[21] The empirical-rational strategy is the oldest and most frequently used. It is based on reason and intelligence.

The *normative–re-educative strategy* is a more active strategy. People do what they do because of norms they hold and a commitment to those norms. Norms come from society, culture, religion, family, and from other sources. Change occurs when commitment to some present norm decreases to a point where a new norm can be adopted. Thus, change resulting from the normative–re-educative strategy is a modification of values and attitudes, as well as of behavior.[21]

The normative–re-educative strategy requires direct intervention by a change agent to aid in the unlearning and relearning process. The individual and the change agent actively work together to produce the change. Behavioral science techniques, such as consciousness-raising, may be used to help individuals become aware of their values and norms so that they may change to new ones.[21]

The *power-coercive strategy* requires some type of legitimate power to force compliance with change. Very simply, those with greater power influence and control those with lesser power.[21] The power-coercive strategy may be used by persons in top-level positions of an organization to effect change that they believe is needed. The group affected by the change is forced to comply, without having any input. There are many disadvantages to the power-coercive strategy; however, combined with another strategy, it may be used to promote acceptance of change by group members.

With any strategy, the change agent must allow time for the group to accept and/or practice the change. Practice time serves as a trial period that allows the group to adjust to and experience the benefits of a new condition. The group is then able to evaluate their new knowledge, attitude, and/or behavior. When group members see that their new knowledge, attitude, or behavior meets their desired goal, they will be reluctant to return to their former ways of thinking and acting.

When selecting a strategy, change agents must take into account both their relationship with the group and the target of change. Change agents will be most effective when the strategy used is consistent with the overall goals of the planned change and does not jeopardize the relationship with group members.

Diffusion of Innovation

Current thought about knowledge utilization in nursing is based on a diffusion of innovation model. Rogers[22] presented a five-stage model of what is called the Innovation-Decision process. Early in the process a search for information occurs. This *knowledge*, or evidence, is communicated to potential "adopters" of the change. The second stage is *persuasion*. Planning is involved in this stage and may include a clinical trial of the proposed innovation. A *decision* to adopt or reject the proposed change or innovation occurs. The fourth stage is the *implementation* of an adopted change. In this stage the APRN would communicate the change to all. This might include formal policy and procedure change in an organization. The final or fifth stage is the *confirmation* stage. Often, more evidence is gathered after the innovation or practice change has been implemented or diffused more broadly. This type of evidence confirms that the innovation or change adequately addressed the practice problem originally identified. It is possible in the confirmation stage that a new decision to discontinue the proposed innovation could occur.

Change in Practice by the APRN

In addition to the theories of Lewin,[20] Chin and Benne,[21] and Rogers,[22] the APRN should be familiar with the processes of evidence-based practice (EBP) and research utilization. EBP is broader than research utilization; EBP encompasses multiple types of evidence, including expert opinion based on actual clinical case experiences, as well as research. APRNs use research to improve practice. Since many practice changes do not have a significant research base, other types of knowledge and experience are used to guide practice change. However, as McCloskey[23] noted, the utilization of research is essential for EBP.

Research utilization is a planned change process. It is important to improving clinical practice, providing a link between problem identification and problem solving that incorporates current research-based knowledge. The research utilization process involves reviewing existing research-based knowledge to determine whether substantive investigations have been conducted that address the practice problem to be solved. Elements of traditional research critique are used in identifying and summarizing the research base. In Stetler's model[24] of research utilization, at least three phases must occur before the decision to use research in practice:

1. Preparation
2. Validation
3. Comparative evaluation

When data are insufficient or when no research base to guide the APRN exists, an original research approach may be needed. The research process and the research utilization process are quite similar (Table 4-2). When a sufficiently strong research base exists, the change or "innovation" can be introduced by the APRN. The innovation should first be introduced on a trial basis to allow group modification and acceptance of the innovation. The APRN should incorporate a sufficient evaluation plan—often a replication study in one's own setting to determine the effectiveness of the innovation to solve the identified practice problem.

The process of research utilization includes the following phases or steps[25]:

1. Identify the patient care problem.
2. Identify and assess research-based knowledge relevant to the specific problem.
3. Adapt and design a research-based practice innovation.
4. Conduct a trial of the innovation.
5. Decide whether to adopt, modify, or reject the innovation.
6. Develop the means to extend or diffuse the adopted innovation.
7. Develop mechanisms to maintain the innovation over time.

Table 4-2 **The Research Process Compared with the Research Utilization Process**

Research ←Interdependent Processes→	Research Utilization
Purpose: To identify and refine solutions to problems through the generation of new knowledge.	Purpose: To get the new solutions used for the good of society; to identify need for refinement.
Delimit problem.	Identify patient-care problem.
Review related literature. Develop conceptual framework.	Identify and assess research-based knowledge to solve problem.
Identify variables.	Design nursing practice innovation and patient outcomes based on research knowledge.
Select design. Formulate hypothesis.	Compare patient outcomes produced by innovation with those of existing practice.
Specify population. Select sample.	Choose patient sample representative of those in original research.
Develop or select instruments.	Use instruments identified in original research.
Collect data.	Conduct clinical trials.
Analyze data.	Analyze data.
Interpret results.	Decide to adopt, alter, or reject full-scale implementation of innovation.
Communicate findings.	Develop means to extend (diffuse) the new practice and maintain it over time.

Source: Firlit, S, Kemp, MG, and Walsh, M. Preparing master's students to develop clinical trials to confirm research findings. *West J Nurs Res* 8:108. Copyright © 1986 by Sage Publications, Inc. Reprinted by permission of Sage Publications, Inc.

As guidelines or standards of practice change, the APRN can use change theory to move a group to accepting and using a new standard of care. The APRN requires a "knowing in practice" to facilitate change[26] and should withhold suggestions to change until well established in the APRN role.

Models of Health Promotion

Advanced nursing practice consists of a variety of skills, but one of the most important for all APRNs is health promotion. Health promotion is a goal of all nurses, but for many APRNs, it is their principal goal. If the best method for predicting people's participation in healthy behaviors can be identified, APRNs can intervene in the best ways with their clients. The following are some of the models and theories that the APRN might use for health education, anticipatory guidance, and health promotion.

Health Belief Model

The health belief model (HBM) was developed in the 1950s to explain people's actions (or lack of actions) regarding preventive health behavior.[27] Through considerable research over the years, the HBM has been clarified and modified, and it is now used to explain or predict people's use of a broad range of health actions.[28]

The underlying assumption of the HBM, represented in Figure 4-4, is that behavior is determined more by a person's perceived reality than by the physical environment. People take actions to screen for or to prevent a disease or health problem, but only to the extent that the disease exists in their perception. Further, people must have incentives for action and feel themselves capable before undertaking a given health action.[29] Sociodemographic variables, such as age or race, are assumed to influence behavior indirectly, through effects on the other components.

The likelihood of action is based on individual perceptions of the threat of disease; modifying factors include cues to action and perceived benefits minus barriers. Threat consists of the individual's perceived susceptibility—that is, an individual's subjective beliefs about his/her own vulnerability to develop a disease or ability to accept the diagnosis of a disease, and the individual perception of the seriousness or severity of the disease and the (medical or social) consequences of the disease should it develop.

Demographic characteristics—for example, sex and socioeconomic status—influence how an individual perceives a threat as well as the benefits of care and barriers to care or behavioral change. Cues to action are triggers that may promote action. Cues may be internal, such as physical symptoms, or external, such as the media or a discussion with someone who has the disease. Cues to action apparently influence how individuals perceive threat, but they have not been studied systematically. The benefits people perceive for a particular action minus the perceived barriers of taking the action directly affect the likelihood of action. Both benefits and barriers are beliefs, rather than objective facts; that is, they are individual perceptions.

Self-efficacy,[30] the belief that a person can actually perform the necessary behavior to achieve the desired outcome, has become an important concept in its own right. Although some have tried to incorporate self-efficacy into the HBM, the originators of the model consider self-efficacy—or the lack thereof—to be a barrier to action.[28]

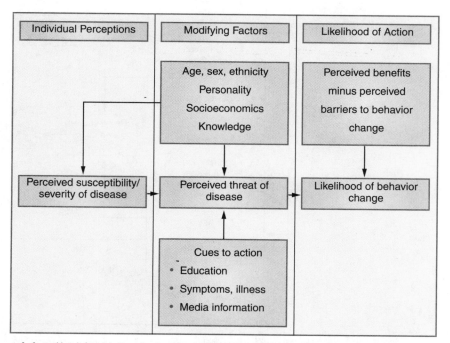

Figure 4-4: Health Belief Model. (From Strecher, VJ, and Rosenstock, IM. The health belief model. In Glanz, K, Lewis, FM, and Riner, BK (eds), *Health Behavior and Health Education*, 2nd ed. Jossey-Bass, San Francisco.)

The most common criticism of the HBM is that the relationship between beliefs and behavior has never been established clearly. Many studies have been conducted using the HBM to explain or predict actions as diverse as having a Pap smear, maintaining a diet, or writing a living will. The amount of variance explained differs considerably, suggesting that factors other than those considered in the HBM model are involved. Still, until other factors are specifically identified, many researchers and APRNs will continue to use the HBM in research and to guide practice.

Health Promotion Model

In an attempt to define additional variables that might explain preventive health behavior, Pender took the HBM, added a number of cognitive variables, and applied it to nursing practice.[31] As she expanded and clarified her thinking, she created the health promotion model (HPM).[32] Pender views the HPM as an organizing framework for theory development and research and acknowledges that it is continually subject to change.

The HPM, now known as the revised HPM, is shown in Figure 4-5. It shows the great complexity involved in explaining the performance of health behaviors, and the model has

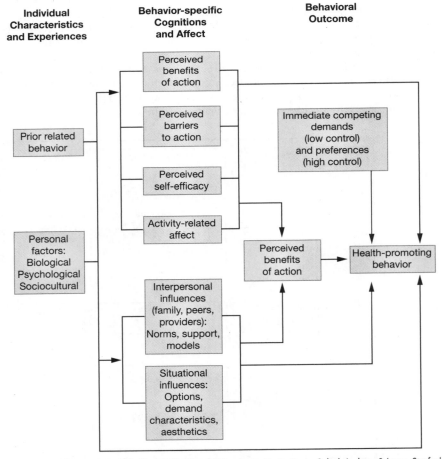

Figure 4-5: Health Promotion Model. (From Pender NJ. *Health Promotion in Nursing Practice*, 3rd ed. Appleton & Lange, Stanford, CT, 1996, p. 67, with permission.)

increased in complexity as it has developed. Most simply, the model shows that an individual's personal biological, psychological, and sociocultural characteristics, as well as certain behavioral and cognitive processes, are responsible for health behaviors. The boxes and arrows in the model demonstrate that the cognitive processes are interrelated and that personal characteristics and cognitive processes may, both directly and indirectly, result in health behavior. The revised HPM includes more variables, but the most important may be a commitment to a plan of action. Researchers have long questioned whether deciding to perform a behavior and actually performing a behavior are the same or different processes.

To facilitate their health promotion research, Walker, Sechrist, and Pender[33] developed the Health-Promoting Lifestyle Profile (HPLP) to be used in research as a predictor variable that represents health action. The HPLP-II is a 52-item questionnaire that has been analyzed to include six factors[32]:

1. Health responsibility
2. Physical activity
3. Nutrition
4. Interpersonal relations
5. Spiritual growth
6. Stress management

Together, these factors represent a balanced and positive approach to healthful living and wellness potential.

Both researchers and practicing APRNs can use the HPM and the HPLP-II. Researchers may use the HPLP-II as either a dependent or an independent variable. APRNs can use the HPLP-II to obtain information about a client's lifestyle and use the HPM more generally as a framework for thinking about health behavior.

The Transtheoretical Model

The transtheoretical model (TTM) is an integrative model that uses stages of change to explain health behaviors.[34] This model has integrated theories of psychotherapy and behavior change, and from its beginnings in the field of smoking cessation,[35] it has been applied to many topics in health behavior change.

The TTM describes the process of change as occurring in six stages:

1. *Precontemplation* occurs when a person has no intention of making a change within the next 6 months.
2. *Contemplation* occurs when a person intends to make a change within the next 6 months.
3. *Preparation* takes place when a person intends to make a change in the next month.
4. *Action* occurs when the person has been involved in making a change within the past 6 months.
5. *Maintenance* takes place when a person still tries to prevent relapsing to the original behavior, but generally feels like she or he can continue with the change.
6. *Termination* occurs when a person is so comfortable in the new behavior that he or she will not return to the original behavior.

Termination was not part of the original theory. Termination is now thought to be achieved when individuals have "total" self-efficacy, so that they will not go back to the original (unhealthy) behavior, regardless of the situation.

In addition to the stages of change, there are 10 processes of change—overt and covert actions that people use as they progress through the stages of change. The processes of change have been strongly supported in research.[35] The 10 processes of change are:

1. Consciousness raising
2. Dramatic relief
3. Self-reevaluation
4. Environmental reevaluation
5. Self-liberation
6. Helping relationships
7. Counterconditioning
8. Contingency management
9. Stimulus control
10. Social liberation

APRNs will tailor interventions to assist persons to move through the stages, using these processes of change.

The TTM continues to evolve. Kelly[36] recently described "commitment to health" as a middle range theory that is derived from the TTM and is used to predict the likelihood of peoples' behavior changes between the action and maintenance stages.

PRECEDE-PROCEED Model

The PRECEDE-PROCEED model is used for comprehensive planning in health education and health promotion with individuals and communities.[37-39] The PRECEDE acronym stands for predisposing, reinforcing, and enabling causes in educational diagnosis and evaluation, and the PROCEED acronym stands for policy, regulatory, and organizational constructs in educational and environmental development (PROCEED). Although PRECEDE was developed and used before PROCEED was added, both are integrated into a single model.

The PRECEDE portion of the model is the diagnostic phase that assists the APRN in considering the many factors that influence health status and in choosing a highly focused subset of factors as the target for a health intervention.[37-39] The PROCEED phase provides steps for developing policy and for initiating the implementation and evaluation processes of the health intervention.[38]

A unique feature of the model is the concept of "beginning at the end." Instead of planning an intervention that promotes outcomes, the APRN looks first at extant outcomes or the quality of life of the designated population or individual. The APRN must ask "why" before "how" and, by thinking deductively, identify consequences before seeking causes. As seen in Figure 4-6, the process is ultimately circular.

In the initial social diagnosis phase, the APRN considers the general hopes or problems of the target population by having them engage in a self-assessment, which, in itself, can be an educational process. In phase 2, epidemiological diagnosis, specific health goals or problems that contribute to the issues or problems identified in phase 1 are identified. During phase 3, specific behavioral or environmental factors that could be linked with the problems established as most important in phase 2 are identified. Because these problems will be the focus of the intervention, they must be described as specifically as possible.

Phase 4 is termed the educational and organizational diagnosis. The large number of potential factors that could influence a given health behavior are identified, sorted, and categorized into three classes:

1. Predisposing factors
2. Enabling factors
3. Reinforcing factors

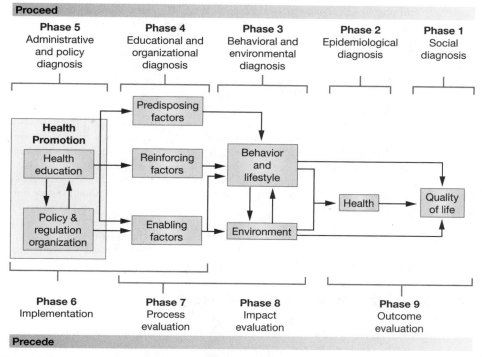

Figure 4-6: PRECEDE-PROCEED Model. (From Green, LW, and Kreuter, MW. *Health Promotion Planning: An Education and Environmental Approach,* 2nd ed. Mayfield Mountain View, CA, 1991, p. 24, with permission.)

Predisposing factors are those attitudes, values, perceptions, and knowledge that foster or inhibit motivation for change. Enabling factors are those skills and resources that make possible behavioral or environmental changes. Barriers to change must also be considered, because some resources (e.g., laws) may either foster or inhibit changes. Reinforcing factors include the rewards, feedback, and support received after adoption of a change. As with enabling factors, there are some reinforcing factors (e.g., weight gain) that can encourage or discourage continuation of a change.

In phase 5, the APRN assesses the resources, policies, abilities, and constraints of the situation or organization and then selects the best combination of methods and strategies to be implemented in phase 6. Although various types of evaluation are noted for phases 7 through 9, evaluation is a continuous process throughout the model.

PRECEDE-PROCEED can be used in a wide variety of community, workplace, and healthcare settings. PRECEDE has been used for health education programs of many types and in numerous settings. PRECEDE-PROCEED has been used in programs to decrease blood pressure and to stop smoking. Green and Kreuter[38] suggested that using the whole model makes planning and evaluation of health promotion programs more efficient and effective. For example, women who quit smoking cigarettes when pregnant tend to believe that smoking cessation will benefit their babies. The APRN who wants to foster continued smoking cessation after delivery might place more emphasis on teaching the mother about the effects of secondhand smoke on infants.

Theory of Care-Seeking Behavior

A more recent theory for health promotion is the theory of care-seeking behavior (CSB) developed by Lauver[40] and based on the concepts from Triandis's theory of behavior, which suggests that behavior results from intentions and habits, modified by facilitating conditions and physiological arousal. According to the CSB theory, engaging in healthcare behavior is a function of the psychosocial variables of affect, utility, norms, and habits, which may be influenced by facilitating conditions (e.g., insurance and having a regular health provider). Clinical and sociodemographic variables, such as the presence of symptoms, do not influence behavior directly but may influence the psychosocial variables (Fig. 4-7). Affect refers to feelings; utility (i.e., expectations and values about outcomes of care) refers to one's own beliefs; norms refer to others' beliefs; and habits refer to one's usual actions concerning a proposed health behavior.[41]

Empirical research findings from a number of studies support the individual relationships proposed in the CSB theory for secondary prevention, such as cancer screening.[40,41] For example, the APRN who wants to teach young adult men about the importance of testicular self-examinations must consider the man's feelings and beliefs about developing testicular cancer and what he hears from his buddies about it as well as the risk because of his age.

The CSB theory is similar to HBM and HPM theories, although it uses fewer variables to explain behavior, which can be an advantage for both research and practice if the CSB can be shown to predict behavior. Still, as with HBM and HPM, there are very few studies that have examined all of the possible variables and all of the relationships within a single study. If APRNs use CSB, HBM, or HPM, their clinical experiences can give support for the theory, which can then be further developed in research.

Models of Advanced Practice Nursing

Models and theories of advanced practice nursing describe primarily who an APRN is and/or what an APRN does. In comparison to leadership and change theories, the models of advanced practice are relatively new and are more descriptive- than predictive-level theories.

Novice to Expert

Benner's novice-to-expert theory[42] may be the most familiar theory of advanced practice nursing. However, what Benner really describes is expert nursing[42] rather than advanced practice nursing. Nonetheless, the expert nurse may very well be an APRN.

Benner's theory[42] was based on Dreyfus's model of skill acquisition, in which increments of change occur with increases in skilled performance, based on education and experience. Three kinds of changes occur with increasing levels of proficiency:

1. There is movement from reliance on abstract principles to the use of past concrete experiences as paradigms.

2. Perception of a situation changes so that it is seen less as a compilation of equally relevant bits and more as a complete whole in which only certain parts are relevant.

3. The person changes from a detached observer to an engaged and involved performer.

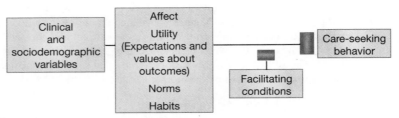

Figure 4-7: Care-Seeking Behavior Mode. (From Lauver, D. A theory of care-seeking behavior. *Image J Nursing Sch* 24:281, 1992, p. 281, with permission.)

Benner identified five levels of performance for nursing:

1. Novice
2. Advanced beginner
3. Competent
4. Proficient
5. Expert

Novices, with no experience in situations in which they are expected to perform, are focused only on rules and are unable to use discretionary judgment. Advanced beginners demonstrate marginally acceptable performance. They have had enough experience to recognize (or to see when pointed out by a mentor or instructor) the recurrent characteristics of a situation but cannot make those characteristics objective nor differentiate importance among them. Advanced beginners operate on general guidelines or standards of care and are beginning to recognize recurrent patterns in clinical practice.

Competent nurses begin to see their actions in terms of long-range goals or plans. They establish plans using considerable conscious, abstract, and analytic consideration of problems. However, their use of plans also limits awareness of the situation because they are focused on the plan rather than on the whole situation. Competent nurses feel a sense of mastery and the ability to cope with and manage the many contingencies of clinical nursing. They become efficient and organized. This level of competence is often viewed as ideal.

Proficient nurses continue to move forward with a vision of what is possible. They perceive situations as wholes rather than as parts, and their performance is guided by maxims, which are developed over time through a deep understanding of the situation. Proficient nurses know what to expect from a given situation, quickly recognize when a situation is different, and know how to modify plans when a situation varies from the expected. They acquire a perspective about the important attributes and characteristics of a situation and use fewer options while developing focus on the most important aspects of situations.

Proficiency marks the transition from competence to expertise.[43] A transformation occurs between the competent nurse and the two higher levels of performance. Proficient and expert nurses use past concrete experiences to guide their analyses of present situations in a way that competent nurses do not. Expert nurses do not rely on analytic principles to connect their understanding of a situation to an appropriate action. Experts use their vast background of experience and intuitive grasp of situations to focus immediately on the accurate range of problems without wasting effort and time on a large range of unlikely possible solutions. Experts see what needs to be accomplished and how to accomplish it. They operate from a deep understanding of situations and often cannot clearly describe the rationale for their actions. What experts can describe with clarity are the goals established and the outcomes achieved.

From the descriptions of nurses about their practices, Benner[42] identified seven domains of nursing practice:

1. The helping role
2. The teaching-coaching function
3. The diagnostic and patient-monitoring function
4. The effective management of rapidly changing situations
5. The administration and monitoring of therapeutic interventions and regimens
6. The monitoring and assuring of quality of healthcare practices
7. The implementation of organizational and work-role competencies

In their continuing research and development of the novice-to-expert theory, Benner and her colleagues explore the complexity of clinical judgment and caring practices.[43] A limitation of Benner's work for APRNs is the fact that the research has been limited to hospital nurses, and particularly critical care nurses.

Brykczynski, one of Benner's students, studied how experienced nurse practitioners (NPs) make clinical judgments.[44] She identified the same domains in NP practice that Benner had identified in hospital nurse practice, with one exception: the diagnostic and patient-monitoring function and the administering and monitoring of therapeutic interventions were combined into a single "management of patient health and illness" function. After Brykczynski[44] presented her results to the National Organization of Nurse Practitioner Faculties (NONPF), educators began to use the domains in their teaching of NPs, and NONPF used them in revising their curriculum guidelines.[45,46] Hence, Benner's model, at least indirectly, has become the framework for the education, and thus the practice, of NPs

Advanced Nursing Practice

In Calkin's[47] model of advanced nursing practice, advanced practice is defined as that enacted by nurses with master's degrees. Calkin used the 1980 American Nurses' Association (ANA) definition of nursing—the "diagnosis and treatment of human responses to actual or potential health problems"—as the basis for differentiating advanced practice from other levels of practice. The three levels of practice are (1) novice, (2) expert-by-experience, and (3) advanced.[47]

Novices, or beginning nurses, can manage only a narrow range of usual or average human responses. Because of the knowledge that they bring to the clinical situation from their educational programs, Calkin suggested that novices have greater knowledge than skill. That is, they are more comfortable with the science of nursing than with the art of nursing.

Experts-by-experience are those nurses who have excelled in their ability to diagnose and treat human responses. They are able to identify and intervene in a much wider range of human responses than novices. Calkin said experts-by-experience may intuit much of their skill and may be unable to explain their actions. Nonetheless, they provide skillful care, having developed skill greater than knowledge.

APRNs are those able to manage the fullest range of human responses that is closest to the actual range of potential responses. This ability develops as a result of the specialized knowledge and skills they acquired through education and experience. They can identify and intervene in the extremes of responses and in unpredictable as well as in predictable situations. Calkin[47] suggested that APRNs use deliberation and reasoning more than intuition when diagnosing and treating. She argued that APRNs articulate about nursing, use reasoning to deal with practice innovations, and develop or contribute to newer forms of practice. They do not focus on tasks and skills.

Differentiated Practice

Differentiated practice is another approach to describing the differences between levels of nursing practice. Koerner[48] described three levels of practice based on education: (1) associate degree, (2) baccalaureate degree, and (3) master's degree. In her integrated model, competency can be achieved at each level of nursing practice, so long as the differentiated roles and functions are clear.

The nurse with an associate degree provides care for a specified period of time and/or in structured settings with established policies and procedures. Care is focused primarily on the client and family. The nurse with a baccalaureate degree provides integrated health care from preadmission through postdischarge in structured and unstructured settings and/or in environments that may not have established policies and procedures. This nurse also collaborates with members of the interdisciplinary healthcare team for a total plan of care. The master's-degreed APRN provides leadership that promotes holistic patient outcomes, functions in a variety of dynamic settings across the entire continuum of care, and uses independent nursing judgment based on theory, research, and specialized knowledge.[49] When all providers function as a team and assume equal accountability for client outcomes, quality of care can improve to a higher level.

Koerner[48] discussed the importance of mutual valuing, partnerships, and collegiality among nurses at all levels and suggested that at each level, the nurse can be an expert. Koerner further suggested that APRNs support professional development by focusing on contextual and environmental issues more than the other levels of nurses do and that APRNs have more career options.

Comparison of Advanced Practice Models

Advanced practice models for nursing practice consider two factors: 1) education and 2) experience. Advanced practice requires a minimum of a master's degree. Both Koerner[48] and Calkin[47] base their models on educational preparation and defined advanced practice as master's preparation. Advanced practice also requires experience in nursing, beyond that of newly graduated registered nurses, even if the experience is limited to that required for completion of the master's educational program. There is no novice APN.

Advanced practice nursing is not the same as expert nursing practice. Although Calkin[47] equated her expert level with that of Benner,[42] we believe that any nurse at any level can be an expert practitioner, but APNs are distinguished by the master's degree. Benner's model[42] was developed through research with practicing clinical nurses and reveals much about what nursing practice includes. Nurses practicing in any setting for a long enough period may become expert in that role. It is our contention that Benner's model can be applied to any nurse in any kind of practice, regardless of educational level. The level of expertise develops with experience as well as with education.

Leadership is not explicitly described by either Benner[42] or Calkin.[47] It is, however, implicit in Benner's domains of nursing practice, especially those dealing with teaching, managing, monitoring, and organizing. Leadership also is inherent in Calkin's advanced nursing practice, because it is based on deliberative action that requires specialized skill and rationale. Leadership is an explicit part of the role of Koerner's APN.[48] APNs use leadership in all of their actions, by making judgments based on theory, research, and specialized knowledge.

Collaborative Practice

Much has been published about collaboration in advanced nursing practice, with some postulating that collaborative practice by APRNs and physicians (or others) is the "ideal" form of implementing the role.[50] Working together, APRNs and other healthcare professionals create a synergy that can result in "a product that is greater than can be produced by the [individual] professionals alone."[51] Roberts[52] described a continuum of interdisciplinary practice, from parallel practice to collaborative practice. She notes that as collaboration increases, the level of professional autonomy decreases.

Parallel practice is the least collaborative, although the most familiar.[52] Communication and functions of the providers are separate; for example, the APRN, physical therapist, and physician are all working with the patient on his pain but do not communicate their plans except in medical records that may or may not be reviewed periodically by other team members. They never see the patient together.

Coordinated practice is the next level on the continuum.[52] There is a structure in place to minimize duplication of effort and to maximize use of client and provider time and resources. Consultation is common in this type of practice, but a primary provider maintains responsibility for care delivery. This type of care is usually the one preferred by third-party payers because the primary provider acts as a gatekeeper to eliminate unnecessary costs and duplication of services.

The collaborative practice model reflects increased interaction among providers. There is direct, usually face-to-face communication and shared responsibility or co-management for patient care. Usually, one provider seeks the expertise of another; for example, a primary care physician may ask the APRN who is a diabetes educator to co-manage the care of a client newly diagnosed with diabetes.

Most of what is written about collaborative practice simply lists components of collaboration and barriers to collaboration, and before any model of collaborative practice can be developed, these elements must be identified. Components of collaborative practice include open communication, mutual trust, professional competence, shared power, joint responsibility and accountability, shared goals and vision, understanding of each other's practice style and scope of practice, and frank discussion of financial issues.[53,54] Barriers tend to be the absence or opposites of these factors, as well as age, gender, and cultural issues, reimbursement issues, and lack of understanding by clients and families.[55]

One comprehensive model of collaborative practice is the Conceptual Model of Collaborative Nurse-Physician Interactions[53] (Fig. 4-8). Although we believe that the model can apply to any health professional collaborators, Corser developed the model for APRN and physician collaboration. Central to the model is the collaborative interaction between APRN and physician. This interaction consists of many of the factors described earlier, which are affected by personal/interpersonal and organizational/professional influences that are experienced by both the APRN and the physician. Finally, this model is the only collaborative practice model that includes outcomes—for both patients and providers—as the purpose or result of collaborative practice. Outcomes should be the focus of practice.

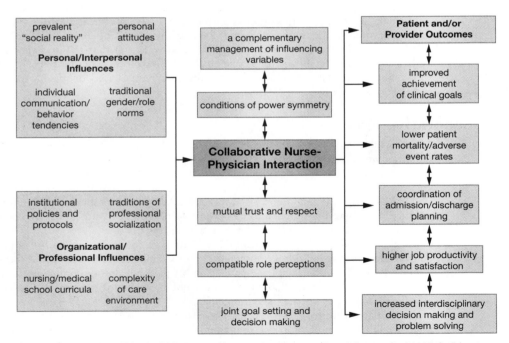

Figure 4-8: Conceptual Model of Collaborative Nurse-Physician Interactions. (From Corser, WD. A conceptual model of collaborative nurse-physician interactions. *Sch Inq Nurs Pract* 12:325, 1998. Copyright Springer Publishing Company, Inc. New York, NY. Used by permission.)

Summary

In each of the leadership and change models and theories, assessment of the group members is key to choosing the specific approach or style the APRN would use. Assessment of the situation or organization is also necessary so that the APRN can focus on goals appropriate for individuals in that setting. Finally, the relationship between the APRN and the group members is critical to achieving any desired goal, such as health promotion.

The models of advanced practice nursing show the importance of both education and experience of the APRN. The model of collaborative practice extends beyond nursing to include interacting with other healthcare professionals for the improvement of client outcomes and greater job satisfaction of the professionals.

SUGGESTED LEARNING EXERCISES

1. Select one of the theories of leadership presented in this chapter. Specify the variables that you would assess to determine an effective style of leadership to enact in your practice.
   Analyze a change that occurred in your organization. Was the change planned or unplanned? Who was the change agent? What strategies were used by the change agent? Evaluate the effectiveness of the strategies and suggest alternatives.

2. Identify a needed change in your organization. What are the driving and restraining forces that will enable or prevent the change? Develop a prospectus for planned change that takes into account the identified forces. Role-play with student colleagues and present your prospectus to them; convince them of the soundness of your plan.

3. Discuss a problem in clinical practice. Plan a course of action to determine if a research base exists that could be used to solve the problem. Propose a clinical trial of the research-based solution.

4. Form into teams. Create a health promotion clinical scenario or describe one in which you were involved. Detail all important factors in one of the health promotion models and describe a plan for implementation. Present your work to your student colleagues and have them critique your interpretation.

5. Analyze the similarities and differences between the Calkin and Benner models. Are these models sequential, and of what importance is this? Describe how you might apply the models to your practice situation.

6. Consider how the Calkin and Benner models relate to the concept of leadership described in this chapter. Sketch the parallels among key ideas. Again, how do the models relate to those of change presented in this chapter? Create a comparison chart.

7. Calkin described the APRN role and compared it to other levels of nursing practice. A nurse colleague declares to you that "there is little or no difference between you and me in the way you practice and what you can capably perform. Just compare my 15 years of practice and experience to your education and credentials." Respond as Calkin would by identifying major characteristics of advanced nursing practice and relate Calkin's ideas to the need and justification for your role.

8. Analyze a practice situation. Determine where it is on the continuum of interdisciplinary practice. What characteristics of collaborative practice are present? What barriers to collaborative practice exist? How can you use change theory to minimize barriers?

References

1. Bernhard, LA, and Walsh, M. (1995). *Leadership: The Key to the Professionalization of Nursing*, 3rd ed. Mosby, St. Louis, MO.

2. McGregor, D. (1960). *The Human Side of Enterprise*. McGraw-Hill, New York.

3. Fleishman, EA (1973). Twenty years of consideration and structure. In Fleishman, EA, and Hunt, JG (eds). *Current Developments in the Study of Leadership.* Southern Illinois University Press, Carbondale, IL.

4. Fleishman, EA, and Harris, EF. (1962). Patterns of leadership behavior related to employee grievances and turnover. *Personnel Psychol* 15:43.

5. Stogdill, RN. (1974). *Handbook of Leadership: A Survey of Theory and Research.* Free Press, New York.

6. Korman, AK. (1966). Consideration, initiating structure, and organizational criteria: A review. *Personnel Psycholy* 19:349.

7. Evans, MG. (1970). The effects of supervisory behavior on the path-goal relationship. *Organizational Behavior and Human Performance* 5:277.

8. Davis, K, and Newstrom, JW. (1985). *Human Behavior at Work: Organizational Behavior,* 7th ed. McGraw-Hill, New York.

9. Fiedler, FE. (1967). *A Theory of Leadership Effectiveness.* McGraw-Hill, New York.

10. Fiedler, FE, and Chemers, MM. (1974). *Leadership and Effective Management.* Scott, Foresman, Glenview, IL.

11. Fiedler, FE. (1973). The trouble with leadership training is that it doesn't train leaders. *Psychol Today* 6:23.

12. Fiedler, FE, and Garcia, JE. (1987). *New Approaches to Effective Leadership: Cognitive Resources and Organizational Performance.* John Wiley & Sons, New York.

13. Hersey, PH, Blanchard, KH, and Johnson, DE. (2007). *Management of Organizational Behavior: Leading Human Resources,* 9th ed. Pearson Prentice Hall, Upper Saddle River, NJ.

14. Haigh, CA. (2008). Using simplified chaos theory to manage nursing services. *J Nurs Mngmt* 16:298.

15. Lawrimore, EW. (2004). The new science of complexity vs. old science. http://www.codynamics.net/science.htm. Accessed August 6, 2008.

16. McConnell, ES, Lekan-Rutledge, D, Neidjon, B, and Anderson, R. (2004). Complexity theory: A long-term care specialty practice exemplar for the education of advanced practice nurses. *J Nurs Educ* 43:84.

17. Burns, JM. (1978). *Leadership.* Harper & Row, New York.

18. Judge, TA, and Piccolo, RF. (2004). Transformational and transactional leadership: A meta-analytic test of their relative validity. *J Applied Psychol* 89:75.

19. Bass, BM. (1985). *Leadership and Performance Beyond Expectations.* Free Press, New York.

20. Lewin, K. (1951). *Field Theory in Social Science.* Harper, New York.

21. Chin, R, and Benne, KD. (1985). General strategies for effecting change in human systems. In Bennis, WG, Benne, KD, and Chin R (eds), *The Planning of Change,* 4th ed. Holt, Rinehart, and Winston, New York.

22. Rogers, EM. (2003). *Diffusion of Innovations,* 5th ed. Free Press, New York.

23. McCloskey, DJ. (2008). Nurses' perceptions of research utilization in a corporate health care system. *J Nurs Scholarship* I 40:39.

24. Stetler, CB. (1994). Refinement of the Stetler/Marram Model for application of research findings to practice. *Nurs Outlook* 42:15.

25. Horsley, J, et al. (1983). *Using Research to Improve Nursing Practice: A Guide.* Grune and Stratton, Orlando, FL.

26. Mantzoukas, S, and Watkinson, S. (2006). Review of advanced nursing practice: The international literature and developing the generic features. *J Clin Nurs* 16:28.

27. Rosenstock, IM. (1966). Why people use health services. *Milbank Memorial Fund Quarterly* 44:94.

28. Strecher, VJ, and Rosenstock, IM. (1997). The health belief model. In Glanz, K, Lewis, FM, and Riner, BK (eds), *Health Behavior and Health Education,* 2nd ed. Jossey-Bass, San Francisco, CA.

29. Rosenstock, IM, Strecher, VJ, and Becker, MH. (1988). Social learning theory and the Health Belief Model. *Health Educ Q* 15:175.

30. Bandura, A. (1997). *Self-Efficacy: The Exercise of Control.* Freeman, New York.

31. Pender, N. (1975). A conceptual model for preventive health behavior. *Nurs Outlook* 23:385.

32. Pender, NJ, Murdaugh, CL, and Parsons, MA. (2006). *Health Promotion in Nursing Practice,* 5th ed. Pearson Prentice Hall, Upper Saddle River, NJ.

33. Walker, SN, Sechrist, KR, and Pender, NJ. (1987). The health-promoting lifestyle profile: Development and psychometric characteristics. *Nurs Res* 36:76.

34. Prochaska, JO, Redding, CA, and Evers, KE. (1997). The transtheoretical model and stages of change. In Glanz, K, Rimer, BK, and Viswanath, K (eds), *Health Behavior and Health Education: Theory, Research, and Practice,* 2nd ed. John Wiley & Sons, San Francisco.

35. Prochaska, JO, and DiClemente, CC. (1983). Stages and processes of self-change of smoking: Toward an integrative model of change, *J Consulting and Clin Psychol* 51:390.

36. Kelly, CW. (2008). Commitment to health theory. *Res and Theory for Nurs Prac: An International J* 22:148.

37. Green, LW, et al. (1980). *Health Education Planning: A Diagnostic Approach.* Mayfield, Palo Alto, CA.

38. Green, LW, and Kreuter, MW. (1991). *Health Promotion Planning: An Educational and Environmental Approach,* 2nd ed. Mayfield, Mountain View, CA.

39. Green, LW, and Kreuter, MW. (1999). *Health Promotion Planning: An Educational and Ecological Approach,* 3rd ed. Mayfield, Mountain View, CA.

40. Lauver, D. (1992). A theory of care-seeking behavior. *Image J Nurs Sch* 24:281.

41. Lauver, D. (1992). Psychosocial variables, race, and intention to seek care for breast cancer symptoms. *Nurs Res* 41:236.

42. Benner, P. (2001). *From Novice to Expert: Excellence and Power in Clinical Nursing Practice,* commemorative ed. Addison-Wesley, Menlo Park, CA.

43. Benner, PA, Tanner, CA, and Chesla, CA. (1996). *Expertise in Nursing Practice.* Springer, New York.

44. Brykczynski, KA. (1999). Reflections on clinical judgment of nurse practitioners. *Sch Inq Nurs Pract* 13:175.

45. National Organization of Nurse Practitioner Faculties. (1995). *Curriculum Guidelines and Program Standards for Nurse Practitioner Education,* 2nd ed. NONPF, Washington, DC.

46. Price, MJ, Martin, AC, Newberry, YG, et al. (1992). Developing national guidelines for nurse practitioner education: An overview of the product and process. *J Nurs Educ* 31:10

47. Calkin, JD. (1984). A model for advanced nursing practice. *J Nurs Adm* 14:24.

48. Koerner, J. (1992). Differentiated practice: The evolution of professional nursing. *J Prof Nurs* 8:335.

49. Nelson, RJ, and Koerner, JG. (1994). Context. In Koerner, JG, and Karpiuk, KL (eds), *Implementing Differentiated Nursing Practice: Transformation By Design.* Aspen, Gaithersburg, MD (pp. 1–21).

50. Bush, NJ, and Watters, T. (2001). The emerging role of the oncology nurse practitioner: A collaborative model within the private practice setting. *Oncol Nurs Forum* 28:1425.

51. Waldman, R. (2002). Collaborative practice—balancing the future. *Obstet Gynecol Surv* 57:1.

52. Roberts, J. (1997). Educational approaches that promote interdisciplinary collaborative practice within academic health centers. *Womens Health Issues* 7:323.

53. Corser, WD. (1998). A conceptual model of collaborative nurse-physician interactions: The management of traditional influences and personal tendencies. *Sch Inq Nurs Pract* 12:325.

54. Stapleton, SR. (1998). Team-building: Making collaborative practice work. *J Nurse Midwifery* 43:12.

55. Neale, J. (1999). Nurse practitioners and physicians: A collaborative practice. *Clin Nurs Spec* 13:252.

Margaret T. Bowers is assistant clinical professor at Duke University School of Nursing and a nurse practitioner (NP) in the Duke Heart Failure Disease Management Program. She earned her master's degree as a critical care clinical nurse specialist (CNS) at Duke University School of Nursing and received a post-master's certificate as a family nurse practitioner (FNP) at Duke as well. She is specialty director for the Acute Care and Cardiovascular Nurse Practitioner programs at Duke University School of Nursing. Ms. Bowers recently completed a Robert Wood Johnson-funded project, *Expecting Success in Cardiac Care: Reducing Racial Disparities,* where she was the lead for the community demonstration project. In this role, she provided cardiology consultations in a local clinic for the medically underserved that did not have access to cardiology specialists. She is principal investigator for an American Association of Critical Care Nurses (AACN)–funded clinical practice grant evaluating daily weight monitoring and early symptom recognition in an outpatient population with heart failure.

Catherine L. Gilliss is professor and dean at the Duke University School of Nursing and vice chancellor of nursing affairs at Duke Medicine. For many years, she directed the FNP specialty program at the University of California at San Francisco (UCSF). She also coordinated UCSF's Primary Care Nurse Practitioner Program, the largest graduate primary care nurse practitioner program in the nation, which, in 1995, was recognized with the Excellence in Primary Care Education Award by the Pew Health Professions Commission. Dr. Gilliss received her undergraduate nursing education at Duke University, her master's degree in psychiatric–mental health nursing at The Catholic University of America, and her post-master's adult nurse practitioner (ANP) certificate at the University of Rochester in New York. Her doctoral and postdoctoral work was completed at the UCSF's School of Nursing. She has been internationally recognized for her research on families and chronic illness. Dr. Gilliss has served on the boards of numerous professional societies and journals. She is currently serving as President of the American Academy of Nursing (2009-2011).

Linda Lindsey Davis is a professor of nursing in the Duke University School of Nursing and a senior fellow in the Center for Aging and Human Development at Duke. Dr. Davis is an adult nurse practitioner who holds a doctorate in nursing from the University of Maryland at Baltimore, a master's of science in nursing from the University of North Carolina at Chapel Hill, and a bachelor's in nursing from Old Dominion University in Norfolk, Virginia. She was one of the first Robert Wood Johnson Nurse Faculty Fellows in Primary Care and completed her nurse practitioner training at the University of Rochester in New York. Dr. Davis has published numerous papers and book chapters on the geographic, social, and financial profiles that place elders at risk for higher levels of morbidity, institutionalization, and early mortality. She maintains an active program of elder care community education and service, and her model for effective elder care (RURAL: Relevance-Unity-Responsiveness-Access-Local Leadership) is used by the U.S. Agency on Aging as an algorithm for elder care program and policy development in rural communities. She currently is the principal investigator for a study funded by the National Institute of Nursing Research on caregiver skill training around home care for an aged family member with Alzheimer's disease or Parkinson's disease.

The authors would like to recognize the contribution of Dennis J. Cheek, PhD, RN, FAHA, and Karol S. Harshaw-Ellis, MSN, RN, A/GNP, ACNP-CS, authors of the chapter "Advanced Practice Nurses in Non-Primary Care Roles: The Evolution of Specialty and Acute Care Practices" in the second edition of *Advanced Practice Nursing: Emphasizing Common Roles.*

CHAPTER 5

Acute and Primary Care Advanced Practice Nursing: Past, Present, and Future

Margaret T. Bowers, MSN, RN, FNP-BC; Catherine L. Gilliss, DNSc, RN, FAAN; and Linda Lindsey Davis, PhD, RN, ANP, DP-NAP, FAAN

CHAPTER OBJECTIVES

After completing this chapter, the reader will be able to:

1. Synthesize the implications of various healthcare workforce projections for primary care and acute care systems in the first half of the 21st century.
2. Analyze socioeconomic and political forces contributing to the emphasis on primary care systems in the United States.
3. Weigh the advantages and disadvantages of using the following methods for evaluating advanced practice nursing in primary care settings:
   a. Classification of patient encounters
   b. Comparison in standards of care
   c. Documentation of functions of primary care
4. Explore factors that facilitate or inhibit advanced practice registered nursing in primary care and acute care systems.

CHAPTER OBJECTIVES

5. Describe the evolution of advanced practice registered nursing in non-primary care roles.
6. Explore the factors influencing advanced practice registered nursing in acute care systems and other non-primary care settings.
7. Discuss interprofessional practice across the continuum of care.

Although governmental efforts in the mid-1990s failed to bring about healthcare reform, the American healthcare system implemented many of the changes proposed. While problems with access and quality and service fragmentation continue to influence healthcare delivery in some areas of the United States, the focus on reducing healthcare system expenditures has fueled continued interest in primary care systems. The future healthcare needs of society depend on how we evaluate those systems with respect to issues such as patient safety, practice gaps, quality of care, and the prevention and treatment of chronic diseases.[1] This chapter provides an overview of the social, political, and economic issues that have influenced primary care and acute care over the past decade. It also discusses the factors that may facilitate or inhibit the participation of advanced practice registered nurses (APRNs) in primary care and acute care systems in the future.

Health Care in the 20th Century

In hierarchical healthcare systems, "primary care" has been the term used to describe basic services on which other more specialized services are built. Presumably, primary care systems can handle as much as 99% of the health problems in a community.[2] In 1978, the World Health Organization (WHO) proposed that primary health care, designed to bring accessible and economical care into communities where people live and work, should be a basic component of every country's healthcare system.[3] Primary care has been accepted as the necessary foundation for health care in the majority of industrialized nations, with the United States being a notable exception. The U.S. healthcare system has been described as a pluralistic, overlapping collection of practitioners providing different aspects of care in a variety of settings.[4] The late 20th century witnessed continued dissatisfaction with U.S. health care, described by many as:

- Disease-focused, concerned more with the technology of the diagnosis and treatment of specific diseases, rather than with holistic health care
- Fragmented, so that patients and their families receive uncoordinated and episodic treatment from various specialists for their health problems
- Inaccessible, in that services and providers are located primarily in urban population centers, creating pockets of unserved or underserved areas in rural towns and inner cities
- Costly, in that many people, particularly elderly persons, minorities, and the poor are unable to afford needed healthcare services, creating growing numbers of underinsured and uninsured Americans

Health Care in the 21st Century

Because healthcare costs continue to account for more than 20% of the U.S. gross national product, solutions to the problems in the American healthcare system continue to be defined in economic terms.[5] Because of the promised cost savings of managed care, the numbers of individuals, families, and communities enrolled in health maintenance organizations (HMOs) have stimulated competition between these organizations (large and small, public and private) to offer various primary care plans. Changes in the system that contributed to this over the past decade have included the following[6–10]:

- Downsizing or closure of many hospitals nationwide
- Increased emphasis on disease prevention and health promotion, both for cost savings and for quality-of-life benefits to consumers
- Development of healthcare partnerships between medical centers and corporate and business entities to deliver the most economical health care for enrolled and prepaid populations
- Use of health outcome data as justification for spending healthcare dollars
- Significant expansion of primary care in ambulatory and community-based settings
- Sweeping changes in the education and practice of health professionals to staff these emerging primary care systems

For more than 35 years, healthcare providers, educators, and policy makers in the United States have described primary care as an economical strategy for increasing consumer access to a broad range of holistic and humanistic services. To many, continued investment in primary care systems in the United States represents a logical solution to long-standing problems that have troubled the U.S. healthcare delivery system in the past, including unequal access, rising costs, fragmentation, and overemphasis on medical technology. The 1998 Pew Report further describes customization and patient control as key factors in the delivery of health care in the future.[11]

The Nature of Primary Care

This section discusses the nature and content of primary care, how it can be evaluated, and the specific roles of the generalist, specialist, and APRN in the delivery of primary health care.

Definitions of Primary Care

Definitions of primary care have evolved. White[12] defined primary care as first-contact care. Alpert and Charney[13] added that primary care medicine involves longitudinal responsibility for a patient, including integration of both health and disease services. In 1978, the Institute of Medicine[14] (IOM) defined primary care as having the functions of improved accessibility, continuity, comprehensiveness, coordination, and accountability. Golden[15] reported that primary care is characterized by long-term, close relationships between practitioner and patient and family. Within this relationship, the primary care provider treats common and acute illnesses and refers patients with less frequently occurring and more complex problems to specialists. Starfield[16] summarized the four key functions of primary care:

1. First contact, in which services are timely, accessible, and available at the point of entry into the system
2. Longitudinal, in that services, organized to focus on the patient and not the illness, are provided to the patient by the same provider over time
3. Comprehensive, in that a broad range of services are offered by the provider
4. Coordinated, in that a single provider organizes information related to patient referral, procedures, and therapies to improve the continuity and quality of care

More recently, the IOM[17] re-examined early definitions of primary care as a first step toward projecting the future of health care in the United States. The revised IOM definition includes many of the elements originally introduced but added a focus on the family and community contexts in which care should be provided:

> Primary care is the provision of integrated, accessible health care services by clinicians who are accountable for addressing a large majority of personal health care needs, developing a sustained partnership with patients, and practicing in the context of family and community.[17] (p. 16)

In fact, there is mounting concern that the very definition of primary care must be challenged.[18] A recent proposal suggests seven core principles to support the renaissance of primary care[19]:

1. Health care must be organized to serve the needs of patients.
2. The goal of primary care systems should be the delivery of the highest-quality care as documented by measurable outcomes.
3. Information and information systems are the backbone of the primary care process.
4. Current healthcare systems must be restructured.
5. The healthcare financing systems must support excellent primary care practice.
6. Primary care education must be revitalized with an emphasis on the new delivery models and training sites that deliver excellent primary care.
7. The value of primary care practice must be continually improved, documented, and communicated. See Table 5-1.

Content of Primary Care

Based on the IOM definition, a number of assumptions can be made about the nature of primary care. Integrated primary care must include consideration of the total person—body

Table 5-1 **Examples of Primary Care Services**
• Preventive care and screening
• Health and nutrition education and counseling
• History taking
• Physical examination
• Diagnostic testing
• Prescription and management of drug therapy
• Prenatal care and delivery of normal pregnancies
• Well-baby care
• Diagnosis and treatment of common health problems and minor injuries
• Diagnosis and treatment of chronic conditions
• Minor surgery
• Coordination of services and referral for specialty care when needed

Adapted from *The Alliance for Health Reform: A Primary Care Primer*. The Alliance for Health Reform, Washington, DC, 1993, p. 14.

and mind—as well as the context in which care occurs. Accessible care must be personalized according to the needs of individuals within their communities. The majority of primary care includes both episodic and ongoing services. A sustained partnership between a primary care provider and patient over the life cycle implies the provider's need to know about biomedical health problems, social sciences (including personal, interpersonal, and larger social systems), and the way to work successfully with other providers in interdisciplinary practice teams. Given the socioeconomic and political contexts in which primary care is practiced today, providers also need to understand expected and desired outcomes of care based on normative evidence and the particular client's situation. The sophistication required to accomplish these expectations cannot be overestimated. Financial incentives and reporting of clinical outcomes and quality data play a large part in the ability of providers to deliver this type of care.[20]

Evaluation of Primary Care

There are numerous approaches to evaluating clinical services. Three methods that have potential for documenting the nature and scope of advanced nursing practice in primary care systems are the classification of patient encounters, comparisons in standards of care, and documentation of the functions of primary care. A brief description of the three methods and an example of a study using each method demonstrates their usefulness for evaluating advanced nursing practice in primary care settings.

CLASSIFICATION OF PATIENT ENCOUNTERS

Patient encounters are classified according to whether visits are first encounters; encounters for continuing care by the same provider; encounters for ongoing, nonspecialized services; or encounters for consultation and referral to a specialist. Alternatively, visits are classified according to whether they are primarily for health screening or prevention, for health promotion, for management of a specific illness (acute or chronic), or for referrals to specialized services not available in the primary care setting.

Most of the information on patient encounters in primary care settings comes from data collected through the periodic National Ambulatory Care Survey (NACS),[21] an ongoing survey of community-based physicians stratified by specialty and by geographic region in the United States conducted annually since 1990. The survey data continue to demonstrate that the majority of visits to U.S. physicians by individuals in all age groups are for management of specific symptoms, the most common being those associated with colds. Screening or preventive services continue to rank below symptom management as the common reason for patient encounters with a primary care physician.[21] The NACS's exclusive focus on physicians does not permit characterization of patient encounters with nonphysician providers. A more widely defined focus would be useful in classifying APRN encounters with patients in primary care settings.

Classification of encounters provides a typology of service needs and of services delivered. Classification of the purposes of patient encounters allows providers and administrators to identify the service needs of individuals and families within a target population. Classification of patient encounters according to the predominant focus of each encounter also enables evaluators in multidisciplinary settings to determine which member of the multidisciplinary team is providing those services. By classifying the encounter, evaluators are able to determine whether physicians are providing most of the illness-management services and/or whether APRNs are providing most of the health screening procedures.

This method also enables evaluators to analyze the nature of service referrals. For example, the evaluator may wish to know whether providers are referring emotional or social problems outside the primary care setting, even though competent care providers are available in that setting. Finally, a frequency count of the types of services offered can assist in determining whether continuing education is needed by the staff. However, classification of patient encounters by service need and service frequency does not assess quality of care.

COMPARISON IN STANDARDS OF CARE

With the standards-of-care method of evaluating primary care, patient encounters are analyzed to determine whether they meet commonly accepted standards for quality of care, such as the appropriate use of diagnostic tests, the accurate recognition of patient problems, the selection and implementation of an acceptable regimen for treatment, and documentation of plans for patient education and follow-up care. Given the current emphasis on patient outcome data, this evaluation method enables evaluators to compare actual patient outcomes with expected patient outcomes.

A good example of a study of compliance with commonly accepted standards of care in primary care practice may be found in the work of Avorn, Everitt, and Baker.[22] These investigators compared 501 practicing physicians and 298 practicing NPs in their approach to a patient presenting with epigastric pain. Using a case of a patient presenting with a history of aspirin, coffee, cigarette, and alcohol use, plus severe psychological stress, and the negative results of an endoscopy, the investigators compared the reported treatment decisions of the two types of providers. Half the physician sample recommended immediate treatment of the hypothetical patient with medication, whereas only 20% of NPs recommended immediate medication as the desirable action. Investigators found that the physician sample more often omitted the standard practice of collecting an adequate medical history. In contrast, the NP group more often recommended a more extensive medical history before making a treatment choice and, when making treatment choices, more frequently began with nonpharmacological interventions. The investigators concluded from these findings that the medical providers were less likely to comply with standard history-taking procedures and that the two types of providers, physicians and NPs, differed significantly regarding their actual practice activities.

Comparing standards of care has great potential for further exploring APRN adherence to quality-of-care standards. An inpatient model used at Vanderbilt Medical Center in 1996 looked at the impact of an NP caring for patients on a heart failure service. Both cost and length of stay were evaluated when comparing NP-managed patients with those treated during the previous year by residents. The cost reduction and decreased length of stay for the NP-managed patients was significant. Since many factors can influence these results, further studies are needed in the current healthcare environment.[23]

Comparing practice activities against commonly accepted standards of care is not only a useful assessment of the quality of patient care, it is also useful in identifying the need for continuing education among providers. The Avorn, Everitt, and Baker study recommended enhanced continuing education for physicians about the importance of extensive history taking before initiating a treatment regimen.

The standards-of-care method would be particularly useful for documenting the quality of care delivered by APRNs in primary care settings. However, this evaluation method does not document whether desirable primary care functions, as described earlier, are present in the practices of providers.

DOCUMENTATION OF FUNCTIONS OF PRIMARY CARE

Documentation can help assess whether selected primary care characteristics are present in the care delivered. For example, patient encounters might be analyzed and given a score based on whether the encounters are longitudinal, comprehensive, or coordinated. Managed care models need to implement evaluation studies that document the existence of functions believed to demonstrate the advantages of primary care. An example of a study of how provider characteristics can influence care delivery demonstrates the potential of this method for documenting the advantages of advanced nursing practice in primary care.

As part of a larger study of medical outcomes in the United States, Safran, Tarlov, and Rogers[24] documented primary care characteristics in the care provided to 1208 patients by physicians. The physicians practiced in either traditional fee-for-service care plans or were employed by HMOs or independent practice associations (IPAs). Patients with one of four conditions—hypertension, diabetes, congestive heart failure, or recent myocardial infarction—were asked to complete a series of questionnaires about whether the care they received over a 2-year period had the characteristics of:

- Accountability (interpersonal and technical)
- Accessibility (financial and organizational)
- Continuity and comprehensiveness
- Coordination

Patients who received care through the HMO or IPA model reported greater financial accessibility and better coordination of care. However, those patients who received care through a traditional fee-for-service (private practice) model reported greater continuity and better organizational access and provider accountability. Investigators concluded from these mixed findings that the orientation of individual practitioners influences the characteristic nature of the services provided.

The documented characteristics evaluation method can also be used to identify the presence of other functions considered examples of high-quality primary care (e.g., the family-centered nature of a patient encounter, the use of existing community-based resources for referrals, and so forth). This method also would be useful in determining whether advanced practice in primary care settings demonstrates the desired function of primary care contacts.

Table 5-2 outlines the three different approaches to evaluation of primary care. Because each of these common approaches to primary care evaluation has both strengths and limitations, some combination of the three likely would provide the best assessment of the nature, scope, and quality of care and the unique characteristics of advanced nursing practice in primary care settings.

Roles: Generalist Versus Specialist Care

The IOM definition of primary care suggests that there are significant distinctions to be made between generalist and specialist care.[17] Primary care involves the delivery of services by generalist practitioners, with referral of patients to specialists for complex health problems. The characteristics, processes, and goals of generalist and specialist care are not the same. The goal of specialty practice is to cure or treat a specific problem, disease, or illness. The goal of generalist care is health promotion, prevention of disease or illness, and amelioration of symptoms.[15] Table 5-3 compares generalist with specialist care.

According to Starfield,[16] the nature of hospital-based education and practice makes it difficult for specialists to provide the key components of primary care described earlier. First-contact primary care typically occurs early in the natural history of a health problem, when evolving signs and symptoms cannot easily be tied to a specific disease or illness. In addition, because many of the presenting problems seen in primary care settings can be traced to stressful personal, familial, or environmental factors, counseling and affective support often are the major treatment components.

Hospital-based training and practice do not provide experiences and necessary skills for managing the physical, psychological, or social problems that commonly are presented in primary care settings (e.g., individual patient problems such as stress reaction, vague anxiety and confusion, family turmoil relating to marital conflict or adolescent crises, alcohol or other substance use, divorce or death or dying of a family member). If specialist providers were to spend the time needed to develop and implement successful interventions for managing these and similar primary care problems, they would often have less time to see specialty patients and to stay current on new knowledge and discoveries in their specialties. Finally, primary care delivery is difficult for a specialist because few specialists have the educational preparation, background experiences, or skills to perform the time-consuming but necessary function of coordinating services provided by others.

Table 5-2 **Approaches to Evaluating Primary Care Services**			
Classification of patient encounters	Determine the nature and scope of services provided.	Classification of patient visits according to a purpose, such as screening, management of disease, or consultation	Helpful for determining needs of target population Useful for determining staffing needs Useful for staff continuing education Not useful in assessing quality of services provided Useful in assessing quality of specific services
Comparison on standards of care	Compare services provided against accepted standards for quality of care.	Comparison of encounter against known standards of care for problem, such as: Problem identification Use of diagnostic tests Treatment regimen Patient education	Useful for staff continuing education Not helpful in considering the unique characteristics of primary care
Documentation of functions of primary care	Document the presence or absence of functional characteristics of high-quality primary care.	Use of setting for first contact Length of relationship with one care provider for longitudinality Documentation of results of referrals in patient records for coordination Evidence that a variety of patient problems are managed for comprehensiveness	Useful in assessing whether key primary care functions are present in patient encounters

Role of APRNs

APRNs complete educational programs that prepare them for generalist practice or specialty practice, and sometimes both. The Consensus Model for APRN Regulation[25] has reaffirmed four APRN roles: certified registered nurse anesthetist (CRNA), certified nurse-midwife (CNM), clinical nurse specialist (CNS), and nurse practitioner (NP). The CRNA provides anesthesia and anesthesia-related care. The CNM is a clinical expert who has knowledge, skills, and clinical reasoning for the care and management of women and newborns. The CNS is an expert clinician who provides comprehensive practice activities in the areas of

Table 5-3 **Specialist Versus Generalist Services**

Service Characteristic	Specialist Care	Generalist Care
Nature of service	**Scope of services:** Management of specific, complex problems	**Scope of services:** Management of varied problems, needs
Focus of service	Problem-focused, short-term, episodic service for diagnosis and treatment of specific problem	Patient-focused, long-term, continuous delivery of services
Role of service provider	Direct-care provider	Direct-care provider, plus plan and coordinate service delivery provided by others

indirect/direct patient care, education, consultation, and research utilization. The NP provides comprehensive health assessments, determines diagnoses, plans and prescribes treatment, and manages healthcare regimens in a variety of settings for individuals, families, and communities. The NP role includes promotion of wellness, prevention of illness and injury, and management of acute and chronic conditions.[26] Early in the evolution of the NP role, most NPs delivered health care from ambulatory care settings, physician practices, or clinics. Few practiced in institutions, the exception being neonatal NPs (NNPs).

Primary Care Providers in the 21st Century

Changing population demographics, the growth of managed care plans, and revitalization of the dialogue regarding healthcare reform have stimulated considerable discussion about who will provide care in the emerging healthcare delivery systems. To a great extent, efforts to build a reformed primary healthcare delivery system depend on the number and types of generalists, the availability and ideal mix of providers, and the incentives for, benefits of, and barriers to practice.

Physicians as Primary Care Providers

Although the need for primary care physicians (i.e., generalist practitioners in family practice, internal medicine, or pediatrics) by the year 2000 was estimated to be as high as 50% of practicing physicians, medical practice continues to focus largely on specialty care.[27] A report on the physician workforce projected that medical and surgical specialists will continue to increase in states where personal income levels are greater. Conversely, general practitioners are in shorter supply in the "richer" states.[28] In 2004, there were 779,772 physicians in the United States, but only 13.6% of them identified themselves as family or general practitioners.[29] These data support the Council on Graduate Medical Education (COGME) projection, set forth in a 2005 report,[30] forecasting a decrease in the numbers of generalist physicians. In fact, changes in healthcare economics have worked in favor of increasing the numbers of nonphysician clinicians and decreasing the numbers of physicians entering primary care. According to McClellan:

> We are seeing more and more evidence that programs led by nurses can improve patient care and outcomes while reducing costs. Meeting the overall needs of each patient as effectively as possible has long been the goal of nursing care, and we need nurses' leadership now more than ever.[31]

This need for primary care clinicians provides fertile ground for APRNs to establish themselves firmly within the medical community and to garner the reimbursement and recognition they deserve.

Over the past several decades, there have been two competing predictions about the supply of primary care physicians for the future: either a deficit or an adequate supply. Although dependent upon a variety of potential influencing factors, the deficit prediction is predominant at this time. Critics have identified several organizational factors that discourage the shift of medical education and practice from hospital-based specialty care to community-based, generalist care.

First, as secondary and tertiary settings, hospitals and health science centers provide the necessary technological support for medical specialist education and practice. Second, mechanisms for medical student education funding have favored specialty practice. The majority of medical student education occurs traditionally in hospitals, with more than 80% of the cost of medical resident training covered by the provision of inpatient clinical services. Last, because primary care residencies typically generate less clinical revenue than specialty residencies, many teaching hospitals have been reluctant to reduce specialty residencies in exchange for an increase in the number of generalist care residencies.[32]

Past efforts to increase the number of medical primary care providers in the United States have concentrated on providing incentives for medical schools to establish more family practice training and residency programs and on encouraging more new physicians to choose the generalist practice option.[13,16,27] Despite incentives that favor medical school applicants with a stated interest in generalist practice and despite offering loan forgiveness to students choosing primary care, the number of new graduates entering specialty practice has remained constant.[33] More than 15 years ago, Levinsky[34] speculated that primary care practice would continue to be unattractive to physicians for several reasons:

■ Lack of financial incentives, because the annual income of generalist physicians is typically 40% to 60% lower than that of specialists

■ Reduced satisfaction with the physician-patient relationship, which many physicians relate to the loss of practice autonomy as physicians become employees of managed care practices

■ The large number of "unsatisfying" patients seen in primary care settings (i.e., elderly, poor, HIV-positive, and substance-use patients and others for whom medical treatment options are limited and long-term, successful medical outcomes are unlikely)

In the early 1990s, the growth of managed care was hailed as an impetus for growth in the number of primary care physicians in the United States. However the opposite occurred, with graduating medical student interest in primary care declining an estimated 8% between 1997 and 2000.[35] In 2008, this concern was highlighted by the fact that only 2% of all new physicians opted for primary care or general medicine residencies.[36] In a widely cited paper published in the *Harvard Business Review*,[37] the reasons given for the decline in new medical school graduates' interest in primary care were defined as the result of an era of "disruptive" innovation that stemmed from the increased production of NPs and physician assistants (PAs) who perform many primary care services faster, better, and (most importantly in the managed care marketplace) in a more cost-effective manner with less salary expense.

Physician Assistants in Primary Care

Since the passage of the Medicare and Medicaid laws in the 1960s, federal efforts in primary care have focused on increasing the numbers of both nonphysician and physician generalists. Early efforts to build a cadre of primary care providers in the United States took place in the 1960s, when physician shortages and maldistribution stimulated the development of various nonphysician primary care provider programs. These programs were focused primarily on providing physician substitutes for rural and underserved areas.[38,39]

The Physician Assistant (PA) program at Duke University and the Medex programs at the University of Washington and University of Utah are early examples of education programs for nonphysician providers. The first PA program opened at Duke under the direction of Eugene Stead, MD. Interestingly, Stead had originally planned to develop this role in conjunction with his nursing colleague, Thelma Ingles. However, the nursing community reacted strongly against the development of a nursing role that appeared to take on medical tasks. Consequently, Stead initiated this first PA program by drawing from the large pool of military corpsmen returning from the Vietnam War.

In 2008, the American Academy of Physician Assistants (AAPA) reported that approximately 79,900 individuals were educated as PAs; their most frequently reported work setting was the hospital (38%).[40] The content of PA practice, as described by Jones and Cawley,[39] includes evaluation, monitoring, diagnostic testing, therapy, counseling, and referral. The scope of PA practice is regulated under state medical practice acts, and thus the activities of PAs in primary care practice vary from state to state. However, PAs are generally licensed as dependent to physicians, in contrast to NPs, whose practices are more independent.

Numerous studies have documented the PA's ability to provide medical services with a high level of patient satisfaction.[39,41,42] PAs are reported to see patient populations similar to those of physicians and are considered capable of providing approximately 75% of physician-specific services.[42] Regan and Harbert[43] reported that depending on his or her particular use in a practice, a PA can reduce overhead and increase the financial productivity of a physician by a total of $72,077 to $332,200 annually. Reports have suggested that managed care organizations are using PAs and APRNs to control costs; roughly, two-thirds of all sampled groups have reported employment of APRNs and PAs.[41–45]

APRNs as Primary Care Providers

To date, APRNs in primary care settings have practiced as NPs or CNMs. The introduction of the NP role occurred simultaneously with that of the PA. Conceived as a primary care generalist, the NP (initially called a pediatric associate) role was originally developed by Loretta Ford, PhD, a nurse, and Henry Silver, a pediatrician, both practicing in Colorado.[46] The role developed over time and extended into adult health, family health, and gerontological health.

In 2004, there were an estimated 109,582 nationally certified NPs and 12,820 nationally certified CNMs in the United States,[47] with 325 graduate nursing programs or postmaster's nursing programs preparing NPs in a variety of specialist practice areas.[47–49] The number of schools offering NP programs has now increased to 343. Most schools offer preparation for FNPs (83%), followed by adult NPs (42%) and pediatric NPs (28%).[50] According to the National Organization of Nurse Practitioner Faculties (NONPF), NPs are educated to practice independently and interdependently in collaborative practice arrangements.[50]

As primary care generalists, NPs employ a population-based perspective to care for individuals, families, and communities. Clinical decision-making, based on critical thinking, is essential to the work of the NP, who must synthesize theoretical, scientific, clinical, and practical knowledge to diagnose and manage actual and potential health problems. Central to the role of the NP is the promotion and maintenance of health. NPs have major roles in health promotion, disease prevention, service coordination, and acute and chronic disease monitoring.[51] Although NPs are expected to use short-term encounters to address the restoration of health, long-term contact and teaching encounters are viewed as more meaningful opportunities to contribute to the long-term health of the patient. Strategies of NP care include patient advocacy, therapy and health education, counseling, service coordination, and treatment evaluation.

According to NONPF, NP practice is not setting-specific but rather is focused on the primary care needs of patients in whatever setting they may occur.[50] In the late 1980s and early 1990s, the numbers of NPs began to increase in acute care settings, where they were taking the place of medical residents in hospitals.[52,53] In addition to ANPs and FNPs, women's health NPs and CNMs provide primary care services to women across the lifespan.

Evolution of APRN Roles

Advanced practice nursing roles and practice evolved almost exclusively within the context of an acute care delivery system. Even when the NP role was created to provide healthcare services in community-based settings, this occurred within a delivery system focused on acute care.

Chapter 1 provided a comprehensive review of the evolution of APRN roles. Modern nurse anesthesia traces its roots to the last two decades of the 1800s, where records indicate that nurses were often asked to administer anesthesia. The first nurse anesthetist, in 1877, was Sister Mary Bernard at St. Vincent's Hospital in Erie, Pennsylvania.[54] Anesthesia practice was so common that, in her 1893 textbook entitled *Nursing: Its Principles and Practices for Hospital and Private Use*, Isabel Adams Hampton Robb included a chapter on the administration of anesthesia.

In 1925, Mary Breckenridge established the Frontier Nursing Service in Kentucky and was the first nurse to practice as a nurse-midwife in the United States. She received her midwifery education in England and returned to the United States with other British nurse-midwives to set up a system of care similar to the one she had observed in Scotland.[55]

Advanced practice nursing has also been successful for over 50 years in creating roles that assisted in solving social, financial, and political healthcare problems. After World War II, nurse educators developed the CNS role to improve the quality of care in hospitals. This was the first advanced practice nursing role that was designed not to provide direct patient care, but rather to support nursing services through education. Although initially, specialization for nurses was primarily limited to the areas of administration and education, the first use of the term "nurse clinician" to designate a specialist in nursing practice occurred in 1943 (credited to Reiter).[56] The development of the first master's program in a clinical nursing specialty is attributed to Hildegarde Peplau at Rutgers University in 1954 to prepare nurses for the role of psychiatric clinical nurse specialist.[57]

Neonatal Nurse Practitioner

In the 1970s, the neonatal nurse practitioner (NNP) role evolved as a way to rectify problems in the delivery of health care for this at-risk population. Pediatric residency slots were being eliminated because of an overabundance and uneven geographic distribution of pediatricians.[58] At the same time, neonates were demanding a higher acuity and complexity of care. In 1973, a group of interested physicians and nurses formed an ad hoc committee known as the Blue Ribbon Panel, funded by the March of Dimes, to discuss educational programs that would prepare nurses to function in intensive perinatal care settings.[58a] The expectation was that the neonatal nurse clinician (NNC) would function primarily in the neonatal intensive care unit and any reassignment tasks would be a collaborative effort between physicians and nurses, requiring reassessment of the functional roles of both professions.[58] In 1974, the University of Arizona also launched a program no different in design or content from the Blue Ribbon guidelines; however, it was called a neonatal nurse practitioner (NNP) program.[58] Most of the original NNC/NNP programs were 4 to 9 months in length and were hospital based. It was not until the 1980s that hospital-based NNP certificate programs began to close down, as the trend moved toward university-based continuing education programs and graduate programs with NNP content integrated into the curricula.

In 1982, groups of NNCs and NNPs met during the American Academy of Pediatrics District meeting to discuss the future role of NNCs and NNPs. The first Neonatal Nurse Clinician, Practitioner, and Specialist (NNCPS) Conference was held in April of 1983 with the primary purpose of promoting the NNC/NNP role.[58] In June 1984, the National Association of Neonatal Nurses (NANN) was established. In spring 1985, the NNCPS joined the newly established NANN. The NANN has provided the organizational support to move the advanced practice of the NNP forward.

The NNP model has continued to evolve for the last 35 years. The NNP diagnoses and treats in collaboration with neonatologists and other pediatric physicians. The NNP makes independent and interdependent decisions in the assessment, diagnosis, management, and evaluation of the healthcare needs of neonates and infants.[59] In addition, the NNP selects and performs clinically indicated advanced diagnostic and therapeutic invasive procedures.[59] This established role provided the foundation and groundwork for the acute care nurse practitioner (ACNP) role in both the adult and pediatric clinical areas.

Acute Care Nurse Practitioner

In the 1990s, the Acute Care Nurse Practitioner (ACNP) began to establish a presence within hospitals. However, as early as the 1970s, the title of ACNP was being used, and the roles were described. The ACNP evolved as a direct result of blending the CNS and primary care NP roles, most likely due to their similar educational preparation. Many of the core classes of ACNP programs parallel those of the CNS programs.[60,61] The differences are that CNSs focus on systems and indirect care, and the ACNPs have a primary focus on direct patient care.[60,61] ACNPs also generally have more in-depth education in the areas of pharmacology, pathophysiology, health assessment, and managing physiologically unstable patients.[60–62]

The ACNPs in the 1970s and 1980s were adult primary care nurse practitioners who were recruited and employed in acute care settings. One early example was the use of an ACNP within the department of cardiac surgery at the University of Rochester Strong Memorial Hospital in a collaborative practice model that incorporated both direct patient care and advanced practice nursing scholarly activities.[63] Spisso and colleagues[64] reported in 1990 the use of NPs on their trauma service at the University of California, Davis, Medical Center. Prepared as primary care NPs with experience in surgical, critical, or acute care, these NPs during the 1980s were being recruited to decrease the patient burden on the available residents, whose residency hours were being reduced.[65,66] The NPs were successful in improving the quality of care and patient satisfaction and in decreasing length of hospital stay.[64,65]

By 1992, the ANA task force on ACNP and the Joint ACNP work group defined the role of the ACNP as one who provides advanced nursing care to patients who are acutely and critically ill. This includes providing direct patient care management by performing in-depth physical assessments, interpreting laboratory and diagnostic tests, and performing therapeutic treatments such as examining and cleaning wounds and inserting arterial or central venous catheters as well as ordering pharmacological agents.[67]

In the 1990s, as ACNP educational programs were developing, some of the first descriptions of the ACNP role came from the University of Pittsburgh, University of Pennsylvania, and Case Western Reserve University. Both Duke University Medical Center and the University of Pittsburgh Medical Center began using ACNPs in neurological intensive care units, where they started by overseeing the care of two or three intensive care unit patients. But as the physicians developed trust and confidence in ACNPs' decision making, their responsibilities increased.[67] Over time, they were permitted to provide care to an increased number of complex critically ill patients, interpret diagnostic studies, and perform procedures such as central line placement.[67]

It did not take long for healthcare leaders to realize that the acute care setting in the current delivery system required changes. As a result, the role of the ACNP began to gather support among physicians and administrators within tertiary healthcare centers across the country.[65,68–71] and in 1995 the American Nurses Association (ANA) and the American Association of Critical-Care Nurses drafted the document "Standards of Clinical Practice and Scope of Practice for the Acute Care Nurse Practitioner."[62] This interest and support have made the ACNP role an evolving career opportunity for critical care nurses. Certification is currently available by passing the adult ACNP examination, administered by the American Nurses Credentialing Center (ANCC), which certifies NPs who care for acutely ill adult patients. The Pediatric Nursing Certification Board (PNCB) provides certification examinations for ACNPs in the pediatric domain. The Consensus Model for Advanced Practice Nursing: Licensure, Accreditation, Certification and Education (2008) bifurcates the NP role into acute care and primary care. The acute care NP can be prepared for practice with the adult-gerontology or the pediatric populations.[25] The opportunities in advanced practice nursing will continue to expand as a result of changes in acute care settings, including the increased acuity of hospitalized patients, the demands of managed care organizations to reduce length of stay, better coordination of patient care, and the regulation of work hours for medical interns and residents.[61,65-67,72-74]

University Hospital of Cleveland, an affiliate of Case Western Reserve University, selected four units in which to place their initial ACNP graduates: the neuroscience unit, general oncology service, medical intensive care unit, and adult internal medicine unit. In each of these acute/critical care units, the ACNP performed the history and physical and some procedures such as arterial line insertion, lumbar punctures, insertion and removal of feeding tubes, and removal of pulmonary artery catheters. The neurology, oncology, and medical intensive care units were staffed with residents and/or fellows and attending physicians on a rotating basis. The ACNP, however, was based on a specific unit for continuity of care. Although the role and responsibilities of the ACNP differed among hospitals and units, there were commonalities, including patient management, leadership, teaching/mentoring, research, and professional development, common to the role of most ACNPs today.[75-77]

The University of Missouri Hospital and Clinics, Columbia, began to use NPs in the areas of general surgery, nephrology, and otolaryngology due to changes in their residency programs. The University of Missouri model was unique since these NPs provided both inpatient and outpatient care. Urban[78] described in-depth APRN roles in cardiovascular surgery. The two key functions were "case management" and "care coordination"; these two functions are also considered important components of the CNS role. Some of the highlights of the ACNP role were performing presurgical assessments, communicating with families and other healthcare team members, and providing patient education and discharge planning.

In contrast, the CNS role has centered around expert clinician, consultant, educator, researcher, administrator, and, in the 1990s, case and outcomes manager.[60] As conceptualized by the National Association of Clinical Nurse Specialists (NACNS), the CNS role involves three spheres of influence: client (direct care); nursing personnel (advancing the practice of nursing); and organization (interdisciplinary).[79] The ACNP role focus has been direct comprehensive care, which includes conducting histories and physicals, diagnosing, and treating.[60]

Sole and colleagues[80] described the role of an ACNP and PA in the care of stable trauma patients in a level I trauma center. The model of care delivery at this particular institution was a collaborative practice model.[80-82] The patients under the care of the ACNP and/or PA were assigned to an intermediate care service (ICS), who managed four to six patients each on a daily basis. The trauma surgeons or surgical intensivists rounded on a weekly basis but were available at any time for urgent issues. The ACNPs' duties included reviewing prior progress notes, diagnostic studies, and laboratory data and developing the plan of care for these patients with specialized needs. They performed history and physicals, wrote orders, and educated staff and families. To evaluate the effectiveness of the ICS, a retrospective chart review on 93 patients was performed. The findings revealed that one-fourth of the patients were discharged to a skilled nursing facility, rehabilitation center, or other hospital. All of the patients on the ICS survived and none required a higher level of care.

The expansion of the ACNP role across inpatient and outpatient settings has become common in the effort to provide continuity of care. Martin and Coniglio described using an ACNP in caring for patients with head and neck cancer in both the inpatient and outpatient setting.[82] Martin outlined the use of the ACNP to provide seamless comprehensive care across the spectrum of health care to complex transplant patients.[83] Evaluating the effectiveness of the ACNP role continues to be a source of research in an era in which quality of care, cost effectiveness, and outcomes are key components of looking at models of practice.[84] An inpatient model was used at Vanderbilt Medical Center in 1996 to look at the impact of an NPs' caring for patients on a heart failure service. Both cost and length of hospital stay were evaluated when comparing NP-managed patients with those treated during the previous year by residents. The cost reduction and decreased length of stay for the NP-managed patients was significant.[23] Changes in Medicare reimbursement have influenced the use of ACNPs: they are used in increasing numbers in acute care, emergency care, and long-term care settings.[85]

As the U.S. population ages, the use of critical care services has increased. Research studies have well established that physicians who received formal training in critical care medicine demonstrated both reduced mortality and reduced length of stay for patients compared to those who do not have this specialty training. At the same time, the supply of qualified physician intensivists has not been able to keep up with the demand for services.[86] ACNPs look beyond the patients' medical needs and incorporate psychosocial assessments and discharge planning into the care they provide. This influences factors such as length of stay and reduction in hospital costs. When they are integrated into a team of care providers who implement evidence-based practice health care, the effectiveness of ACNPs is obvious.[87]

Hospitalist/ACNP Model

The ACNP continues to move into many areas of the healthcare delivery system, but opportunities are now available for yet another model of practice. This model involves working with a hospitalist team. Hospitalists are internists who specialize in inpatient medicine and work in academic and nonacademic healthcare settings. The hospitalist movement emerged in California as a way to deal with the demands of managed care and decreased funding of residents[88] and evolved for many of the same reasons as did the ACNP. Both the ACNP and hospitalist are being used as solutions to address many of the problems that plague the current healthcare system. As a result, ACNPs and hospitalists are establishing yet another model of healthcare delivery: the ACNP/Hospitalist Model. Howie[89] and colleagues described the implementation of an ACNP/Hospitalist Model at the University of San Francisco Medical Center. Job opportunities and role descriptions for ACNPs working with hospitalists have become much more common.[90,91] The Hospitalist Model is not without flaws, however, because there is a break in the continuity of care when patients are transitioned from their primary care provider to another provider who is unfamiliar with them.[92]

In one practice, an ACNP was employed by a group of 12 internists to assist them in delivering care to their hospitalized patients. Prior to hiring the ACNP, each internist was responsible for rounding on his or her own patients. Each internist had a primary care patient panel of at least 2500 patients and was responsible for the total spectrum of care for each patient. Traditionally about 25% of the patients in the practice were hospitalized for a variety of reasons at some point in time. As one solution, the group decided that each physician would independently rotate on a weekly basis in the hospital. As patients became more complex, it was no longer cost-effective or efficient to continue this traditional care model. In addition, patients were experiencing longer lengths of stay, duplication of services, and dissatisfaction. At this point, the physician group decided to hire an ACNP.

The ACNP was brought into the practice to provide care for the patients hospitalized at a 400-bed community hospital owned by a large teaching medical center. The physicians, through their insight, sought an NP to provide continuity of care. Together, the ACNP/internist team covered an average census of 5 to 30 patients per week. Patients generally were admitted to the general medicine service but could be admitted to the medical intensive care, surgical intensive care, coronary intensive care, telemetry, or surgical units. The ACNP also evaluated and admitted patients through the emergency department. The duties of the ACNP included performing histories and physicals, writing orders, prescribing pharmacological and nonpharmacological treatment modalities, interpreting laboratory and diagnostic data, family counseling and teaching, performing medical procedures and consults, consulting with specialists, discharge planning, preparing discharge or transfer summaries, communicating with managed care companies and case managers, and serving as a consultant to the hospital nursing staff.

Non-Primary Care Roles: Growing Specialties

In 2008, schools of nursing reported having 189 APRN programs (CNS and NP programs only) with an acute or critical care focus.[49] Seventy schools reported having an acute care NP-adult master's program. In addition, 46 schools reported having a master's NNP program. A small number of schools (11) reported having a master's pediatric ACNP program.[49] In addition, 47 acute and critical CNS-adult programs and 8 acute and critical care CNS-pediatric programs were reported. Finally, seven schools reported having an acute or critical care CNS-neonatal program.[49] National certifying examinations for acute care CNS and NP areas of practice are offered by the ANCC, the National Certification Corporation (NCC), the American Association of Critical Care Nurses and the PNCB.

Research on Advanced Nursing Practice

An extensive body of literature is available documenting the effectiveness of APRNs (in particular NPs). These studies focus on NPs working in primary care and in acute care settings.

Primary Care Studies

Three reviews of APRN practice in primary care are considered definitive. The first, a study commissioned by the U.S. Congress and conducted by the Office of Technology Assessment (OTA),[93] reviewed the published reports of NP practice. The OTA study findings demonstrated that NP care is of *equal* quality to that of physicians in the areas of history taking; diagnosing of minor, acute illnesses; and managing stable, chronic diseases; and *superior* in the areas of communication and preventive care.

In the second literature synthesis, Crosby, Ventura, and Feldman[94] reviewed 248 published reports on NP practice from the period 1963 to 1983. The review included 187 reports judged to be methodologically sound and summarized the findings in relation to NP utilization, delivery of patient care services, short-term patient outcomes, and long-term patient outcomes. On the basis of their analysis of the reports, Crosby, Ventura, and Feldman concluded that NPs:

- Work primarily in ambulatory settings and physicians' offices
- Perform a range of services, including both physician-substitute services (history taking, physical and diagnostic examinations, and management of chronic illnesses) as well as complementary services (patient teaching and counseling) comparable or superior to that of other providers
- Have positive short-term patient outcomes (patient knowledge, compliance, return for health maintenance and follow-up visits) equal to, or better than, those of other providers

Long-term patient outcomes were described in only 14% of the reports and, therefore, were not analyzed.[94]

Brown and Grimes[95] provided a synopsis of both NP and CNM practice. The strength of their report is found in its use of rigorous statistical techniques that combined the probability values (*P* values) and arrived at standard mean differences across statistical comparison studies of APN providers (experimental groups) and physicians (control group). To be included in the review, the report had to describe:

- Practice in U.S. or Canadian settings
- An intervention provided by an NP-CNM or an NP-CNM-physician team
- Data on a control group of patients managed by a physician
- Outcomes related to process of care, clinical (patient) outcomes, or utilization and cost effectiveness
- Use of a traditional research design (i.e., experimental, quasi-experimental, or ex post facto)
- Statistical data sufficient to compare the experimental and control groups

More than 900 reports were reviewed and 38 NP and 15 CNM studies met the methodological requirements for inclusion. From the review of the 38 NP studies, the investigators concluded that NPs[95]:

- Provide more health promotion care and ordered more diagnostic tests than the physician group
- Have comparable scores on patient knowledge but higher scores than their physician counterparts on patient compliance, functional outcomes, resolution of pathological conditions, and satisfaction with care
- Spend more time with patients and have lower laboratory costs and fewer hospitalizations than their physician counterparts

While costs per NP visit were lower, the investigators noted this finding was confounded by salary differentials between NPs and physicians. Though small, effect sizes demonstrated statistically significant findings indicating that for the variables listed, NP care was comparable or better than physician care.

CNMs, individuals educated in both nursing and midwifery, are considered to be well-qualified primary care providers for women and newborns.[95] In the CNM studies reported by Brown and Grimes,[95] only those in which CNMs and physicians had patients with comparable risks were compared. These nine studies demonstrated that CNMs[95]:

- Used less analgesia and intravenous fluids and performed less fetal monitoring, episiotomies, and forceps deliveries
- Induced labor less frequently than physicians
- Had patients who more often delivered in sites other than delivery rooms (process of care)
- Had infant outcomes (incidence of low birth weight, fetal distress, 1-minute Apgar scores, and neonatal mortality) comparable to their physician counterparts (clinical outcomes)
- Had shorter hospital lengths of stay and more postpartum visits than their physician counterparts

CNMs and physicians differed most in the process-of-care variables, reflecting the midwives' tendency to provide less technology-oriented care.

Critics of these three reports cite lack of control for differences in the complexity of patients managed by physicians and NPs-CNMs. However, Brown and Grimes, who selected for analysis only those randomized clinical trials where patient complexity was comparable for NPs and physicians, still found results indicating that NP-CNM care is comparable or superior to that of physicians.

Nurse practitioners can provide 80% to 90% of the services provided by physicians. Because the cost of educating NPs and CNMs is approximately 20% to 25% less than the cost of educating physicians, these two types of APRNs were determined to be economical sources for primary care providers.[96] In a more recent study of NP and physician practice, Mundinger [97] reported outcomes from a study of NPs in primary care settings. Patients who received care from either a physician or an NP reported the same level of satisfaction and had the same health outcomes. This study is important because it was a prospective study of NP outcomes in a practice where NPs had the same authority, responsibility, and type of patient population as physicians in comparable practice settings.

Acute Care Studies

Studies on the practice of ACNPs have focused not only on quality-of-care issues but also on evaluating their autonomy in an acute care setting as well as cost-reduction strategies. In a systematic review of the literature by Kleinpell, Ely, and Grabenkort,[98] they identified only two randomized control trials on the impact of PAs and NPs in acute and critical care settings. This low level of evidence demonstrates the need for further research in this area.

Previous work by Almost and Laschinger[99] had endorsed the fact that primary care NPs had more collaborative practice within their work environment, which resulted in a higher degree of autonomy and less job strain. More recently, Cajulis and Fitzpatrick[100] sought to describe the level of autonomy of 54 ACNPs in a variety of specialty areas in a large metropolitan hospital. The results of the study revealed that NPs working in specialized settings in an acute care environment practiced with a high level of autonomy, with over half the sample indicating very high levels of empowerment. The extent of empowerment did not, however, equate to certain practice patterns, and the ACNPs did not have admitting privileges, nor were they reimbursed for their services at this particular institution.

In a multicenter survey of 74 NPs working in a pediatric intensive care or step-down unit, Verger and colleagues[101] attempted to describe the evolution of the pediatric acute care NP role since its introduction almost 15 years earlier. Although all respondents to the survey had undergone master's-level education, only 54% had received academic preparation in pediatric critical or acute care. The remaining respondents were primary care PNPs, FNPs, and even one adult ACNP. Increased acuity in the pediatric critical care population supports the need for providing NPs who have the clinical expertise and skills to manage these patients and families. The survey results mirrored studies completed with adult acute care and NNPs describing clinical practice, research, and role development.

Policy Issues Influencing Advanced Practice in Emerging Care Systems

Policy issues in advanced practice nursing systems include barriers to advanced practice in primary care settings (the regulation of advanced nursing practice, prescriptive authority for APRNs, reimbursement of APRN services) and the need for a mix of providers for a primary care system that meets the needs of target populations, uses providers' skills and services in the most efficient and cost-effective way, and provides incentives for interdisciplinary practice teams.

Barriers to Advanced Practice in Primary Care

Given that NP and CNM outcomes are comparable to physician outcomes, the lower health-care education and delivery costs associated with APRNs should result in more APRNs in primary care settings. Yet advanced nursing practice continues to face professional barriers. Despite the increased number of nurses completing programs preparing them for primary care practice, the number of APRNs actively involved in practice is far smaller. Safriet[5] identified three major barriers to advanced nursing practice in primary care settings: regulation of advanced practice nursing, prescriptive authority for APRNs, and reimbursement for APRN services.

REGULATION OF ADVANCED NURSING PRACTICE

Every state has licensing laws designed to protect the public. State practice acts govern the nature and scope of the services of physicians, nurses, and other health professionals. Physicians were the first practitioners to receive legislative approval for their activities, and state medical practice acts are all-encompassing in reserving for physicians the legal right to diagnose, prescribe, treat, and cure health problems. Because medical practice acts deny these functions to anyone not licensed as a physician, other health professionals seeking to perform these functions are compelled to negotiate changes in their own practice acts to include diagnosis, prescriptive, and curative functions.[102,103]

PRESCRIPTIVE AUTHORITY FOR ADVANCED PRACTICE REGISTERED NURSES

The ability to prescribe drugs and therapeutic agents is a second requisite for comprehensive primary care. In the past, APRNs used numerous strategies to prescribe medications in primary care settings, even in the absence of legal authority. These included choosing a medication for a patient and then having a physician write and sign a prescription, using a physician's name to call in a prescription to a pharmacy, cosigning (with a physician) a prescription, and using written protocols to allow the nurse to prescribe medications with the type and dosage determined by formulary. Although these strategies enabled APRNs to manage medication regimens, APRNs became, as a result, "hidden" providers of this important primary care service. Throughout recent years, the ability of APRNs to have some level of prescriptive authority has increased, including the right to prescribe controlled substances. Only two U.S. states,* Alabama and Florida, do not allow APRNs to prescribe controlled substances.* However, 38 states still require some degree of physician involvement or delegation in writing prescriptions.[104,105]

REIMBURSEMENT FOR APRNS' SERVICES

Perhaps the greatest barrier to advanced nursing practice in primary care settings has been the uneven success nurses have experienced in receiving reimbursement for their services. Because reimbursement decisions rest almost exclusively with states (where third-party insurers are regulated), the issue of reimbursement for APRNs' services depends on individual state statutes. Where state statutes permit reimbursement for APRNs' services, Medicaid-approved nurse provider rates range from 60% to 100% of what physicians are paid for the same services.[104–107]

Removing Barriers to Advanced Practice

Progress on resolving these three barriers to primary practice by APRNs has been slow. Using economic projection techniques, in the early 1990s Nichols[105] estimated that barriers to practice, which prevented APRNs from providing the full range of services they are educated to provide, cost the nation $9 billion annually, or much more in today's economy. Progress in achieving legislative authority in all 50 states and the District of Columbia to allow APRNs to perform the functions they are educated to provide has been slow but successful.[104]

In a study of practice barriers among a sample of practicing California NPs,[103] those reporting the greatest barriers were NPs whose practices addressed the needs of underserved

---

* Legislation allowing prescription of controlled substances was passed in Missouri; regulations are being promulgated.

populations (prisoners, psychiatric patients, rural communities), thus documenting the fact that advanced nursing practice barriers continue to limit access for those groups who can least afford the denial of primary health care. Removal of practice barriers is necessary if APRNs are to be major providers of primary care in the future. In a 1994 report, the Pew Health Professions Commission[106] specifically called for removal of barriers to the expansion of NP practice. In its 1995 report, the commission called for changes in the regulatory system for the health professions to permit standardized regulation, where appropriate, to support optimal access to a competent workforce.[107] The 1998 Pew report focused on preparing advanced practice nursing to translate a core set of skills across diverse practice settings and to manage persons with healthcare problems regardless of their location.[11]

The Balanced Budget Act of 1997 had a significant impact on the reimbursement of ACNPs by allowing them to bill for direct care provided to hospitalized Medicare patients.[108] Previously, APRN services were only reimbursed if provided in a rural area or within a skilled nursing facility. This opportunity to be directly reimbursed for care delivered also posed challenges to NPs to learn the complex system of Medicare billing for inpatient care. Documentation of inpatient NP services allows for measurement of productivity and quality of care. Both of these factors elevate the professional worth of the NP and demonstrate the impact of care to patients and to other health professionals as well as policy makers. In early 2009, the Medicaid Advanced Practice Nurses and Physician Assistants Access Act was introduced in Congress requesting removal of language from the Balanced Budget Act of 1997 that required states to "determine whether they wished to recognize NPs, nurse-midwives and PAs as primary care providers in the Medicaid managed care primary care provider system."[109] As of January 6, 2009, this bill was introduced and then referred to the Committee on Finance (http://www.govtrack.us/congress/bill.xpd?bill=s111-63).

Another factor that has had a significant impact on the increasing importance of APRNs billing separately for their services is the reduction in work hours for medical residents. Many institutions are using APRNs as care providers to fill in the gap this has created. As patient acuity increases so does the demand for healthcare providers who can function as part of an interdisciplinary team with positive outcomes.[110] The previously mentioned complexity of inpatient billing practices forces hospitals to look at implementing models that provide the most significant impact on patient outcomes as well as generate revenue.[110]

The Need for a Mix of Providers in Primary Healthcare Systems

Health care over the life span requires services ranging from health promotion and disease prevention to management of chronic or life-threatening illness to end-stage, palliative care. This broad range of services cannot likely be delivered by a single health professional. Thus, a major issue for future primary healthcare systems is creating an ideal mix of interprofessional providers to provide the broadest range of needed services with the greatest economy.

The value of interprofessional teams is often praised in the literature.[111–115] According to the Pew Commission,[107] interprofessional collaborative practice is necessary for integrated clinical care. It requires providers conversant in team concepts who can respectfully engage in open communication with other team members. Practice situations that favor collaborative teamwork are those characterized by situational complexity requiring more than one set of skills, clinical knowledge too great for one clinician to possess, and team members willing to sacrifice some degree of autonomy in order to achieve the best quality of care. Despite the philosophical support for team practice, there is little literature on organizing the most efficient and effective team of healthcare clinicians. At least three factors will likely influence the mix of team providers for emerging primary care systems:

1. The needs of the target population
2. The provider's skills and services
3. Incentives for interprofessional practice teams

THE NEEDS OF THE TARGET POPULATION

The characteristics of the target population to be served by a primary care system are a decisive factor in developing a mix of providers. For example, communities with a high proportion of families with school-age children will need a group of primary care providers with a set of skills and services different from those of communities with a large proportion of retired senior citizens. Primary care systems that serve homeless people would need to have providers with skills in managing chronic and infectious diseases and in finding and using social services. Farm communities would require a primary care system of providers skilled in accident prevention and management and controlling occupational toxic exposures. The skill base and expertise of providers in a primary care setting must vary depending on the target population's needs.

The acute care system is also evolving in terms of both its mix of providers as well as models of delivering care. The target population's characteristics include an aging population with multiple chronic illnesses. The level of care required for these older adults posthospitalization may include rehabilitation, skilled nursing care, or home care. Technological advances and market pressures have also impacted acuity of hospitalized patients by discharging them to the outpatient area more quickly, thereby increasing the acuity level of those in the inpatient settings.[11] In addition to the previously mentioned hospitalist model, Ettner and colleagues evaluated a multidisciplinary doctor-nurse practitioner (MDNP) model that focused on maintaining quality and continuity of care while reducing costs.[114] In the MDNP study, of the 1207 patients enrolled, 581 received the intervention and 626 received usual care. The NPs who provided the intervention used clinical guidelines to minimize redundancy of services, and the intervention group received weekly phone calls from the NPs to assess symptoms, medical compliance, and follow-up plans. A unique aspect of this study was that nonintervention services (rehospitalization and emergency department visits) were also calculated and evaluated at 30 days and 4 months postdischarge. The implications of these findings for the increasing utilization of ACNPs in the future are significant, and replication studies will be vital to supporting this type of model in nonacademic centers.

THE PROVIDER'S SKILLS AND SERVICES

There are three approaches to multiprofessional service delivery that have implications for APRNs who seek to practice in primary care systems:

Under a **provider-substitution model,** all providers in the setting offer the same set of services. Thus, APRNs, physicians, and PAs in the setting offer the same diagnostic, disease prevention, health promotion, and disease management services.

With a **supplemental model,** multiprofessional providers offer a core set of services, with each team member also offering supplemental services. Under this model, all APRNs, physicians, and PAs in a setting might provide first-contact services (taking a health history, performing diagnostic tests, and identifying the priority health problem). However, only the physician would manage patients diagnosed with chronic illnesses. The PA would manage acute illnesses and trauma, and the APRN would provide health promotion services.

Finally, in a **complementary model,** providers in a setting offer only those services for which they are uniquely prepared by education, experience, or legal statute. Using the complementary model for primary care services, the PA might do all initial, first-contact patient encounters, the physician might see patients with illnesses, and the APRN might provide health screening and disease prevention programs for individuals and families.

The decision to use a substitute, supplemental, or complementary model of provider practice in a setting will influence recruiting and employment decisions. Under a substitution model, the decision to employ APRNs, physicians, PAs, or other service providers would be influenced *only* by the availability and costs of employing those different types of providers. If there is an adequate and economical supply of physician generalists, exclusive focus on a physician substitution model may have negative connotations for APRNs who want to work in primary care settings. Under the provider supplement model, each provider offers the same core set of services plus a skill-specific service. However, in a system increasingly concerned with costs, the connotation that any provider's services are *supplemental* in nature could have negative implications for APRNs, unless the need for and cost justification of those services is successfully marketed to consumers. Settings driven by economical concerns may elect not to offer supplemental services. Exclusive emphasis on complementary services, such as those offered by physicians or by APRNs, increases the risk of fragmentation of services in a system already criticized for lack of service articulation. However, if complementary interprofessional practice is thoughtfully implemented, it can result in each provider offering those services for which they are qualified. Complementary interdependent team practice has great promise for primary care settings.

First introduced in 1967 by the American Academy of Pediatrics, the "medical home" is a concept of care delivery that continues to evolve but remains focused on a continuous comprehensive model of care.[115] By 2007, four professional medical organizations focusing on primary care—the American Academy of Family Physicians, the American Academy of Pediatrics, the American College of Physicians, and the American Osteopathic Association—released a statement on the Joint Principles of the Patient-Centered Medical Home.[115] Some of the primary tenets of this model of the patient-centered medical home include ease of access, whole-person care directed by a primary medical provider, and care coordinated across the healthcare system with quality and safety as hallmarks. APRNs have the clinical and professional skills to become part of this type of model of care. Because the broad range of needed primary care services cannot likely be provided by a single professional, the manner in which primary care systems conceptualize and implement service delivery has great implications for new APRNs who will enter practice in the next decade.

Table 5-4 summarizes advantages and disadvantages of each method of allocating skills and services among providers. Although proponents of emerging primary care systems emphasize the need for collaboration and service coordination, little attention has been given to mechanisms for articulating the services of multiprofessional providers. As changes in the healthcare system evolve, APRNs must be clear when marketing their services whether their skills and services substitute, supplement, or complement those services offered by other providers and on the costs and benefits and related quality outcomes of the services. The question remains, will APRNs have the chance to be the primary provider in a patient-centered medical home or, more appropriately, a patient-centered health home?

◦ INCENTIVES FOR INTERPROFESSIONAL PRACTICE TEAMS

Gatekeeping, patient ownership, and control of service delivery by selected professionals have been identified as deterrents to the delivery of economical primary care services. Efforts to limit patient access to the services of other providers are often seen in the "turf battles" regularly played out between medical specialists and generalists, between physicians and nurses, and between nurses and PAs. In its recommendations for the future education of all health professionals, the IOM concluded that future healthcare systems must have practitioners who are able to work effectively as team members in settings that emphasize "integrated services." The American College of Physicians (ACP) 2009 policy monograph on Nurse Practitioners in Primary Care[116] acknowledges the need for effective interprofessional collaboration in order to provide quality care. In order for this collaboration to be most effective, it must be efficient and timely. In an era of electronic health information it will be

Table 5-4 **Advantages and Disadvantages of Substitutive, Supplemental, And Complementary Service Delivery In Primary Care**

Provider Services	Potential Advantages	Potential Disadvantages
Substitutive: multidisciplinary providers who offer the same services	Standardization of services offered Reimbursement tied to services, not to discipline of provider	Provider competition Little or no collaborative, interdependent team practice
Supplemental: multidisciplinary providers who offer a core set of services, plus additional, or supplemental, services	Standardization of core set of services offered Utilization of unique practice strengths of multidisciplinary providers for supplemental services	Services of some providers considered supplemental "extras" Collaborative, interdependent team practice around supplemental services only
Complementary: multidisciplinary providers, who offer different services	Utilization of interdependent collaborative practice to offer coordinated, comprehensive services Utilization of unique practice strengths of multidisciplinary providers	Potential fragmentation in service delivery Lack of service coordination

vital to ensure there is an infrastructure to support these technologies in primary care practices in all regions. In addition, demonstrating successful interprofessional collaboration must be initiated in the academic setting, both didactic and clinical, in order for it to be sustained in clinical practice [112, 117]

However, current organizational and service reimbursement characteristics serve as strong disincentives to the development of interprofessional teams. Academic health centers, considered by many health policy planners to represent the best hope for the practice education of future primary care providers, continue to emphasize the separate education of physicians, nurses, pharmacists, and other health professionals.[113, 114] Healthcare delivery models continue to emphasize the compartmentalization of services, organized around the single provider-patient encounter. Existing reimbursement patterns continue to be based on reimbursement of a single provider without considering the unique skills and services of different providers or the specific health needs of individuals and families.[104,106,110,115]

Because existing professional education models continue to favor one-on-one provider-patient relationships, the development of productive interprofessional team practices for primary care will require the redesign of the education of health professionals as well as service delivery and reimbursement models. A novel approach to changing the behavior of practicing clinicians is one proposed by Scheffler, an economist.[111] He suggests that financial incentives be offered to primary care teams who will work together to enhance the quality of care. Changes in reimbursement patterns that promote team-practice reimbursement must occur as well. The broad-scale implementation of patient-centered health homes may provide the necessary shift in these relationships and encourage interprofessional academic preparation. The 2009 ACP policy statement[116] also suggested that an NP-led, patient-centered "medical" home should be evaluated and subject to the same standards of recognition and evaluation as physician-led practices. In addition, it recommended that payments for both models be based on differences in the case mix of patients seen.

Policies related to healthcare reform continue to lag behind the ever-changing needs of the patients in our healthcare system.

Summary

The continuing turmoil in health care, sweeping changes in funding and reimbursement, growing dissatisfaction and crisis in managed care, decreasing number of available physician residency positions, and decreasing numbers of physicians selecting primary care practice have led to growing opportunities for APRNs in both acute and primary care.[91,101,108] These opportunities have led to the emergence and resurgence of APRN roles in acute and critical care settings, including the NNP, adult ACNP, pediatric ACNP, and pediatric and adult acute care CNS. The future holds tremendous potential for these acute care NP and CNS roles in terms of addressing many of the current problems that plague the healthcare delivery system.

Providing high-quality, hospital-based care through a permanent team of health-care providers who view the patient, family, and community in a holistic manner will be the task undertaken by the evolving APRN cohort. As the population ages, NPs and CNSs will play even larger roles in the care of patients with multiple, complex problems across the life span. Improvements in quality of care, patient outcomes, and patient satisfaction are key aspects of APRN care in all settings, including the acute care setting. Therefore, future opportunities for APRNs in specialty and acute care settings have the potential for unlimited growth as advanced practice nursing meets the patient care challenges of today's healthcare system.

High-quality healthcare systems are those that provide accessible, economical, and effective services to specific target populations. Spiraling costs and consumer dissatisfaction with unequal access and fragmented services have generated renewed interest in primary care systems and primary care providers. The most recent IOM definition of primary care manifests the wide-ranging expectation that the primary care system of the future must be staffed by generalists who are capable of providing comprehensive, holistic care that addresses a wide range of individual and family health problems.

Because no single provider can be expected to possess the knowledge and skills to address the complete range of episodic and chronic health problems commonly experienced across the life span, multiprofessional team practice is a necessity. This interprofessional team approach must include a group of professionals who have received the academic preparation to be able to collaborate successfully in a patient-centered care model. Whether the future primary care systems achieve their expected goals of first-contact, longitudinal, and coordinated and comprehensive care, will depend, to a great extent, on whether interprofessional practice teams successfully collaborate in balancing substitutive, supplemental, and complementary services for target populations. The purpose of this chapter has been to explore the social, political, and economic issues that will facilitate or inhibit the participation of APRNs in these future practice endeavors.

SUGGESTED LEARNING EXERCISES

1. Analyze the nurse practice act in the state in which you intend to practice. How might nurses work to amend the state nurse-practice act to allow APRNs to better meet the primary care and acute care needs of underserved and unserved population groups in the state? In the United States?

2. What do you believe is the ideal provider mix for an interprofessional team in primary care and in acute care? Design an interprofessional team to meet the primary care needs in your community.

3. Discuss incentives for developing and supporting multiprofessional practice teams in an acute care setting.

4. Design a hospitalist, interprofessional team for one service in a community hospital. Explain your rationale.

5. How might health policy planners ensure an adequate supply of advanced practice providers for both the acute and primary care settings for the next decade?

6. Which model of practice do you believe offers the greatest opportunity for the APRN in non-primary care settings? Justify your answer.

7. Discuss the differences in the ACNP and critical care CNS roles.

8. Prepare a presentation to be made to a physician group practice explaining the positive impact an APRN can have on patient care outcomes and the practice as a whole.

References

1. Towers, J. (2003). NP practice in 2012. *JAANP* 15:12.

2. Starfield, B. (1993). Roles and functions of non-physician practitioners in primary care. In Clawson, D, and Osterwels, M (eds), *The Role of Physician Assistants and Nurse Practitioners in Primary Care.* Association of Academic Health Centers, Washington, DC.

3. World Health Organization. (1978). *Primary Health Care.* Geneva, Switzerland.

4. Franks, P, Nutting, P, and Clancy, C. (1993). Health care reform, primary care, and the need for research. *Acad Med* 270:1449.

5. Safriet, B. (1992). Health care dollars and regulatory sense: The role of advanced practice nursing. *Yale J Regulation* 9:417.

6. American Nurses Association. (1991). *Nursing's Agenda for Health Care Reform.* American Nurses' Association, Washington, DC.

7. Pew Health Professions Commission. (1991). *Healthy America: Practitioners for 2005.* Pew Health Professions Commission, San Francisco, CA.

8. Council on Graduate Medical Education. (1992). *Third Report: Improving Access to Health Care through Physician Workforce Reform: Directions for the 21st Century.* U.S. Department of Health and Human Services, Washington, DC.

9. Public Health Service. (1993*). Health Professions Report.* U.S. Department of Health and Human Services, Washington, DC.

10. The Alliance for Health Reform. (1993). *A Primary Care Primer.* The Alliance for Health Reform, Washington, DC.

11. Pew Health Professions Commission. (1998). *Recreating Health Professional Practice for a New Century: The Fourth Report of the Pew Health Professions Commission.* San Francisco, CA.

12. White, K. (1967). Primary medical care for families. *N Engl J Med* 277:847.

13. Alpert, J, and Charney, E. (1973). *The Education of Physicians for Primary Care.* U.S. Department of Health, Education and Welfare, Public Health Service, Health Resources Administration, Rockville, MD. HRA publication 74–3113.

14. Institute of Medicine. (1978). *Report of a Study: A Manpower Policy for Primary Health Care.* National Academy of Science, Washington, DC.

15. Golden, A. (1982). A definition of primary care for educational purposes. In Golden, A, Carlson, D, and Hagan, J (eds), *The Art of Teaching Primary Care.* Springer, New York.

16. Starfield, B. (1992). *Primary Care: Concept, Evaluation and Policy.* Oxford University Press, New York.

17. Institute of Medicine. (1994). *Defining Primary Care: An Interim Report.* National Academy Press, Washington, DC.

18. Showstack, J, Rothman, A, and Hassmiller, S. (2003). Primary care at a crossroads. *Ann Intern Med* 138:242.

19. Showstack, J, Lurie, N, Larson, E, Rothman, A, and Hassmiller, S. (2003). Primary care: The next renaissance. *Ann Intern Med* 138:268.

20. Premier Hospital Quality Incentive Demonstration: Rewarding Superior Quality Care, June 2008. Can be accessed at http://www.cms.hhs.gov/HospitalQualityInits/Downloads/HospitalPremier FactSheet200806.pdf.

21. National Medical Care Survey Data. (2000). Can be accessed at http://www.cdc.gov/nchs/about/major/ahcd/ambucare.htm.

22. Avorn, J, Everitt, D, and Baker, M. (1991). The neglected medical history and therapeutic choices for abdominal pain. *Arch Intern Med* 151:694.

23. Dahle, K, et al. (1998). Impact of a nurse practitioner on the cost of managing inpatients with heart failure. *Am. J of Cardiol* 82(5), 686.

24. Safran, D, Tarlov, A, and Rogers, W. (1994). Primary care performance in fee-for-service and prepaid health care systems. *JAMA* 271:1579.

25. APRN Consensus Work Group & National Council of State Boards of Nursing APRN Advisory Committee. (2008). Consensus Model for APRN Regulation: Licensure, Accreditation, Certification & Education. Can be accessed at http://www.aacn.nche.edu/education/pdf/APRNReport.pdf.

26. American Nurses Association. (1996). *Scope and Standards of Advanced Practice Nursing,* Washington, DC.

27. Rivo, M, and Satcher, D. (1993). Improving access to health care through physician workforce reform. *JAMA* 270:1074.

28. Cooper, R, Getzen, T, McKee, H, and Laud, P. (2002). Economic and demographic trends signal an impending physician shortage. *Health Affairs* 21(1):140–154.

29. Phillips, R, Jr., Dodoo, M, Jaen, C, and Green, L. (2005). COGME's 16th Report to Congress: Too Many Physicians Could Be Worse Than Wasted. *Ann Fam Med* 3:268.

30. Council on Graduate Medical Education. (2005). COGME Physician Workforce Policy Guidelines for the U.S. for 2000–2020. U.S. Department of Health and Human Services, Rockville, MD.

31. McClellan, M. (2008). Advisory Council for the American Academy of Nursing Raise the Voice Campaign.

32. Barnett, P, and Midtling, J. (1989). Public policy and the supply of primary care physicians. *JAMA* 262:2864.

33. Kassebaum, D, Szenas, P, and Ruffin, A. (1993). The declining interest of medical school graduates in generalist specialties: students abandonment of earlier inclinations. *Acad Med* 68:278.

34. Levinsky, N. (1993). Recruiting for primary care. *N Engl J Med* 328:656.

35. Sandy, L, and Schroeder, S. (2003). Primary care in a new era: Disillusion and dissolution? *Ann Intern Med* 138:262–267.

36. Hauer, K, Durning, S, Kernan, W, Fagan, M, Mintz, M, O'Sullivan, P, et al. (2008). Factors associated with medical students' career choices regarding internal medicine. *JAMA* 300(10):1154–1164.

37. Christensen, C, Bohmer, R, and Kenagy, J. (2002). Will disruptive innovations cure health care? *Harvard Business Review* 78:102–112, 199.

38. Fowkes, V. (1993). Meeting the needs of the underserved: The roles of physician assistant and nurse practitioners. In Clawson, D, and Osterweis, M (eds), *The Role of Physician Assistants and Nurse Practitioners in Primary Care.* Association of Academic Health Centers, Washington, DC.

39. Jones, P, and Cawley, J. (1994). Physician assistants and health system reform: Clinical capabilities, practice activities, and potential roles. *JAMA* 272:725.

40. American Academy of Physician Assistants. Accessed at www.aapa.org/research.

41. Hooker, R. (1993). The role of physician assistants and nurse practitioners in a managed organization. In Clawson, D, and Osterweis, M (eds), *The Role of Physician Assistants and Nurse Practitioners in Primary Care.* Association of Academic Health Centers, Washington, DC.

42. Cawley, J. (1993). Physician assistants in the health care workforce. In Clawson, D, and Osterweis, M (eds), *The Role of Physician Assistants and Nurse Practitioners in Primary Care.* Association of Academic Health Centers, Washington, DC.

43. Regan, D, and Harbert, K. (1991). Measuring the financial productivity of physician assistants. *Med Group Manage J* 38(6):46.

44. Cooper, R. (2007). New directions for nurse practitioners and physician assistants in the era of physician shortages. *Acadc Med* 82(9):827–828.

45. Dial, T, Palsbo, S, Bergsten, C, Gabel, J, and Weiner, J. (1995). Clinical staffing in staff- and group-model HMOs. *Health Affairs* 14:168.

46. Ford, L. (1983). Practice perspectives in primary care: Nursing. In Miller, R (ed), *Primary Health Care: More Than Medicine*. Prentice-Hall, Englewood Cliffs, NJ.

47. Health Resources and Services Administration. (2004). *The Registered Nurse Population: Findings from the March 2004 National Sample Survey of Registered Nurses*. Can be accessed at http://bhpr.hrsa.gov/healthworkforce/rnsurvey04/tables.htm.

48. Berlin, L, Stennet, J, and Bednash, G. (2003). *2002–2003 Enrollment and Graduations in Baccalaureate and Graduate Programs in Nursing*. American Association of Colleges of Nursing, Washington, DC.

49. Fang, D, Tracy, C, and Bednash, G. (2009). *2008–2009 Enrollment and Graduations in Baccalaureate and Graduate Programs in Nursing*. American Association of Colleges of Nursing, Washington, DC.

50. National Organization of Nurse Practitioner Faculties Curriculum Guidelines Task Force (NONPF). (1995). *Advanced Nursing Practice: Curriculum Guidelines and Program Standards for Nurse Practitioner Education*. NONPF, Washington, DC.

51. Booth, R. (1994). Leadership challenges for nurse practitioner faculty. Keynote address presented at the Twentieth Annual Conference of the National Organization of Nurse Practitioner Faculties, Portland, OR.

52. Genet, C, et al. (1995). Nurse practitioners in a teaching hospital. *Nurse Pract* 20:47.

53. Goskel, D, Harrison, C, Morrison, R, and Miller, S. (1993). Description of a nurse practitioner inpatient service in a public teaching hospital. *J Gen Intern Med* 8:29.

54. Bankert, M. (1989). *Watchful Care: A History of America's Nurse Anesthetists*. Continuum, New York.

55. Varney, H. (1997). *Varney's Midwifery*, 3rd ed. Jones and Bartlett, Sudbury, MA.

56. Reiter, F. (1966). The nurse-clinician. *A J Nurs* 66:274.

57. Sheehy, C, and McCarthy, M. (1998). *Advanced Practice Nursing—Emphasizing Common Roles*. F.A Davis, Philadelphia.

58. Johnson, P. (2002). The history of the neonatal nurse practitioner: Reflections from "under the looking glass." *Neonatal Network* 21:51.

58a. Bellflower, B, and Carter, M. (2006). Primer on the Practice Doctorate for Neonatal Nurse Practitioners. *Advances in Neonatal Care* 6:6.

59. National Association of Neonatal Nurses. (2001). *Position Statement on Advanced Practice Neonatal Nurse Role*. NANN, Petaluma, CA.

60. Mick, D, and Ackerman, M. (2000). Advance practice nursing role delineation in acute and critical care: Application of the strong model of advanced practice. *Heart and Lung: The Acute and Crit Care* 29:210.

61. Daly, B. (1997). *Acute Care Nurse Practitioner*. Springer Publishing Co., New York.

62. American Nurses Association and the American Association of Critical Care Nurses. (1995). *Standards of Clinical Practice and Scope of Practice for the Acute Care Nurse Practitioner*. Washington, DC.

63. Parinello, K. (1995). Advanced practice nursing. *Crit Care Nursing Clinics of North Amer* 7:9.

64. Spisso, J, O'Callaghan, C, McKennan, M, and Holcroft, J. (1990). Improved quality care and reduction of housestaff workload using trauma nurse practitioners. *J of Trauma* 30:660.

65. Ingersoll, G. (1995). Evaluation of the advanced practice nurse role in acute and specialty care. *Crit Care Nurs Clinics of North Amer* 7:25.

66. Kindig, D, and Libby, D. (1994). How will graduate medical education reform affect specialties and geographic areas? *JAMA* 272:37.

67. Kelso, L, and Massaro, L. (1994). Implementation of the acute care nurse practitioner role. *AACN Clin Issues* 5:404.

68. Kleinpell, R. (1997). The acute care nurse practitioner: An expanding opportunity for critical care nurses. *Critical Care Nurse* 17:66.

69. Knaus, V, Felton, S, Burton, S, Fobes, P, and Davis, K. (1997). The use of nurse practitioners in acute care settings. *J Nurs Admin* 27:20.

70. Hicks, G. (1998). Cardiac surgery and the acute care nurse practitioner—"the perfect link." *Heart and Lung: The J Acute and Crit Care* 27:283.

71. Shah, S, Bruttomesso, K, Sullivan, D, and Lattanzio, J. (1997). An evaluation of the role and practices of the acute-care nurse practitioner. *AACN Clin Issues* 8:147.

72. Rudisill, P. (1995). Unit-based advanced practice nurse in critical care. *Crit Care Nurse Clinics North Amer* 7:1.

73. Whitcomb, R, Wilson, S, Chang-Dawkins, S, Durand, J, Pitcher, D, Lauzon, C, and Aleman, D. (2002). Advanced practice nursing: Acute care model in progress. *J Nurs Admin* 32:123.

74. Zaidel, L. (2003). Acute care NPs: What does the future hold? *The Nurse Practitioner Journal.*

75. Kleinpell, R. (1998) Reports of role descriptions of acute care nurse practitioners. *AACN Clin Issues* 9:290.

76. Richmond, T, and Keane, A. (1992). The nurse practitioner in tertiary care. *J Nurs Admin* 22:11.

77. Gates, S. (1993). Continuity of care: The orthopaedic nurse practitioner in tertiary care. *Orthopaedic Nursing* 12:48.

78. Urban, N. (1997). Managed care challenges and opportunities for cardiovascular advanced practice nurses. *AACN Clin Issues* 8:78.

79. National Association of Clinical Nurse Specialists. (2003). NACNS position paper: Regulatory credentialing of clinical nurse specialists. *Clinical Nurse Specialist* 17:3.

80. Sole, M, Hunkar-Huie, A, Schille, J, and Cheatham, M. (2001). Comprehensive trauma patient care by nonphysician providers. *AACN Clin Issues* 12:438.

81. Buchanan, L. (1996). The acute care nurse practitioner in collaborative practice. *Journal of the Academy of Nurse Practitioners* 8:13.

82. Martin, B, and Coniglio, J. (1996). The acute care nurse practitioner in collaborative practice. *AACN Clin Isssues* 7:309.

83. Martin, R. (1999). Organ transplantation: The role of the acute care nurse practitioner across the spectrum of health care. *AACN Clin Issues* 10:285.

84. Kleinpell, R, and Gawlinski, A. (2005). Assessing outcomes in advanced practice. AACN clinical issues: advanced practice in acute & critical care. *Advanced Practice Nursing* 16(1):43–57.

85. McMullen, M, et al. (2001). Dimensions of Critical Care Nursing, "Evaluating a nurse practitioner service. The use of quality indicators and evidence-based practice."

86. Ewart, G, Marcus, L, Gaba, M, Bradner, R, Medina, J, and Chandler, E. (2004). The critical care medicine crisis: A call for federal action. A white paper from the Critical Care Professional Societies. *Chest* 125:1518–1521.

87. Larkin, H. (2003). The case for nurse practitioners: Used correctly, they can improve outcomes, lower costs and make up for reduced residents' hours. *Hospital & Health Networks* 77(8):54–56, 58.

88. Wachter, R, and Goldman, L. (1996). The emerging role of "hospitalist" in the American hospital system. *N Eng J Med* 335:7.

89. Howie, J, and Erickson, M. (2002). Acute care nurse practitioners: Creating and implementing a model of care for an inpatient general medicine service. *Amer J Crit Care* 11:448.

90. Wolfe, S. (2000) Hospitalists. Good news or bad news for nurses? *RN* 63:3.

91. Diamond, H, Goldberg, E, and Janosky, J. (1992). The effect of full-time faculty hospitalist on the efficiency of care at a community teaching hospital. *Ann Intern Med* 129:3.

92. Moore, G, and Showstack, J. (2003). Primary care medicine in crisis: Toward reconstruction and renewal. *Ann Intern Med* 138(3):244.

93. Congress and Office of Technology Assessment. (1986). *Nurse Practitioners, Physician Assistants and Certified Nurse Midwives: A Policy Analysis.* U.S. Government Printing Office, OTA-HCS publication, Washington, DC.

94. Crosby, F, Ventura, M, and Feldman, M. (1987). Future research recommendations for establishing NP effectiveness. *Nurse Pract* 12:75.

95. Brown, S, and Grimes, D. (1992). *Executive Summary: A Meta-Analysis of Process of Care, Clinical Outcomes, and Cost-Effectiveness of Nurses in Primary Care Roles: Nurse Practitioners and Nurse-Midwives.* University of Texas, Houston.

96. American College of Nurse-Midwives. (1992). *Position Statement.* American College of Nurse-Midwives, Washington, DC.

97. Mundinger, M, et al. (2000). Primary care outcomes in patients treated by nurse practitioners or physicians: A randomized trial. *JAMA* 283(1):59.

98. Kleinpell, R, Ely, E, and Grabenkort, R. (2008). Nurse practitioners and physician assistants in the intensive care unit: an evidence-based review. *Crit Care Med* 36:2888–2897.

99. Almost, J, and Laschinger, H. (2002). Workplace empowerment, collaborative work relationship and job strain nurse practitioners. *Journal of the American Academy of Nurse Practitioners* 14(9):408–420.

100. Cajulis, C, and Fitzpatrick, J. (2007). Levels of autonomy of nurse practitioners in an acute care setting. *Journal of the American Academy of Nurse Practitioners* 19:500.

101. Verger, J, Marcoux, K, Madden, M, Bojko, T, and Barnsteiner, J. (2005). Nurse practitioners in pediatric critical care: Results of a national survey. *AACN Clin Issues* 16(3):396–408.

102. Phillips, S. (2008). Legislative update: After 20 years, APNs are still standing together. *The NP* 33(1):10–34.

103. Anderson, A, Gilliss, C, and Yoder, L. (2006). Practice environment for nurse practitioners in California: Identifying barriers. *West J Med* 165(3):209.

104. Pearson, L. (2009). Pearson Report. *The American Journal for Nurse Practitioners* 13(2). Can be accessed at http://www.webnp.net/downloads/pearson_report09/pearson09_maryland-nhampshire.pdf.

105. Nichols, L. (1992). Estimating costs of underusing advanced practice nurses. *Nursing Economics* 10:343.

106. Pew Health Professions Commission. (1994). Nurse practitioners: Doubling the graduates by the year 2000. In *Commission Policy Papers.* Pew Health Professions Commission, San Francisco.

107. Pew Health Professions Commission. (1995). *Critical Challenges: Revitalizing the Health Professions for the Twenty-First Century.* Pew Health Professions Commission, San Francisco.

108. Richmond, T, Thompson, H, and Sullivan-Marx, E. (2000). Reimbursement for acute care nurse practitioner services. *American Journal of Critical Care.* 9(1):52–61.

109. American College of Physicians. (2009). Nurse practitioners in primary care. Policy Monograph. American College of Physicians, Philadelphia.

110. Ellis, E, Mackey, T, Buppert, C, and Klingensmith, K. (2008). Acute care nurse practitioner billing model development. *Clinical Scholars Review* 1(2):125–128.

111. Scheffler, R. (1996). Life in the kaleidoscope: The impact of managed care on the US health care work force and a new model for the delivery of primary care. In Institute of Medicine (Donaldson, M, Yordy, K, Lohr, K, and Vanselow, N, eds), *Primary Care: America's Health in a New Era.* National Academy Press, Washington, DC, pp. 312–340.

112. Grumbach, K, and Bodenheimer, T. (2004). Can health care teams improve primary care practice? *JAMA*, 291:1246–1251.

113. Low, D. (1994). Commentary. In Larson, P, Osterweis, M, and Rubin, E (eds), *Health Workforce Issues in the 21st Century*. Association of Academic Health Centers, Washington, DC.

114. Ettner, S, Kotlerman, J, Afifi, A, Vazirani, S, Hays, R, Shapiro, M, and Cowan, M. (2006). An alternative to reducing the costs of patient care? A controlled trial of the multi-disciplinary doctor-nurse practitioner (MDNP) model. *Medical Decision Making 9–17.*

115. American Academy of Family Physicians (AAFP), American Academy of Pediatrics (AAP), American College of Physicians (ACP), and American Osteopathic Association (AOA). (2007). *Joint Principles of the Patient-Centered Medical Home.*

116. American College of Physicians. (2009). *Nurse Practitioners in Primary Care.* American College of Physicians Policy Monograph, Philadelphia.

117. American Association of Colleges of Nursing and Association of American Medical Colleges. (2010). Lifelong learning: A report of an expert panel. Washington, DC: Author

Geraldine "Polly" Bednash was appointed Chief Executive Officer and Executive Director of the American Association of Colleges of Nursing (AACN) in December 1989. Dr. Bednash oversees the educational, research, governmental affairs, research and data bank, publications, and other programs of the only national organization dedicated exclusively to furthering nursing education in America's universities and 4-year colleges. From 1986 to 1989, Dr. Bednash headed the association's legislative and regulatory advocacy programs as director of government affairs. Dr. Bednash currently serves as a member of the Organizational Affiliates Council of the Association of Academic Health Centers. Her publications and research presentations cover a range of critical issues in nursing education, nursing research, clinical practice, and legislative policy. Before joining the AACN, Dr. Bednash was assistant professor at the School of Nursing at George Mason University and a Robert Wood Johnson Nurse Faculty Fellow in Primary Care at the University of Maryland. Her experience includes developing resource policy for the Geriatric Research, Evaluation, and Clinical Centers of the Veterans Administration and serving as nurse practitioner and consultant to the family practice residency program at DeWitt Army Hospital at Fort Belvoir, Virginia, and as an Army Nurse Corps (ANC) staff nurse in Vung Tau, Vietnam. Dr. Bednash received her bachelor's of science in nursing from Texas Woman's University, her master's of science in nursing from the Catholic University of America, and her doctorate from the University of Maryland. She is a fellow of the American Academy of Nursing and a member of Sigma Theta Tau.

Leo A. Le Bel is a retired ANC officer who received his anesthesia education at Walter Reed Army Medical Center and later served tours of duty in Vietnam, Europe, and various U.S. military posts. He now practices in Connecticut. Leo has held a variety of positions in both the military and civilian sectors, including clinical, administrative, and academic positions in hospitals ranging from rural community facilities to level-one trauma centers. He has been an independent anesthesia provider, consultant, and instructor in both clinical and didactic settings; director of two nurse anesthesia educational programs; and a staff member of the American Association of Nurse Anesthetists (AANA). He has served on two anesthesia journal editorial boards; published in various journals, textbooks, and trade publications; and been involved in clinical research. He has served as a committee member or officer in numerous local, state, and national professional organizations, including positions as an AANA Regional Director, as AANA Vice-President, and as a member of the AANA Foundation Board of Trustees. He is also co-owner of a Connecticut healthcare consulting company. Leo obtained his diploma in nursing in 1965 from a three-year, hospital-based program, his BSN degree from St. Anselm College (NH), his M.Ed. degree from Boston University, and his JD degree from Seattle University.

CHAPTER 6

Formulation and Approval of Credentialing and Clinical Privileges

Geraldine "Polly" Bednash, PhD, RN, FAAN; and Leo A. Le Bel, M.Ed, JD, APRN, CRNA

CHAPTER OBJECTIVES

After completing this chapter, the reader will be able to:

1. Analyze the roles played by education, accreditation, certification, and licensure in the regulation of advanced practice and the impact of the advanced practice registered nurse (APRN) consensus statement.

2. Engage in a dialogue regarding the issues surrounding regulation of the roles of APRNs.

3. Compare and contrast the scope of each of the four APRN roles authorized by the nurse practice act in the state in which an APRN intends to practice, including barriers to practice.

4. Discuss the differences between clinical and full staff privileges.

5. Contact a local hospital and obtain information and materials necessary for applying for clinical privileges.

Licensure, certification, and clinical privileges are all interwoven components of advanced nursing practice. Increasingly, licensure and certification of APRNs are being linked directly to other forms of regulation related to APRN education and the accreditation of APRN programs. Additionally, licensure and certification will be explicitly connected as elements of the regulatory processes that grant both the authority and the recognition for practice. Clinical privileges can be an obstacle or a pathway for extending practice and functioning as a comprehensive clinical provider. Unfortunately, acquiring national certification and state recognition to practice through licensure does not always automatically provide APRNs with the authority to acquire clinical privileges to practice in nursing homes, hospitals, clinics, and a variety of other settings. However, APRNs must be well versed in how to acquire these professional standings or to challenge barriers placed in their way.

This chapter discusses professional and public regulation of APRN practice, professional certification for APRNs, and clinical practice and institutional privileges for APRNs.

Regulation: Professional and Public

The regulation of APRN practice is accomplished in a variety of ways. Licensure, certification, and professional standards of practice represent variations on the regulation of practice. Each is structured on the basis of a different set of values to control safety and quality in practice.

External regulation can occur through licensure or certification of the individual practitioner. Licensure is a publicly controlled operation in which the state or governing authority sets minimum standards for safe practice. The individual must meet these standards in order to be granted the privilege of practicing in a particular jurisdiction.[1] Licensure is a public function that the Constitution delegates to the states and territories. Certification, on the other hand, is, in most instances, voluntarily sought by the professional. The professional agrees that certification has value and undergoes a process of testing to establish that the professional meets the standards developed by the certifying body, which is usually a nongovernmental and professionally monitored organization. In contrast to licensure, which validates the clinician's minimum level of competence, certification is usually designed as a mechanism for documenting that the clinician has achieved a higher level of competence and perhaps specialization.[2] However, APRN certification is playing an increasingly significant role in granting a license to practice as an APRN, and, thus, APRN certification exams have emerged as distinctly different types of certification exams given their use as a regulatory mechanism rather than solely as a mechanism for defining excellence.

Standards of practice are internally directed and professionally controlled. Professions such as nursing, medicine, law, and others engage in thoughtful deliberation regarding the standards that the profession must meet; they represent the profession's efforts to self-regulate.[1] Professional self-regulation provides accountability to the society served by the profession and acknowledges that the profession will engage in efforts to protect the public from either unscrupulous or unsafe practice. Professional nursing organizations, such as the American Nurses Association (ANA), the American College of Nurse-Midwives (ACNM), the American Association of Nurse Anesthetists (AANA), and others establish professional standards of practice through their collective members. These professional standards may be used as a mechanism for judging the practice of an individual APRN and may also serve as a measure of quality of practice in legal assessments of a clinician's capabilities.

For APRNs, public regulation and professional certification have become intertwined as employers and regulators increasingly seek APRNs to deliver safe, appropriate, and cost-effective care. Additionally, APRN education and the accreditation processes designed to ensure quality in the APRN educational process have undergone significant review as fundamentally important components of regulation. This chapter provides a comprehensive assessment of these issues in this period of rapid change. A focus on current issues in regulation, the confusion and lack of regulation standardization among the states, and emerging issues in the licensure process begin the discussion.

Current Issues in Regulation

The regulation of advanced practice nursing will be transformed significantly in the coming decade. A number of factors have led policy makers to question the appropriateness or adequacy of the current systems of regulation for APRNs, including regulatory barriers to practice, difficulties with interstate mobility, the lack of uniformity in public regulation of APRNs, and the increased confusion regarding advanced practice roles and specialties. In addition, growing concerns over the adequacy of the current workforce in the health professions have increased interest in expanding the numbers of APRNs and the roles they will play in what may become a dramatically reformed healthcare delivery system.

Over the past two decades, a number of commissions or advisory bodies have engaged in reviews of the entire spectrum of licensure and certification activities for health professionals.[3-5] The Pew Health Professions Commission report, *Reforming Health Care Workforce Regulation: Policy Considerations for the 21st Century*,[6] is one of the most comprehensive overviews of regulation in all the health professions. This review raised concerns regarding a number of regulatory issues that have affected, and will continue to affect, advanced practice in nursing. The Pew report was the result of a year-long review of public regulation systems and their usefulness in protecting the public. The commission task force recommended 10 reforms in regulatory systems (Table 6-1) and strongly urged their implementation in order to achieve standardized, accountable, flexible, effective, and efficient regulatory structures.

One issue reviewed by the Pew commissioners and others was the complex array of issues affecting access to health care. They identified a growing concern that the regulation of professional practice often decreases access to health care, rather than protects it. Regulations very often serve professional interests and are used to draw regulatory lines around practice domains and to limit the care activities in which professionals can "legally" engage. The authors of the Pew report recommended expansion of authority to practice based on clear standards of competence and safety, rather than on professionally designed boundaries to the scope of practice.

The Pew report provides an important backdrop to policy discussions regarding the current evolution of healthcare delivery. The report makes clear that the regulation of practice should be based on demonstrated competencies, not on the ability of one clinical group to draw territorial lines around a domain and proclaim dominance. APRNs, who have experienced limits on their practice that were either politically or professionally motivated, rather than factually based, have very widely supported this recommendation. More recently, policy makers and other health professionals have joined with nurses in their opposition to artificial barriers to full practice. As policy makers seek to address concerns over the growing costs of delivering healthcare services through reform of the current U.S. healthcare systems, these issues have become more prominent. This has enhanced the willingness of both employers and the public to seek care from APRNs and has fostered an interest in reconceptualizing how care is delivered and who is capable of delivering it.

Today, "bottom-line" concerns drive much of the decision making in health care and shape how healthcare professionals are used. These new dynamics have created a marked and growing demand for APRNs. The rapid growth of commercially based acute care clinics, such as the CVS pharmacy "Minute Clinics," designed to provide consumers quick access to high-quality primary care services, has become a powerful force in increasing the demand for one specific APRN provider—the family nurse practitioner. Additionally, an enhanced focus on the need for care coordination and expanded access to primary and acute care services has created strong interest in the important role APRNs can play in providing care. This awareness, coupled with the decreased interest in primary care practice among physicians, has increased the demand for all APRNs.

Much of the interest in using APRNs has been based on their ability to substitute for more costly providers, such as physicians. Evidence has supported the conclusion that APRNs are safe, competent, and cost-effective providers of healthcare services who are able to operate

Table 6-1 **Reforming Healthcare Workforce Regulation: Policy Considerations for the 21st Century**

Statement of Recommendations

1. States should use standardized and understandable language for health professions' regulation and its functions to describe them clearly for consumers, provider organizations, businesses, and the professions.

2. States should standardize entry-to-practice requirements and limit them to competence assessments for health professions to facilitate the physical and professional mobility of the health professions.

3. States should base practice acts on demonstrated initial and continuing competence. This process must allow and expect different professions to share overlapping scopes of practice. States should explore pathways to allow all professionals to provide services to the full extent of their current knowledge, training, experience, and skills.

4. States should redesign health professional boards and their functions to reflect the interdisciplinary and public accountability demands of the changing healthcare delivery system.

5. Boards should educate consumers to assist them in obtaining the information necessary to make decisions about practitioners and to improve the board's public accountability.

6. Boards should cooperate with other public and private organizations in collecting data on regulated health professions to support effective workforce planning.

7. States should require each board to develop, implement, and evaluate continuing competency requirements to ensure the continuing competence of regulated healthcare professionals.

8. States should maintain a fair, cost-effective, and uniform disciplinary process to exclude incompetent practitioners to protect and promote the public's health.

9. States should develop evaluation tools that assess the objectives, successes, and shortcomings of their regulatory systems and bodies to best protect and promote the public's health.

10. States should understand the links, overlaps, and conflicts between their healthcare workforce regulatory systems and other systems that affect the education, regulation, and practice of healthcare practitioners and work to develop partnerships to streamline regulatory structures and processes.

Report of the Taskforce on Health Care Workforce Regulation. (1995). *Reforming Health Care Workforce Regulation: Policy Considerations for the 21st Century.* Pew Health Professions Commission, San Francisco.

within an appropriate independent practice domain and therefore can play an important role in the delivery of a wide range of care services. Finally, a growing body of research has documented the different, and enhanced, outcomes achieved by APRNs: more cost-effective interventions, higher patient satisfaction, and increased compliance with therapeutic regimens, to name just a few. Increasingly, these enhanced outcomes have caused policy makers and employers to question the logic or appropriateness of regulatory policies that limit the practice of APRNs.[7–9]

Regulation of Advanced Practice Registered Nursing: Variety and Confusion

Every APRN must initially acquire the basic registered nurse (RN) license by passing the National Council Licensure Exam (NCLEX) administered by the National Council of State Boards of Nursing (NCSBN). However, unlike the uniform standard for licensing of entry-level

RNs, there is no uniform standard for licensing APRNs. Those wishing to be licensed as APRNs face a panoply of state requirements for licensure with a wide variety of specifications regarding scope-of-practice authority and titling.

LACK OF STANDARDIZATION AMONG STATE REGULATORY BOARDS

Each state or territory of the United States maintains some form of regulatory oversight over APRNs. In all 50 states and in 4 American territories, APRNs are specifically regulated as a separate group within that state.[10] In some states, APRNs are granted a second license for practice.[10–12] In other states, APRNs are granted some form of state authority to practice in an advanced role, which may be called "recognition" or "certification."[11,12] Unfortunately, these state regulatory initiatives lack consistency in terms of titling, practice privileges, or prescriptive authority,[11,12] and which regulatory boards are involved differs significantly. APRNs are almost uniformly licensed, certified, or recognized by state boards of nursing (BONs), but in some states, the board of medicine plays a role in oversight or regulation. For example, in North Carolina the boards of nursing and medicine are jointly responsible for the regulation of NP practice.

In all states, NPs have achieved statutory recognition and some form of state authority to write prescriptions.[12,13] Certified registered nurse anesthetists (CRNAs) and certified nurse-midwives (CNMs) are recognized as APRNs in almost all states, but in some states the CNS is recognized only in particular areas of specialization or populations (e.g., psychiatric–mental health nursing or pediatrics) or is not recognized as an APRN. Even states that recognize CRNAs, CNMs, and CNSs as APRNs, frequently have laws or regulations that limit their prescriptive authority. For example, in Utah, CRNAs are prohibited from writing prescriptions that may be filled at a pharmacy, but they are allowed to order the use of drugs in a care setting as a component of anesthesia. An analysis of state regulatory environments, *The Scope of Practice and Reimbursement for Advanced Practice Registered Nurses: A State by State Analysis*,[13] conducted by the George Washington University Intergovernmental Health Policy Institute, concluded:

> The lack of standardization among states' scopes of practice provisions for [advanced practice registered nurses] APRNs causes confusions for APRNs, other health care providers, insurance companies and consumers, and inhibits national unity among APRNs.[13(p3)]

In addition to the regulatory variety and inconsistencies among states, a major criticism of current APRN regulation has involved the great array of titles that states recognize. Pearson[14] provides an annual update of the recognized state authorities, prescriptive limitations, and titles for nurse practitioners. The NCSBN also produces what they call a Member Board Profile[10] on its Web site, which is a comprehensive listing of state board regulatory structures and frameworks for APRNs (see http://www.ncsbn.org). The array of titles (and acronyms) reported has created tremendous confusion for employers, other health professionals, policy makers, and APRNs. Safriet[15] was harshly critical of this inconsistent titling, seeing it, because of the confusion it causes, as enhancing the potential for regulators to limit APRNs' practice authority.

For many groups, both nursing and non-nursing, Safriet's work on the confusing array of regulatory authorities and their sometimes illogical word choices has highlighted the failure of public regulation. Safriet noted that these often illogical regulatory structures most often are based on a concept of advanced practice nursing as a purely substitutive professional role that is secondary to physician practice. This concept is not based on fact or experience, and it fails to take into account the large body of research documenting the efficacy of advanced practice nursing. However, Safriet's seminal report on APRN regulation has been instrumental in effecting a great deal of change in public regulatory structures, as evidenced by the increasing number of states that have expanded APRNs' authority to practice and prescribe.

Moreover, the work of Sekscenski and colleagues,[16] documented that those states with the most restrictive APRN regulatory structures have the lowest per capita APRN ratios.

APRN OPPOSITION TO INSTITUTIONAL OVERSIGHT OF PRACTICE

Sekscenski and colleagues[16] noted that the mobility of APRNs is also severely hindered by the lack of consistency in practice regulation. This inconsistency inhibits intrasystem mobility in the emerging large corporate healthcare structures. Integrated networks can span state lines in their scope-of-care responsibilities. However, neighboring states can have markedly different policies regulating the practice of APRNs. In addition, in many instances, APRNs living along the borders of states often may have practice sites in several states. Finally, with the growing use of telehealth and distance-mediated health care, it is often not clear to regulators if the care provider is covered under the laws of the state in which the provider is located or by the laws of the state in which the patient is receiving care. The "brave new world" of cyberspace has created new modes of care delivery, such as computer- and video-transmitted patient-care experiences, that can create uncertainty about where care is being delivered and who has authority for oversight of the professional's authority to practice.

Some employers argue that if organizations were charged with oversight, the issue of practice location would not be defined by state boundaries. Proponents of corporate-controlled regulation of APRNs and other health professionals note that such a licensure procedure would provide organizations with more flexibility in the use of APRNs, thus overcoming the artificial or inappropriate barriers to their full utilization. Historically, the nursing profession has been vocally and visibly opposed to the notion of institutional licensure for professional nurses. Opponents of the institutional approach to the regulation of APRNs contend that quality of care could be hindered by inadequately prepared clinicians who are educated by the corporation and are authorized to practice in a system that is more concerned with cost than quality. Questions also arise about the ability of these corporate structures to engage in the expensive processes of testing and evaluation necessary to ensure competence for advanced practice.[17]

Emerging Issues in the Advanced Practice Licensure Process

The regulation of advanced practice nursing is still a subject of debate; several different proposals have been advanced in an effort to make the regulations standardized and consistent.

PROPOSAL FOR SECOND LICENSURE

The NCSBN, a national membership organization that represents individual state or territorial boards of nursing, has engaged in a variety of efforts that have brought more urgency to the issue of the regulation of advanced practice. In 1993, the NCSBN House of Delegates approved a position statement mandating that all APRNs be granted a second license for practice and be required to hold a master's degree to be eligible.[18] The position statement noted that second licensure already existed in a number of states, that APRN practice was markedly different from that authorized through the RN licensure process, and thus, that advanced practice required a new regulatory mechanism and a second licensure exam. The second-licensure issue was opposed by a number of nursing organizations, including a variety of specialty certifying organizations, the ANA, and the American Association of Colleges of Nursing (AACN). These groups argued that the use of two levels of licensure was both confusing and unnecessary and that the existing professional certification was adequate to ensure the skills and competence of APRNs. Most nursing organizations, however, did not oppose the proposed graduate degree requirement also included in the 1993 NCSBN position statement. They did, however, voice some concern about the second licensure requirement and the graduate degree requirement being tied to each other.

As significant factors in the proposal for a second license, the NCSBN cited inconsistent requirements and the limitations to mobility that resulted from them. The second license was an attempt to bring uniformity to titling and educational requirements, and the NCSBN House of Delegates adopted this position at its 1993 meeting.[18] However, because all states grant some type of recognition equivalent to the pure definition of licensure, the requirement that this additional recognition be termed a "license" to practice would not expand states' authority to regulate, a right already granted to the states through the Tenth Amendment of the Constitution. The APRN *Consensus Model* (2008) does stipulate that a second license be issued to APRNs. (See the section "Development of the APRN Consensus Model" later in this chapter for more information on this topic.)

DEVELOPMENT OF MULTISTATE COMPACTS

One of the overarching issues that drove the NCSBN to consider a uniform licensure exam and process for regulation of advanced practice was the emerging awareness that state boundaries were no longer defining the practice domains of APRNs and their consequent exposure to an array of regulatory requirements. As noted above, large, multifaceted healthcare organizations have created practice domains that stretch beyond state boundaries, the customary limit defining practice regulations. This multistate expansion, in turn, has created among APRNs an interest in greater mobility and in greater consistency in public regulatory requirements. As has been mentioned, currently the APRN practices in a regulatory environment that varies widely, is sometimes conflicting, and often is very limiting.

This interest in facilitating interstate practice by APRNs—and RNs—led the NCSBN to create a licensure compact, which allows individuals to practice in a state in which they do not have a license if the state of residence and the state of practice have joined the multistate compact. The compact is modeled after those that control driving privileges. Individual drivers are not required to hold a driver's license in each state in which they drive, but instead are granted this privilege through agreements across states. The first step in creating a multistate licensure compact focused on basic RN practice, and currently 23 states have passed legislation and joined the multistate compact for basic RN practice.[19] Because APRNs commonly engage in either telehealth or multistate practice and face a confusing array of advanced practice licensure mechanisms, titles, and authorities, there is a similar need for a multistate APRN compact. To date, three states—Utah, Iowa, and Texas—have passed laws authorizing an APRN compact, but no date has been set for implementing it.[20]

As part of the development of a multistate compact for advanced practice, multiple nursing organizations worked with and gave consultative advice to the NCSBN on uniform standards for advanced practice education and regulation. The organizations represented the full spectrum of practice, credentialing, and education for advanced practice as a nurse practitioner, nurse anesthetist, nurse-midwife, or clinical nurse specialist. In developing the compact, consensus was sought on multiple logistical or standard issues, such as the basic level of education necessary to be covered under the compact or the types of certification that would be mandated for coverage. This process resulted in the development of an NCSBN statement on *Uniform Advanced Practice Registered Nurse Licensure/Authority to Practice Requirements.*[21] This agreement and additional work among the national organizations that represent APRNs changed the nature of certification exams and strengthened their role as a central element of the licensure process for APRNs.

EXTERNAL REVIEW OF CERTIFYING BODIES

Certification exams have historically been viewed as mechanisms to test and signify expanded knowledge and expert competence in a specific area or practice specialty. The agreement within the APRN community and among the state regulators of APRN practice to use nationally recognized certification exams as a mechanism to validate eligibility for state recognition required a reconceptualization of these exams. They were to become a measurement of the entry-level competence of APRNs, not a measure of expanded competence or expertise. The major certification bodies that administer these exams agreed to national review by an external entity that accredits certification bodies to provide assurance that their APRN certification exams were psychometrically sound, were legally defensible, and did test entry-level competence to practice.

The two national organizations that review and validate (accredit) the certifying organizations' capabilities are the Accreditation Board for Specialty Nursing Certification (ABSNC), formerly the American Board of Nursing Specialties Accrediting Council (ABNS), and the National Commission for Certifying Agencies of the Institute for Credentialing Excellence (NCCA-ICE), formerly the National Organization for Competency Assurance. See Tables 6-2 and 6-3 for information on these organizations.

Nursing regulators, who had previously questioned these organizations' ability to ensure the competence of recently graduated APRNs, agreed that the certifying bodies, after undergoing an extensive review and validation process through these two agencies, could validate APRN safety for practice. The NCSBN Delegate Assembly agreed that the nursing certification bodies had made significant changes in the standardization of the exams and uniformity of expectations across the NP certification organizations, thus creating what the NCSBN termed "legally defensible, psychometrically sound, nurse practitioner examinations that are sufficient for regulatory purposes."[21]

Table 6-2 Accreditation Board for Specialty Nursing Certification

The Accreditation Board for Specialty Nursing Certification (ABSNC), formerly known as the American Board of Nursing Specialties Accreditation Council (ABNS), is the peer review body in nursing that oversees development of national professional certification processes. The ABNS, established in 1991, was the result of a 3-year project funded by the Macy Foundation to bring uniformity to professional certification in nursing and to ensure that certification was a mechanism for enhancing the quality of care delivered. The purposes of the ABSNC are to:

1. Provide a forum for nursing certification collaboration;

2. Promote the value of nursing certification to various publics;

3. Provide a mechanism for accreditation and recognition of quality nursing specialty certification accreditation.

The ABSNC has established 19 standards that must be met in order for a certification program to be recognized by the ABSNC. Individuals who successfully complete professional certification exams from an organization that is ABSNC-recognized are considered "board certified." The following APRN certification organizations have been accredited by the ABSNC:

1. American Nurses Credentialing Center

2. National Board on Certification and Recertification of Nurse Anesthetists (NBCRNA)

3. Oncology Nursing Certification Corporation

For information on ABSNC standards, contact:

American Board of Nursing Specialties (the parent organization).
610 Thornhill Lane
Aurora, OH 44202
Phone: 330-995-9172
Fax: 330-995-9743
E-mail: ABNSCEO@aol.com
Web site: http://nursingcertification.org

Table 6-3 **National Commission for Certifying Agencies**

National Commission for Certifying Agencies (NCCA) is the accreditation body of the Institute for Credentialing Excellence (ICE), formerly the National Organization on Competency Assurance. The mission of the NCCA is to:

1. Establish accreditation standards,

2. Evaluate compliance with the standards,

3. Recognize organizations/programs that demonstrate compliance, and

4. Serve as a resource on quality certification.

NCCA has established 21 standards that an organization must demonstrate compliance with in order to be recognized. The following APRN certification organizations have been recognized by NCCA:

- American Academy of Nurse Practitioners Certification Program

- American Association of Critical-Care Nurses Certification Corporation

- American Nurses Credentialing Center

- American Midwifery Certification Board

- National Board on Certification and Recertification of Nurse Anesthetists (NBCRNA)

- National Certification Corporation for the Obstetric, Gynecologic, and Neonatal Nursing Specialties

- Oncology Nursing Certification Corporation

- Pediatric Nursing Certification Board

For information on ICE-NCCA standards, contact:

ICE
2025 M Street, N.W., Suite 800
Washington, DC 20036
Phone: 202-367-1165
Web site: http://www.noca.org

DEVELOPMENT OF THE APRN CONSENSUS MODEL

Recently, additional discussion by the NCSBN to consider again the development of a uniform licensure exam for validation of competence created a good deal of dissention and controversy among the advanced practice community. Given the previously agreed-to understanding among the certification bodies and the NCSBN, representatives of the national APRN certification bodies asserted that certification exams should continue to serve as the appropriate mechanism to ensure entry-level competence for practice. Moreover, organizations asserted that they had complied with the required changes in their certification exams to provide a legally defensible, entry-level advanced practice licensure proxy. State boards and the NCSBN representatives, however, expressed concern regarding the tremendous diversity in advanced practice specialization and in role definitions, a diversity that presented state boards with a confusing list of recognition concerns. For example, in a number of states, individuals were bringing requests to state boards for recognition as an APRN in what was considered a very discrete subspecialty for which there was no nationally recognized certification exam. Additionally, many states did not require the APRN to prove he or she had successfully passed a certification exam and thus were required to review each individual's transcript, educational program experiences, and clinical training activities before granting licensure or recognition. These states asked the NCSBN to consider developing a national licensure exam for APRNs that would then provide each state board with a uniform process for approving individual licensure.

As a result of the re-emergence of interest in the development of a national APRN licensure exam among state regulators and growing concerns over the confusing number of specialties in which APRNs were being prepared and seeking approval to practice, the American Association of Colleges of Nursing (AACN) and the National Organization of Nurse Practitioner Faculties (NONPF) recommended that a process of national consensus be convened to address these issues. Organizations that represent APRN education, practice, licensure, and accreditation then came together to develop a model, called the APRN Consensus Model, regarding APRN education, roles, specialties, titles, and so on. This model delineates the specific APRN roles and populations for which the APRN will be educated and granted authority to practice (Fig. 6-1). Additionally, it designated the official title for all advanced practice nurses as Advanced Practice Registered Nurse (APRN). Accreditation expectations for the educational programs were developed, including the agreement that all APRN programs must be accredited by a nationally recognized nursing accrediting body and that all new APRN programs must undergo a preapproval review prior to admitting students. Additionally, the consensus agreement included a continued endorsement of the use of the nationally recognized certification exams as proxy exams for licensure.

The most significant component of this agreement was the consensus regarding the roles and populations for which individuals would be educated and granted authority to provide care in the four APRN roles. Additionally, the agreement stated that regulation at the state level would focus only on the role and population for which the APRN was prepared to

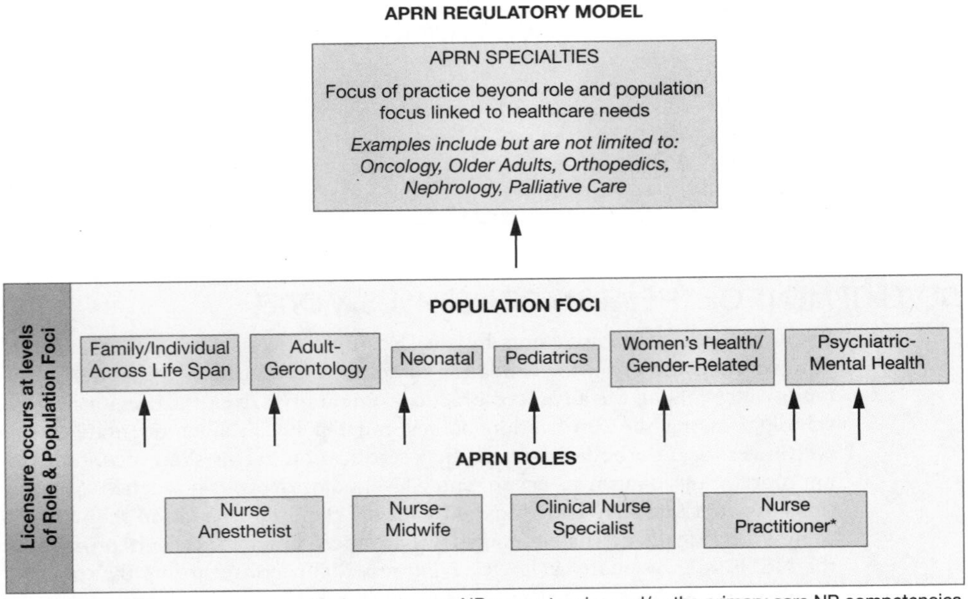

*The nurse practitioner is prepared with the acute care NP competencies and/or the primary care NP competencies. The ACNP and PCNP delineation applies only to the pediatric and adult gerontology NP population foci.

Figure 6-1: APRN Regulatory Model.

provide care. Specialization could occur beyond this, but this level of practice would not be regulated by the state board of nursing. For example, an APRN could be prepared to function as a certified nurse practitioner (CNP) (role designation) who would provide care to children (pediatric population focus). State boards would authorize practice for these individuals as CNPs. Should the pediatric CNP desire to focus on the care of children with cardiac disorders, that would require additional specialty preparation and would not be regulated by the state board. The Consensus Model strongly recommends professional certification in the specialty, although it is not mandated. One major change in population foci was the agreement that adult and geriatric care would be merged to create one focus titled adult-gerontology, a decision resulting from the growing awareness that the largest users of healthcare services are part of the older adult population and that all clinicians caring for adults should have a comprehensive understanding of the healthcare needs of older adults, including the frail elderly. This decision has significant implications, and will create dramatically different education programs and certification exams, for this new, expanded population focus.

The Consensus Model for APRN Regulation, hereafter referred to as the Consensus Model, has been endorsed by APRN organizations representing all four APRN roles (NP, CNS, CNM, CRNA) and all regulatory entities (licensure, accreditation, certification, and education). The Consensus Model established a target date of 2015 for final and complete implementation. Currently, discussion continues regarding the creation of a network known as LACE—licensure, accreditation, certification, education—that will facilitate the implementation of the Model over time. Full information about the Consensus Model and a list of the endorsing organizations can be accessed on the AACN Web site (http://www.aacn.nche.edu), under Education Policy. Meanwhile, states continue to use a variety of measures for assessing eligibility for practice, including education or training, the passage of a certification exam, or some other state requirements. When these qualifications can be validated by the state board, the APRN is granted authority to practice. In many states, the regulatory agencies governing advanced nursing practice have agreed to accept proof of successful completion of professional APRN certification as validation of eligibility for the advanced practice role.

Professional Certification for Advanced Practice Registered Nursing

Professional certification is the process by which an organization, based on predetermined standards, validates a nurse's qualifications, knowledge, and practice in a defined functional or clinical area of nursing. Professional certification is reserved for those nurses who have met the requirements for clinical or functional practice in a specialized field, have pursued education beyond basic nursing preparation, and have received the endorsement of their peers. On satisfying these criteria, nurses are eligible to take certification examinations based on nationally recognized standards of nursing practice that demonstrate special knowledge and skills surpassing those required for state licensure.[21]

The use of professional certification to validate the public authority to practice intermingles the domains of professional certification and public regulation. The credentialing organization, separate and distinct from the professional membership or specialty organization, bases its credentialing examination on the definitions of standards and scope of practice set by the membership of the professional organization. After an in-depth job analysis of practicing clinicians, a test development committee composed of individuals who by their education and experience are recognized as experts in the specific area of practice, identifies relevant content, areas of focus, and the professional competencies to be measured. Next, examination questions are solicited from an identified panel of nurses certified in the specialty area and other experts throughout the country. The submitted questions undergo rigorous review, critique, and rating for accuracy and relevancy by a psychometrician. Using a predetermined blueprint or test plan, the panel of experts or test development committee then selects a representative sample of the questions for inclusion on the certifying examination.

Many professions also require practical tests and oral reviews to supplement written examinations in determining a candidate's qualifications for certification. Written examinations are the most frequently used form of evaluation, with 47% of certification organizations using written examinations only; an additional 28% use written examinations in combination with practical tests and/or oral reviews. The means of testing depends on the occupation or profession. Written examinations can effectively evaluate knowledge, but manual or verbal skills often must be demonstrated through a practical test or oral presentation. Approximately 25% of certification programs use a practical test, and 11% use an oral review.[22]

Prior to the agreement by the NCSBN to recognize certification exams as a proxy for a license to practice as an APRN, the states varied greatly in their use of national certifying examinations as precursors to state recognition. Member boards of the NCSBN expressed concerns regarding the psychometric properties of the testing mechanisms used by certifying bodies and questioned their abilities to ensure the competence of an individual to serve in the expanded APRN role. Other critics of state reliance on professional certification processes pointed to the inconsistencies in the criteria the certifying bodies set for allowing an individual to sit for APRN certification. Educational requirements, graduate degree requirements, and precertification practice requirements varied among these organizations. Some reportedly applied varying degrees of scrutiny to the educational credentials of applicants and allowed some applicants to waive such requirements. In 1993, the collaborative efforts of the NCSBN and the four primary organizations that certify NPs created a laudable agreement that would ensure both professional accountability in setting standards of practice and public oversight of practice authority. This 1993 agreement set the stage for later development of the APRN Consensus Model. The NCSBN delegates began their work by focusing on NP practice, but there is widespread understanding that the regulation of advanced practice extends to concerns about the preparation of CNSs for advanced practice. In fact, current requirements in the NCSBN's *Uniform Advanced Practice Registered Nurse Licensure/Authority to Practice Requirements* apply to all APRNs. And, as this issue has evolved, the relationship between public regulation and private credentialing has become more widely understood and debated.

Other concerns regarding the regulation of APRNs have also been discussed. One is how to ensure and evaluate that the credentialed provider remains competent and current in both the skills and knowledge needed to practice safely and effectively. Moreover, as noted previously, the development of new specialties or populations for which national certification examinations do not yet exist for some APRN roles has created unintended barriers to practice in states that require national certification for practice authority. Continuing discussions of these issues are driven by concerns about protecting the public and allowing APRNs to function to their fullest capacity. These issues bear watching in each state. In any event, it appears certain that the regulation process will continue to evolve as issues related to multistate practice and the definition of specialty practice are addressed by regulators and as the APRN Consensus Model is implemented.

Master's Requirement for NPs

A variety of professional organizations offer certification for APRNs. (A list of the professional organizations and the roles and populations they certify is provided in Table 6-4.) Some variation in philosophy, criteria, and requirements exists among the certifying organizations, particularly those that certify NPs. In the past, the most obvious difference has been the requirement for a master's or higher degree in nursing. Now, all of the organizations that certify NPs require that a candidate have a master's or higher degree in order to be eligible for the certification examination.

Table 6-4 **Professional Organizations That Certify Advanced Practice Registered Nurses**

Certifying Body	Areas of Certification
American Academy of Nurse Practitioners Certification Program	Adult NP Family NP Gerontological NP
American Association of Critical-Care Nurses Certification Corporation	Acute Care-Adult CNS Acute Care-Pediatric CNS Acute Care-Neonatal CNS Acute Care Nurse Practitioner (Adult)
American Midwifery Certification Board	Certified Midwife Certified Nurse-Midwife
American Nurses Credentialing Center	Acute Care NP Adult NP Family NP Gerontological NP Pediatric NP Adult Psychiatric and Mental Health NP Family Psychiatric and Mental Health NP School NP Public/Community Health CNS Gerontological CNS Adult Health CNS Adult Psychiatric & Mental Health CNS Child/Adolescent Psychiatric and Mental Health CNS Pediatric CNS Home Health CNS
National Board on Certification and Recertification of Nurse Anesthetists	Certified Registered Nurse Anesthetist
National Certification Corporation for Women's Health, Obstetric and Neonatal Nurses	Neonatal NP Women's Health NP
Pediatric Nursing Certification Board	Pediatric NP—Acute Care Pediatric NP—Primary Care
Oncology Nurse Certification Corporation	Oncology CNS Oncology NP

The National Certification Corporation on Women's Health and Neonatal Nursing (NCC) was the only organization, until 2007, without a master's degree requirement for NP certification. Representatives of all women's health NP and education organizations examined this issue and developed a plan to require a master's degree for certification. A consensus statement issued in September 1995 recognized a national trend toward graduate education for NPs and the need to identify and support mechanisms for an orderly transition of women's health care NP education from certificate to graduate education.[23,24] Starting on January 1, 2007, the NCC began to require individuals desiring certification as a women's health care or neonatal NP to hold either a master's degree in nursing or a post-master's certificate.

Increasing Need for Doctor of Nursing Practice Degree

In 2004, members of the AACN approved the recommendation that all APRNs should be educated in a graduate program designed to grant a Doctor of Nursing Practice (DNP) degree.[25] As a result of several years of study and consensus development regarding the emerging demands of the complex healthcare system, there is a growing consensus that this requirement should become the standard for APRN education. Additionally, a clear understanding has developed that the credits required for advanced practice master's degree programs had expanded beyond the level usually required for a master's degree due to the growing demand for APRNs with additional skills in our increasingly complex healthcare system. Currently, no certification body requires the APRN to hold a DNP; however, the National Board on Certification and Recertification of Nurse Anesthetists (NBCRNA) has indicated that in 2025 all new applicants for certification must hold a doctoral degree. Other certification representatives indicate that as APRN practice evolves in response to the expanded knowledge base in health care, the certification exams will also change and the DNP requirement for new applicants will emerge.

Certification Requirements for Different APRN Roles

The continued evolution of advanced practice and the lag period necessary for the development of new certification exams will continue to create challenges for those wishing to practice as certified APRNs. However, given the national consensus regarding the educational requirements for recognition across the states, individuals who seek a graduate degree for APRN practice should make sure that the program they enroll in follows or meets the Consensus Model and that graduates of the program are eligible to take the appropriate certification exam. Individuals seeking entry into an advanced practice nursing program are encouraged to document whether the program they are considering has met the requirements of the certifying body from which they plan to seek certification. In addition, prior to entering an APRN program, individuals should determine state and national certification requirements and document that the program and certification will allow them to follow their chosen career path. In some instances, two or more organizations offer exams for the same role and practice area but hold different expectations of the educational program.

The requirements for initial and continued certification vary among the professional certifying organizations. The lengths of certification terms also vary, usually ranging from 1 to 8 years, after which time recertification is necessary. In addition, requirements for certification are revised regularly. Therefore, APRNs should stay informed about the terms and requirements for certification in their particular role and population. The following four sections provide overviews and comparisons of the certification requirements for each of the APRN roles; a fifth section discusses recertification. For more detailed and current information regarding eligibility requirements for certification or recertification in each of the roles and practice areas, the APRN should contact the professional organization named.

NP CERTIFICATION

NP certification is provided through a number of organizations, including the American Academy of Nurse Practitioners (AANP) Certification Program, the American Association of Critical-Care Nurses (AACN), the American Nurses Credentialing Center (ANCC), the National Certification Corporation (NCC), the Pediatric Nursing Certification Board (PNCB), and the Oncology Nursing Certification Corporation (ONCC). (Currently, certification is offered in a number of population foci and/or specialties, including adult acute care NP, adult NP, family NP, gerontological NP, neonatal NP, pediatric NP, psychiatric/mental health NP, women's health care NP, advanced oncology nursing, and others.)

The ONCC offers certification in advanced nursing oncology for both NPs and CNSs. As noted, the APRN Consensus process has created a clear framework for the future regarding the use of specialty certifications, and NP certification and state regulation for practice will undergo significant revisions. As a result, the ONCC certification exam will most likely not be recognized for granting state authority to practice unless a separate exam that tests the role and population competencies (e.g., pediatric or adult/gerontology) separate from the oncology specialty is developed. In the future, the NP would be licensed as an adult/gerontology CNP with a specialty in oncology (see Fig. 6-1). Additionally, in the future adult and gerontology education programs and certification examinations will be merged to prepare and certify individuals as primary care adult/gerontology NPs or acute care adult/gerontology NPs. The American Association of Colleges of Nursing (AACN) is leading a national effort to develop competencies for the new adult/gerontology population foci for primary care and acute care NPs that will reshape the education programs and certification exams for individuals seeking state licensure to care for adult populations.

CLINICAL NURSE SPECIALIST CERTIFICATION

Clinical nurse specialist (CNS) certification is offered by the ANCC, the American Association of Critical-Care Nurses Certification Corporation (AACN-CC), and the ONCC (see Table 6-4). Each of these certification programs requires that candidates have a minimum number of hours in direct patient care in their area of specialization. ANCC certification as an adult or child and adolescent psychiatric and mental health CNS requires not only documentation of a specified number of hours in direct patient care but also a minimum number of hours of consultation and supervision by a nurse who is ANCC certified or eligible for certification in psychiatric and mental health nursing.[22]

The AACN-CC offers certification programs in adult, neonatal, and pediatric critical-care nursing. To qualify for these examinations, an individual must hold a current RN license, have a master's or higher degree in nursing with specific preparation as a CNS, and document that the educational program followed the standards delineated in the AACN's *Essentials of Master's Education for Advanced Practice Nursing*.[26] Additionally, as with NP certification for care of adults, as the Consensus Model is implemented, the CNS seeking a state license to practice in the care of adults will be required to pass a certification exam that has combined the competencies for both adult and gerontology practice. This requirement will dramatically reshape the education and certification of both NPs and CNSs. Competencies for the adult/gerontology CNS are also being developed through the national initiative led by AACN.

NURSE-MIDWIFE CERTIFICATION

The American Midwifery Certification Board (AMCB) is the only professional organization that offers certification for nurse-midwifery. To be eligible for the national certification examination, the individual must hold a current RN license to practice in the United States and must document satisfactory completion of a nurse-midwifery program or a midwifery program for non-nurses that is either accredited or pre-accredited by the Accreditation Commission for Midwifery Education (ACME), formerly the American College of Nurse-Midwives Division of Accreditation (http://www.acnm.org/acme/cfm). Core competencies for basic nurse-midwifery are clearly delineated by the ACNM for each of the components of nurse-midwifery care: preconception, antepartum, intrapartum, postpartum, neonatal, and family planning and gynecological care.[27] Like certification organizations for the other APRN roles, the AMCB has now moved to require completion of a master's degree to become a certified nurse-midwife (CNM). Until recently, the individual seeking this certification had only to complete either a post-baccalaureate certificate program in nurse-midwifery or the nurse-midwifery component of a master's-level nursing program. All nurse-midwifery programs must be accredited or pre-accredited by the ACME.

NURSE ANESTHETIST CERTIFICATION

Professional certification for nurse anesthetists is offered solely by the National Board for Certification and Recertification of Nurse Anesthetists, an arm of AANA. To be eligible to take the certification examination for certified registered nurse anesthetist (CRNA), candidates must hold a current and unrestricted RN license in the states in which they practice and must have completed a nurse anesthesia educational program accredited by the Council on Accreditation of Nurse Anesthesia Educational Programs (http://www.aana.com).[28] In its requirements for program accreditation, the Council on Accreditation of Nurse Anesthesia Educational Programs delineates the number and type of patient experiences required for graduation. In addition, it defines the number of required experiences, specific types of anesthesia, and the methods used to administer the anesthesia.[28]

REQUIREMENTS FOR RECERTIFICATION

After the period of initial or subsequent certification has expired, recertification is required. Commonly, recertification includes either re-examination or documentation of a specified number of hours in direct patient care in one's role and area of specialization and a specified number of hours of continuing education. A number of states now require the individual to have a specified number of continuing education hours annually in pharmacology to maintain one's prescriptive privileges. (However, the adequacy of continuing education requirements in ensuring practitioner competence was seriously questioned by the 1995 Pew report *Reforming Health Care Workforce Regulation*.[6])

Recertification requirements have changed significantly over time, so the certified APRN is encouraged to review carefully the expectations of each certification body. For example, for many years, midwifery certification was granted for the life of the midwife. Recently, the American Midwifery Certification Board (AMCB) changed its certification requirements. Individuals who were certified for midwifery practice after 1996 must now apply for recertification every 8 years and must meet the same recertification criteria as all other CNMs.[27] The term of certification provided by certification bodies can also vary. The reader is advised to seek information from the certifying board to determine its unique terms or requirements.

Clinical Practice and Institutional Privileges

As the United States enters the beginning of the second decade of the 21st century, its healthcare system faces numerous challenges, including declining reimbursements, large numbers of uninsured, many near-bankrupt health facilities, a weak economy, and declining numbers of providers. These problems have resulted in consumers experiencing a critical lack of access to appropriate practitioners, especially to practitioners capable of providing quality primary care services in a cost-effective, comprehensive, and timely fashion. APRNs, by virtue of their education, experience, and growing numbers, are increasingly being asked to fill this void. To do this successfully, APRNs must be capable of:

- Providing their full scope of legally authorized practice
- Providing their services in all practice settings, both traditional (e.g., acute care hospitals) and nontraditional (e.g., health clinics located in commercial establishments, such as the Minute Clinics)
- Providing their services under federal, state, and institutional regulations and policies that facilitate the full utilization of their APRN skills

The following section addresses issues of clinical practice and privileging that allow for the maximum utilization of APRNs in a variety of clinical settings.

State and Institutional Control of the Practice of Healthcare Providers

State (statutory) control of the professional practice of healthcare providers such as nurses and physicians began in the early 1900s (approximately, 1911) and became nearly universal by the mid-1940s. By the latter period, almost all states had enacted legislation to control physicians, nurses, and other types of providers.[29] As a consequence of those laws, institutions such as hospitals began exerting their own internal control over providers. Initially, clinical privileges (i.e., the right to practice in a given healthcare facility) were reserved to the physician medical staff; other providers were excluded. Even today, medical staffs exert the dominant influence in a facility's credentialing process, although, over time, most facilities have established an ancillary (or auxiliary) medical staff to encompass such nonphysician providers as APRNs, dentists, speech and occupational therapists, and others whose activities require licensure and/or credentialing in order to practice. In a few individual instances, nonphysicians have been allowed to be part of the "full" medical staff. This occurs generally in small, rural hospitals that have a very small staff, and such situations remain rare.

All providers in healthcare facilities must be credentialed, either through the medical staff process or another mechanism. The granting of clinical privileges authorizes a practitioner to provide professional services to patients within the institution. One significant aspect of those privileges is the ability to admit and discharge patients from the facility, an authority traditionally reserved to physicians. Over the years, APRNs have battled successfully to gain for themselves admitting privileges. Although the number of APRNs with admitting privileges is currently small, it continues to grow, and it is these APRNs who have laid the foundation for today's level of APRN practice. Admission privileges are a key aspect of a provider's scope of practice since they allow the provider—in this discussion, an APRN—to provide needed care without having to rely on another provider, such as a physician. The privilege expedites the speed with which care can be provided and allows for quick response to emergencies or patient conditions that occur outside the facility and for which immediate care and treatment are necessary.

Clinical Practice Settings for APRNs

APRNs are increasingly found in diverse practice settings and in a variety of practice specialties. Their practices are expanding into new areas that range from acute care hospitals to community-based settings. Because of general societal concerns regarding safety, quality of care, and the capabilities of providers, APRNs can expect that increased emphasis and oversight will be given to their professional credentialing. It behooves all APRNs, therefore, to familiarize themselves with credentialing processes as these can have a profound impact on clinical practice.

The current total number of APRNs nationwide is unknown, but it is thought to be several hundred thousand.[30] The number of APRNs holding clinical privileges in the facilities in which they practice is also unknown, but their numbers are growing as more facilities recognize APRNs as highly competent providers who require appropriate credentialing. As mentioned earlier, the four main groups of advance practice registered nurses (APRNs) typically regulated by state boards of nursing are nurse anesthetists, nurse-midwives, clinical nurse specialists, and nurse practitioners. These groups are briefly described in subsequent sections. These four provider groups are regulated by nursing boards or midwifery boards in part because they render critical services directly to patients on a "one-on-one" basis. Many other nurses who have graduate degrees are not regulated as APRNs because they do not have direct, one-to-one contact with patients. They typically work in areas such as administration and public health, which require advanced knowledge and skills, but it is felt that they do not require the same level of state oversight and they may not use the title APRN or APN. However, depending on their practice setting, these individuals may require credentialing by their facility.

The remainder of this section discusses the typical credentialing processes for the four types of APRNs in clinical practice settings.

CERTIFIED REGISTERED NURSE ANESTHETISTS

According to the AANA, the number of certified registered nurse anesthetists (CRNAs) is now approaching 40,000.[31] A recent internal survey indicated that approximately 70% of CRNAs are credentialed through a facility's medical staff process; the remainder are credentialed through other mechanisms. The majority of CRNAs practice clinically in conjunction with physician anesthesiologists and are often employed by anesthesiology groups. Others practice in CRNA-only groups, as per diem or *locum tenens* providers through staffing agencies, and still others are employed by hospitals. CRNAs also practice in all branches of the military and in the Veteran's Administration system. Regardless of practice setting, virtually all CRNAs are credentialed by their facility in some manner.

CERTIFIED NURSE-MIDWIVES

According to ACNM, most certified nurse-midwives (CNMs) work in an office or clinic setting and are employed by either individual physicians or a hospital. According to 2002 data, nearly 99% of births attended by CNMs occurred in a hospital; the remainder occurred in either a free-standing birthing center or at the patient's home.[32,33] A recent resurgence of demand for CNMs has come about due to the combination of high malpractice insurance premiums for obstetricians (the highest, on average, of any medical specialty), decreased reimbursements that have forced hospitals to close obstetrical units, a decline in the numbers of obstetric physicians, a growing preference for the services provided by a CNM, and other societal factors. As a result CNMs have taken on a greater role in the management of obstetrical and gynecological patients. In addition, the care provided by CNMs has, over time, expanded to new areas, such as genetic counseling, providing information on infertility treatments, and the public health aspects of containing the spread of sexually transmitted diseases (STDs).

CLINICAL NURSE SPECIALISTS AND NURSE PRACTITIONERS

The practice settings and scope of practice of clinical nurse specialists (CNSs) and nurse practitioners (NPs) are considerably more diverse than those of CRNAs or CNMs. As the demand for new services has grown in the past decade, the diversity has also grown. Less hard information is therefore available regarding the current practice arrangements of NPs and CNSs.

In 1992, approximately 1.8% of NPs were not working with a physician or psychologist, the implication (by extrapolation) being that these NPs were in independent practice as solo practitioners. An additional 2.1% had a contractual arrangement whereby they paid a consultation fee to either a physician or psychologist. Another 3.4% received a "fee for service" but were otherwise not paid a salary.[34] These statistics imply that more than 90% of NPs were salaried in some way at this time.

Data concerning CNSs showed that 18.4% did not work with a physician or psychologist, an estimated 8.6% paid a consulting fee to either a physician or psychologist, and 27.8% received only a "fee for service."[34] The fee-for-service group, however, accounted for only 2.3% if psychiatric–mental health CNSs were excluded from the sample. This finding is not entirely surprising since, at that time (1992 survey) psychiatric–mental health CNS practitioners were nearly the only APRN group significantly engaged in fee-for-service practices as independent providers. Few other CNS practitioners had such practices.

Increased APRN Role in Acute Care Hospital Settings

In recent years, the number of APRNs, particularly NPs, working in acute care hospital settings has steadily increased. APRNs have taken on a greater portion of the in-house care of hospitalized patients, not unlike physician hospitalists. The numbers of patients who, while hospitalized, continue to be cared for by a physician as their primary care provider are decreasing, mostly due to a shift in the numbers and types of providers, to the economic realities that force providers to relinquish a greater portion of the patient's hospital care to others, and to the growing complexity of health care. APRNs have shown they can contribute to the efficient care of hospitalized patients without a sacrifice in safety or quality.

Neonatal NPs are the largest group of NPs in hospital-based settings, which employ 94% of neonatal NPs. Adult NPs comprise the second-largest group of NPs in hospital-based practices (11.5%). Nearly two-thirds—62.9%—of medical-surgical CNSs also work in hospital settings. By comparison, more than 34.3% of gerontology NPs are employed in nursing homes or extended care facilities, and adult psychiatric CNSs work primarily outside hospital settings, with only 22% practicing in hospitals.[34]

The shifting dynamics of health care are driving major changes in how care is provided and by whom. APRNs are increasingly working more independently from physicians, a change driven by the baby-boomer generation that has come to expect a high standard of health care but is now becoming an aging population with increased healthcare needs at a time when there are dwindling numbers of providers, especially physicians. APRNs are therefore taking on greater responsibility for the total care delivered to their patients. Their ability to do so, however, is often compromised by institutional policies that limit their ability to coordinate and provide needed services. The lack of admitting privileges, for one example, continues to be a major obstacle to the full utilization of APRNs.

Factors Governing Institutional Privileges

In order for an individual APRN to obtain clinical privileges within a facility, he or she must first meet the requirements of three categories of regulatory oversight: state laws and regulations, facility accreditation standards, and institutional bylaws.

STATE LAWS AND REGULATIONS

State statutes (laws) set out the legal requirements for practice as a particular type of practitioner (e.g., nurse, physician) within the state. Requirements for APRNs may be set out in the Nurse Practice Act (NPA), in a separate Advanced Practice Nursing Act (APNA), or in the rules and other guidelines established by the state's nursing regulatory board, which is typically the state BON. What a practitioner may and may not do is specified in these acts and/or rules and is referred to as one's "scope of practice."

It is essential that all APRNs be familiar with the contents of their state's nurse practice act(s) and be aware of requirements that restrict or limit them. The APRN should not assume that he or she has the same scope of practice in State A as he or she has in state B. For example, the prescriptive authority of an APRN may be limited to particular classes of drugs in one state, but not in another, so the APRN needs to be familiar with the scope of practice under the laws of each state. Care providers also need to know whether the clinical privileges awarded by a facility are in accord with the requirements of the nurse practice act(s) and other regulations of the state in which they practice.

FACILITY ACCREDITATION STANDARDS

Some, but not all, states require that hospitals, clinics, surgical centers, and/or physician offices comply with standards set out by an appropriate accrediting organization. In other states, accreditation can be a voluntary process. Individual practitioners are "certified" in a particular specialty or area of practice; facilities are "accredited." Facilities meeting accreditation standards are recognized as functioning within generally accepted standards of safety and quality. Organizations that accredit facilities typically require standards concerning the clinical privileging of practitioners providing services in the facility. These requirements must be met before a practitioner, such as an APRN, can be granted clinical privileges.

Recognized accrediting bodies are granted "deeming" authority by the Centers for Medicare and Medicaid Services (CMS) of the U.S. Department of Health and Human Services (DHHS). Facilities that are inspected and approved by the accrediting organization are "deemed" to have met CMS requirements (although CMS does conduct some follow-up inspections of its own to ensure compliance). To be approved for deeming authority, an accrediting organization must demonstrate that its program meets or exceeds the CMS requirements for which it seeks authority to deem compliance. The accrediting standards must comply with CMS's Medicare conditions of participation (COP), that is, the conditions required to be met in order to participate in the Medicare program.

The most prominent and major accrediting organization of health-care facilities in the United States is the Joint Commission (JC), known previously as the Joint Commission on Accreditation of Healthcare Organizations (JCAHO). It is the largest accreditor of hospitals in the United States and is, therefore, the accrediting agency most familiar to nurses. JC also accredits other types of health-care facilities, such as ambulatory surgery centers, home care services, laboratory services, long-term care facilities, critical access hospitals, and office-based surgeries. In total, JC accredits more than 15,000 facilities and programs in the United States. It also accredits facilities in other countries through its international arm.

In 1983, JC revised its medical staff standards to provide for clinical privileging of nonmedical practitioners.[35] The change was driven by legal antitrust cases, greater emphasis on cost controls, alterations in reimbursement, and expanding numbers of new nonphysician providers. JC's 1984 standards allowed hospitals to grant medical staff membership to other licensed providers permitted by state law.[36] The current standards of JC are available, at a cost, in both print and online formats. Frequently asked questions about its standards and other accreditation issues can be found at The Joint Commission's Web site (http://www.jointcommission.org/).

Hospitals also may be accredited through the Healthcare Facilities Accreditation Program (HFAP) of the American Osteopathic Association (AOA). Though not as well known or as large as JC, the HFAP program has been in existence since 1945 and is recognized by federal and state governments, insurance carriers, and managed care organizations. Its accreditation reviews are not limited to osteopathic hospitals, but also include other types of hospitals as well as nonhospital facilities.[37]

A third accreditation organization, DNV Healthcare, Inc., was recently approved by CMS (on September 26, 2008) as the third hospital accrediting organization with deeming authority, making it the first new accrediting organization in more than 30 years. DNV Healthcare is a subsidiary of the DNV (Det Norske Veritas) corporation, a multinational company headquartered in Oslo, Norway, which dates to 1867 and now operates in more than 100 countries. The company is involved in risk management to safeguard life, property, and the environment. DNV Healthcare is a division of Houston, Texas–based DNV USA. DNV's accreditation program differs from that of JC and HFAP programs in several ways. The accreditations are done annually, rather than every several years as with JC and HFAP. In addition, its accreditation program, called the National Integrated Accreditation for Healthcare Organizations (NIAHO[SM]) is based on the ISO-9001 quality assurance and improvement standards of the International Organization for Standardization. At the time of obtaining CMS approval, DNV had accredited 27 hospitals in 22 states using the NIAHO process.[38]

Although the JC, HFAP, and NIAHO programs are the only ones dealing with hospitals, they are not the only organizations that accredit healthcare facilities. Similar organizations focus on accrediting ambulatory clinics or other facilities. One, the American Association for Accreditation of Ambulatory Surgery Facilities, Inc. (AAAASF), formed in 1980, now accredits more than 1000 facilities nationwide.[39] Another is the Accreditation Association for Ambulatory Health Care (AAAHC), which was formed in 1979.[40] These organizations set standards for care in ambulatory surgery clinics, offices that perform plastic surgery, ophthalmology clinics, and other free-standing facilities. In addition, California has its own accreditation program, called the Institute for Medical Quality (IMQ). It accredits only in-state facilities.

All the foregoing organizations (JC, HFAP, DNV, AAAASF, AAAHC, IMQ) have standards that, to a lesser or greater extent, set criteria for the issuing of clinical privileges. APRNs should, therefore, familiarize themselves with the clinical privileging requirements of the organization that accredits the facility in which they work. Requirements are not the same for all accrediting organizations, and some are stringent. Failure to adhere to accreditation standards, including those dealing with clinical privileging, could, in some circumstances, threaten the facility's accreditation status and perhaps even its state licensure. It is incumbent on each APRN to inquire about the credentialing requirements for any facility in which they will provide care to patients.

INSTITUTIONAL BYLAWS AND POLICIES

A hospital's legal authority is vested in its governing board. In turn, the board grants membership to the medical staff and determines what credentials are acceptable for given providers. It is the governance body that decides what activities and functions may be performed by individual practitioners who independently provide patient care services within the facility. The board's delineation of functions extends even to determining the functions of providers who are not members of the physician medical staff. It is important to note that the governance board (either itself or through its medical staff process) can restrict a provider's functions even if those functions are permitted by state law, accreditation standards, or case law. Facilities cannot grant a provider clinical privileges greater than those specified by state law, but they can limit or restrict those privileges.

APRNs who have clinical privileges in a hospital are usually part of the ancillary medical staff (also called allied, associate, or affiliate medical staff), rather than the "full" medical staff, which typically is restricted to physicians. As mentioned earlier, APRNs (with some exceptions) do not typically have admitting or discharging privileges under their own authority, a major difference from the privileges granted to physicians. Another major difference is that nonphysician allied medical staff members typically are not allowed to serve on various committees of the physician medical staff. Neither do providers such as APRNs have medical staff voting privileges or disciplinary due-process appeal rights. The functions delineated for allied medical staff members can limit the circumstances under which they can render a service and limit the specific acts (functions) that may be performed. Generally, allied medical staff privileges are subject to oversight by the medical staff and are subject to medical staff and department bylaws, rules, and regulations.

Types of Institutional Privileges

All licensed providers (physicians, APRNs, and others) must be credentialed for privileges by the facility within which they render services (Table 6-5). Credentialing can be viewed as of two types: clinical, which allows the provider to render professional services to patients; and admitting, which allows a provider to admit or discharge a patient to or from the facility. Providers can request admitting privileges when applying to a facility for clinical privileges. Privileges are based on the credentials—academic, licensure, and other—that a practitioner possesses. The application for, and awarding of, privileges is, therefore, referred to as the "credentialing process."

The credentialing process generally consists of verifying four key elements:

- The individual's license and legal status
- The person's relevant education
- The individual's training and work experience
- The person's current competence to practice

Verifying these elements involves soliciting and collecting the needed data and preparing it for review by the designated medical staff committee that awards or denies the application.

Table 6-5 **The Institutional Credentialing Process**

What Is "Credentialing"?

Credentialing is the process by which hospitals and other facilities authorize what functions a healthcare professional can provide to persons treated by the facility. The term is sometimes used as a shorthand reference to a provider's "scope of practice," but this is inaccurate. Legal authority for an individual's "scope of practice" is set by the applicable state practice act and regulations of a state oversight board. For APRNs, this authority is typically found in state nurse practice acts and state board of nursing regulations. A hospital, however, can restrict or limit what a practitioner may do within the facility. For example, the APRN may be prohibited from carrying out particular procedures in the facility even though she or he has received the appropriate education and training, has the applicable professional certifications, and is legally authorized to perform those procedures under state laws and regulations. While a facility can limit or totally bar what a particular provider can do within the facility, it cannot allow an individual to perform procedures or other acts beyond the individual's legally authorized scope of practice.

Why Have Credentialing?

The core purpose of a hospital or facility credentialing process is to reassure patients, the public, the facility, and other healthcare professionals of the quality and competence of individual practitioners. Because of the need to obtain, verify, and evaluate a practitioner's past history of education and experience, the process can be complicated, cumbersome, and costly. Some of the difficulties apt to be encountered are detailed below.

Who Controls the Credentialing Process?

The governance body for the hospital or clinic facility controls the credentialing processes and procedures. Credentialing is generally conducted in conjunction with the medical staff, which may actually set the specific procedures to be used, approves individual applications, and provides for any required oversight. For this reason, the process is often referred to as "medical staff credentialing or privileging." Yet, the process may not be the same for everyone. (See below.)

Who Actually Carries Out the Credentialing Process?

Hospitals typically have a specific department called the Medical Staff Office that handles applications for credentials. They provide the application forms for those seeking clinical appointments, gather all the necessary background documents, verify their authenticity from original sources, validate work experiences, confirm any past disciplinary actions the individual may have, and prepare the application for review and a determination by the medical staff.

Is the Process the Same for Everyone?

The answer to this question can be both "Yes" and "No," depending on the circumstances. Some providers are credentialed in the same manner as are the physicians on the medical staff. However, in some instances, a person may be credentialed through the hospital's Human Resources (HR) division. Nursing staff members are sometimes credentialed in this way, especially non-APRNs. A few facilities credential (or grant privileges) to their nursing staff directly through the department of nursing (DON). Some believe credentialing through an HR or DON process is less efficient than using a medical staff process. Because the persons carrying out the investigatory and other aspects of the credentialing process (see below) may not have the same expertise as those involved full-time with medical staff credentialing, HR and DON privileging can be more problematic. Others think using a full medical staff privileging process for credentialing of nonphysician staff is unnecessary and costly. The differences in the HR, DON, and medical staff credentialing processes are more a matter of degree than reflective of substantive differences since the aims of each of these approaches require similar procedures. All of them aim to ensure patient safety and the quality of the care provided.

Table 6-5 **The Institutional Credentialing Process—cont'd**

Who Can Be Credentialed?

Traditionally, credentialing applied only to physicians on a hospital's medical staff. In recent years, under growing pressure from the public, government agencies, and others concerned with maintaining patient safety and quality care, the trend has been to require credentialing of other providers. APRNs are more and more being included in the hospital's credentialing process. Other providers who are not physicians (e.g., psychologists, dentists, speech therapists) also are increasingly required to undergo credentialing. Typically, these are persons who provide specialized, direct care to patients. For example, one APRN group—CRNAs—often are required to be credentialed by the same process as physicians on the medical staff. Information gathered by the American Association of Nurse Anesthetists (AANA) indicates that approximately 70% of practicing CRNAs are currently credentialed through a medical staff process. AANA is the national professional organization for CRNAs and represents more than 90% of the nation's nurse anesthetists.

Does Credentialing Mean Providers Who Are Not Physicians Become Members of the Medical Staff?

In general, only physicians are members of the medical staff. Providers who are not physicians, while they undergo the same credentialing process, are usually assigned an "allied" or "associate" medical staff designation. However, in smaller hospitals, some providers who are not physicians are eligible for membership in the "full" medical staff. Due to the limited number of providers in such facilities, it is often more convenient to have a single staff structure so as to better coordinate services between physicians and those providers who are not physicians. So, in some instances, APRNs and others can be found as members of the "full" medical staff. Physicians, especially those in primary care, are expected to decrease in number in the foreseeable future. This and other changes in health care are signs that, in the future, it will be helpful and prudent for larger hospital facilities to include nonphysician providers on their "full" medical staffs.

Are There Differences Between Medical Staff and Allied/Associate Medical Staff Membership?

There are two important differences between "full" medical staff membership and allied medical staff membership. The first is that allied medical staff members have virtually no vote in setting the rules regarding practice within the facility. That power resides with the "full" medical staff. Members of the allied staff may be able informally to influence medical staff members about a particular point of view on an issue, but they otherwise do not have a say on important issues.

Another major, sometimes critical, difference is that "full" medical staff members are accorded full "due-process" safeguards, while those on the allied medical staff generally have no such protections. This means that should a dispute arise over the clinical performance of an allied staff member, the individual may be terminated without any opportunity for a full hearing in which to defend his or her actions. This, obviously, can have a catastrophic impact on that individual's career. While the hospital can grant that individual a hearing or other due-process rights, there is no requirement (in most cases) that they do so. This leaves the individual without recourse except, perhaps, through legal channels.

Members of the "full" medical staff, on the other hand, are accorded due process as a matter of right and are entitled to a fair hearing before they can be dismissed or otherwise disciplined. As the healthcare system increasingly focuses on individual clinical competence, there will be more questions about individual clinical performance that will need to be resolved. Allied medical staff members, therefore, will be disadvantaged in defending themselves against charges of sub-par clinical performance if they have no opportunity for a fair and impartial hearing.

Continued

Table 6-5 **The Institutional Credentialing Process—cont'd**

How Does One Apply for Hospital Privileges?

The process for applying for clinical privileges varies with each hospital but generally follows the process described here. Specific information and an application packet can be obtained from the hospital's medical staff office. Be aware, however, that the entire process for completing an application for privileges can be lengthy—often approaching 3 to 4 months. During this time, the individual is usually not allowed to practice in the facility, though some may provide for temporary employment that is limited to a specific time frame or restricted in terms of the interim clinical practice allowed.

What Information Do Applications Require?

The typical application packet includes a formal application form requesting clinical privileges in a specific role, a checklist setting out the requested specific clinical privileges (especially procedures to be performed) that may need to be reviewed and approved by a department head, and forms by which the applicant attests to his or her state of health and current competency to practice. The individual must also provide academic and work histories, documentation of all licenses, certifications and evidence of any specialty training. A photo may be requested but is often not asked for until the applicant is awarded privileges since a photo can bias the privileging decision on the basis of ethnicity or other factors. Application packets must be complete before the medical staff office will forward the application to the medical staff for review and a decision.

What Problems Can Delay Finalization of an Application?

Increasingly, applicants for clinical privileges must undergo criminal background and credit history checks. These slow down the application process but, by far, the greatest delays come from the need for the hospital to obtain "primary source verification" for all submitted documents and information. For example, this means the medical staff office must obtain verification of a nursing school diploma directly from the school. Obtaining a photocopy of the diploma directly from the applicant or any other "secondary" source is unacceptable. Obviously, schools get many such requests and are not always quick to respond. Similarly, past employment must be verified, and hospitals where the applicant has worked also may not have adequate staff to respond quickly. The problem of obtaining quick verification of data from primary sources is complicated further when the individual has practiced in many locales, over many years, and been licensed in multiple states. Many data must be gathered. Furthermore, any unexplained breaks in practice or negative reports, disciplinary actions, etc. need to be fully vetted and resolved before the application is submitted to the medical staff for action. Again, the application will not be acted upon until all application issues are resolved.

Does Being Credentialed by the Hospital Allow Practitioners Who Are Not Physicians the Right to Admit Patients to the Facility?

It has not generally been the case that the clinical privileges awarded to APRNs include the ability to admit patients to the facility for care. More often, the APRN must collaborate with a physician with admitting privileges in order to admit a patient. Not having admitting privileges can be problematic when a patient being treated in, for example, a clinic facility develops a problem requiring additional observation and care. Time can be wasted in contacting a collaborating physician to effect the admission. It is true, however, that a few facilities have begun giving admitting privileges to some APRNs. While APRN admitting privileges are presently the "cutting edge" of APRN practice, there clearly is emerging a growing trend to allowing the practice.

> ## Table 6-5 **The Institutional Credentialing Process—cont'd**
>
> ### What Can Applicants Do to Facilitate Their Credentialing Application?
> An applicant can decrease the likelihood of delays by ensuring that all necessary information is provided quickly, that it is accurate, and that the addresses and phone numbers of schools, prior places of employment, etc. are correct and current. Some of this information can be updated by an Internet search. The military services have central contact points for tracking down information related to military education and work experiences. These too can be located via the Internet.
>
> An applicant should also be up front about any past problems that have occurred, including drug dependence issues, hospital or state regulatory board disciplinary actions, malpractice actions, and similar issues. Any attempt to cover up such past incidents will likely result in a negative credentialing decision.
>
> Doing a good job of facilitating the initial application for hospital credentials will also be helpful when the time comes for the practitioner to be recertified. This generally occurs every 2 years.
>
> ### What Benefits Are Conferred by Credentialing (and Recredentialing)?
> Hospital credentials and the awarding of clinical privileges help to legitimize a person in his or her profession. It provides assurance that the individual is competent and capable of rendering high-quality care. A positive history over many years adds to one's professional credibility and enhances a person's career and work opportunities.

The collection of data is usually performed by a medical staff office charged with obtaining and maintaining credentialing records for all providers currently on staff at the facility. Whenever possible, verification of data is to be obtained from primary sources. This means, for example, that academic transcripts must be obtained directly from a university registrar. It is not acceptable for the person applying for privileges to submit photocopies as part of the official application. Photocopies can be provided to expedite the work of the medical staff office, which then must obtain primary verification from the original sources. There are accepted standard procedures for dealing with situations such as lost records, records from foreign countries, schools that have closed, and so on. APRNs should be aware that the credentialing process can take months to complete. The initial application for privileges is typically the most arduous, but each time the individual has to undergo recertification, typically every two years, the entire application process is nearly fully repeated.

CLINICAL PRIVILEGES

APRNs who are employed by a health-care facility must apply for and be granted clinical privileges prior to caring for patients. Although most will obtain their clinical privileges through the medical staff process of the facility, some will be credentialed through another entity, such as the department of nursing, special privileging committees, or the human resources department.

APRNs who are not employed by an institution and who are licensed independent practitioners (LIPs) must be credentialed through the medical staff privileging process at the facility where they seek to practice. A LIP is defined as an individual permitted by law and by the hospital to provide patient care services without direction or supervision, within the scope of the individual's license and consistent with individually granted clinical privileges. (See, for example, the Glossary section of the JC's *Accreditation Manual for Hospitals*.) Status as an LIP depends on state and federal laws and hospital bylaws and policies. Among APRNs often recognized as LIPs are CRNAs, CNMs, and NPs.

ADMITTING PRIVILEGES

APRNs practicing outside a hospital facility can, as part of their request for clinical privileges, ask to be granted admitting privileges. Having admission privileges allows the APRN to provide patients a continuity of care that would not otherwise be possible. A 1983 District of Columbia law prohibited hospitals there from denying clinical privileges or medical staff membership to CRNAs, CNMs, and certified NPs, as well as to other providers. The legislation was expanded in 1985 to include CNSs. At least five states—Alaska, Arizona, Arkansas, Oregon, and Wisconsin—allow APRNs to admit patients. Most states do not regulate the granting of hospital admission privileges for APRNs; the decision rests with the facility itself. Some states grant privileges only when the APRN's collaborating physician has medical staff privileges at the hospital.

The advantages of the APRN's having hospital admitting privileges are well recognized. They include:

- Allowing the APRN to direct the care a patient receives
- Allowing the APRN to deal more effectively with a patient's emergent condition since no time is lost gaining physician approval for the admission
- Ensuring that the patient can be discharged back to the APRN's care, thus ensuring the patient's continuity of care
- The ability to obtain reimbursement from third-party payers
- The ability to refer the patient to specialty providers
- The ability to be economically competitive with other healthcare providers

Obtaining privileges necessarily entails that the APRN assume greater professional accountability and responsibility. The APRN must fully participate in patient care decisions and ensure that the patient is rendered appropriate care 24 hours a day. He or she becomes legally liable for any personal acts of negligence or omission, just as a physician or hospital is under the same circumstances. Similarly, the APRN may be liable for failing to refer a patient to another provider when the patient's condition is beyond the APRN's competence. The professional demands on the APRN can be heavy and substantially reduce the time and energy available to engage in other activities or to meet personal or family commitments.

Appeal for Denial of Privileges

Applications for hospital credentials can be denied and often are upon the initial application. Initial denials can happen because the institution wants to avoid having the provider on its staff. These exclusions are sometimes derogatorily referred to as "economic credentialing," since there is economic harm to the person denied the credentials. Denials of this type may be couched in terms intended to give the decision legitimacy, but although facilities have considerable discretion in granting or denying privileges, denying an applicant for exclusionary purposes can expose it to legal liability if an applicant can show the exclusion was for prohibited discriminatory purposes.

Reasons for denial of privileges vary but are most often due to the inadequacy of a candidate's credentials, which can include a lack of demonstrated current competency (e.g., a person who has been out of practice for an extended period); the lack of, or weakness of, academic or performance records; or evidence the individual has experienced prior problems related to his or her professional practice. Privileges can also be denied at the time of recredentialing, but this is rarer and usually occurs because of serious changes in the practitioner's ability to demonstrate continued competence, such as a physical impairment or an addiction problem.

When privileges are denied, the applicant may choose to appeal the decision of the medical staff committee. The appeal must adhere to the processes set out in the medical staff bylaws, and the individual must exhaust due-process rights under the appeal process before electing to take an alternative action such as a lawsuit. Courts usually grant hospitals considerable latitude in dealing with medical staff matters, and a person who seeks legal redress without first having exhausted the hospital's appeal process is likely to be unsuccessful in initiating a lawsuit. Sometimes, the person denied privileges elects not to appeal but rather to reapply at a later date, using the interim time to correct identified deficiencies.

As a last resort, an APRN can look to the court system when he or she has been denied privileges, but this process is lengthy (perhaps as long as a dozen years or more), costly, and difficult. In bringing a suit against a hospital, the APRN may engender hostility in the community and damage his or her reputation in a way that has long-term negative consequences. Thus, the decision to bring a lawsuit to obtain clinical privileges is a difficult one, especially since there is no guarantee of success. The APRN considering this option should seek the counsel of a competent attorney with expertise in this area. Bringing a lawsuit to obtain clinical privileges can be an emotionally draining experience. Many faced with the decision have, instead, opted to seek credentials and employment at other facilities, but this can be difficult when practice options in a locale are limited.

Other ways an APRN may appeal the denial of privileges or other actions they feel discriminate against them are through complaints to the Federal Trade Commission (FTC) or through evoking antitrust laws.

COMPLAINTS TO THE FTC

APRNs (individuals or groups) who feel they have been discriminated against can file a complaint with the FTC. The basis for these cases is usually charges of anticompetitive behavior on the part of the hospital. For example, in a case involving nurse-midwives and the medical staff at the Memorial Medical Center of Savannah, Georgia, the nurse-midwives alleged that, in 1983, the hospital medical staff credentials committee voted to allow a nurse-midwife to perform deliveries at the center in the presence of a physician, a practice allowed by Georgia law. Subsequently, the medical staff protested the decision and threatened to take their patients to another hospital. The credentials committee then reversed its decision and denied the midwife hospital privileges and did this without stating any sound basis for the reversal. The FTC issued a consent order in the case on January 28, 1988. Under the consent agreement, the medical staff agreed not to deny or restrict nurse-midwife hospital privileges unless it could show a reasonable basis for such a decision and that denial of privileges would serve the interest of the hospital in providing healthcare services.[41]

As APRNs gain more recognition and acceptance on hospital staffs, discrimination issues will become less problematic. This, and the cost associated with pursuing legal remedies, makes it likely that fewer APRNs will advance FTC claims.

ANTITRUST RULINGS

APRNs who are denied hospital privileges or medical staff membership may be able to take legal action in federal court under the Sherman Antitrust Act. The U.S. Supreme Court acknowledged that health care is a commercial enterprise operated for economic benefit in the case of *Hospital Building Company v. Trustees of Rex Hospital*, 428 US 738 (1976).[42] The court ruled that health care is subject to the Sherman Act, which prohibits conspiracies "in restraint of trade or commerce among the several states" (Section 1) and also "prohibits the monopolization of "any part of the trade among the several states."[43,44] Both provisions have been the basis of lawsuits brought by healthcare practitioners who were denied hospital privileges. Certain types of providers, or those affected by "exclusive" contracts between a hospital and a group providing services (e.g., pediatric care), have used these two sections of the Sherman Act as the basis on which to bring their claims. Additionally, a number of states have passed legislation, similar to the Sherman Act, that provides for state remedies for aggrieved parties.

Two requirements must be met preliminarily in order to advance a Sherman Act claim successfully. First, the claimant must show that the controversy involves interstate trade or commerce.[44] This sometimes can be demonstrated by a very tenuous, and often implied, connection between the hospital and interstate trade (e.g., a showing that the hospital has out-of-state shareholders or purchases equipment from another state). In other instances, the court requires a tighter nexus of connection between the hospital's action and interstate trade or commerce. In these cases, it may require a more direct connection between the denial of privileges and interstate commerce. Second, an individual bringing the suit must show there has been a conspiracy in restraint of trade. This may amount to no more than a joint understanding that creates a restraint for the claimant. Determining whether the needed "restraint" is sufficient depends on the facts of the case. In one case (*Bhan v. NME Hospitals*) brought by a CRNA, the court found no restraint of trade because all NME hospitals operating in a given area had policies that did not allow nurse anesthetists to practice.[44] Yet, in another case (*Oltz v. St. Peter's Hospital*), a nurse anesthetist obtained a favorable decision because the defendant hospital was the only hospital in the area equipped to do general surgery.[45]

In the *Bhan v. NME Hospitals* case, several precedents relevant to advanced nursing practice and antitrust case law were established. Mr. Bhan, a CRNA, had worked for one of the NME hospitals on a fee-for-service basis for several years. Under a contract with the hospital, he and an anesthesiologist had provided all of the hospital's anesthesia services until the time that the hospital hired a second anesthesiologist. At that time, Bhan's anesthesiologist associate urged the hospital to drop Bhan from the staff and to rely on himself and the newly hired anesthesiologist. The hospital followed this recommendation. Mr. Bhan claimed that the all-anesthesiologist policy was adopted as part of a conspiracy to eliminate competition. The federal trial court dismissed the lawsuit on the grounds that nurses and doctors do not compete, because in California, CRNAs were not authorized to write orders and were required to work under a supervising physician. The U.S. District Court of Appeals reversed this decision, stating that although the legal restrictions on CRNAs create a functional distinction between them and anesthesiologists, such restrictions did not preclude their reasonable interchangeability. In effect, the court held that nurses have standing to sue under the antitrust laws when they are excluded from practicing as the result of anticompetitive arrangements between hospitals and physicians.

In the *Oltz v. St Peter's Community Hospital* case, a federal trial court and the federal court of appeals agreed that the hospital had conspired with anesthesiologists to restrain the nurse anesthetist's practice. Mr. Oltz was an independent contractor providing anesthesia services, primarily for obstetric cases. The facts demonstrated that Mr. Oltz was popular with the obstetricians, who preferred his services to those of the anesthesiologists. When the hospital decided to organize an anesthesia department, Mr. Oltz's contract was terminated. The contract was reinstated when the hospital received correspondence from Oltz's attorney and the state attorney general's office. Subsequently, three of the hospital's four anesthesiologists threatened to quit if Oltz's services were retained, and so his contract was once again terminated. After Oltz's departure, each anesthesiologist received a 40% to 50% salary increase. A monetary pretrial settlement was negotiated with the anesthesiologists, and Oltz proceeded successfully in obtaining a jury verdict against the hospital. This is one of the few cases in which a healthcare provider has been able to prove that the installation of an exclusive contract violated the Sherman Act and caused economic damages.[45]

In *Nurse-Midwifery Associates v. Hibbett,* midwives used the Sherman Antitrust Act and the Tennessee state antitrust laws to keep the defendants from denying staff privileges to nurse-midwives.[46] The defendants included three hospitals, three obstetricians, a pediatrician, and an insurance provider. The midwives claimed their denial of privileges had put them out of business. One obstetrician, Hibbett, was a member of the insurance company board of trustees. The court, for various reasons, denied the midwives' claim regarding one hospital and concluded that the claim against the other two hospitals and Hibbett required a trial. An out-of-court settlement was reached by the parties after 13 years of legal wrangling.

The foregoing cases are meant to illustrate the principles and problems with which APRNs must contend whenever they seek practice credentials and clinical privileges from hospitals. The cases are not, however, intended as a comprehensive or definitive review of the legal implications of being denied hospital privileges. APRNs faced with antitrust issues are urged to consult with a competent attorney in the state in which they practice.

Primary Care Provider Status for APRNs

Some, but not all, APRNs are involved with providing primary care services to patients. Such services can be rendered in a variety of clinical settings and under numerous practice arrangements. Though primary care providers (PCPs), as a group, tend to offer the same kind of comprehensive assessment and diagnostic services, there is as yet no universally accepted definition or credential that uniquely identifies a provider as a PCP. However, given the growing numbers of NPs and CNMs who offer such care (and the significantly diminished numbers of physicians entering primary care medical specialties), it may be that PCP NPs will become a more distinguishable entity in the future.

APRN Access to Reimbursement Panels

As APRNs increasingly move into "independent" practice arrangements, reimbursement for professional services becomes a greater priority and, in turn, a major obstacle. APRNS must deal with the issue of accessing provider reimbursement panels. Healthcare management organizations and other insurance providers who pay for healthcare services traditionally have restricted membership on their reimbursement panels exclusively to physicians. The panels determine what the insurer will pay for services, so physicians have a vested interest in increasing their payments to the detriment of other providers, such as APRNs. Nurses have been requesting representation on these panels for many years but have generally been unsuccessful.

The importance of having APRNs represented on payer panels cannot be overemphasized. Such panels determine which professionals get reimbursed for services and at what level. Many APRN providers are not recognized by these panels, and those who are are frequently paid less than a physician for providing the same service. In addition to this economic inequity, the situation harms APRNs in other ways, including lower professional esteem, lack of recognition by other professional groups, and decreased competitiveness in the marketplace. The stumbling block to changing this situation is that insurance companies are proprietary organizations that, alone, determine who will be represented on their payer panels.

It is incumbent upon APRNs to continue applying for a "seat at the table" and to continue to inform insurers about the safe, high-quality, cost-effective array of services with excellent outcomes that they provide. Healthcare changes currently being considered under the Obama administration may provide new opportunities for APRNs to be included in more reimbursement decisions.

Summary

Regulation of advanced nursing practice will undergo tremendous change over the next decade, and the consensus-based recommendations regarding APRN education, accreditation, certification, and licensure have the potential to create clarity and uniformity that will benefit both APRNs and patients in the future.

The growing awareness that a reformed healthcare system will require a strong and vibrant supply of APRNs to deliver the full range of care to patients with acute and chronic conditions has dramatically increased the call for expanding the numbers of APRNs. Additionally, the view that clinical prevention and health promotion will be central components of any reform initiatives will also increase opportunities for using the skills of nurses prepared with advanced clinical skills and knowledge.

APRNs have a responsibility to respond to concerns regarding confusion over their expanded number of practice specialties through strong support of consensus-based recommendations. Changes in the healthcare delivery system, increased consumer involvement in health care, and public demand for accountability in providing high-quality, cost-effective care, have, and will continue to have, a significant impact on the regulation and credentialing of APRNS. Thus, APRNs must assume a leadership role not only in the delivery of healthcare services but also in the professional and public regulation of nursing practice. To assume such a role, APRNs must be able to understand and articulate the authorized scope of their practice. The ability to understand the interrelationships among the processes used by the public and the profession to regulate advanced nursing practice and to respond appropriately to these processes is crucial.

SUGGESTED LEARNING EXERCISES

1. Review the statutory and regulatory standards for advanced nursing practice in the state in which you expect to practice after graduation. Determine which is the correct state regulatory agency, and obtain from it the state authority-to-practice guidelines.

2. Identify the APRN-certifying organization that administers the examination most relevant to your expected area of practice, and obtain information regarding the standards for practice, the process of application for certification, and the process for renewal of certification.

3. Access the Consensus Model for Advanced Practice Registered Nurse Regulation: Licensure, Accreditation, Certification and Education (http://www.aacn.nche.edu/education/pdf/APRNReport.pdf); analyze the proposed changes in the regulation of advanced practice education, accreditation, certification, and licensure; and determine its impact on your area of advanced practice.

4. Obtain a copy of the bylaws of a hospital to determine the process used to delineate and grant clinical and admitting privileges. Based on the hospital's bylaws, determine whether an APRN is eligible for membership on the medical staff.

5. Review the annual update on licensure and prescriptive privileges and the NCSBN Member Board Profiles to identify changes that have occurred from the previous year. How does the state in which you practice compare to other states in the area of independent practice, scope of practice, prescriptive authority, and reimbursement for all APRNs?

References

1. American Nurses Association. (1995). *Nursing's Social Policy Statement.* American Nurses Association, Washington, DC.

2. Malson, LP. (1989). *Credentialing in Nursing: Contemporary Developments and Trends.* American Nurses Association, Kansas City, MO.

3. Cox, C, and Foster, S. (1990). *The Costs and Benefits of Occupational Regulation.* Bureau of the Federal Trade Commission, Washington, DC.

4. Friedland, B, and Valachovic, R. (1991). The regulation of dental licensing: the dark ages? *Am J Law Med* 17:249.

5. Maine Health Professions Regulation Taskforce. (1995). *Toward a More Rational State Licensure System for Maine's Health Professionals: A Report to the Governor and Maine Legislature. Medical Care Development, Maine Health Professions Regulation Task Force,* Medical Care Department, Maine Health Professions Regulation Task Force, Augusta, ME.

6. Pew Health Professions Commission. (1995). *Reforming Health Care Workforce Regulation: Policy Considerations for the 21st Century.* Pew Health Professions Commission, San Francisco, CA.

7. Burl, JB, and Bonner, A. (1994). Demonstration of the cost-effectiveness of a NP/physician team in long-term care facilities. *HMO Practice* 8(4):157.

8. Frampton, J, and Wall, S. (1994). Exploring the use of NPs and PAs in primary care. *HMO Practice* 8(4):164.

9. Schultz, JM, Liptak, GS, and Fioravanti, J. (1994). Nurse practitioners' effectiveness in NICU. *Nurs Mngmnt* 25(10):50.

10. National Council of State Boards of Nursing. *Member Board Profiles.* https://www.ncsbn.org/983.htm. Accessed May 4, 2010.

11. NCSBN. (2003). *Using Nurse Practitioner Certification for State Nursing Regulation: A Historical Perspective.* Chicago, IL. Can be accessed at ncsbn.org/public/regulation/licensure_aprn_practitioner.html.

12. King, CS. (1995). Second licensure. *Adv Practice Nurs Quarterly* 1(1):7.

13. Henderson, T, Fox-Grage, W, and Lewis, S. (1995). *Scope of Practice and Reimbursement for Advanced Practice Registered Nurses: A State-by-State Analysis.* Intergovernmental Health Policy Project, Washington, DC.

14. Pearson, L. (2008, February). The Pearson Report: the annual state-by-state national overview of nurse practitioner legislation and health care issues. *AJNP.*

15. Safriet, BJ. (1992). Health care dollars and regulatory sense: the role of advanced practice nursing. *Yale J Regulation* 9(2).

16. Sekscenski, E, et al. (1994). State practice environments and the supply of physician assistants, NPs, and certified nurse-midwives. *N Engl J Med* 331:1266.

17. American Nurses Association. *Institutional Licensure: An Historical Perspective. House of Directors Action Report.* (1995). American Nurses Association, Washington DC.

18. National Council of State Boards of Nursing. (1993). What regulation of advanced practice can offer health care reform. (1993). *Issues* 14(3):4.

19. National Council of State Boards of Nursing. *Map of NLC States.* http://www.ncsbn.org/158.htm. Accessed April 25, 2009.

20. National Council of State Boards of Nursing. *APRN Multistate Compact.* http://www.ncsbn.org/917.htm. Accessed April 25, 2009.

21. National Council of State Boards of Nursing. (2000). *Uniform Advanced Practice Registered Nurse Licensure/Authority to Practice Requirements*. National Council of State Boards of Nursing, Chicago, IL.

22. American Nurses Certification Corporation. (1995). *1996 Certification Catalog*. American Nurses Certification Corporation, Washington DC.

23. National Certification Corporation. (1995). *Certification Committee Newsletter*. National Certification Corporation, Chevy Chase, MD.

24. Association of Women's Health Organizations and Neonatal Nurses, National Association of Nurses in Reproductive Health, and Planned Parenthood Federation of America. (1995, Sept 15). *Consensus Statement on Women's Health Care Nurse Practitioner Education*. Washington, DC. pp. 19–35.

25. American Association of Colleges of Nursing (2004). *Position Statement on the Practice Doctorate in Nursing*. American Association of Colleges of Nursing, Washington DC.

26. American Association of Colleges of Nursing. (1997). *Essentials of Master's Education for Advanced Practice Nursing*. American Association of Colleges of Nursing, Washington DC.

27. American Midwifery Certification Board. *Certificate Maintenance*. http://www.amcbmidwife.org/c/97/certificate-maintenance. Accessed October 15, 2009.

28. American Association of Nurse Anesthetists. http://www.aana.org/credentialing. Accessed October 15, 2009.

29. Cooke, M, Irby, DM, Sullivan, W, and Ludmerer, KM. (2006, Sept 28). American Medical Education 100 Years after the Flexner Report, *NEJM* 355:1339–1344.

30. American Nurses Association. *More About RNs and Advanced Practice RNs*. http://nursingworld.org/EspeciallyForYou/StudentNurses/RNsAPNs.aspx. Accessed May 3, 2009.

31. American Association of Nurse Anesthetists (AANA). *Certified Registered Nurse Anesthetists (CRNAs) at a Glance*. http://www.aana.com/aboutaana.aspx?ucNavMenu_TSMenuTargetID=179&ucNavMenu_TSMenuTargetType=4&ucNavMenu_TSMenuID=6&id=265. Accessed May 3, 2009.

32. National Vital Statistics Report. (2002, February 12). 50(5). http://74.125.47.132/search?q=cache:sGdqXA99IMYJ:www.cdc.gov/nchs/data/erratas/nvsr50_05_t10.pdf+National+Vital+Statistics+Report,+Vol.+50,+No+5,+February+12,+2002&cd=2&hl=en&ct=clnk&gl=us. Accessed May 3, 2009.

33. Readership and practice profile of the ACNM: findings of a direct mail survey. *J Nurse-Midwifery* 39(1). http://www.sciencedirect.com/science?_ob=ArticleURL&_udi=B6T8N-4G0105T-37&_user=10&_rdoc=1&_fmt=&_orig=search&_sort=d&view=c&_acct=C000050221&_version=1&_urlVersion=0&_userid=10&md5=3815e55cb848228e152e545a6b7cfa41. Accessed May 3, 2009.

34. Department of Health and Human Services. (1994). *Survey of Certified Nurse Practitioners and Clinical Nurse Specialists: December 1992*. Department of Health and Human Services, Public Health Service, Health Resources and Services Administration, Bureau of Health Professions, Division of Nursing, Rockville, MD.

35. Joint Commission on Accreditation of Healthcare Organizations. (1994). *1995 Accreditation Manual for Hospitals*, Vols. 1 and 2, 1992. The Joint Commission (now), Oakbrook Terrace, IL.

36. Stevens, JE. (1984). The question of hospital privileges for allied health professionals. *Quality Review Bulletin* 10(1):17.

37. Healthcare Facilities Accreditation Program (HFAP). Information at: https://www.do-online.org/index.cfm?PageID=edu_main&au=D&SubPageID=acc_main&SubSubPageID=acc_hfmain. Accessed May 3, 2009.

38. Zieger, A. (2008, Sept 26). CMS gives DNV Healthcare authority to accredit U.S. hospitals. *FierceHealthcare Newsletter*. http://www.fiercehealthcare.com/story/cms-gives-dnv-healthcare-authority-accredit-u-s-hospitals/2008-09-26. Accessed May 3, 2009.

39. Information about the American Association for Accreditation of Ambulatory Surgery Facilities (AAAASF) can be accessed at: http://www.aaaasf.org/. Accessed May 3, 2009.

40. Information about the Accreditation Association for Ambulatory Health Care (AAAHC) can be accessed at: http://www.aaahc.org/eweb/StartPage.aspx. Accessed May 3, 2009.

41. American College of Nurse-Midwives. (1988). Hospital staff settling charges they illegally denied hospital privileges to nurse-midwife. *J. Nurse-Midwifery* 33:152.

42. Cushing, M. (1989). Safeguarding the spirit of competition. *Am J Nurs* 89:1035.

43. Sherman Act, 15 USC 1 and 2.

44. Blumenreich, GA. (1998). Antitrust protection against a hospital's denial of access. *JAANA 56* (5):383.

45. Brent, Nancy J. (2001). *Nurses and the Law: A Guide to Principles and Applications,* 2nd ed. Elseveier Health Sciences, p. 502. A synopsis of this case can be accessed at: http://books.google.com/books?id=sSBqMss0mPAC&pg=PA500&lpg=PA500&dq=Oltz+v.+St.+Peter's+Community+Hospitall&source=bl&ots=obTtIMzHfo&sig=4OorTTRFuG7S-vSdY1g60SEmF1A&hl=en&ei=-l_-SfT5KsfBtwfViLjFCg&sa=X&oi=book_result&ct=result&resnum=3#PPR14,M1. Accessed May 3, 2009.

46. *Nurse Midwifery Associates v. Hibbett,* 918 F2d 605 (6th Cir 1990).

Michael Kremer received his doctorate from the Rush University College of Nursing. His master's of science in nursing degree is from Seattle Pacific University, and he received his nurse anesthesia education at the University of Illinois-Springfield and undergraduate psychology and nursing degrees from Northern Illinois University. He is an associate professor in adult health nursing and Director of the Nurse Anesthesia Program in the Rush University College of Nursing. Dr. Kremer also served as an associate professor and nurse anesthesia program director at Rosalind Franklin University in North Chicago, Illinois. He has held numerous elected and appointed positions at the state and national levels.

Margaret Faut-Callahan received her master's and doctoral degrees from the Rush University College of Nursing and attended Loyola University in Chicago, Illinois for her undergraduate education. She is Dean of the Marquette University School of Nursing, Milwaukee, Wisconsin, and previously served as Professor and Chair of Adult Health Nursing and Director of the Nurse Anesthesia Program in the Rush University College of Nursing. She is a leader in nursing and advanced practice nursing education and was an early proponent of graduate-level education for nurse anesthetists, including master's and doctoral programs with a nurse anesthesia emphasis. She has held many elected and appointed positions at the state and national levels and as primary investigator on a National Cancer Institute Palliative Care Grant.

CHAPTER 7

Reimbursement for Expanded Professional Nursing Practice Services

Michael J. Kremer, PhD, CRNA, FAAN; Margaret Faut-Callahan, PhD, CRNA, FAAN

CHAPTER OBJECTIVES

After completing this chapter, the reader will be able to:

1. Discuss the components of a traditional economic system.
2. Describe the criteria for an economic system in relation to health care.
3. Note the effect of changes in price, supply, and demand for health care.
4. Discuss cost considerations in the provision of health care by and reimbursement for physicians and APRNs.
5. Demonstrate familiarity with key terms in finance and reimbursement.
6. Describe the development of federal reimbursement policies for APRN reimbursement.

Market-driven factors, policy decisions, and political factors have influenced the payment of nonphysician providers. The genesis of the nurse practitioner (NP) role in the mid-1960s included advocacy by nursing leaders for reimbursement mechanisms for NPs.[1] However, it was not until 1997 that all advanced practice registered nurses (APRNs) had billing rights under Medicare and other payers.

A policy shift in health care that emerged in the 1980s was the adoption of traditional market forces in an attempt to achieve greater efficiency in the production of healthcare services. Reliance on regulatory control of healthcare financing, such as the certificate of need (CON) system imposed in the 1970s, failed to contain healthcare costs. Regulatory control was advocated ostensibly from a quality standpoint, but healthcare providers favored the weakest mechanisms to ensure quality while supporting regulations that advanced their economic self-interests and enabled them to create monopolistic positions in their respective markets.[2] The monopolies that were created determined the type and amount of health care provided and obtained regulatory barriers to prevent others from seeking to enter markets over which they had control. It was posited that if health care had been governed less by regulations and more by traditional market forces, the genesis of monopolistic forces would have been stifled. In that case, market forces would have predominated, and professionals would have been forced to compete on the basis of price, quality, and the extent to which they provided services that were responsive to the preferences of consumers.[3] This chapter discusses these economic trends in the context of the components of the economic system.

Rising healthcare costs in a time of economic constraints require APRNs to be cost-effective and knowledgeable regarding reimbursement for their services. Rapid changes in reimbursement legislation, policies, and procedures make these daunting tasks. The current American healthcare system does not resemble its antecedents. Managed care and preferred provider organizations (PPOs) dominate health care, and large provider networks have emerged as a result of consolidations and mergers. As patient care has moved from inpatient to outpatient settings, managed care organizations (MCOs) have increasingly stressed the importance of health maintenance, preventive services, chronic illness management, and patient education. From an economic standpoint, improved client health translated into MCO cost savings. Since 1996, public and legislative pressure has led state legislatures to enact more than 100 laws that restrict managed care administrative or clinical practices. At the federal level,

Congress has grappled with legislation calling for improved access, quality assurance, and provider choice for patients.[4]

APRNs cannot rely on administrators, office managers, and physician employers to protect and promote their interests. Effective strategies to surmount APRN reimbursement barriers require concerted efforts from nurse educators, professional nursing organizations, and savvy practicing nurses to lobby elected bodies and MCOs to ensure full APRN participation in available reimbursement mechanisms.[4]

The Economic System

The economic system consists of the network of institutions, laws, and rules created by society to answer the following universal economic questions:

- What goods and services shall be produced?
- How shall they be produced?
- For whom shall they be produced?

Every society needs an economic system because human, natural, and artificial resources are scarce relative to human wants and because these resources have alternative uses and there are multiple competing wants. Decisions must be made about the use of these resources in production and the distribution of the resulting output among members of society.[5]

The United States spends more on health care per capita than any other nation. Healthcare spending in the United States comprises 16% of the gross domestic product (GDP) and is expected to reach 19.5% of the GDP by 2017. In 2007, the United States spent $7439 per person on health care, or $2.26 trillion. As of this writing, the federal government is proposing unprecedented steps, including $1 trillion in support, to address fiscal instability attributed to subprime mortgages and financial market deregulation.[6] Difficult decisions must be made regarding the allocation of healthcare resources, and the difficulty of these decisions is compounded by the uncertain state of the global economic future. Some relevant questions raised in this regard include:

- Who will receive healthcare services?
- By whom will these services be provided?
- At what cost will these services be provided?

Criteria for an Economic System Related to Health Care

Given the increasing scarcity of resources along with competing goals, the healthcare economic system should result in:

- An optimum amount of resources devoted to health care;
- The optimal combination of these resources; and
- An appropriate allocation of resources between current provision of health care and investment in future health care through research, education, and implementation of evidence-based practices

The general rule for reaching such optima is "equity at the margin."[5(p13)] For instance, the first criterion would be met if the last dollar's worth of resources devoted to health care increased human satisfaction by exactly the same amount as the last dollar's worth devoted to other goods.[5] The contrast between this view of a social optimum and the notion of optimum as used in health care requires discussion. The relationship between health and healthcare inputs can be described by a curve that may initially rise at an increasing rate but then levels off or declines. Optimal care can be defined as Point A, where no further increment in health is possible. The social optimum requires that resource inputs do not exceed the point at which the value of an additional increment to health equals the cost of inputs required to obtain that increment, or Point B. At Point C, where the ratio of benefits to costs is at maximum, additional inputs add more to benefits than to costs. See Figure 7-1.

Types of Economic Systems

Economists have identified three "pure types" of economic systems:

1. Traditional
2. Centrally directed
3. Market price

Every economy is a blend of types, but the relative importance of the different types varies. Primitive and feudal societies relied on basic economic decisions that were made by one person or a small group of people. The former Soviet Union was an example of such a system. The United States, Canada, and most countries of Western Europe have relied on market systems for more than 100 years.[5]

A market system contains decision-making units called households and firms. Households own all the productive resources in society and make these resources available to firms. The firm transforms these resources into goods and services that are distributed back to the households. The flow of resources and of goods and services is facilitated by a counterflow of money.[5]

In a market system as shown in Figure 7-2 the exchanges of resources and services for money take place in markets where prices and quantities are determined. These prices are the signals or controls that trigger behavioral changes related to technology or preferences. The market system is sometimes referred to as the price system.[5]

In the markets for resources, households are the suppliers and firms provide the demand. In the markets for goods and services, the firms are the suppliers and the households are the sources of demand. In each market, the interaction between demand and supply determines the quantities and prices of the various resources and the various goods and services.

Figure 7-3 demonstrates a typical market. The income of each household depends on the quantity and quality of resources available to it and the prices of those resources. The amount of household income determines its share of the total flow of goods and services.

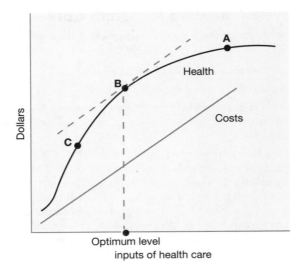

Figure 7-1: Determination of optimum level of healthcare utilization.

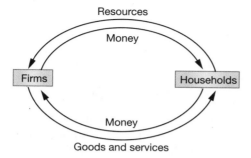

Figure 7-2: Elementary model of a market system.

The household is assumed to spend its income to maximize its utility, or satisfaction. This occurs according to the principle of "equality at the margin." It adjusts its purchases so that marginal utility, or the satisfaction added by the last unit purchased of each commodity, is proportional to its price.[5]

It is assumed that firms attempt to maximize profits, or the difference between what they must pay households for the use of resources and what they get from the households for the goods and services they produce. To maximize profits, firms must also follow the equality at the margin rule, adjusting their use of different types of resources so that the marginal products, or the addition to output obtained from one additional unit of input, are proportional to the price.[5]

The essence of a competitive market is that:

- There are many well-informed buyers and sellers, but no one of them influences price.
- The buyers and sellers act independently.
- There is free entry for other buyers and sellers not currently in the market.

The U.S. economy departs in many respects from the competitive market model. This departure is especially noticeable in the healthcare sector. Most health-care markets depart substantially from competitive conditions, sometimes inevitably and sometimes as a result of deliberate public or private policy.[5]

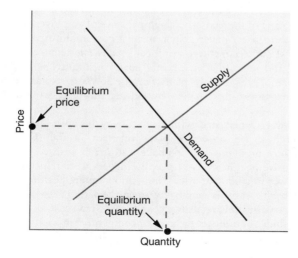

Figure 7-3: A typical market.

Market Competition

In a competitive industry, firms have strong economic incentives to minimize the costs of producing their products and services so they can be priced competitively and sold in the marketplace. To minimize production costs, firms must be innovative in their use of capital and labor, endeavoring to find the least costly number and combination of resources to produce their goods. Because consumers consider both the price and quality of goods and services when making purchases, firms attempt to improve the quality of their products without causing significant price increases. Firms conduct market research to determine consumer preferences and initiate promotional activities to inform the public on the price and quality of their products, as well as to differentiate their products from those of their competitors.[3]

A competitive marketplace is characterized by consumers being provided with a variety of choices in the goods and services available for purchase. Influenced by their income, tastes, and preferences and by the amount of information available about the product, consumers consider the trade-off between price and quality and purchase those items that are most satisfying to them. Those in control of supply and demand in competitive markets are in touch with each other. Satisfying the consumer is the only way that firms can sell their products and earn profits.[3]

Cost-Unconscious Demand

Much of the healthcare system has been built on what has been termed "cost-unconscious demand."[7] The lack of sensitivity to the price of health care has occurred for multiple reasons. Tax laws permit the exclusion of employer-paid health insurance premiums from the taxable income of employees. This has led to the purchase of more health insurance coverage than would be the case if employees bought the insurance directly using after-tax income. This tax policy has resulted in overconsumption of health care because employees are not conscious of the price of the services they consume. Similarly, providers, who know that an insurance company will pay for the services, have no economic incentive to restrain the cost of providing a treatment or the amount of care provided.[8] As long as the patient and provider are insensitive to price and are spared from fiscal accountability for their actions, patients will continue to demand more health care than they may require, and providers will continue to supply that care. Under this system, neither party has economic incentives to consider the costs or benefits of consuming additional amounts of health care, but behave as if more is better.

Employers, in most instances, also have fostered cost-unconsciousness by constructing their health insurance offerings so that the employee who chooses the lowest-priced health plan is not permitted to keep any of the savings.[5] The prevalence of employers subsidizing the more costly fee-for-service third-party-payer system against cost-minimizing health maintenance organizations (HMOs) and competitive healthcare plans has removed incentives for employees to shop around and select the least costly health insurance plan. This practice stymied price competition among healthcare plans because lower-cost plans cannot "take business away from the next-lowest-priced plan by cutting the price paid to the people actually making the choice."[5]

It was thought that employers persisted with this strategy because, in addition to the perverse incentives to purchase fee-for-service plans inherent in the tax treatment of employer-paid health insurance premiums, unions have historically insisted that their members have 100% comprehensive healthcare coverage. Employers were reluctant to use their considerable purchasing power to stimulate price competition among healthcare plans.[3]

The increasing cost of health care to employers since the late 1980s became a major economic force that impacted healthcare delivery and cost. The cost of health care to employers undermined the ability of industry to be price competitive in a global marketplace. Employers became motivated to adopt reforms demanding health services that stimulate greater price competition among healthcare plans and other supply-side providers. It is in the best interest of the nursing profession to become involved in research and management efforts seeking to find solutions to some of these supply, demand, and cost problems in health care and to prepare for a far more competitive healthcare system.[3]

Attempts to Reduce Costs

One recent example of public economic policy having an impact on reimbursement in health care is the Medicare payment policies affecting physicians. In 1996, the federal government completed the 4-year phase-in of the resource-based relative value scale (RBRVS) as its payment system for physicians under Part B of the Medicare program. Although the program seemed to accomplish one of its primary objectives—to transfer payments from tests and procedures to evaluation and management services—physicians were dissatisfied with the program in a number of ways. The Physician Payment Review Commission (PPRC), which monitors the implementation of the fee schedule, has expressed concern that low Medicare RBRVS payments may negatively affect the access that beneficiaries have to physicians. Other investigators[9,10] have shown that low Medicaid fees hamper access to office-based physicians and encourage the use of hospital outpatient department and emergency services, both of which reinforce PPRC concerns about the link between physician payments and decreased access to care. Should federal budget deficit pressures result in prolongation of inadequate RBRVS payments (approximately 75% of Medicare physician payments are financed using general tax dollars) and should physicians respond by reducing medical care provided to an increasing number of Medicare beneficiaries, then additional demand for APRNs could develop.[11]

The use of market forces in health care has stimulated discussion of the nature of competition in the healthcare marketplace. Managed care transformed the organization and delivery of health care, but some of those changes were transient. The previously espoused vision for integrated healthcare delivery has been supplanted by mandates for more active roles for consumers of health care. A current impetus for reduced healthcare costs is putting competitive pressure on providers to improve the quality of care and concomitantly to reduce costs.[12]

However, the role of consumer decision making relative to healthcare cost and quality has been questioned. During the development of managed care, it was believed that market competition would create a system that offered excellent care at low cost. The goal was for providers to compete on the basis of the quality of services provided. More than 20 years later, an early leader in managed care noted, "until recently, I was convinced that consumers, given adequate information about their choices, could effectively influence both the cost of health insurance and the quality of health care. I was wrong! . . . Studies show that despite greater public access to sound health information, market forces . . . do not exert sufficient influence over the quality of health services."[13] The American Nurses Association (ANA) notes that "despite 15 years of incremental, market-based approaches to reform healthcare payment and delivery systems in the United States, systematic transformation remains elusive. The healthcare system continues to be inequitable, fragmented, ineffective, costly, and often fraught with errors."[14]

In 1998, NPs and clinical nurse specialists (CNSs) entered the realm of U.S. healthcare financing as Medicare providers, the culmination of more than 30 years of attempts to attain this status.[15] This achievement over the long term may help decrease healthcare costs as NPs and CNSs are typically paid less than physicians.

Medicare Payment Systems

In 2007, there were 43.9 million citizens enrolled in Medicare.[16] The diagnostic-related group (DRG) approach was used in the Medicare program to quantify and limit hospital costs via Medicare Part A and other third-party payers. With this approach, payment is made to hospitals based on the average cost of care and length of stay for specific medical diagnoses. Investigators have described issues in measuring nursing work and variability in nursing care intensity based on hospital payment and DRG.[17,18]

Medicare Part B provides payment to clinicians, including physicians, APRNs, physician assistants (PAs), psychologists, and podiatrists, for services provided in inpatient and outpatient settings. Payment for Part B services is based on the RBRVS in which billing codes, often Current Procedural Terminology (CPT) codes, are assigned a relative value for work, practice expense, and professional liability; this number is then multiplied by a dollar amount conversion factor that provides a billable amount for each billed code. Billing and coding functions are typically performed by billing services that employ professionals with expertise in these areas. It is important to realize that 100% of what is billed is not collected, but working with billers and coders helps to bolster the providers' collection rates.

Covered nursing services in Medicare Part B include direct payment to an APRN, along with indirect payments to Medicare providers, for nursing care provided by staff employees. APRNs are Part B Medicare providers and can be directly reimbursed for identified services in Medicare claims.

Growth of Retail Health Clinics

An emerging trend in NP practice has been the growth of retail healthcare clinics located in major retail chain stores, including Target and Wal-Mart, and drugstore chains such as CVS and Walgreens. Most of these retail clinics, also known as the "Convenient Care Industry," are staffed by NPs, who provide patients with fast and affordable treatment for common medical conditions as well as with preventive care. They use their skills to diagnose, treat, and prescribe medications as well as to provide healthcare screenings, diagnostic tests, vaccinations, immunizations, and in some locations physical examinations.[19] Retail clinics provide significant cost savings for nonemergent care that might otherwise be provided in hospital emergency departments, and consumers have expressed satisfaction with them. However, some physicians have expressed doubts about the quality of care provided in these settings.[20]

APRN Autonomy and Reimbursement

Groups such as the American Medical Association (AMA) and their component societies lobby state legislatures, Congress, and the Center for Medicare and Medicaid Services (CMS) to restrict the definition of primary care provider (PCP) to physicians and to limit reimbursement laws and regulations to an equally narrow providership. However, their success has been mixed. In response to the increasing acceptability of APRNs in the workforce, numerous state legislatures have legitimized the autonomy of APRN practice in laws and regulations. As of 2009, 24 states including the District of Columbia had statutes granting APRNs the right to practice without physician supervision or collaboration.[21] Eighteen states have mandated direct reimbursement to APRNs by private insurers, HMOs, MCOs, and Medicaid.[22] Little change has been made in reimbursement laws over the past several years except for the recent increase in certified nurse-midwife reimbursement rate from 65% to 100% under Medicare. This change was part of the Patient Protection and Affordable Care Act signed into law March 2010.

The most common statutory language pertaining to APRNs grants NPs title protection and the board of nursing (BON) sole authority in scope of practice, with no statutory or regulatory requirements for physician collaboration, direction, or supervision. As of 2009, in 20 states, NPs had title protection with the BON as the sole authority in scope of practice; however, scope of practice required physician collaboration in those states. In three states, NPs had title protection and the BON was the sole authority for scope of practice, but there was some requirement for physician supervision. In four other states, NPs had title protection but their scope of practice was jointly authorized by the BON and the board of medicine.[22]

A recent analysis demonstrated that in states in which APRNs had greater amounts of professional independence they had substantially lower earnings compared with higher rates of compensation for PAs. As PAs and NPs compete economically, it is interesting to note that the principal operational difference between these two groups is that the PAs are salaried employees who must work under physician supervision, which implies that physicians have responded to increased APRN professional independence with the employment of fewer APRNs and more PAs.[23]

The 1997 Balanced Budget Act guaranteed Medicare reimbursement for nonphysician providers (e.g., NPs, CNSs, and PAs) regardless of setting and became a model for reimbursement practices adopted by states and other health plans. Although this act authorizes direct APRN reimbursement, it also requires collaboration with physicians.[24] This requirement is a problem in states in which collaboration is not required because APRNs in those states who have established independent practice are not able to bill Medicare without changing their practices and obtaining physician collaboration.[4]

The potential economic consequences of the pricing decisions of an advanced nursing practice, including the anticipated effects on physicians and consumers, are discussed later in this chapter. To describe these consequences adequately, it is first necessary to discuss key economic terms and concepts that underpin the relationship between price and the firm's demand, the amount of total revenues, profitability, and economic responses by physicians or consumers.[11]

Current healthcare economic conditions include obstacles to the involvement of APRNs in reimbursement strategies, including limitations on scope of practice and exclusion of nursing diagnoses and interventions from payment. The key to rectifying this inequity is understanding and participating in current reimbursement processes. At the same time, there is significant impetus for change related to reimbursement. The expanded knowledge, abilities, and skills of APRNs provide opportunities for the increased substitution of APRN services for those services traditionally provided by physicians.[25]

Disequilibrium

One disturbing characteristic of some healthcare markets is the failure of price to reach a level of equilibrium, or the level at which the quantity demanded and the quantity supplied are equal.[5] Most recently, payers have provided greater incentives for primary care services than for specialty care services, leading to an economic disincentive for the use of specialty services. The persistence of price disequilibrium is a clear indication that the healthcare market departs substantially from the competitive norm. In the case of excess demand, rationing ensues. Services such as hemodialysis or major organ transplantation may not be available to all members of society.

Supplier-Induced Demand

Figures 7-4 and 7-5 illustrate excess demand and supply, assuming constant initial supply, demand, price, and quantity conditions. An increase in the number of physicians in this market shifts the supply curve, resulting in a reduction in price and an increase in the quantity of care. Assuming that demand is inelastic with respect to price, the incomes of physicians will decline, which, in turn, will induce physicians to recommend additional units of service. This results in a shift to the demand curve. In this case, both price and quantity increase in response to the physician-induced demand. In contrast to the theoretical expectation that an increase in supply raises quantity and reduces price in a competitive market, findings suggest that an increase in the supply of physicians is accompanied by an increase in quantity and constant or rising price.[26]

Such results are consistent with the demand-shift hypothesis. The healthcare provider is hypothesized to shift demand to attain a target income. The target income is the amount of

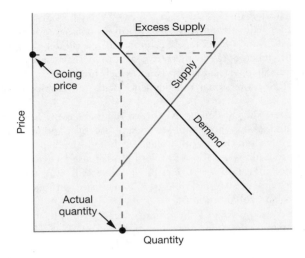

Figure 7-4: Excess supply.

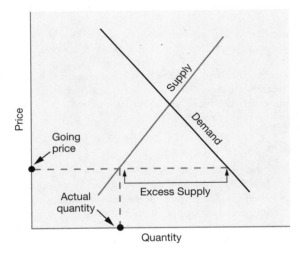

Figure 7-5: Excess demand.

money earned by comparison with other physicians of the same specialty training and geographic location. Empirical studies of the impact of increases in the physician-population ratio on utilization indicated no decline in utilization associated with increases in physician supply. A modest positive relationship has been found between utilization and the physician–population ratio, with estimated elasticities ranging from 0.03 to 0.80.[26]

The inducement hypothesis questions the appropriateness of increased cost sharing by consumers as an approach to controlling utilization and moderating growth in healthcare expenditures. Additional cost sharing and the concomitant decrease in consumer-initiated demand not only reduces physician earnings but also induces providers to increase demand, reducing the impact of higher net prices on total healthcare spending. The inducement hypothesis suggests that controls placed on fees charged by physicians are unlikely to be successful in constraining total spending on health services. Rather, price controls may be more widely applied, inducing the substitution of more expensive services for less costly ones.[26]

Conducting empirical studies on the demand for health care is challenging. Challenges include the questionable adequacy of health insurance information to obtain estimates of the price of health services. Another issue is the effect of provider influence on demand, including the extent to which supply creates its own demand. Health status is another issue that impacts demand, but exclusion of health status variables biases the results related to the importance of other independent variables. Empirical studies demonstrate that the demand for health services is inelastic related to price and income. The demand-for-health model recognizes that health services are purchased to obtain better health. Other items purchased, such as tobacco products, fatty foods, or alcoholic beverages also have impacts on health status. An example of this model occurs when older persons, in an effort to retard the depreciation in health caused by advancing age, increase their purchase of health services.[11, 26]

The Effects of Changes in Price, Supply, and Demand for Health Care

The hospital sector is the most inflationary component of the health services industry. As with other aspects of the healthcare industry, general inflation is responsible for the bulk of the increase in hospital expenditures. However, increased intensity, or acuity per visit, accounts for more of the increase in hospital expenditures than do the services of physicians or nursing homes.[26]

Increasing Hospital Inpatient Expenses

Since 1998, the United States has experienced ongoing increases in the growth of hospital inpatient expenses. Pharmaceutical and outpatient expenses have also grown, but because hospital inpatient care represents the largest single component of healthcare expenditures, even small growth rates in inpatient expenses have large effects on healthcare expenditures overall.

In 2004, inpatient hospital expenditures comprised about 34% of the growth in total healthcare expenditures. Private insurance (43.7%) and Medicare (38.3%) paid for the majority of inpatient hospital expenses, with 2.2% of payments coming from individuals and their families.[27] From 1998 through 2001, inpatient expenditures increased by an average of 5.9% annually, twice the overall annual rate of inflation during this time period.[28] See Figure 7-6.

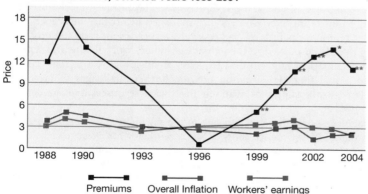

Increases in Employer Health Insurance Premiums Compared With Other Indicators, Selected Years 1988-2004

Premiums   Overall Inflation   Workers' earnings

SOURCES: Henry J. Kaiser Family Foundation/Health Research and Educational Trust Survey of Employer-Sponsored Health Benefits, 1999-2004; KPMG Survey of Employer-Sponsored Health Benefits, 1993 and 1996; Health Insurance Association of America, 1988-1990; Bureau of Labor Statistics, Consumer Price Index(U.S. City Average Net Annual Inflation, April to April), 1988-2004; and Bureau of Labor Statistics, seasonally adjusted data from the Current Employer Statistics Survey, 1988-2004.

NOTES: Data on premium increases reflect the cost of health insurance premiums for a family of four. Statistical significance indicators denote that premium estimates are statistically different from the previous year shown.
*$p < .10$ **$p < .05$

Figure 7-6: Increases in employer health insurance.

The mean expenditure for a hospital stay in the United States in 2004 was $10,300.[27] The average expense per night for a hospitalization in 2004 was approximately $3000, and the median per diem cost was about $1800. Total hospital expenses increased with the length of stay. Hospital stays when surgery was performed (about one-third of inpatient discharges in 2004) were more expensive than stays for nonsurgical reasons. In 2004, the average expense per stay was $14,279 for patients who underwent surgery, nearly double the average for other hospital stays. The average per diem expense was more than twice as large for surgical admissions ($5059) than for nonsurgical admissions ($1954).[27,28]

The key drivers of inpatient expenditures, based on state-level healthcare and inpatient expenditure data, are:

- The overall level of economic activity—for example, disposable income, local prices, and wages.
- Level of hospital technology, including cost of technology, consumer demand, and backlash against managed care.
- Hospital market and financial structure—for example, competitive markets, hospital closures, and profit versus nonprofit status.
- Healthcare labor force, particularly nursing supply shortages.
- Prescription drugs and medication errors.[29]

More than 800 financially distressed hospitals closed or merged between 2000 and 2005.[29,30] The combination of a highly competitive marketplace, hospital specialization, and heavy regulatory and legislative burdens were the causes of these widespread hospital closures during this time frame.[29,30] Despite original projections that the now-documented increase in growth of hospital costs would be short-lived and that technological change would support a trend away from hospitalization towards outpatient care,[31] evidence indicates that inpatient costs have continued to escalate because of the ongoing adoption of evolving medical technology.[32]

Because there is a strong relationship between economic activity and hospital inpatient expenditures, economic slowdowns such as the recession occurring at this writing may relieve some of the pressure for cost increases. An economic slowdown in the early 1990s triggered multiple aggressive healthcare and hospital cost-containment strategies that held the rate of growth in healthcare expenditure in check for several years. The primary mechanism employed at that time was to move more consumers into managed healthcare insurance plans and to discount provider reimbursement levels aggressively. Insurance industry experts speculate that these options have been pushed to the extent consumers will tolerate and will not substantially alter future inpatient and healthcare cost trends.[33] However, the current economic recession and global financial situation provide further challenges to providers, payers, and patients related to the supply of available healthcare resources and the demand for those goods and services.

The issues of the magnitude of economies of scale in the production of hospital services have been extensively studied. Past evidence shows a slight tendency for average costs to decline as output increases. However, there is stronger evidence of scale economies for particular types of medical services. For example, case mix, patient acuity, and type of payer are important factors that must be taken into account when considering the effect of hospital size on average costs.[26]

Public and Private Efforts to Control Costs

In the 1980s, the federal government began to accrue annual budget deficits in excess of $200 billion. As the amount of the national debt grew, a greater portion of the federal government budget each year was required to pay interest on the debt, which reduced the amount of dollars available for other discretionary spending. The current national debt is over $9 trillion and growing.[34] Since the inception of the Medicare and Medicaid programs in 1966, total public spending on health care has increased tremendously, reaching $507 billion in 1997[35] and $2.3 trillion in 2007, or $7600 per person. U.S. healthcare spending is expected to reach $4.2 trillion, or 20% of GDP, by 2016.[36] Healthcare spending currently is 4.3 times greater than the amount spent on national defense. Even though almost 47 million Americans are uninsured, the United States spends more on health care than other industrialized nations with universal health care. Healthcare spending comprises 10.9% of the Swiss GDP, 9.7% of the German, and 9.5% of the French.[36]

In the early 1980s, several private and public sector initiatives were introduced to stimulate economic competition among hospitals and physicians. The first of these efforts arose from the double-digit inflation during the Carter administration, followed by a sharp economic recession during the years of the Reagan administration. The volume of lower-priced imported goods rose significantly, as did competition from Japan and other countries. Many American businesses became aware of and concerned about the effects of steadily increasing healthcare premiums, which increased labor costs. Employers feared that if left unchecked, rising healthcare costs would thwart their ability to price products competitively in a global market. Businesses sought to reduce costly inpatient medical stays by instituting programs that mandated prehospital testing and screening, utilization review, and second opinions for surgery, and they pressured insurance carriers to cover the expenses of less costly outpatient settings. Before Medicare implemented DRGs, these private sector actions caused declines in hospital admissions and occupancy rates.[8]

State regulation of hospital costs has become increasingly widespread. Rate regulation has had a moderate impact on cost per admission, cost per patient day, and per capita expenditures. In addition, the growth in labor costs have been shown to slow with prospective payment.[26] Prospective payment may have helped moderate the growth in current healthcare expenditures, but there is little evidence that regulations designed to limit capital formation have succeeded. In situations where regulation of capital expenditures was successful in limiting growth in the number of beds, hospitals substituted investment in new services. Declining government support for capital regulation and industry have been advanced as possible reasons for the ineffectiveness of attempted controls on hospital capital formation.[26]

Cost Considerations in Provision of Care and Reimbursement for Physicians and APRNs

Several factors must be considered in providing healthcare services—the price of the services, access to care, the role of healthcare plans and health insurance, competition, and antitrust issues.

Price of Services

Greater availability of primary and preventive care has been tied to cost savings and improved quality. Nonphysician providers are cost-effective with regard to the expense of their education and in their practice patterns and fees. How these professionals are paid and which of their services are covered have been contentious issues for more than two decades. This is evidenced by the patchwork of policies governing payment for their services, even with a single-payer system like Medicare, and by substantial variation in payment rates among state Medicaid services.[37]

The extraordinary rise in healthcare costs and the inability of nursing to show cost savings have been barriers to adopting direct payment. Despite the breakdown of public and private spending on health care, health care's portion of the gross national product (GNP) grew from 5.3% in 1960 to 12.5% in 1990, increasing from $42 billion to almost $647 billion.[38] Congress has shown its concern about the rise in the healthcare budget by enacting new cost-containing Medicare payment systems for the services of hospitals and physicians.

Congress has also exhibited restraint in the annual funding of other health programs, frequently only increasing funding to cover inflationary costs. Reimbursement legislation for the services of APRNs is almost always evaluated as a cost item. APRNs are defined as nurse practitioners (NPs), clinical nurse specialists (CNSs), certified nurse-midwives (CNMs) and certified registered nurse anesthetists (CRNAs).[37] A summary of federal reimbursement for APRNs is shown in Table 7-1. The Congressional Budget Office (CBO) has consistently supported the notion that if the number of providers is increased, the costs for health care will increase because of the greater number of services provided.[39]

Access Issues

Paying APRNs directly allows them to provide care and improve needed access to care. Changes in federal health programs enacted by Congress were made to improve access to healthcare services to medically underserved populations, such as nursing home residents, low-income women and children, and people in rural areas. Direct reimbursement gives APRNs recognition and visibility as PCPs.[39] More than 47 million U.S. citizens lack health insurance, and most of these people lack access to primary care.[40,41] Additional PCPs will be needed to meet the needs of this uninsured population. Direct reimbursement of APRNs eliminated one of the most significant barriers to the utilization of these nurses.[39]

The Omnibus Budget Reconciliation Act (OBRA), enacted by Congress in 1990, allowed the services of NPs and CNSs to be reimbursed when provided in rural areas. This law was enacted because Congress wanted to improve access to care for rural Medicare beneficiaries. Although physician collaboration was required for NPs and CNSs, these providers were not required to submit claims through their employer, but were allowed to submit claims directly. The payment level authorized was 85% of the physician fee schedule for outpatient services and 75% of the physician fee for inpatient services.[41]

The Balanced Budget Act (BBA) of 1997 further removed economic disincentives for the utilization of APRNs by authorizing direct Medicare reimbursement for NP and CNS services in all settings. NPs who wish to submit claims for services must apply for a Unique Physician Identification Number (UPIN) number under their own name. Under BBA terms, both urban- and rural-based NPs can practice in all valid phases of services. NPs are required to work collaboratively with a physician. However, because NPs do not need the immediate availability of a supervising physician, they have more latitude in where and how they practice than PAs have. Prior to the BBA, urban-based NPs were reimbursed 85% of physician fee schedules for all services, and rural NPs were reimbursed at 75% of physician fee schedules for hospital services and 85% of physician fee schedules for other services. After BBA implementation, both urban and rural NPs were compensated at 85% of physician fee schedules across the board and could be employed or

Table 7-1 **Current Status of Federal Reimbursement for Nurses in Advanced Practice**				
Federal Programs	NP	CNM	CRNA	CNS
Medicare Part B	Yes	Yes	Yes	Yes
Medicaid	Yes[1]	Yes	State discretion	State
CHAMPUS[2]	Yes	Yes	Yes	Yes[3]
FEHBP[4]	Yes	Yes	Yes	Yes

[1] Limited to pediatric NPs and family NPs.
[2] Civilian Health and Medical Program of the Uniformed Services.
[3] Limited to certified psychiatric nurse specialists.
[4] Federal Employee Health Benefit Program.

self-employed. In addition, before the BBA, rural-based NPs were reimbursed at 65% of physician assist-at-surgery fees. With BBA provision, urban- and rural-based NPs are reimbursed at 85% of physician assist-at-surgery fees.[41,42]

Healthcare Plans and Health Insurance Policies

The forces that evolved through the 1980s and 1990s culminated in the development of healthcare price competition because cost-conscious purchasers of health care sought to obtain greater value for each dollar spent. The development of managed health care became a significant force with which APRNs rapidly gained familiarity.

Managed care involves applying standard business practices to healthcare delivery and purports to represent the elements of the American free enterprise system. Newer methods of providing financing and reimbursement for health services have required hospitals and healthcare providers to transition to new business models. Today, providers are confronted with price competition and the need to control costs while at the same time facing increasing demands for data documenting the quality of clinical outcomes.[43] In 1993, for the first time, 51% of employees with employer-sponsored health insurance were enrolled in managed care plans. In addition, many traditional insurance plans had incorporated managed care features, including subjecting provider services to external utilization reviews, second opinions, and so forth. By 2001, 93% of Americans with health insurance coverage were in some form of managed care plan.[44,45]

In 2007, the percentage of citizens covered by private health insurance was 67%, and people covered by employment-based health insurance comprised 59% of the insured. Of the insured in 2007, 28% were covered by government health insurance, with 13% of those receiving benefits under Medicaid. The percentage of children under 18 years old without health insurance was 11% in this time period.[46] As policy makers, payers, providers, and consumers of health care seek solutions to ever-increasing costs, managed care in the United States has experienced continued growth and possibly renewed interest. The purchasers of health care, including private and public payers, as well as patients, have become particularly interested in managed care as a flexible means for reducing healthcare expenditures while preserving high-quality patient care. Insurers are under intense pressure from employers to reduce premiums. Accomplishing this without reducing profits means decreasing costs, which, in turn, requires insurers to limit expenditures, generally by controlling provider services.

The growth of prepaid and capitated networks has been aided by continuing regulatory- and market-based adjustments designed to ensure that providers compete fairly, on the basis of price and quality. APRNs have found, as predicted, that more of the clinical and economic forces that shape their practices and determine their incomes are driven by the impersonal, unambiguous incentives that govern price-competitive industries. Providers and health professionals are rewarded economically to the extent that they keep prices low and quality high.[11]

APRNs AS ECONOMIC COMPLEMENTS OR ECONOMIC SUBSTITUTES

The evolution of prepaid capitated firms and the managed care industry has been a positive development for APRNs, whether they are employed by managed care firms, compete independently as solo providers, or are employed in group practices. Economically, the major difference between practicing as an HMO employee versus independently is that as an employee, the APRN functions as an economic complement. In independent practice, APRNs function largely as economic substitutes to an HMO or medical group practice.[11]

APRNs are an economic complement as long as their services increase the productivity of the managed care firm and the profits of the owners. The complementary role is similar to that of a hospital-employed RN, whose nursing practice increases physician productivity by allowing the physicians to both treat inpatients and maintain an office practice. Because HMOs operate according to a prepaid capitated budget, there are economic incentives to keep the total costs of providing health care as low as possible. In this way, any amount of unspent dollars can be retained as profit. Thus, HMOs have an economic interest in providing enrollees with more preventive care and health education so that future consumption of HMO resources is reduced. HMOs attempt to reduce the need for hospital admissions, negotiate discounts on pharmaceuticals and medical equipment, and pursue other cost-reduction strategies.[11] However, there is a tendency for participants of one managed care plan to jump to another plan when premiums rise or employer options change.

It has been suggested that adequately educated APRNs have proven competence and are capable of working without physician supervision.[47] Many of the clinical services provided by APRNs closely substitute for those rendered by physicians. Because APRNs are less costly to an HMO in terms of salary and benefits—although this differential has shrunk in recent years—it is intuitive that APRNs represent an economic opportunity for HMOs to fill gate keeping and other provider roles. As purchasers increasingly demand that HMOs lower the premiums charged per enrollee to prevent employees from enrolling in different and lower-cost HMOs, price competition between HMOs is significant. HMOs have faced pressures to keep costs low, which would arguably increase the demand for APRNs. Ultimately, MCOs need to foster competitive pricing but at the same time increase enrollment satisfaction and attain desired clinical outcomes for enrollees.[11]

With the ongoing economic recession, anticipated healthcare costs for 2009 are expected to increase by 10%. Costs are passed on to employees by adding alternative health plans and by increasing deductibles. Employee wellness programs are offered to foster wellness and decrease utilization of healthcare services. There may be some slowing in cost increases owing to these measures. However, the health-care system may be "fundamentally broken . . . and employers, stressed by rising healthcare costs, are once again seeking to shift a larger share of the cost burden to employees. Rising deductibles, co-pays, and out-of-pocket spending limits put painful pressure on many workers and their families."[48]

EXPECTED CONTINUED RESISTANCE TO APRNs IN MANAGED CARE

For at least two economic reasons, APRNs must anticipate that physicians and PAs will resist the increasing employment of APRNs. As more APRNs become available, the total supply of health professionals will increase relative to the available number of managed care positions. Consequently, this will place downward pressure on the salaries that managed care firms are able to offer and still hire all the providers they want. If the supply of PCPs increases, additional physicians will seek employment with managed care firms and compete for available positions with APRNs, who have a comparative cost advantage.[11] In contrast, if the number of primary care positions decreases and more PCPs are available, physicians will continue to be forced to accept lower levels of compensation, coming into direct competition with APRNs who have sought higher salaries.

A second reason to expect physician resistance to the expansion of APRNs in managed care is that many firms might adopt policies that direct the caseloads of APRNs to include lower-acuity patients. By having to care for higher-acuity patients, primary care physicians may not be able to obtain desired clinical outcomes or levels of patient satisfaction to qualify for a year-end bonus. A study of the Kaiser Permanente HMO system determined that more than 80% of the care provided by HMO physicians could be provided by an APRN or PA. In primary care, the percentage exceeds 90%. In any healthcare system, the highest cost is labor. If an APRN or PA is able to provide the same services as a physician, with similar quality and outcomes, the only barrier to the utilization of these nonphysician providers is physician attitudes.[45]

In the 1990s, research showed that PAs and APRNs could see as many or more patients per day as physicians at 50% less than the cost of a physician. From a workload standpoint, adult medicine physicians, PAs, and APRNs at Kaiser Permanente Northwest appeared to see similar numbers of patients on hourly, daily, and annual bases. In addition, the types of patients seen by PAs and APRNs in adult ambulatory settings were generally similar to those seen by physicians. From this standpoint, it was concluded that APRNs and PAs were substitutes for, rather than complements to, physician services.[45–47]

It is important for APRNs to understand that while they represent cost savings to owners of prepaid health plans, they also pose an economic threat to primary care and specialist physicians. Thus, organized medicine has taken action aimed at monitoring any expansion of the APRN scope of practice.[48,49] The organized-medicine policy position is that APRNs must practice under the supervision of a physician.[36] The lack of direct reimbursement for APRN services in the past decreased the overall effectiveness of these nursing professionals. Before direct reimbursement, NPs billed patients under the title of physicians.[49] In group practices, services provided by APRNs are often billed under physician provider numbers or "incident" to physician services. This practice has promoted the economic dependence of the APRN on the physician and can make the APRN a "ghost" provider in the healthcare system. In addition, if APRN services are billed as "incident to," very strict criteria and conditions are mandated for their services.

The legality and ethics of billing for APRN services under physician provider numbers must be questioned, particularly in states where APRN reimbursement is permitted by statute. APRNs must be proactive to ensure that their employers use billing practices that include direct reimbursement for APRN services. Direct billing enables the tracking of revenue generated by APRNs. APRNs' fiscal data, patient outcomes, and performance indicators are necessary to negotiate contracts and assess cost-effectiveness. Failure to link APRN provider numbers to their patient care encounters makes accurate compilation of data and evaluation of APRN cost-effectiveness impossible.[4]

Competition

APRNs need to understand who their competitors are, how many of them exist, where they are located, what services they offer, how much they charge, and how they are paid. This information will tell APRNs a great deal about what other providers have found effective or ineffective, sparing practicing APRNs from making time-consuming and costly mistakes. Knowing as much as possible about the competition also enables APRNs to determine how they can fill service gaps, take advantage of market niches, and provide care creatively at a lower cost.[11] This type of knowledge can be obtained through contracting with health marketing research firms, by developing a strategic plan with consultation as necessary, and by formulating an appropriate business plan based on the information gathered in this process.[50–53]

Marketers take a heterogeneous group of prospective buyers and divide them into smaller, homogenous groups who want approximately the same thing. This process is called market segmentation, and each subgroup is called a market segment. Markets are segmented by variables such as age, sex, and income. Each segment is evaluated using a set of predetermined criteria. If two or more target markets are chosen, the organization is practicing a multisegment strategy. The process of gathering the information necessary to operate any business is called market research. Formal research techniques rely on systematic gathering of information from sources inside and outside the firm. Surveys, experimental designs, expert panels, and subscriptions to proprietary or syndicated research reports are typical of the formal research effort. Information that is routinely gathered, codified, analyzed, and stored is part of a marketing information system, which becomes a ready information source for decision makers.[53]

A marketing mix includes the following components:

- Product
- Branding
- Packaging
- Price

- Place
- Promotion
- Product positioning[53]

Branding is important from the standpoint of professional identification. Clients must realize that healthcare services are available from appropriately prepared and credentialed APRNs. **Packaging** is a function of the image projected by the product—in this case, the image projected by the APRN. Clinical competence, affability, availability, and a professional demeanor help to prepare an appealing package when APRNs market their services. **Price** is another important consideration with multiple objectives. Nearly all objectives will have to be related to long-term profitability. The marketer must estimate demand at the price level and forecast the response of competitors. Marketers typically create channels of distribution to move the product from producer to user.

Promotion informs, persuades, or reminds customers about a product, such as advanced practice nursing services. Promotion management begins with an understanding of the target markets the firm has chosen to serve. This means one must know which media (newspapers, television, and Web sites) the market uses to get information and understand how it processes information and makes decisions. A promotion plan includes some combination of promotion tools, referred to as the promotion mix. Like the marketing mix, it is a synergistic blend of elements. The four groups of promotion tools are:

- Advertising
- Sales promotion
- Public relations and publicity
- Personal selling[53]

Advertising is the use of impersonal messages sent through paid media, such as television, radio, newspapers, magazines, Web sites, transit and highway billboards, telephone and business directories, and direct advertisements. **Public relations activities** are designed to foster goodwill, understanding, forgiveness, or acceptance. Publicity is not always favorable.[54] As the marketplace for healthcare providers contracts, a mixture of conciliatory and defensive posturing is seen in published interviews, as described in the following paragraph.

A newspaper interview with two APRNs and a physician was titled "Nurse Practitioner Supervision at Issue: RNs Push for Collegial Practice."[54] The physician commented that nurses had the ability to "treat a sore throat but lacked the medical education, judgment, and hours of supervised experience that will allow them to look at the entire differential of what [a] sore throat may be"[54] (p. 3). In this article, the perception of the physician was that nurses and physicians should "be a team" and that patients should know whether they are seeing "a board certified physician or a board certified advanced practice nurse." Despite some positive comments from the NPs interviewed for this story, the physician was able to cast doubt on the capabilities of APRNs. The impression left for consumers was that NPs may not be able to provide quality care without physician supervision.

Antitrust Issues

The economic competition between physicians and APRNs leads to occasional difficulties with antitrust issues. The ANA and APRN organizations carefully monitor the potential development of antitrust issues. The ANA has indicated that regulations are necessary to prevent any of the following possible events:

- Use of practice arrangements that prohibit nurses from performing patient care activities within the scope of state nurse practice acts;
- Use of practice arrangements that limit the activities of nurses recognized as advanced practitioners;

■ Imposition of insurer limits on the availability and accessibility of liability coverage for nurses or the requirement for physician supervision as a prerequisite for coverage;

■ Use of insurance surcharges to increase malpractice premium coverage and other insurance-related impediments to physician-nurse collaboration;

■ Subjective or arbitrary insurance reimbursement policies, such as denial of reimbursement for services performed within the scope of practice for any licensed provider if there is coverage for that service provided by the physician; and

■ Denial of staff privileges at healthcare facilities, including prescriptive authority for those authorized by state law to prescribe.[52]

Without federal protection and clearer guidelines, every time APRNs are denied basic practice rights, they would have to enter into lengthy litigation to demonstrate their legal right to compete. Case law exists that states some specialty nurses and physicians compete. (See *Oltz v. St. Peter's Community Hospital,* 861 F2d 1440, 1443 [9th Cir. 1988] and *Bahn v. NME Hospital,* 772 F2d 1467, 1471 [9th Cir. 1975]). Not only is this an issue of paramount importance to nurses, it is a priority issue of the Coalition for Quality Care and Competition, which represents more than 400,000 nonphysician providers. Issues important to this coalition include:

■ Prohibition of any entity or plan from discriminating against a class of healthcare professionals;

■ Elimination of restrictions in current law that pose barriers for nonphysician providers to practice in accord with state licensing acts;

■ Federal provisions guaranteeing nondiscriminatory access to qualified health providers being uniformly applied to all states, entities, and plans; and

■ Replacement of the term "physician" with the term "qualified professional" in healthcare regulatory language.[52]

These positions significantly qualify the needs of nonphysician providers in regulatory arenas. Without federal protection and a mandate that states must adopt these provisions, the nonphysician provider will be in the situation of fighting for practice privileges and the right to provide care.

If APRNs in solo or group practice arrangements are to survive in a competitive market, they will need to be alert, seek ways to innovate and keep their costs as low as possible, and be willing to make frequent adjustments in the quality, pricing, and marketing of their services. On recommendation is that APRNs set their prices below the prevailing market price of services provided by physicians or their nearest competitors.[11] In addition, identifying services not provided or inadequately provided in a given market, such as ongoing management of clients with chronic conditions or health education services, will make the APRN viable in an extremely competitive environment.

Many policy makers and researchers argue that there are problems with physician oversupply and imbalance in specialty mix. Some have argued that these problems would be resolved as a more competitive healthcare market developed; they predicted that cost-conscious integrated systems would change the demand for the services of physicians. As a result, physicians would experience lower incomes or potential unemployment, sending a signal to students and educators to change behavior. A systematic analysis has not been done to assess the impact of changes in the organizing and financing of health care on the physician labor market. However, two types of changes have been predicted for medical education: (1) the effect of increasing demand for generalists on the changing specialty mix and (2) the question of whether the market would create incentives to train fewer physicians.[55,56]

Although there have been marketplace changes, it is difficult to know whether these changes signal a departure from previous trends. Positions in generalist fields have become slightly more attractive, but income changes have been modest, and the number of specialists continues to increase. In 2008, the average income for primary care physicians was $186,044, while the mean income of all specialist physicians was $339,738.[55] See Figure 7-7.

Recent data from the Government Accounting Office indicate that graduating medical students prefer surgical and procedural specialties and that physician subspecialization is increasing. Given the number of available residency positions, more medical students have chosen surgical and procedural specialties over primary care specialties since 1999. Therefore, surgical and procedural specialties have been more competitive than primary care specialties. Graduates of U.S. allopathic medical schools fill higher numbers of the more competitive and procedural residency positions than do graduates of osteopathic or international medical schools. The percentage of physicians who chose subspecialty training increased from 2002 to 2007. This trend was seen in orthopedic surgery (a surgical subspecialty), and anesthesiology (a procedural specialty). Multiple factors and demographic characteristics influence the specialty choices of graduating medical students. The desire for a controllable lifestyle with a predictable schedule and fewer hours on call combined with a high salary may lead them to pursue procedural specialties like anesthesiology and avoid other specialties such as primary care.[56]

Key Terms in Finance and Reimbursement

In order to participate fully in efforts to change the financing of the healthcare system and improve reimbursement schedules and cost-benefit ratios, providers must understand some key terms in finance. This section helps to explain some of these terms.

Fee-for-Service, Capitation, and Other Models of Reimbursement

The traditional healthcare billing system in which a provider charges a patient separately for each service is the **fee-for-service** system. This type of system allows patients to have free choice in healthcare providers and does not require providers to assume risk for the provision of care. For example, providers are more likely to be reimbursed proportionally for providing care in a fee-for-service system than in a managed care system.

Using nurse anesthesia as an example, we will describe fee-for-service and traditional indemnity insurance plans in the context of reimbursement for services provided by these

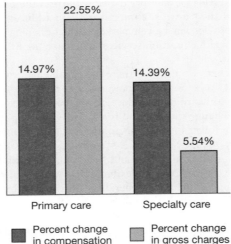

Figure 7-7: Five-year change in compensation and production, 2004–2008.

APRNs. From the early to mid-20th century, CRNAs were usually paid employees of either a surgeon or a hospital. In rural areas, CRNAs often contracted with hospitals to provide services based on fee-for-service structures, that is, a set amount of compensation per case rather than straight salary for hours worked.[57]

Blue Cross and Blue Shield were among the first private payers to emerge during the 1930s. Early insurance plans paid only for physician or hospital charges, and they would not directly reimburse other healthcare providers, such as CRNAs, psychologists, and physical therapists. To obtain payment for their services, these providers would submit charges to the hospital or physician. The hospital or physician would then obtain reimbursement for the services of these providers as "incident to" their own services and pass the money on to the nonreimbursed provider.[57]

Healthcare costs escalated under the private-payer systems of reimbursement, often due to the failure of payers to reimburse lower-cost providers such as non-physicians; the preferential reimbursement of higher-cost systems, such as hospitals, rather than ambulatory or outpatient services; and the insistence of physicians that harm would come to the physician-patient relationship if the fee-for-service structure was not maintained and strengthened.[57] In an effort to control escalating costs, Medicare instituted a prospective payment system (PPS) in 1983. Initially, this legislation affected only Medicare Part A (hospital costs). Subsequently, Medicare Part B (physician and nonphysician costs) was also included in the PPS. Before 1983, Medicare reimbursed hospitals for CRNAs on a cost-based system in which the hospital passed along the actual costs of providing the Medicare portion of CRNA services directly to Medicare.[57]

As a result of the OBRA of 1986, all CRNAs, regardless of their practice setting, were able to receive reimbursement from Medicare directly or to assign their billing rights to their employer. All CRNA services are subject to Medicare assignment (no balance billing). A subsequent law allowed rural hospitals with 500 or fewer surgical cases annually and one full-time CRNA to "pass through" the costs of anesthesia services. In 1992, the final regulations were published that detailed procedural definitions of the 1986 legislation.[57]

Most health insurance plans have undergone rapid change in an attempt to control spiraling costs. APRNs can expect reimbursement rates to decrease or remain flat, affecting APRNs in all types of practice settings. Global economic conditions at this time contribute to this flattening. In many markets, fee-for-service reimbursement no longer exists; it has been supplanted by managed care plans, where all providers, including physicians, are salaried. Despite this, organized medicine continues to advocate for the fee-for-service system on the basis of the physician-patient relationship.[57]

The penetration of managed care in major markets involves other operational components that contribute to the ubiquity of this model of healthcare delivery. **Capitation,** or prepayment for services on a per-member monthly basis, is one of these components. Providers are paid the same monthly amount regardless of whether members receive services and regardless of the costs for those services. To determine an appropriate capitation, it is important first to determine what will be covered in the scope of services, including all services that the provider will be expected to deliver. Certain services are difficult to define, such as diagnostic testing, prescriptions, and surgical procedures. Services such as immunizations and office care are easier to define. Providers need to be able to estimate costs for each capitated service.

Pay for performance (P4P) is a reimbursement model that seeks to align financial incentives with improved outcomes and value versus the current system, which rewards quantity and intensity of care delivered. Most performance-based compensation systems hold the PCP accountable for non-primary care services, either through risk programs or through positive incentive programs. P4P has been implemented in other countries and may be most advanced in the United Kingdom. Measurement for P4P is evolving, as are the types of incentives. For this model to succeed, all healthcare stakeholders would need to embrace P4P.[58]

Health plans and healthcare purchasers and provider organizations throughout the United States are developing P4P programs, with the intention of improving the quality of care while containing costs. Health plans and large, self-insured employers have used quality scorecards to measure hospital and physician performance combined with financial incentives geared toward hospitals, physician group practices, and individual physician and practice teams. Variables involved in developing a positive incentive program include quality metrics, units of accountability, size of incentive, data and measurement systems, payout formulas, and collaboration among payers. Similar programs, known as pay-for-quality (P4Q) programs, include the Bridges to Excellence and Rewarding Results programs.[59]

A **point-of-service (POS)** plan is a type of managed care group health insurance with characteristics of both an HMO and a PPO. There is more flexibility with a POS plan than in an HMO and less than in a PPO. In a POS plan, consumers select a primary care physician from a list of participating providers, similar to an HMO. All health care for that patient is directed by this physician, so he or she is the "point of service." This physician refers patients to other in-network physicians if there is a need for specialty care. The network typically has a broad base of healthcare providers and covers a wide geographic area.[60]

Point-of-service plans provide a difference in benefits depending on whether or not the member chooses the plan and its providers or chooses to comply with the authorization system to go outside the plan and choose an out-of-network provider for services.[60] For example, the plan may provide 100% coverage for costs using a network provider but only 70% coverage if an out-of-network provider is chosen. Increasing co-payments and deductibles are two mechanisms health plans and purchasers of health insurance use to control rising costs of health insurance premiums.

Co-payment, Coinsurance, and Deductibles

A **co-payment** is the portion of a claim or medical expense that a member must pay out of pocket. This is usually a fixed amount, such as $15 in many HMOs and PPOs. **Coinsurance** describes a provision in a member's coverage that limits the amount of coverage the plan will provide to a certain percentage of the costs, often 80%. Any additional costs are paid by the member out-of-pocket. It is a significant challenge for clinicians to provide services to clients with varying degrees of insurance coverage. A **deductible** is that portion of a subscriber's healthcare expenses that must be paid out-of-pocket before any insurance coverage applies, commonly $100 to $300. Deductibles are common in indemnity insurance plans and PPOs but are uncommon in HMOs. Deductibles may apply to only the out-of-network portion of a point-of-service plan.

Adverse Selection

Adverse selection is a situation in which an insurance carrier or benefit plan has a disproportionate enrollment of adverse risks, such as an impaired or older population, with a potential for higher healthcare utilization than budgeted for an average population. Adverse selection occurs when premiums do not cover the cost of providing services.[61] Therefore, insurers may indicate that it is fiscally essential for them to avoid providing health insurance coverage to higher-risk individuals.

Community Rating

Community rating involves setting health insurance premiums based on the average cost of services for all covered people in a geographic area, regardless of their history or potential for using health services. Community rating is a method of calculating health insurance premiums that sets the same price for the same health benefit coverage for all individuals in a pool of insured and does not take into account such variables as the claims experience of the group, age, sex, or health status. Community rating helps to spread the cost of illness evenly over all health plan enrollees, rather than charging the sick more for health insurance.[61]

Experience Rating

Another method of determining the cost of health insurance to consumers is experience rating. With experience rating, health insurance premiums are based on the average cost of actual or anticipated health care used by various groups and takes into account such variables as previous claims experience, age, sex, and health status. It is the most common method used to establish premiums for health insurance in private programs.[62-64] With increasing managed care penetration in many markets and the move toward fully capitated systems, competition between insurance plans has intensified. Underbidding for contracts between competing managed care plans may be part of that process, regardless of the methods used to derive premium costs.

Global Budgeting

Global budgeting is an overall budget limit on healthcare services, regardless of where the funds originate. Global budgets can take the form of a state or federal maximum limit on total healthcare expenditures but usually imply federal limits. In some contexts, global budgeting has come to mean setting a limit on spending within sectors. For example, specific allocations for physicians, APRNs, or hospitals may be specified.[65] Canada has used global healthcare budgeting with varying results. The National Health Service in Great Britain coexists with private indemnity insurance carriers. Clinicians working for salaries under global budgets or in capitated systems have less financial incentive to provide services than under traditional fee-for-service care delivery.

Issues to Be Considered by APRNs

Even when APRNs are employed by large HMOs, it is important for them to be aware of issues such as fluctuations in the numbers of enrollees because the current healthcare marketplace is dynamic and competing provider groups bid vigorously for contracts. APRNs seeking to affiliate themselves with HMOs and PPOs need to consider what type of plan structure is employed. The plan may be a corporation, a partnership for profit, or a not-for-profit plan. The sponsorship of HMOs and PPOs provides a key to the underlying philosophy and initial purpose of the plan. The sponsorship could also reflect the receptivity of the plan to discussion regarding APRN services. Typical sponsors include insurance companies, providers, investor ownership, consumer ownership, third-party administrators (PPOs), and entrepreneurial arrangements.[63-65]

APRNs must ascertain the current arrangement between MCOs and providers. To some degree, this is determined by the model of the HMO or PPO. The current arrangements will affect the approach APRNs should take in the negotiating process. The following information should be gathered:

- Who are the existing providers for the plan and what hospitals are they associated with? What is the size of the network? How long have the providers been participating? How many new providers are added each year? How many providers have left the plan?

- Are the providers contracted with as a physician association, a joint venture, or as individual physicians or physician groups? If the plan contracts with one large association of physicians, providers may have to subcontract with this organization before contracting with the plan. Even if contracting directly with the plan is possible, the physician association usually has more influence than in less-centralized organizations and may have to be included in discussions between APRNs and the plan. If the plan contracts with groups or with individual physicians, the ability for new provider groups to contract directly with the plan is improved.

- Does the plan contract with other healthcare providers, such as nurse anesthetists, podiatrists, optometrists, chiropractors, and mental health professionals? To the extent that a plan has already broadened its panel of providers beyond that of medical doctors, some of the groundbreaking work has already been achieved. Such plans already appreciate the quality of service and cost-containment ability of contracting with nonphysician providers. The doorway probably is open for nonphysician providers who can demonstrate the efficacy and cost-effectiveness of their services.

■ What are the reimbursement arrangements with providers? As much information about the current reimbursement and risk arrangements with the existing providers should be gathered. Such information will help determine the feasibility of various arrangements (e.g., discounted, capitated, fee schedule), which a group of APRNs might consider, as well as the extent to which the plan typically shifts the risk to providers.[66]

Entrepreneurial APRNs need to be prepared to accept risk when contracting with managed care entities. If the clinical services performed by APRNs cost less to provide than the contracted amount per member per month, profit is attained. However, if APRNs provide services beyond the contracted amount, they, not the MCO, incur loss.

Reimbursement for Specific APRN Roles

The failure of many MCOs to recognize APRNs as reimbursable care providers has been a significant concern. Lack of provider status may result in denial of payment for services rendered by APRNs even if the services are delivered within the legal scope of APRN practice. Laws in each state vary in their definitions and processes for APRN reimbursement.[65-67] Laws in several states require Medicaid agencies to recognize APRNs as PCPs, but these laws do not apply to all third-party payers. Some states leave the decision about APRN recognition up to individual MCOs, and other states have no nursing reimbursement laws.[4] Current information on state reimbursement laws and regulations is provided in the annual Legislative Update published in *The Nurse Practitioner* [21] or the Pearson Report now published in *The American Journal for Nurse Practitioners*.[65]

Many APRNs who deliver services within physician or group practices are frustrated that their patient encounters are billed under physician provider numbers or "incident to" the services of the physician. Practices may choose to bill for APRN services in this manner to ensure that the practice receives 100% of a typical physician fee reimbursement rate for services. Unless the APRN service was truly delivered under the specific criteria for "incident to" service, reimbursement for the service should be billed under the provider number of the APRN. Medicare and Medicaid reimbursement rates for services provided by APRNs vary from state to state and differ among nongovernmental third-party payers, ranging from 70% to 100% of a typical physician fee. Physicians and office managers may be unfamiliar with state laws pertaining to APRN reimbursement, causing APRN employers to bill inadequately and not receive appropriate payment from third-party payers.[4] The following sections discuss reimbursement issues for specific APRN groups.

Certified Nurse-Midwives

A study of certified nurse-midwives (CNMs) practicing in the United States reported that more than 77% of respondents were reimbursed by salary, 14% received hourly wages, and 17% were compensated on the basis of productivity. Profit sharing was available to 17% of respondents.[68] The majority of CNMs work as physician (21%) or hospital (18%) employees, while 18% were in solo or private practice.[68]

Current CNM salary data show salaries at the 25th and 75th percentiles, ranging from $86,125 to $101,727 in the Midwest, with some regional variations.[69] In one study, CNMs were asked to categorize the types of reimbursement mechanisms in place for them. These research findings are shown in Table 7-2. (The reimbursement percentages may vary from state to state particularly for Medicaid.) Respondents were also asked to identify data needed to apply for a provider contract (Table 7-3). More than 75% of CNMs indicated they needed to produce their CNM/RN licenses, certification, and professional liability coverage to apply for a provider contract.[68]

When asked who had primary responsibility for obtaining and/or maintaining provider contracts in their practices, 51% said their business manager, 22% said the CNM director, and 14% indicated the physician director, while 7% stated someone else. Other persons with primary responsibility included the hospital administration, the marketing department, an outside agency, office staff, or a university department. Of the responding CNMs, 5% said this question did not apply to them.[68]

Table 7-2 **CNM Reimbursement Data by Reimbursement Type**[62]

Reimbursement Type	% Physician Fee	Average Contract Negotiation Time (mo)	Capitated or Global Fee
Medicare	100	2	Global
Managed care Medicare	80	2	Global
Managed care Medicaid	100	6	Global
CHAMPUS	100	1.5	Global
Managed care CHAMPUS	75	9	Capitated
FEHBP*	100	3	Global
Managed care FEHBP	100	3	Global
Primary care FEHBP	80	9	Global
Commercial carriers	100	2	Global

*FEHBP = Federal Employee Health Benefit Plan.

Table 7-3 **Evidence Needed for CNMs to Apply for a Provider Contract**[62]

Document	Frequency (%)
CNM/RN license	86
Evidence of certification	82
Evidence of professional liability coverage	77
Physician name and number	62
Curriculum vitae	57
Evidence of independent hospital privileges	17
Evidence of dependent hospital privileges	23
Evidence of courtesy hospital privileges	5
Evidence of prescriptive authority/DEA* number	48
Physician practice agreement	47

*DEA = Drug Enforcement Administration.

A paper on CNM economics described practice arrangements for nurse-midwives. In one type of practice, the obstetrician/gynecologist had 65% of the patients in the practice, while the CNM performed 60% of the deliveries, delivering all her own patients and splitting calls with the physician. The CNM in this practice assisted with C-sections, performed circumcisions, co-managed diabetic patients, and provided public lectures on an array of topics, which increased the size of the practice. In another practice, the CNM described a 4% to 5% lower C-section rate in her practice compared with the national rate of 21%. Lower professional fees collected for vaginal deliveries, versus the costs associated with cesarean sections, may present a real economic consideration for some practices.[70]

Malpractice premiums for obstetricians and other specialty physicians have increased over time. The economic impact has been profound, with some hospitals discontinuing obstetrical services. Implications for CNMs are twofold: Collaborating physicians may become scarce, while the demand for CNM services may increase. The entire specialty of obstetrics and gynecology has been profoundly affected by the increased costs associated with malpractice premiums.[71]

Certified Registered Nurse Anesthetists

Anesthesia care is a highly contested terrain in advanced practice. The supply of anesthesiologists has grown rapidly despite evidence that nurse anesthetists provide equally good care at a fraction of the cost.[72] Attempts by the federal government to make Medicare payments more efficient and equitable by lowering the economic return to physicians specializing in anesthesia has created a hostile work environment.

WORKFORCE OF EQUALLY QUALIFIED BUT LESS EXPENSIVE PROVIDERS DIMINISHING

Anesthesia is an example of the choices and challenges facing society regarding the future workforce mix. Two providers currently administer anesthesia in the United States: physician anesthesiologists and certified registered nurse anesthetists (CRNAs). Over the past 30 years, the supply of anesthesiologists has tripled while the number of CRNAs has grown 75%. The growth in anesthesia providers has outpaced the growth in demand for their services. A rapid influx of anesthesiologists into what had been predominantly a nursing domain ran counter to the trend in managed care plans to place a priority on the use of nonphysician providers.[72]

The ongoing emphasis on healthcare cost-containment would likely fuel a less costly anesthesia workforce, but this has not uniformly been the case. Competitive market theory predicts that rapidly rising anesthesia costs combined with increased public and private efforts to control outlays would result in the hiring of more CRNAs and fewer anesthesiologists. In 2007, the median salary for anesthesiologists was $352,959 while the median salary for CRNAs was $140,000.[73] CRNAs and anesthesiologists are highly substitutable, as evidenced by the distribution of these two types of providers across hospitals and regions.[72,74,75]

Because of their more extensive medical training and higher hourly cost, the role of the anesthesiologist in the perioperative setting is logically one of medical supervision or consultation. It does not make economic sense for anesthesiologists to displace CRNAs and take over the myriad tasks they already perform ably at less than half the cost. In addition to these economics, outcome studies do not demonstrate significant differences between the two provider groups.[74,75] The Joint Commission does not require the presence of an anesthesiologist on the staff in order to accredit hospitals.[76] Despite the evidence of substitutability and lower costs over the past 30 years, CRNAs have seen their clinical role in some settings diminish to the point where they are the minority provider.[72] If efficient payment policies, unhampered by hospital organizational and state licensing rigidities, were put into place, this current trend of a diminishing CRNA workforce (and an increasing number of anesthesiologists) would be far different. Now, anesthesiologists (43,000) outnumber CRNAs (35,000) in the United States.

INFLATIONARY PAYMENT SYSTEMS

Historically, insurers have paid either on the basis of discounted charges or actual costs, both highly inflationary. Payers almost always divide their payments between two components, the hospital payment and physician payment. Many private payers cannot report what average total outlays are for a particular surgery across different hospital settings. Bifurcated payments for anesthesia have been problematic due to the degree of substitution between CRNAs and anesthesiologists and opportunities for "double billing." Hospitals bill only for the anesthesia costs that they incur. Until recently, CRNAs, like other nurses, were predominantly hospital-employed, in which case the institution billed for their services, sometimes directly but more often indirectly as an overhead support cost to surgery. Anesthesiologists nearly always bill directly for their professional services. With CRNA costs sometimes hidden in hospital bills, it has been difficult for payers to isolate the true full costs of anesthesia and make comparisons of costs and workforce mix across institutions.[77] The most inflationary aspect of anesthesia billing is supervision by anesthesiologists. This state exists because of the close substitution of CRNAs for physicians. Private insurers have allowed anesthesiologists to double-, triple-, or quadruple-bill for their time in overseeing CRNAs without significant prorating to account for the modest time they personally spend with each patient.[72]

Medicare reimbursement for anesthesiologists has always been different from that for other physicians because it is based on a dollar "conversion factor" multiplied by corresponding base and time units for a given case. In the early years of this reimbursement program, anesthesiologists who directly employed and supervised CRNAs were paid their full allowable charge under Part B with no separate CRNA charge. There were no limits to the number of concurrent cases the physicians could bill for. The program made a distinction when the CRNA was hospital-employed, in which case the billable time units, but not the base units, were halved. The rationale was that the Medicare program was also paying the salary of the nurse anesthetist to the hospital under Part A. When Congress passed the OBRA of 1987, it corrected this problem by reducing base units from 10% to 40%, depending on the number of cases concurrently supervised by the anesthesiologist.[72]

Medicare changes implemented in 1998 removed economic incentives for anesthesiologists to medically direct two CRNAs concurrently. For CRNAs employed by physicians, the practice must still bill 50–50 for the two providers on concurrent cases. When the practice receives the full Medicare allowable payment in two components, it can reimburse CRNAs at the going wage, which is usually less than half the Medicare allowable fee. While Medicare implicitly recognizes the two providers as equal in terms of payment on a per-case basis, the potential impact on existing CRNA employment arrangements is not neutral.[72]

The Medicare program established a set of conflicting incentives antithetical to the most efficient anesthesia team arrangement through a set of well-meaning but shortsighted policy changes. Medicare mandates that the anesthesiologist be personally involved in seven key tasks throughout the anesthetic procedure. The bill-splitting rule described earlier established an effective pay rate for the CRNA comparable to that of physician anesthesiologists who have several more years of medical education. From the inception of the program, Medicare has struggled with anesthesiologist reimbursement. CRNAs dominated the specialty in the mid-1960s and the program stipulated that an anesthesiologist need not be present for nurse anesthetists to provide anesthesia under the direction of the collaborating surgeon. At the same time, Medicare recognized the value added from anesthesiologist supervision through additional direct payment to this one specialty, instead of treating the whole service as hospital-based and falling under Part A. By allowing direct billing by anesthesiologists under Part B, the program failed to grasp the fact that delivery of anesthesia is fundamentally a Part A, hospital-based service.[72]

ANESTHESIOLOGISTS' OPPOSITION TO CRNAs

The rapid growth in the supply of anesthesiologists, coupled with changes in Medicare reimbursement policies that are economic disincentives for team anesthesia, has resulted in occupational licensure becoming a major area of conflict. In the growing competition for hospital-based anesthesia positions, the American Society of Anesthesiologists (ASA) has portrayed nurse anesthetists as "not quite professionals" encroaching on their domain. But anesthesia historically has been a nursing function. For example, in 1949, there were 3678 active CRNAs in the United States versus 1837 anesthesiologists. Anesthesiologists have justified increases in their ranks by making a fine distinction between practicing medicine as physicians and practicing nursing. By historic and legal precedent, anesthesia is the practice of nursing when practiced by nurses.[57]

A healthcare economist who has extensively studied anesthesia reimbursement believes that until payers change the way anesthesia services are reimbursed, unproductive incentives will drive the system in the wrong direction.[72] Payers, especially Medicare, must stop paying anesthesiologists directly for their services if they want them to move into more supervisory and collaborative roles. While split billing by Medicare caps the outlays of the program at what a solo anesthesiologist would cost, the payment is still far greater than what the program would pay under an optimal workforce mix at competitive salaries for the two providers. Split billing does not foster team anesthesia.[72]

POSSIBLE SOLUTIONS

Payers can achieve lower costs and a better workforce mix by negotiating a global payment for inpatient surgery that includes both the hospital and all physician services. For example, a small number of insurers, including Medicare, carve out global bundles for specialized inpatient services, such as cardiac and orthopedic surgery, which puts the medical staff at increased risk for most physician services. Defining anesthesia as a Part A hospital service would accomplish more. If anesthesiologists were unable to bill Medicare and private payers directly, they would have to take salaried positions in the hospital or negotiate less favorable contract relationships. In either case, the hospital would be responsible for how much the anesthesiologists are being paid. If anesthesiologists refused to take lower salaries or discounted fees, institutions would use fewer of them and in more supervisory roles. Some hospitals have begun to do this by encouraging competition for their anesthesia contracts due to high charges and the policies of managed care payers. The staff model HMO, where all anesthesia costs are internalized, also results in higher CRNA–anesthesiologist ratios than in competing institutions where anesthesiologists are "free inputs" to the facility.[72,77] If Medicare persists in its split-billing arrangement and pays both providers equally, CRNA displacement will continue.

Various novel capitation arrangements are currently being used. In fully capitated, staff-model HMOs that own their own hospitals, incentives for using the optimal anesthesia workforce are strongest, because all provider costs are internalized. A Kaiser Permanente internal study concluded that a one-to-four anesthesiologist-to-CRNA ratio was more cost-effective than the then common one-to-two ratio. As anesthesia costs are often a small part of the overall cost, private insurers, however, that are building a hospital network pay scant attention to the cost or the workforce mix in this specialty.[72,77]

An estimated 80% of nurse anesthetists practice in the team mode, working collaboratively with anesthesiologists. Definitive outcomes data derived from prospective multicenter studies demonstrating an optimal provider mix in terms of cost and quality are lacking however. But there are clear incentives to dismantling bifurcated anesthesia payments while optimizing the use of nurse anesthetists and defining anesthesia as a Medicare Part A hospital-based service.[72] However, the gains attained by CRNAs and other APRNs in achieving Medicare Part B billing rights mitigate against such a policy move.[78]

Clinical Nurse Specialists and Nurse Practitioners

A study of psychiatric–mental health clinical nurse specialists (CNSs) and nurse practitioners (NPs) identified these barriers to practice:

- Lack of recognition by MCOs and other payers. Patient access to high-quality care provided by APRNs is limited when health-care systems fail to specifically designate them as providers of care. APRNs often are not identified in advertising and promotional materials published by MCOs, and they may not receive information regarding reimbursement regulations even when they are credentialed by the payers and have their own provider numbers. Credentialing of APRNs frequently is a slow process. MCOs may be unfamiliar with the APRN scope of practice and national certification. As a result, some APRNs practice without their own provider numbers and are employed by practices that do not attempt to obtain APRN provider numbers.

- APRNs lack of knowledge and education about reimbursement, especially NPs and CNSs. APRNs recognize their limited knowledge of reimbursement rules, regulations, and policies; of coding, billing, and insurance coverage; and of how their patient visits are being billed. They have also been unclear about the reimbursement they were actually receiving. This lack of knowledge has affected the ability of APRNs to work effectively within the system and has wasted valuable time.

- Difficulty in coping with rapid changes in reimbursement policies and procedures. The pace of change within the healthcare system necessitates that APRNs frequently update their knowledge and understanding of reimbursement issues and policies. APRNs may react to the rapid pace of change by claiming disinterest or a lack of understanding. Lack of understanding is not an excuse for inappropriate billing or an option for APRNs who are committed to a favorable professional future.[4]

Following the implementation of the BBA of 1997, organized medicine attempted to use several strategies to restrict the ability of NPs and CNSs to bill for Medicare reimbursement. The American Medical Association (AMA) developed a citizens' petition to be filed with the CMS. The petition demanded the implementation of a system that would ensure that only APRNs who provided their services collaboratively with a physician and were within the scope of practice for APRNs in that state would receive Medicare reimbursement. The petition was circulated and endorsements sought from all national medical specialty organizations and state medical associations.[78]

Since the BBA expanded opportunities for direct reimbursement to APRNs, the appropriate relationship between physicians and APRNs, along with the meaning of collaboration, have been hotly contested. The AMA submitted extensive comments to CMS that supported restrictive definitions of collaboration and relationships of APRNs and physicians. But during the comment period, the AMA and other medical organizations failed to achieve their aims, leading the CMS to develop a final rule defining collaboration. The authority of states to determine the appropriate relationship between APRNs and physicians is recognized by federal statute, which defers to state law. States vary in their requirements for APRN-physician relationships, and change is ongoing in the legislative arena. Collaborative physician-APRN relationships are not consistently required in statutory and regulatory language across the states. In states that do not require collaboration, federal regulations require APRNs to document their scope of practice and indicate the relationships they have to deal with issues outside their scope of practice.[78]

The AMA has stated that the CMS has no system to assess and review the hundreds of claims made by APRNs and suggested that a system be developed to determine whether each APRN complied with state law. The AMA asked CMS to limit the distribution and renewal of Medicare billing numbers to APRNs who complied with its collaboration and scope-of-practice requirements. They also asked CMS to conduct audits ensuring that Medicare payments to APRNs were limited to services provided collaboratively with a physician and within APRNs scope of practice allowed by state law.[78]

The arguments used by the AMA are one strategy to retain medical authority for patient care [and] to "recognize . . . APRNs, under physician leadership, as effective physician extenders."[79] An active Medicare fraud and abuse program that covers all providers already exists. If the actions demanded in the petition or similar restrictions were to be implemented, fiscal and other barriers to the full scope of APRN practice would be created. This would "have a chilling effect on Medicare reimbursement opportunities for nurses."[78]

Economic Comparisons of APRNs, PAs, and Physicians

APRNs and PAs often command 80% to 100% of what physicians receive from commercial insurers, and NPs and CNMs have had success in persuading managed care panels to allow enrollees to choose them as PCPs. However, their compensation is not on a par with that of physicians. PAs who provide primary care services in multispecialty groups gross slightly more than $3 for every $1 they receive in compensation, according to the Medical Group Management Association (MGMA). Research has shown that NPs generate median gross charges 300% greater than their median compensation. Similar findings have been reported for CNMs. In contrast, internists gross slightly more than twice their compensation. If an NP or PA produces $30,000 in annual profit, which is an attainable figure according to MGMA, the physician or practice group partners can divide those funds among themselves.[78,79] As this discrepancy between gross income generated and compensation continues, APRNs and PAs remain less costly to the healthcare system.[67]

PAs and NPs increase practice incomes by other means. In managed care markets, they allow physicians to handle larger patient panels and to receive a larger capitation check. In the fee-for-service realm, they free physicians to concentrate on more complex, better-paying cases.[73] Both PAs and NPs have often been categorized as cost centers (areas generating costs but not concomitant revenue) by hospitals and other employers, but they actually represent sources of professional fee income. Both providers generate net revenues per day for their employers.[67] And because of increased reimbursement levels mandated by the BBA, the net revenue generated by NPs and PAs has increased. Many hospitals and other employers of APRNs and PAs continue to realize these providers do generate revenue. See Table 7-4.

For physicians and medical groups, NPs and PAs offer a less expensive means to expand their practices. By hiring these clinicians, a physician group can increase its capacity for a higher volume of patients or expand into new markets without incurring the risks associated with employing a new physician or with practice mergers. The broad expansion of covered service sites the BBA mandated offers an affordable way to grow areas of a practice that may have been unprofitable or less attractive if a physician had to provide the services. In addition, medical groups that take on managed care risk can provide services less expensively and remain within global per-member, per-month budgets.[73]

Because the BBA has expanded market parameters from rural settings to all practice arenas, APRNs need to be aware of the market segmentation and competition that can affect

Table 7-4 **2008 Provider Salary Comparisons**[68]	
Provider	**Annual Salary**
Internal Medicine Physician	$199,886
Nurse Practitioner	$80,322
Physician Assistant	$79,072
Obstetrician-Gynecologist	$283,110
Certified Nurse-Midwife	$86,125

their practices, especially since the BBA has leveled the playing field in reimbursement for NPs and PAs. Market competition between physicians and APRNs was intensified by the BBA provisions that described "midlevel" providers as acceptable lower-cost practitioners, in direct economic competition with physicians. When hospitals hire increased numbers of PAs and NPs, some physicians view this as a threat. However, many physicians have learned to incorporate APRNs and PAs into their practices, to complement their services. Other physicians see APRNs as part of a rising tide of providers threatening their position as the main contact or entry point into the healthcare system. An additional competitive factor is the increasing number of NPs and PAs entering the market.[63,64]

A New Reimbursement Model—Pay for Performance

Pay-for-performance (P4P) is a newer development in health insurance. Under this arrangement, providers are rewarded for attaining pre-established targets for the delivery of healthcare services. This is significantly different from the traditional fee-for-service reimbursement model.[80]

P4P is also known as value-based purchasing. This payment model rewards health-care providers who meet established performance criteria for quality and efficiency. Disincentives, such as elimination of payments for untoward outcomes or "never events," are being implemented. The rapidly aging population and rising healthcare costs have driven the implementation of P4P, but pilot studies underway in several large healthcare systems have demonstrated only slight improvements in specific outcomes and inefficiency. Cost savings in these settings have been limited because of added administrative requirements. Organizations representing healthcare providers have been somewhat supportive of incentive programs to increase quality, but they express concern about the validity of quality indicators, patient and provider autonomy and privacy, and additional administrative burdens.[81]

P4P systems attach compensation to measures of work quality. Current reimbursement methods in health care might reward less-safe care, as some insurance carriers will not pay for new practices geared at error reduction, while providers can still bill for additional services that are needed when patients are injured by mistakes.[81] Currently, P4P systems assess satisfactory performance based on specific clinical measurements, such as glycohemoglobin testing for diabetics.[81] However, the reality is that clinicians who are monitored by narrow criteria have potent incentives to dismiss or refuse to accept patients whose outcome measures fall below the established quality standard and who would worsen the external assessment of the provider, that is, they have a significant incentive to deselect (dismiss or refuse to accept) patients whose outcome parameters are below an established quality standard.[82] Patients with low health literacy, inadequate financial resources for expensive medications or treatments, and ethnic groups historically vulnerable to healthcare inequities may also be deselected by providers who seek improved performance measures.[83,84]

Improving Quality—Never Events

"Never events" are 28 occurrences (and more are being discussed) described by the National Quality Forum (NQF) as inexcusable outcomes in a healthcare setting—these events should never occur. They are "adverse events that are serious, largely preventable, and of concern to both the public and healthcare providers for the purpose of public accountability."[85] Some states have statutes that require disclosure of never events at hospitals, along with associated remunerative or punitive measures for such events. A recent study found that almost 50% of 1285 hospitals responding to a survey waived fees for never events, and those hospitals not waiving fees were more likely to have perfect scores on a safe practices score survey.[86]

As defined by the NQF and commonly agreed upon by healthcare providers, the 28 never events are:

1. Artificial insemination with the wrong donor sperm or donor egg
2. Unintended retention of a foreign object in a patient after surgery or another procedure
3. Patient death or serious disability associated with patient elopement (disappearance)
4. Patient death or serious disability associated with a medication error, that is, errors involving the wrong drug, wrong dose, wrong patient, wrong time, wrong rate, wrong preparation, or wrong route of administration
5. Patient death or serious disability associated with a hemolytic reaction due to the administration of ABO/HLA-incompatible blood or blood products
6. Patient death or serious disability associated with an electric shock or elective cardioversion while being cared for in a healthcare facility
7. Patient death or serious disability associated with a fall while being cared for in a healthcare facility
8. Surgery performed on the wrong body part
9. Surgery performed on the wrong patient
10. Wrong surgical procedure performed on a patient
11. Intraoperative or immediate postoperative death in a physical status 1 patient
12. Patient death or serious disability associated with the use of contaminated drugs, devices, or biologicals provided by the healthcare facility
13. Patient death or serious disability associated with the use or function of a device in patient care, in which the device is used or functions other than as intended
14. Patient death or serious disability associated with intravascular air embolism that occurs while being cared for in a healthcare facility
15. Infant discharged to wrong person
16. Patient suicide or attempted suicide resulting in serious disability while being cared for in a healthcare facility
17. Maternal death or serious disability associated with labor or delivery in a low-risk pregnancy while being cared for in a healthcare facility
18. Patient death or serious disability associated with labor or delivery in a low-risk pregnancy while being cared for in a healthcare facility
19. Patient death or serious disability associated with hypoglycemia, the onset of which occurs while the patient is being cared for in a healthcare facility
20. Deaths or serious disability (kernicterus) associated with failure to identify and treat hyperbilirubin in neonates
21. Stage 3 or 4 pressure ulcers acquired after admission to a healthcare facility
22. Patient death or serious disability due to spinal manipulative therapy
23. Any incident in which a line designated to deliver oxygen or other gas to a patient contains the wrong gas or is contaminated by toxic substances
24. Patient death or serious disability associated with a burn incurred from any source while being cared for in a healthcare facility
25. Patient death or serious disability associated with the use of restraints or bedrails while being cared for in a healthcare facility

26. Any instance of care order by or care provided by someone impersonating a physician, nurse, pharmacist, or other licensed healthcare provider

27. Abduction of a patient of any age

28. Sexual assault on a patient within or on the grounds of the healthcare facility[86]

Four actions have been suggested as industry standards after the occurrence of a never event. These actions include:

1. Apologizing to the patient;

2. Reporting the event;

3. Performing a root cause analysis (RCA); and

4. Waiving costs directly related to the event.[86]

Challenges that confront the healthcare system and that affect APRN reimbursement include:

- The growing demand for APRNs in hospitals, particularly in academic medical centers, to fill gaps left by a shortage of and limited hours of physician trainees[87];

- Access to chronic care services, establishment of meaningful primary care incentives, and payment to ensure sustainable access to care, instead of reliance on emergency departments;

- Providing relevant and evidence-based data on nurse work and nurse outcomes for the P4P mechanisms in healthcare payment; and

- The lack of healthcare dollars and resources to accomplish expectations in both developed and developing countries.

These are all challenges that APRNs can help to address.[15]

Summary

Faltering job and income security creates fear in working families that they may be one catastrophic illness or accident away from economic demise. While insurance companies and the pharmaceutical industry spend billions of dollars trying to influence Congress and the administration on healthcare issues, they cannot obscure the consequences of rising healthcare costs. APRNs can help educate the public and lawmakers about how the economy and health care are inextricably linked.[88] As of this writing, ongoing federal legislative efforts to create additional options for healthcare coverage, such as a coexisting public health coverage system or healthcare cooperatives, have been met with vigorous opposition from citizen and special-interest groups.

Remedies to provide equitable, safe, cost-effective healthcare services can be a contentious topic among providers. The ANA believes a single-payer system is the most desirable structure for financing a reformed system. Clearly, any well-designed interventions that improve access to health care, and improve the quality, equity, and cost-effectiveness of health care, should be considered.[88] It is clear that advanced practice nurses provide safe and cost-effective patient care services that can continue to improve access to health care at a time when resources are scarce.

This chapter discussed reimbursement for APRNs in the context of traditional economic theory and evolving developments in global finance and described the economic system as it relates to health care. It described concepts such as market competition, disequilibrium, and supplier-induced demand and discussed cost considerations in the provision of services by, and reimbursement for, physicians and APRNs in relation to the price of service, access issues, healthcare plans, competition, and antitrust issues. Included were definitions of key terms in finance and reimbursement.

Reimbursement is a challenging component of APRN practice. APRNs should be aware of market economics; use appropriate marketing strategies; and strive to provide high-quality, cost-effective services. As healthcare providers assume more financial risk, fiscal rewards may be less predictable than in the past. However, APRNs are equipped with the necessary knowledge and skills to fill unmet healthcare needs, practicing independently or collaboratively with physicians. Whether APRNs will flourish depends not only on the quality and cost-effectiveness of the care they provide but also on financial, organizational, and legal obstacles to their scope of practice.

SUGGESTED LEARNING EXERCISES

1. An NP who has been employed for 15 years is told that her position is being eliminated, that it is "too expensive" for the proposed practice group budget following review by a business consultant. The owners of her group have been told to decrease fixed costs, such as payroll. The panel of patients seen by this NP would be given the option of being seen by other healthcare providers in the community. How might the NP retain her practice while capturing the income stream generated by her services?

2. A nurse educator who is active in professional organization activities repeatedly cites the benefits of care provided by APRNs, benefits that include safety and cost-effectiveness. At one forum, the educator is closely questioned regarding the availability of data substantiating these benefits. How might the educator respond to these questions, based on the evolving healthcare marketplace?

3. An NP employed by an HMO contemplates relocating from an urban setting to a rural practice, where she thinks about entering a joint practice arrangement with a physician who is motivated to collaborate with the NP. However, both the physician and the NP are unfamiliar with reimbursement mechanisms for services provided by NPs. What resources should these professionals consult to maximize reimbursement from their joint practice arrangement?

References

1. American Nurses Association (ANA). (1977). *Reimbursement for Nursing Services: Position Statement of the Commission on Economic and General Welfare*. ANA, Kansas City, MO.

2. Felstein, P. (1988). The politics of health legislation: an economic perspective. Health Administration Press Perspectives, Ann Arbor, MI.

3. Buerhaus, P. (1992). Nursing, competition, and quality. *Nurs Econ* 10:21.

4. Lindeke, L, and Chesney M. (1999). Reimbursement realities of advanced nursing practice. *Nursing Outlook* 47:6.

5. Fuchs, V. (1986). *The Health Economy*. Harvard University Press, Cambridge, MA.

6. Barr, C. (2008, Sept 28). How it got this bad. Can be accessed at http://money.cnn.com/2008/09/26/news/leverage.fortune/index.htm?postversion=2008092614.

7. Enthoven, A. (1988). Managed competition: an agenda for action. *Health Affairs* 7:25.

8. Feldstein, P. (1993). *Health Care Economics*. 4th ed. Delmar, Albany, NY.

9. Cohen, I. (1993). Medicaid physician fees and use of physician and hospital services. *Inquiry* 30:281.

10. Lee, D, and Gillis, K. (1993). Physician responses to Medicare physician on access to care. *Inquiry* 30:417.

11. Buerhaus, P. (1996). Economics and health care financing. In Hickey, J, Ouimette, R, and Venegoni, S (eds), *Advanced Practice Nursing*. Lippincott, Philadelphia.

12. Ginsburg, P. (2005). Competition in healthcare: its evolution over the past decade. *Health Affairs* 24:1512–1522.

13. Mahar, M. (2007, February). Why market competition will not mend our health care system. *Managed Care Magazine*. http://www.managedcaremag.com/archives/0/02/0/02.collaboration.html. Accessed September 15, 2008.

14. American Nurses Association. Health system reform. http://www.nursingworld.org/MainMenuCategories/HealthcareandPolicyIssues/HSR.aspx. Accessed September 15, 2008.

15. Sullivan-Marx, E. (2008). Lessons learned from advanced practice nursing payment. *Policy, Politics and Nursing Practice* 9:121. http://ppn.sagepub.com/cgi/content/abstract/9/2/121. Accessed September 22, 2008.

16. Author. Health insurance coverage: 2007. http://www.census/gov/hhes/www/hlthins/hlthin07/hlth07asc.html. Accessed September 6, 2008.

17. Welton, J, and Dismuke, C. (2008). Testing an inpatient nursing intensity billing model. *Policy, Politics and Nursing Practice* 9:103–111.

18. Laport, N, Semeus, W, VandenBoer, G, and Van Herck, P. (2008). Adjusting reimbursement for nursing care. *Policy, Politics and Nursing Practice* 9:94–102.

19. American College of Nurse Practitioners. AMA meeting summary, June, 2006. http://www.acnpweb.org/i4a/pages/Index.cfm?pageID=3273. Accessed September 6, 2008.

20. Schmit, J. Could walk-in retail clinics help slow rising health costs? http://www.usatoday.com/money/industries/health/2006-08-24-walk-in-clinic-usat_x.htm. Accessed September 15, 2008.

21. Phillips, S.J. (2010). Twenty-second annual legislative update. *The Nurse Practitioner* 35:1, 24-47.

22. Phillips, S. (2007). Nineteenth annual legislative update. *The Nurse Practitioner* 32:1.

23. Dueker, M, Spurr, S, and Kalist, D. (2005, November). The practice boundaries of advanced practice nurses: an economic and legal analysis. *Social Science Research Network*. Can be accessed at http://papers.ssrn.com/sol3/papers.cfm?abstract_id=869451.

24. Department of Health and Human Services Office of the Inspector General. Medicare Coverage of Non-Physician Practitioner Services, OEI-02-00-00290, June 2001.

25. Hanson, M, and Bennett, S. Business planning and reimbursement mechanisms. In Hamric, A, Spross, J, and Hanson, C (eds), *Advanced Nursing Practice: An Integrative Approach*. 4th ed. Saunders Elsevier, St. Louis, MO, pp. 543–574.

26. Sorkin, A. (1992). *Health Economics*, 3rd ed. Macmillan, New York.

27. Maclin, S, and Carper, K. (2007, March). Expenses for hospital inpatient stays, 2004. http://www.meps.ahrq.gov/mepsweb/data_files/publications/st164/stat164.pdf. Accessed September 6, 2008.

28. Gabel, J, Claxton, G, Gil, I, et al. (2004). Health benefits in 2004: four years of double-digit premium increases take their toll on coverage. *Health Affairs* 23(5):200–209.

29. Prince, T, and Sullivan, J. (2000). Financial viability, medical technology and hospital closures. *J Health Care Finance* 26(4):1–18.

30. Author. Hospital closure *Data*. http://www.appam.org/conferences/fall/dc03. Accessed November 24, 2003.

31. Strunk, B, Ginsburg, P, and Gabel, J. (2002, September). Tracking health care costs: growth accelerates again in 2001. *Health Affairs*. http://content.healthaffairs.org/cgi/content/abstract/hlthaff.w2.299. Accessed September 30, 2009.

32. Costs of medical technology. http//www.sciencedaily.com. Accessed November 24, 2003.

33. Blue Cross Blue Shield. Reimbursement issues. http://bcbshealthissues.com. Accessed June 28, 2003.

34. Treasury Direct. Debt to the penny and who holds it. http://www.treasurydirect.gov/NP/BPDLogin?application=np. Accessed September 6, 2008.

35. EBRI. Online facts from EBRI. National Health Care Expenditures, 1997. http://www.ebri.org/facts/0199atact.htm. Accessed July 6, 2003.

36. National Coalition on Health Care. Health insurance costs. http://www.nchc.org/facts/cost.shtml. Accessed September 6, 2008.

37. Hoffman, C. (1994). Medicaid payment for nonphysician practitioners: an access issue. *Health Affairs* 13:140.

38. *Alliance for Health Reform Sourcebook for Journalists 2003*, Chapter 8, "Health Care Costs." http://www.allhealth.org/sourcebook2002/ch8_8.html. Accessed July 3, 2003.

39. Mittelstadt, P. (1993). Federal reimbursement of advanced practice nurses' services empowers the profession. *Nurse Pract* 18:46.

40. Alliance for Health Care Reform. (2003, March 10–16). Cover the *Uninsured Week on Campus Resource Guide*. Robert Wood Johnson Foundation, Washington, DC.

41. National Coalition on Health Care. Health insurance costs. Available at: http://www.nchc.org/facts/cost.shtml. Accessed September 6, 2008.

42. Lewin, I. (2003). To the rescue: toward solving America's health care crisis. Families USA Foundation, Washington, DC.

43. Faut-Callahan, M. (1995). Economics of anesthesia. Unpublished manuscript.

44. Pryor, C. (1999). Balanced budget act enhances value of physician assistant, nurse practitioners. *Health Care Strategic Management* 17:12–13.

45. Kaiser Family Foundation. (2002). *Trends and Indicators in the Changing Health Care Marketplace.*

46. Author. Health insurance coverage: 2007. http//:www.census.gov/hhes/www/hlthins/hlthin07/hlth07asc.html. Accessed September 6, 2008.

47. Fagin, C. (1992). The cost-effectiveness of nursing care. In Aiken L., and Fagin C (eds), Charting *Nursing's Future: Agenda for the 1990s.* JB Lippincott, Philadelphia.

48. Frontera, J. 2009 health care costs to increase the lowest in years. ThomasNet Industrial News Room. http://news.thomasnet.com/IMT/archives/2008/09-health-care-cost-increase-the-lowest-in-years-pwc-aon-mercer-reports.html. Accessed September 15, 2008.

49. Hooker, R. (1993). The role of physician assistants and nurse practitioners in a managed care organization. Association of Academic Health Centers, Kaiser Permanente Center for Health Research, Sacramento, CA.

50. American Medical Association (AMA). AMA Young Physicians Section Interim 2003 Delegate's Report. http://www.ama-assn.org/ama/pub/category/9982.html. Accessed June 3, 2003.

51. American College of Nurse Practitioners. *AMA Meeting Summary 06/2006.* http://www.acnpweb.org/i4a/pages/Index.cfm?pageID=3723. Accessed May 4, 2010.

52. Timmons, G, and Ridenour, N. (1994). Legal approaches to the restraint of trade of nurse practitioners: disparate reimbursement patterns. *J Amer Acad of Nurse Prac* 6:55.

53. Fugate, D, and Freese, G. (1992). Nursing marketing. In Decker P, and Sullivan E (eds), *Nursing Administration.* Appleton & Lange, Norwalk, CT.

54. Petrakos, C. (1996). Nurse practitioner supervision at issue: RNs push for collegial practice. *The Chicago Tribune*, Nursing News, p. 3.

55. Author. Generalist and specialist physician salaries. http://www.mgma.com/press/article.aspx?id=29318. Accessed September 1, 2009.

56. Author. Trends in medical education. http://www.gao.gov/products/GAO-09-438R. Accessed September 1, 2009.

57. Simonson, D, and Garde, J. (1994). Reimbursement for clinical services. In Foster, S, and Jordan, L (eds.), *Professional Aspects of Nurse Anesthesia Practice.* FA Davis, Philadelphia.

58. Harbaugh, N. (2009). Pay for performance: quality- and valued-based reimbursement. *Pediatr Clin North Am* 56(4):997–1007.

59. Young, G, and Conrad, D. (2007). Practical issues in the design and implementation of pay-for-quality programs. *J Healthc Manag* 52(1):10–18.

60. Author. Point of service plan defined. http://www.medhealthinsurance.com/posplan.htm. Accessed September 1, 2009.

61. Schwartz, A. (1996). Will competition change physician workforce? Early signals from the market. *Academic Medicine* 71:15.

62. Brotherton, S, Simon, F, and Etzel, S. (2005). U.S. graduate medical education 2004–2005: trends in primary care specialties. *JAMA* 294:1075–1082.

63. Michels, K. (1994). Health care reform glossary of terms. *AANA Journal* 62:19.

64. Kongstvedt, P. (1993). Compensation of primary care physicians in open panels. *The Managed Care Handbook*, 2nd ed. Aspen, Gaithersburg, MD.

65. Pearson, L. (2008). The Pearson report. *The American Journal for Nurse Practitioners* 12:2.

66. AANA. (1994). *Practice Management in Changing Environments*, Sections 4-1 and 4-2. American Association of Nurse Anesthetists, Park Ridge, IL.

67. Kennerly, S. (2007). The impending reimbursement revolution: how to prepare for future APN reimbursement. *Nursing Economics* 25(2):81–84.

68. Ament, L. (1998). Reimbursement, employment and hospital privilege data of certified nurse midwifery services. *Journal of Nurse Midwifery* 43:305–307.

69. Salary.com. CNM salaries. http://www.salary.com. Accessed September 20, 2008.

70. Slomski, A. (2000). "We don't just catch babies." *Medical Economics* 77:186–188.

71. Gazella, K. High cost of malpractice insurance threatens supply of ob/gyns, especially in some urban areas. http://www.eurekalert.org/pub_releases/2005-06/uomh_hco053105.php. Accessed October 13, 2008.

72. Cromwell, J. (1999). Barriers to achieving a cost-effective workforce mix: lessons from anesthesiology. *Journal of Health Politics, Policy and Law* 24:1331–1361.

73. Medical Group Management Association. (2008, July 14). Specialty physician compensation barely keeps up with inflation. www.mgma.com/press/article.aspx?id=20662. Accessed October 13, 2008.

74. Simonson, D, Ahern, N, and Hendryx, M. (2007). Anesthesia staffing and anesthetic complications during cesarean delivery: a retrospective analysis. *Nursing Research* 56(1):9–17.

75. Pine, M, Holt, K, and Lou, Y. (2003). Surgical mortality and type of anesthesia provider. *AANA Journal* 71:109–116.

76. The Joint Commission. http://www.jointcommission.org?NR?rdonlyres/76E44364-418D-4347-0E61-BA9CA350F225/0/08_CAH_New_Requirements.pdf. Accessed October 13, 2008.

77. Kaiser Permanente. (1995). An inter-regional examination of operating room best practices. Unpublished report.

78. Minark, P. (2000). Alert! Strategy initiated to restrict advanced practice nurses' ability to bill Medicare. *Clinical Nurse Specialist* 14:250–251.

79. Guglielmo, W. (2000). In the trenches, it's cooperation that matters. *Medical Economics* 77:194–196.

80. Centers for Medicare and Medicaid Services. (2005, Jan 31). Medicare "Pay for Performance (P4P)" initiatives, 2007. http://www.cms.hhs.gov/apps/media/press/release.asp?counter=1343. Accessed May 4, 2010.

81. American Medical Association. Principles for Pay for Performance programs. http://www.ama.com. Accessed September 22, 2008.

82. The Commonwealth Fund. Five years after to err is human: what have we learned? http://www.commonwealthfund.org. Accessed September 22, 2008.

83. Leichter, S. Pay for performance: is Medicare a good candidate? The Cato Institute. http://www.cato.org/pubs/papers/cannon_p4p.pdf. Accessed September 22, 2008.

84. Snyder, L, and Neubaurer, R. (2007). Pay for performance principles that promote patient-centered care: an ethics manifesto (Abstract). *Annals of Internal Medicine* 147:792–794.

85. CMS. Eliminating serious, preventable, and cost medical errors—never events, 2006. http://www.cms.hhs.gov/apps/media/press/release.asp?Counter=1863. Accessed September 22, 2008.

86. Leapfrog Group. Leapfrog group position statement on never events. http://www.leapfroggroup.org/for_hospitals/leapfrog_hospital_quality_and_safety_survey_copy/never_events. Accessed September 22, 2008.

87. Accreditation Council for Graduate Medical Education. The ACGME's approach to limit resident duty hours 12 months after implementation: a summary of achievements, 2003. http://www.acgme.net/acWebsite/duty/Hours/dh_dutyhoursummary2003-04.pdf. Accessed September 22, 2008.

88. The American Nurse. (2008, September/October). Health reform: the 2008 election and beyond. *The American Nurse* 1.

89. American College of Nurse-Midwives. Landmark health reform law to improve access to midwifery, benefit women's health., March 23, 2010. http://www.midwife.org/siteFiles/news/HR3590.pdf. Accessed June 14, 2010.

Christine (Tina) E. Burke has had a clinical practice in nurse-midwifery since 1976, when she earned her master's degree in nursing from Yale University. Dr. Burke is an educator whose teaching credentials include positions at the University of Colorado, Georgetown University, George Mason University, and Yale University. Pentimento Praxis, Dr. Burke's consultation practice, was established in 1992 after completion of her doctorate in nursing from the University of Colorado. The scope of her work and consultations include creating caring communities, training teachers and community members in moral development and character education, working with culturally diverse populations in an inner-city clinic, providing prenatal and gynecological health care, and nurturing the perceptual palette. Dr. Burke lives in Denver, Colorado, where she currently works for The Denver Health Authority.

CHAPTER 8

Marketing the Role: Formulating, Articulating, and Negotiating Advanced Practice Nursing Positions

Christine E. Burke, PhD, CNM

CHAPTER OUTLINE

CHAPTER OBJECTIVES

After completing this chapter, the reader will be able to:

1. Communicate the benefits that accrue to the target population or employer from utilization of the services that advanced practice registered nurses (APRNs) offer through use of the four Ps.

2. Create a personal mission statement after reflecting on personal values, beliefs, and quality-of-life issues that will influence your career pathways.

3. Interpret facts from major documents about cost, outcomes, and use of health services provided by APRNs.

4. Create a marketing plan for an APRN's service.

CHAPTER OBJECTIVES

5. Create a succinct position statement for an APRN's service that differentiates their services from alternatives and links them to target consumer needs and wants.
6. Demonstrate techniques and considerations in negotiating an advanced practice position from initial contact through the interview process to the contractual agreement.
7. Analyze one's existing network and use marketing techniques to further enhance and strengthen the network resources.

Marketing, as a coordinated style of communicating information, is an essential skill for APRNs. Success in the age of pay-for-performance, managed care, and autonomous private practices and businesses demands an appreciation of market theories. APRNs must understand a business plan as well as a nursing care plan to accomplish the goals of independent practice. This chapter is bifocal in its presentation. The information shared is useful from either the employer's or employee's perspective. The skills necessary to gather and interpret marketing data, formulate marketing plans, and create essential written documents for the acquisition and development of APRNs' services are presented through a marketing lens.

The Traditional Marketing Approach: The Four Ps

The marketing process is guided by the four Ps:

- Product
- Price
- Place
- Promotion

These concepts help to assess the needs and available resources to be used in the promotion of the APRN service.

The first P, the **product,** is interpreted in an APRN's business plan not as material goods, but rather as human services. Unlike material products, these services lack tangibility and efficient storage capability for later use and cannot be exactly replicated with each client; these factors pose some of the challenges of creating a marketing plan that accurately projects the future of an APRN's service. The difference of human service is important because it is at the core of patient satisfaction. The development of an APRN's service as a product includes the consideration of the **market segmentation,** or **target markets,** which describe who will be served; **product integrity,** or the balance of needs and resources; and the **competition,** or the other available healthcare services in the community.

Price, the second P, is the identification of the right cost for the services. This price must be neither too high nor too low and also must meet the existing financial mandates of insurance companies, managed care facilities, and federally funded Medicaid and Medicare plans.

APRNs can support their price for services from marketing research based on utilization and cost-effectiveness. Proof that the services meet the needs of the patients and are financially efficient has been determined through research, which is discussed later in this chapter.

The third P is for **place,** or where these services are delivered. The demands of consumers direct this marketing concern. The geographic location and physical convenience of the APRN service play heavily into the clients' decision-making among competitive healthcare services. The more accessible and more easily usable a service is, the more healthcare consumers it attracts. The simple matters of accessibility by public transportation, parking, and physically pleasant office spaces can ultimately lure potential clients from one service to another.

The final P is for **promotion,** or the ability to increase consumers' awareness of the services the APRN offers and communicate information that may attract consumers. The modes of promotion include advertisement, publicity, community presentations, and correspondence. In addition, promotion also includes the manner in which the APRN reflects the quality of the service in speech, dress, and the conduct of the business. The best method of promotion is word of mouth by satisfied consumers. By its nature, this method of promotion is grounded in familiarity and trust, and a good word from a previous employer or consumer can do more for successful marketing than many costly advertising promotions.[1]

In the early 1990s, the marketing firm of Burson-Marsteller introduced a fifth P; it relates to the **perception management** of the target audience. The customer perception of the advanced practice nurse as a capable, knowledgeable healthcare provider is as important as the other four Ps of marketing services. For the consumer, the perception of the provider's skills becomes the reality; when an APRN is marketing to attract business, the need to create a good perception is then obvious. According to Burson-Marsteller, the perceptions motivate behaviors that create the business results. They further believe that the perceptions are built on the societal values that guide the formation of attitudes and, ultimately, behavior. Woods and Cardin,[2] in their discussion of this aspect of perception, further discuss the need to consider the recognition of the emotional and the rational messages we send to our consumers. These messages pass on the value of feeling safe with APRN care and this connects to the universal value we seek—peace of mind.[2]

Marketing has changed some of its point of view. The four Ps are an old standard for creating marketing plans, but a new point of view has emerged that expands this to include the four Cs:

- Customer value
- Cost
- Convenience
- Communication

Dr. Rick Crandall, a noted authority on marketing services rather than products, has stated that for service providers these four areas may prove to be more important than the traditional four Ps.[3]

Employment is one of the obvious goals of APRN education. This goal is met through one of three pathways:

1. Employment in an established healthcare service that already employs APRNs.
2. Creation of new employment opportunities within a healthcare system that has the potential for expansion to include APRNs.
3. Development of a private practice in the clinical or consultation arenas.

In general terms, marketing is the activity that supports the buying and selling of products and services. The key to success in attaining employment involves matching the professional skills necessary for a job and the APRN. By analyzing the healthcare needs of the target population and setting up a research-based plan to meet those needs, APRNs are likely to create employment opportunities or, in marketing terms, to set up voluntary exchanges of goods and services.

A prerequisite to the successful marketing of an APRN is knowledge. Each professional must spend time considering and developing self-knowledge and knowledge about the profession. Attention should be given to the following areas:

- Knowledge of personal values, professional skills, and practical necessities
- Knowledge of practice regulations
- Knowledge of existing services
- Knowledge of clients' healthcare needs and desires
- Knowledge of the target population's understanding of the role and scope of practice of the APRN
- Knowledge of the utilization and cost-effectiveness of, and satisfaction with, advanced practice registered nursing services
- Knowledge of specific marketing elements

Knowledge of Personal Values, Professional Skills, and Practical Necessities

Developing a personal mission statement, or a statement of one's values, beliefs, and goals of practice, can assist in successfully communicating and selling one's view of health care. This statement will explain who one is. The personal mission statement typically includes one's values or guiding principles (e.g., trust, honesty, respect, responsibility, and caring) and one's professional skills and scope of services. Most important, it reveals the vision of the quality of life one needs (time for family, hobbies, political activity, and educational opportunities). This knowledge is usually acquired by introspection, by review of previous employment, and by consideration of personal needs, which are necessary for a reasonable life.

An example of guiding principles that have strongly affected the business community is Stephen Covey's *The Seven Habits of Highly Effective People*.[4] Covey developed a theory regarding the restoration of the character ethic. The habits are the intersection of knowledge, skill, and desire. Knowledge is the theoretical paradigm, or the what to do; skill is the how to do; and desire is the motivation. Covey divides these habits into three arenas:

1. The Private Victory
   - Be proactive based on principles of personal vision.
   - Begin with the end in mind guided by principles of leadership.
   - Put first things first guided by principles of personal management.
2. The Public Victory
   - Think win–win guided by principles of interpersonal leadership.
   - Seek first to understand and then to be understood guided by principles of empathic communication.
   - Synergize, guided by principles of cooperation.
3. The Renewal
   - Sharpen the saw, guided by principles of balanced self-renewal.

The importance of this work is its universal message about human effectiveness. The translation of these theories into nursing practice will help create a stronger, more professional vision.

Questions helpful in the introspective process are:

- What about your work do you enjoy the most?
- What other interests do you have?
- What skills do you do well?
- Which need improvement?
- What support do you need to attain a proficient level of practice?
- What made you leave jobs in the past?
- How will this affect your future employment?
- Do you prefer to work alone or on a team?
- What about your team members is necessary for good working relationships?
- How do you see your role in relation to the healthcare system: What is your need for power or shared power?
- How do you handle stress?
- Will the job you are creating or applying for allow for some stress-reduction management, such as exercise?
- What are your family needs (child care issues and emergency coverage, flexibility of hours to allow for family events)?
- How do you best communicate with others?

The time spent on a personal mission statement can help avoid major career-related frustrations and problems. A considered mission statement can guide the job search with a clarity of purpose by defining both the professional and personal motivating factors. If salary and status hold greater value than free time and an active social life, focus the marketing efforts on demanding a financially fulfilling position. In all cases, be true to yourself. Ask these four questions to help create the foundation for the personal mission statement. Who am I? Where am I going? Who's going with me? What will I do when I get there? Spending time with these questions will help clarify values and make one's personal marketing much more genuine. Authenticity in this endeavor is essential for the pursuit of happiness in vocational life.

Job satisfaction is also to be considered when developing the right relationship to a job. Debra Tri[5] states that there are three basic criteria for APRN job satisfaction: autonomy, a sense of accomplishment, and time to spend on patient care. Consider asking questions about these areas when considering a job.

Fisher and Brown, of the Harvard Negotiation Project, in discussing the role of shared values with employers and employees, remind us that the fewer the differences in shared values the more likely the basis for dealing with issues fairly. The opposite is not true, however; differences are not good for negotiations. It is often enriching for the work at hand to have some value differences that force the creation of new partnerships.[6]

Life coach and author Fiona Harrold offers seven rules of success for professional and personal fulfillment. She believes that if you apply this thinking and follow her strategies, it will help modify personal behavior in a way that will lead to success. These seven rules are:

- Be passionate.
- Practice self-belief.
- Do more.
- Take more risks.
- Inspire others.
- Persevere.
- Be generous.[7]

Success is defined by one's values, beliefs, and life goals. Look for "signature strengths," as discussed by Dr. Martin Seligman, whose extensive research on the blueprint of happiness conceives of it as learned optimism.[8] Harrold also stated that this learned optimism is part of her notion of passion and a key to her rules for success.[7]

Knowledge of Practice Regulations

The legal issues concerning advanced practice nursing are discussed in Chapter 11. Review this chapter and all related statutes and regulations, and include the documents that will support an advanced nursing practice in a marketing portfolio. Typically, these documents include:

- State nurse-practice act
- State board of nursing regulations
- Prescriptive authority legislation
- Third-party reimbursement rules and regulations
- Practice protocols from similar APRNs' services

An excellent resource for regulatory issues is the annual legislative update compiled by *The Nurse Practitioner* and the *American Journal for Nurse Practitioners*. The journal *Nursing Economics* is another that keeps an eye on the legislative changes affecting APRN services. In-depth explanations and evaluations of healthcare policy issues are examined in the segment now called *Health Policy and Politics*.

Knowledge of Existing Services

Investigate the target market with an eye toward answering the following questions:

- What services already exist in the community?
- Who uses the services?
- What are the needs for these services based on the demographic data and the socio-economic mix of the population (e.g., age, employment, unemployment, insured and uninsured)?
- Most importantly, what is not working with these services that an APRN might be able to change (e.g., access to care, cost-effective care, patient education)?

Knowing the competition is the first step in creating a marketing strategy. Deciding how to position the service is the next. Positioning is a marketing strategy that works to separate the uniqueness of a product or service from the generic pack. It begins with knowing one's own service and the competition's service and then finding a niche that allows your service to stand out.[9]

The APRN should ask not what she or he has to offer, but what is needed by the consumer that an APRN can provide. Knowing one's abilities and marketable skills is important, but it is more important to be in a position in which someone desires to use those services. This goal can be best accomplished by recommendations from people already highly respected by the target population or community. In a world full of well-qualified professionals, with strong recommendations the APRN or APRN's service will often rise above the competition and be sought out.

Creating this **market niche,** or the narrow market segment, that the APRN can fulfill can be accomplished by using a reverse marketing strategy. This consumer-driven process creates partnerships between the APRN and the potential clients with the common goal of healthcare satisfaction. The positioning process, therefore, demands a needs assessment of the actual or perceived consumer needs. This is accomplished through the use of interviews, surveys, and questionnaires.

Knowledge of Clients' Healthcare Needs and Desires

Knowledge of the needs and desires of the clients involves watching and reaching people. Mark McCormack, in *What They Don't Teach You at Harvard Business School*,[10] described seven fundamental steps to reading people:

1. Listen aggressively to the what and how someone speaks.
2. Observe aggressively and make note of all body language.
3. Talk less and you will learn more, see more, and hear more.
4. Take a second look at first impressions by reviewing what you first thought about a person or an idea.
5. Take time to use what you have learned by reviewing what you know about your job and the clients and then consider how you will present your services.
6. Be discreet about what you have perceived about others and how they learn about your qualifications. Whenever possible, let others tell how great you are.
7. Be detached enough to step back from a heated business deal and watch what is happening so that your reaction is not overreaction. Always try to act rather than react since this has more power.

Researching the healthcare needs of a target population includes McCormack's ideas of reading people on the interpersonal level and the more global tools for reading a community, such as surveys. These surveys should offer a broader perspective of the healthcare needs from a mix of socioeconomic groups as well as from a variety of community members, consumers, healthcare administrators, insurance agents, and peer professionals.

Knowledge of the Target Population's Understanding of the Role and Scope of Practice of the APRN

By survey, questionnaire, or personal contacts, the APRN can determine the target market's level of understanding of the APRN role. Talking to prospective clients, employers, community leaders, insurance salespersons, hospital employees, and the medical community can help determine what, if any, previous experiences prospective employers have had with APRNs. Once the level of appreciation of the APRN role has been determined, the APRN can formulate a plan for educating or increasing the awareness of the target population regarding the potential benefits of hiring an APRN and their specific skills.

Consider the consultancy roles involved in the job. Liz Benagin's research suggests that APRNs have external and internal consulting roles. The external consulting role is the focused point of the job; the internal consultancy role is an integral part of the APRN role within the job description. Inherent in the use of one's knowledge and skills is the respect for the expertise of the APRN as a consultant to others within the organization or as an external expert brought in to help advise on the work within a healthcare system.[11]

Knowledge of the Utilization and Cost-Effectiveness of and Satisfaction with APRN Services

The APRN should review and collect current literature that supports the role of the APRN. Resource assessment and use are at the core of every economic strategy plan, and a marketing plan should respect not only the fiscal and structural resources of the healthcare system but also the human resources necessary for the provision of health care. Research has shown that nonphysician healthcare professionals provide high-quality primary care and increased consumer access to care. Prospective employers or consumers should be encouraged to read the literature on utilization and take the time to evaluate what APRN services they might substitute for costly physicians' services.

Research in primary care has described the level of productivity and cost associated with patient encounters with nonphysician health providers (NHP), such as nurse practitioners (NPs) and physician assistants (PAs), and with physician providers. At the most basic level, APRNs earn smaller salaries and, therefore, solely on the basis of salary and benefits, they cost less than physicians. More importantly, APRNs are more likely to prescribe improved nutrition, exercise, stress-management techniques, and health promotion, all of which are modalities that are less likely to directly affect the clinic, hospital, or institutional budget. In addition, APRNs are less likely to send each patient home with a prescription, potentially saving healthcare dollars.

Studies reveal that four NHPs can replace two to three physicians. The addition of a NHP to an office or clinic setting can increase total office visits by 40% to 50%, and the substitution of one NHP for one physician resulted in an average savings of more than $34,000 per year.[12] Greenfield and colleagues[13] similarly found that in a healthcare setting in which protocols were used, a NHP system realized a reduction of 20% in visit costs. A meta-analysis of studies on NPs and CNMs provided the nursing profession with excellent support for the use of APRNs in these roles. The Office of Technology Assessment (OTA)[14] concluded in a 1986 study that NPs and CNMs provided a quality of care equivalent to the care given by physicians. This study also concluded that in the areas of communication and preventive care, the nurses were much more adept than physicians. A second study conducted in 1987 by Crosby, Ventura, and Feldman[15] reported findings similar to the OTA study. Their study concluded that:

- Patients are satisfied with their care from NPs.
- The interpersonal skills of APRNs are better than those of physicians.
- The technical quality of APRNs' care is equivalent to that of physicians' care.
- APRNs' patient outcomes are equivalent or superior to physicians' patient outcomes.
- APRNs facilitate continuity of patient care and improved access to care in rural and other settings and provide care to underserved populations.

In November 1995, The Health Research Group of Ralph Nader's Public Citizen released a unique consumer guide to CNM practices in the United States. The report concluded that CNMs will play an increasing role in American obstetric care because of the quality of care, cost-effectiveness, and overall patient satisfaction described by CNM clients.[16] The Nader group found that 87% of CNMs serve low-risk clients, that 92% provide obstetric and gynecological care, that cesarean section rate for CNM clients was half that of the overall rate in the United States, and that CNMs use less technology and more patient education in prenatal visits. The endorsement of the use of CNMs by this prestigious research group can help all CNMs support their place in a healthcare system. In addition, Deonne Brown's descriptive study has demonstrated widespread acceptance of APRNs.[17] These and other research findings can be incorporated into the APRN's marketing plan. Gathering research studies such as these for the marketing portfolio will provide a strong base of support, especially in systems that appreciate statistical proof of healthcare outcomes.

Green and Davis,[18] in their investigation of patient satisfaction with APRN care, cited several implications for APRN practice. These implications for enhancing patient satisfaction include the sociodemographics and health variables of patients, the healthcare system, and characteristics of APRNs. Balancing the patients' needs, the skill sets and knowledge of the providers, and the system's healthcare options are the keys to increasing patients' satisfaction.

Knowledge of Specific Marketing Elements

An understanding of specific marketing elements, such as the difference between substitution and complement functions and the specific roles of the different types of APRNs, is necessary in developing the all-important marketing plan.

Substitution and Complement Functions

In this changing healthcare climate, many physicians are concerned about their power, their income, and even their jobs. The rules are changing too quickly and too dramatically, causing discomfort for many providers, physician and nonphysician alike. APRNs have frequently found employment in areas the physicians regard as less desirable, typically rural areas or underserved inner-city clinics, which may not be financially lucrative and therefore underserved by physicians.

There is little argument about how APRNs can be used in these settings, both as substitutes for, and as complements to, physician providers. For clarity, it helps to define these terms in the context of this chapter. *Complement* is defined as:

- Something that completes, makes up a whole, or brings to perfection.
- The quantity or number needed to make up a whole. Either of two parts that complete the whole or mutually complete each other.

Substitute is defined as something that takes the place of something else, a replacement.[19] (See Chapter 5 by Bowers, Gilliss, and Davis for additional discussion on complement versus substitute roles.)

In an underserved area any competent healthcare provider can reasonably argue for establishing services to provide care that otherwise would be unavailable. This could take the form of working with a physician or physician group to "mutually complete" a healthcare partnership. It also could mean acting as a substitute for a physician, "taking the place of" a physician in an area without one. The arguments for APRN positions in more competitive areas often are more difficult to make and may be less well received. In these areas, it is wise to focus on how APRNs are different rather than how they are the same. If APRNs are "the same as" physicians, it is often more difficult to break into the healthcare system where physicians are abundant. Practitioners may be more marketable if they "mutually complete" a healthcare partnership than attempt to replace one. In marketing in these settings, it is important to stress that APRNs provide similar services but with an emphasis on chronic disease management and health promotion and prevention, which will decrease long-term healthcare costs. .

In the ever-changing healthcare environment, APRNs can no longer afford to be just clinicians. Marketing has become crucial to survival. Defined as the act or process of selling or purchasing in a market, marketing involves an aggregate of functions in moving goods from producer to consumer. Some factors to consider in the marketing process include:

- What is the product or service?
- How is it different from others?
- How is it better?
- Are APRNs more consumer-oriented, more cost-effective, and so forth?

The Product or Service

The product or service generally is the APRN, but the individuation depends on the particular area of practice. APRNs are professionals with specialized knowledge or skills that are applied within a broad range of patient populations in a variety of practice settings.[20]

- Certified nurse-midwives (CNMs) are individuals educated in the two disciplines of nursing and midwifery who are certified according to the requirements of the American Midwifery Certification Board (AMCB). Nurse-midwifery practice is the independent management of the care of essentially normal newborns and women occurring within a healthcare system that provides for medical consultation, collaboration, or referral.[21]
- Certified registered nurse anesthetists (CRNAs) are registered nurses who have completed a nurse anesthesia program accredited by the Council on the Accreditation of Nurse Anesthesia Education Programs and have been certified by the National Board

on Certification and Recertification of Nurse Anesthetists (NBCRNA). CRNAs provide the full range of anesthesia services in a wide variety of settings, including acute care, ambulatory surgical centers, and physician offices.[22]

- Clinical nurse specialists (CNSs) serve as role models in the delivery of high-quality nursing care to patients. The CNS's client is the individual, nurse, other health professional, or system and the focus is on nursing staff education, system analysis, and the provision of direct and indirect nursing care.[23]

- Nurse practitioners (NPs) provide a full range of primary and acute care services with a holistic focus on the patient and family and on providing direct patient care.[24]

The Marketing Plan

After the APRN has collected all the information available from introspection, research data, personal communications, and target population surveys, he or she can create a marketing plan, or outline of strategies for promotion of services. Marketing plans contain five major elements:

1. A statement of purpose and the main objectives

2. The product description or what the APRN's service has to offer

3. The big picture: where the APRN and APRN's service will be in 5 years

4. The immediate action plan or steps for getting to the big picture

5. The marketing tools and strategies to be used. These include interviews, networking, and advertisement.

Figure 8-1 is an example of a marketing plan adapted for CNM practice.[25]

A. Describe your market: _____
   Age: _____
   Family size:_____
   Annual family income: _____
   Location:_____
   Healthcare decision patterns: _____
   Reason to seek CNM care: _____
   Other: _____
   (Geographically describe your service area)
   (Describe your client base economically)
   How large is your market?_____
   Women of childbearing age or birth rate: _____
   Growing _____ Steady _____ Decreasing_____
   If growing, annual growth rate _____
B. Describe the service you will provide: _____
C. Describe your pricing/billing practices: _____
D. Describe the place you will provide services: _____
E. Describe referral sources: _____
F. Describe your competition: _____
G. Describe plans for practice promotion and continued marketing:
   _____
H. Describe any barriers to practice that might exist: _____

I. Describe any consumer or professional networking that will be done:
   _____

Figure 8-1: Developing a marketing plan. (Adapted from Collins-Fulea, C, ed., 1996, *An Administrative Manual for Nurse-Midwifery Services,* Kendall-Hunt Publishing, Dubuque, IA, p. 25.)

A marketing plan should not be considered as fixed in concrete, but rather, as an ever-changing plan. It should be reviewed routinely and revised as needed to reflect changes in professional development or the needs of the target market. The possibility of healthcare and welfare reform in our country, for example, could change access to care. APRNs must be ready to adapt to that change.

Communication Skills

Communication skills are important for networking, job descriptions, writing a cover letter and résumés, and interviewing.

Networking

APRNs are ideally positioned to accommodate the radical changes sweeping the healthcare field, but they will surely experience much struggle in the process. One way to cope with the inevitable struggle is through networking.

Networking is not new! It has been done on both an informal and a formal basis since the beginning of civilization. A network is simply a group of individuals with similar interests and/or problems who join together to provide support and to exchange information. With the advent of computer technology, contacts are no longer limited by geography or phone bills. Networks easily span incredible distances, allowing even the most rural practitioners ready access to a peer group.

INFORMAL NETWORK

An informal network has traditionally been part of the male-dominated business world, especially in the upper levels of certain disciplines. The network comprises acquaintances, colleagues, and friends from school, church, family, sports, and business. When a man needed a favor, he contacted someone in his network. Men grow up knowing how to network, partially because of the influence of team sports. They learn quickly that they need one another in order to win the game, to get ahead.[26]

FORMAL NETWORK

Professional organizations are a good example of a formal network. Through their membership, these organizations are able to quickly disseminate information and take action. When federal legislation is proposed that might have a negative impact on the public's health, the American Nurses Association (ANA) is able to contact its network of state associations and request that they enlist the support of their membership in opposing the bill. Networking through formal organizations can be of immeasurable benefit in achieving success and happiness in an advanced practice role. Through it, one can:

- Build support systems
- Share resources and avoid reinventing the wheel
- Identify similar practice issues, such as restraint of trade; credentialing difficulties; and physician opposition, direct or subtle[27]

A major advantage of networking comes from the fact that the best place to learn about job opportunities is through one's network of friends and acquaintances. Networking, as it relates to job searches, is the process of enlisting other people to help one find employment. Most job openings are filled by word of mouth.[28] One never knows who can help! To help in a job search:

- Build a base of contacts with alumni groups, professional organizations, PTA, and children's sports leagues.
- Expand this contact base.

- Get and use referrals.
- Follow up on all leads.

All leads are worth pursuing. When contacting someone from the network, the job seeker should let that person know about the job search and ask for advice, suggestions, or ideas. (The job seeker should probably not ask directly for a job; a direct request can put people off and decrease the probability of assistance.) The most important information to get is names of other people, because word of mouth is the most effective way to find a job. Other methods include:

- Newspaper advertisements (note: only 10% to 15% of job openings are advertised in newspapers)
- Professional organizations' media
- Large-scale mailing of résumés (note: the success rate for receiving a call for an interview is only 2%)
- Temporary work, which can be a foot in the door and an opportunity for permanent work
- Executive recruiters (headhunters)
- Employment agencies
- Recruiting databases
- Posting the résumé online
- Browsing through job listings

The APRN can get indirect knowledge of changes in job markets by reading the business pages and local business journals for hints of the "hidden" job market. These are found in news of promotions, transfers, retirements, company expansions, company relocations, announcements, awards, mergers, and takeovers.[29]

Online marketing is another approach to networking. Web sites, one's own and others', as well as e-mail and Internet searches have broadened our capabilities for reaching possible employment opportunities and sharing our services with a broader audience.[30]

The Academic Job Search Handbook, written by Vick and Furlong, suggests that networking is crucial in job searching, maintaining your employment, and for professional research.[31] The goal is to create a mutually beneficial relationship with other members of your profession. These relationships are excellent for stimulating ideas and sharing perspectives. The first step in creating these networks is to simply introduce yourself to colleagues. Conferences offer one venue for making these connections. In addition, practice these rules: the shy person should work on courageous acts of vocalization, and those more outgoing and possibly more verbose should regulate contributions to allow for more interpersonal exchanges.

The following 17 suggestions for better networking come from Rick Crandall:

1. Keep track of who you know.
2. Regularly visit groups and join the best.
3. Remember names better.
4. Make notes on business cards.
5. Pay attention.
6. Do research.
7. Project sincerity.
8. Do cold calling.
9. Improve your self-introduction.
10. Do online searches.
11. Listen more than you talk.

12. Follow up.

13. Ask for referrals.

14. Become a star.

15. Read the Monday business calendars.

16. Give a lot.

17. Volunteer.[30]

The Job Description

The purpose of the job description is to clarify the scope of practice and expectations of a professional position (Fig. 8-2). The job analysis previously mentioned helps create the framework for defining the skills, educational requirements, licensure, reporting relationships,

---

POSITION TITLE: Certified Nurse-Midwife (CNM)

DEPARTMENT: OB/GYN   **GRADE:** 15a

JOB SUMMARY: Provides comprehensive, primary health care to a select population of essentially healthy women. Participates in the care of women with medical complications in collaboration with Obstetricians-Gynecologists.

Principal Functions and Responsibilities:

1. Performs accurate history and physical examinations on essentially healthy women.
2. Provides primary care in an ambulatory setting to women, including ordering and evaluating of diagnostic tests and management of minor complications.
3. Provides inpatient obstetrical care for essentially healthy women, including labor management, delivery of infant, repair of lacerations/episiotomies, and management of minor complications. Initiates emergency care as needed.
4. Provides individualized client teaching and counseling utilizing the nurse-midwifery philosophy.
5. Identifies deviations from normal and consults, co-manages, or refers as appropriate.
6. Completes necessary documentation.
7. Participates in research and continuing education activities.
8. Instructs and supervises nurse-midwifery students as assigned.
9. Performs other duties as assigned.

Principal Functions and Responsibilities:

1. Considerable degree of independent judgment, to monitor and respond to changes of a client's condition.
2. Interpersonal skills to work effectively with clients and other members of the health-care team.

Work Conditions:
Normal client-care environment with some exposure to biological hazards and infectious diseases.

Education and Experience Requirements:
Graduation from an accredited school of nurse-midwifery
Certification by ACNM or AMCB
State licensure

Reporting Relationships:

1. Reports to the Director, Nurse-Midwifery Services
2. Indirectly supervises personnel involved with the care of assigned clients.

APPROVED BY:_____ **DATE:**_____

Figure 8-2: The job description. (From Collins-Fulea, C, ed., 1996, *An Administrative Manual for Nurse-Midwifery Services*, Kendall-Hunt Publishing, Dubuque, IA, p. 114, with permission.)

working conditions, and specific functions and responsibilities needed to fulfill job responsibilities and is thus a guide for the prospective employee regarding these issues of practice.

The components of the job description are:

- The job identification, which includes the official title, the salary, and the department of operations, if applicable.
- The job summary, which gives an overview of the scope of the job. The who, what, when, where, and why questions regarding the position should be succinctly answered in this summary.
- The functions and principal responsibilities, which should be described precisely. These include such functions as physical assessment, laboratory results reviews, patient education, documentation, student teaching, clinic maintenance, community outreach, staff development, and research.
- The list of skills required, which should describe attributes such as good judgment, good interpersonal skills, and ethical practice.
- The working conditions, which should describe physical or time and space issues, including hours of patient care, on-call requirements, office space, clinic or hospital locations, and potential occupational hazards.
- The education and experience required, which should state the minimum preparation necessary to practice and often the education and experience preferred for the position.
- The reporting relationship, which is the key to the power structure in the job. This section should accurately describe who reports to whom and if anyone reports to the APRN.

The job description will act as the template for the cover letters, résumés, and the interviewing process.

The Cover Letter

The cover letter accompanies a résumé as a request to be considered for a job. It is the first impression one will make on a potential employer. The letter should be addressed to the appropriate person, be clearly written, and have no spelling or grammatical errors. It needs to describe the specific job one is interested in, the time frame of one's availability, and contact information (i.e., a phone number, fax number, e-mail and street address); and it should be written in a professional business style. The proper business format for the cover letter is as follows:

- The applicant's name and address
- The date
- The name and address of the person to whom one is sending the résumé
- The salutation (i.e., "Dear Dr. . . .")
- The opening statement, which gives the reason one is writing and indicates the job of interest
- A brief paragraph stating why one is interested in the specific clinic or healthcare facility
- A closing paragraph, which includes a request for an interview and offers references if desired
- The complimentary closing (i.e., "Sincerely" or another acceptable closing, with a signature and a typed name beneath the signature)
- If the résumé is enclosed, the word "enclosure" at the bottom left side of the letter

Remember, keep copies of all correspondence.

The cover letter is typically only one typewritten page (Fig. 8-3). This brevity requires the writer to consider what is most essential to entice the prospective employer to read the résumé and to communicate that information in a well-written and clear manner. The cover letter should be written individually for each potential position. It should be printed on good-quality bond paper and proofread carefully for any errors in grammar, spelling, and format.

The Résumé

Résumés vary in length and style, but all function to give a detailed outline of one's professional credentials, education, and experience. A résumé should be tailored to meet the needs and requirements of a specific job. Federal government positions generally require very short résumés (one to three pages), but the applications are very detailed. Academic résumés, or curriculum vitae, are typically fairly lengthy. The educational demands of an academic position are supported by previously given lectures, courses, and publications. Therefore, it is essential to list more fully all of these data.

There are two basic types of résumés: the chronological résumé and the outcome or functional résumé. The chronological résumé provides a brief description of one's job history. This type is best suited to those with a stable job history, with no more than one month between jobs. The outcome résumé does not describe the job history, but rather focuses on areas of proficiency and expertise. This type is best suited to APRNs who have changed fields or are reentering the job market.

C. Brenda Penburke, PhD, CNM
4 Yale Street
New Haven, CN 40511
Telephone: 203-455-1267

November 12, 2010

Dr. Lilly Sen
Walrus Woman's Center
4563 Utopia Way
Astoria, Oregon 46042

Dear Dr. Sen:

I am a certified nurse-midwife presently employed at Planned Parenthood of New Haven, Connecticut. I am considering a move to Astoria and am very interested in the position of Advanced Practice Registered Nurse in your family planning clinic.

I have twenty years' experience in all aspects of nurse-midwifery, most particularly in the areas of well-woman gynecology and family planning.

I have enclosed my résumé for your review. Please feel free to contact me if you require additional information or references. I am looking forward to hearing from you.

Sincerely,

C. Brenda Penburke, PhD, CNM

Figure 8-3: An example of a cover letter.

Sharing résumés with others in the nursing profession as part of the networking process may give some perspectives on how to support a job candidacy. In creating a résumé, consider the essential components of the job being sought and present previous employment or education in this light. Be sure that the résumé accurately describes one's skills and does not mislead a potential employer. Have a colleague read the résumé and job description for the position being sought. This peer pal can comment on its accuracy and presentation.

The general components of a résumé include:

- Name
- Address, phone, fax, e-mail address
- Educational background and degrees earned
- Professional employment; other previous employment, if applicable
- Community service
- Research interests
- Grants written
- Publications
- Speaking engagements
- Honors and awards
- Consulting activities
- Professional memberships
- Military history

Demographic data (i.e., age, children, marital status, dates completed school) should be kept out of a résumé to prevent the possibility of being screened out by any of these noncontributing factors.

Résumés are fundamentally an organized written communication of one's skills, education, and experience. To more effectively stress your previous experience, use action words to generate images of a "doer," or a person who takes the initiative to get a job done. Some of these action words are "administered," "assumed responsibility," "supervised," "designed," "handled," "managed," "prepared," and "taught." Consider reviewing specific health career résumé texts or using a professional résumé-writing service to increase the potential power of the document. Writing good résumés is like any other skill that is developed through good modeling and persistent practice. An excellent resource is *Résumés for Health and Medical Careers.*[32]

Consider also the online résumé services, such as Monster.com, which is a free information program that offers help in all aspects of résumé creation and has a specific section just for healthcare résumés.[33] The Monster Résumé Center can be reached by any Internet search engine. In fact, over the past five years, there has been a remarkable increase in Internet job searching and résumé writing sites.[34] Helpful Web sites include those of most professional organizations, which have created their own career centers for résumé building and job listings. One great example is http://www.MidwifeJobs.com, set up by the American College of Nurse Midwives and the Health Career Network. The number of fee-based résumé writing services has also exploded; simply Google job résumés to find them. These services are often career-specific and their cost is contingent on the complexity of the product desired.

The new graduate or the APRN on a budget may prefer to use books rather than the Internet or professional résumé services. One of these is *Résumé and Personal Statements for the Health Professional,* by Dr. James Tysinger, which is particularly relevant to the APRN.[35] This guide offers a step-by-step approach to writing the documents needed for professional job searches and applications.

The Interview

The interview is the active phase of the exchange of information between an APRN and a potential employer. The applicant and the interviewer create a purposeful relationship to discuss the persons involved in, and the expectations of, a specific job. During this process, both parties have an opportunity to gather information to support the correctness of the applicant's "fit" to the position.

Simple cues such as one's attire, manner of speech, body language, demeanor, and timeliness create the first impression. If the applicant is well groomed, comfortable, dressed appropriately in business attire, prepared to answer questions to demonstrate the skills and educational preparation for the job, and has arrived on time, the applicant will appear in a good light. The current trend towards more casual work attire has made some impact on the expectations of suitable dress for an interview. The best advice is to dress in business attire (suits or dresses) that has a professional appearance. Although pants are acceptable for women in most circumstances, leave the jeans and the casual shirts and sweaters at home. Whenever possible, attempt to dress in the manner that is considered the code for the particular office or institution.

Prepare for the interview by finding out as much as possible about the position, the organization, the location, and the actual job requirements. Develop a list of questions to help clarify areas of concern. Review the personal mission statement and ask questions related to issues that enhance job satisfaction (i.e., salaries and benefits, educational support, vacation and holiday time, local professional networks, and personal relationship needs). Consider personal strengths and weaknesses and how personal growth can be achieved in the position. Ask what mutual benefits might be gained from the relationship. Prepare to answer questions about educational background, human relationship skills, communication style, teaching skills, and leadership roles. Do not hesitate to ask for some of this same information from a potential employer. Remember, the goal of the interview is to match people to positions and to other people. What one gives and what one gets are the basis for marketing as a voluntary exchange of goods and services.

Planning for the interview is the key to success. Consider these eight keys to getting a job offer suggested by Dorothy Leeds in *Marketing Yourself*[36]:

1. Be prepared.
2. Be ready to turn negatives into positives.
3. Ask questions to keep control.
4. Listen actively to the content and intent of questions asked.
5. Do not answer any questions not fully understood.
6. Ask for the job.
7. Follow up.
8. Practice enough to be relaxed and comfortable to allow your best self to shine through.[36]

After each interview, the APRN should make a dated summary of the scope of questions, the perceived responses to the answers, and all promised follow-up and write a thank-you note that includes any follow-up information and a clear statement of the desire for the job. An excellent Web site for job interview follow-up and guides for the postinterview thank-you note is http://www.Quintcareers.com.[37] Tips for boosting interviewing success and excellent examples of thank-you notes for all interviewing situations can also be found on the Monster Interview Center. [38]

Andrea Santiago, writing for http://www.About.com, [39] has described the seven deadly sins of job interviewing:

1. Bringing a list of demands prior to having the job offer.
2. Surprising the potential employer with a significant fact regarding your professional or criminal background. This information should be stated ahead of time with a request to discuss its possible implications concerning your being hired.

3. Never play hard to get. Enthusiasm is a more positive marketing tool.

4. Do not dress down for the interview. Suits are still preferred attire for professional jobs. Cover all tattoos and piercings.

5. Do not show up late.

6. If your interview is during a meal and alcohol is served, drink modestly.

7. Watch your language. Do not use inappropriate or offensive words or jokes.

Avoiding these errors will help frame even a nervous applicant's interview responses and help ensure that the applicant does not make a negative impression on the potential employer.

Evaluation of Job Opportunities

When assessing a job offer, it is important to look at three factors:

1. The company
2. The position
3. The salary and benefits package

The Company

Many resources are available for research on companies that may be of interest. Local libraries have business directories that provide detailed information about specific businesses. Included in these directories are the name of the business, names and titles of key personnel, complete address, phone number, number of employees, kind of business, type of location, and number of years in business.

The Position

It is helpful to get a written job description when negotiating for any position. If the job description is available before the interview, it can serve as a useful guide for questions and clarification of the position. If a job description is not available, request that one be written before accepting the position. Minimally, get a definition of what duties will be performed, who will supervise the position, and where the job will be. Find out what orientation or on-the-job training will be provided.

The Salary and Benefits Package

The salary offered or requested should meet or exceed the salary for similar positions in the area. It should be a salary with which one feels comfortable. Beware of salaries that are much higher or much lower than the norm for the area. If the salary is high, this may indicate the job is undesirable for some reason and therefore hard to fill. If the salary is unusually low, this may indicate a lack of financial stability in the company or perhaps an undervaluing of the position by the company. A good benefits package is worth 20% to 40% of the salary. While successful negotiation is crucial to survival and growth in the profession, not many APRNs possess these important skills.

Before beginning contract negotiations, it is important to have a clear goal. Negotiate from strength. Know the product. Know the negotiators, be familiar with the company, and reaffirm the personal mission statement previously devised.

SALARY

Before beginning negotiations, know what salaries are typical for similar positions in the community. If a salary range is discussed, such as $75,000 to $80,000, simply state that $80,000 would be acceptable. It is probably best not to quote a specific figure unless the limits of the salary range for the job are known. The employer might be willing to offer more than is requested. A counteroffer can always be made if the salary quoted is unacceptably low.

BENEFITS

Items to negotiate include:
- Full family medical and dental insurance
- Indemnity plan or managed care
- Acceptable panel of providers
- Point-of-service clause
- Pregnancy coverage
- Prescription plan
- Vision plan
- Orthodontics
- Preexisting conditions clause
- Vacation days
- Paid holidays
- Sick days
- Retirement benefits
- Time required for vesting
- Safety of investments in the pension plan
- Life insurance
- Long-term disability plan
- Optional short-term disability
- Optional long-term care insurance
- Dependent-care reimbursement account
- Healthcare reimbursement account
- Tax-deferred annuities
- Malpractice insurance
- Opportunities for advancement and career development
- Corporate cellular phone rates
- E-mail access
- Tuition waivers
- Continuing education: travel and registration fee
- Professional dues
- Subscriptions to professional journals
- Payment of consulting physician
- Provision of office space, supplies, personnel, and computers
- Payment of answering service and/or pagers

Close of the Deal

Important things to remember in accepting a job and closing the deal is the necessity for a contract or letter of agreement, a confirmation letter, a letter of acceptance, and a noncompete agreement, if one is required.

Contracts

Defining the parameters of the job through formal contracts, letters of agreement, memoranda, or even verbal agreements is a necessity. Employees without written contracts can legally be considered "at-will" employees. At-will employees are those who may be fired without cause at any time. Likewise, an at-will employee can quit at any time. A **contract** is defined as:[19]

- An agreement between two or more parties, especially one that is written and enforceable by law
- The writing or document containing such an agreement

An **employment agreement,** like the one in Figure 8-4, is a type of contract describing an agreement between an employer and an employee that specifies duties and compensation, as well as the rights and responsibilities of each party. Contracts or employment agreements are

---

EMPLOYMENT AGREEMENT

This Employment Agreement ("Agreement"), effective as of_____ (date), by and between _____ (name) of _____ (address), "the Employer," and _____ (name) of _____ (address), "the Employee."

1. EMPLOYMENT. Employee agrees to provide to Employer the services described in attached job description.

2. PAYMENT. The Employer agrees to provide Employee with an annual salary of $_____.

3. MALPRACTICE. The Employer agrees to provide institutional malpractice insurance coverage for any duties performed within the scope of the Employee's job description. The Employee is not covered by this policy for any activities not specified in the job description.

4. VACATION/SICK DAYS. After completing the probationary period of not more than 90 days, each Employee accrues 0.8 sick days/month and 1.5 vacation days/month. Sick days may be accumulated up to 60 days. Vacation days must be used by the Employee's anniversary date each year.

5. CONTINUING EDUCATION. The Employer agrees to provide 7 days and $ _____ annually for continuing education, to be effective after completion of one year of employment.

6. COMMUNICATIONS. The Employer agrees to provide pagers and answering service to the Employee at no cost. Employee is entitled to corporate cellular phone rates (Employee provides cellular phone). Employee will be reimbursed for work-related calls by submitting an annotated monthly voucher.

This Agreement may be terminated for any reason by either party with a 14-day notice during the probationary period. After achieving Permanent Employee status, either party must give at least 30 days' notice prior to termination.

This Agreement is rendered null and void by falsification of information provided during the application process.

_____   _____
Signature of Employee   Signature of Employer

_____
Date

Figure 8-4: An example of an employee agreement.

legally binding documents that spell out the employer's expectations of the employee. Careful analysis of these complex documents can avoid problems in the future. Pay particular attention to any restrictive covenants, bonus formulas, and termination clauses. [40]

If not offered a contract by the prospective employer, one approach is to supply one. This may seem like a formidable task, but there are many sources of assistance—computer software programs, such as Family Lawyer by Quicken, for example.[41] Basic contract forms can also be purchased at many office supply stores. These resources provide a basic framework with which to begin.

Most employment contracts are fairly straightforward. If you are negotiating phased-in compensation or a partial buy-in of a practice, have an attorney review the contract to ensure adequate protection. Contracts typically have similar areas of content. A basic employment contract should include date of agreement, name and address of the employee and employer, specific duties of the agreement, salary and fringe benefits, a termination of employment agreement, and the signatures of both the employer and employee.

Employment Confirmation Letter

The applicant should get the employment offer in writing. If a verbal agreement is offered, request that the employer "clarify the job" in a written memorandum. If no written offer is made, it is advisable to send a letter to confirm the understanding. The letter should include a clause stating that the job will be defined by the letter unless the employer responds in writing.

Letter of Acceptance

A **letter of acceptance** is used by prospective employees to confirm the employee's understanding of the terms and conditions of the employer's offer of employment and to formally accept the offer.

Noncompete Agreement

A **noncompete agreement** is an agreement made by an employee (the noncompeting party) to not leave the current employer (the protected party) and become a competitor in the same market.[41] See Figure 8-5 for an example of a noncompete agreement. Frequently, these agreements

---

NONCOMPETE AGREEMENT

This Agreement ("Agreement"), effective as of_____ (date), by and between _____ (name and address), "the Employer," and _____ (name and address), "the Employee."

For a period of _____ (specify amount of time) after leaving the employment of _____ , the Employee will not directly or indirectly engage in _____ (area of practice) within a _____ (specify a distance or specific geographical area) of _____ (address of employer).

In addition, the Employee agrees not to directly solicit transfer of care of any clients of Employer for a period of _____ (specify amount of time).

_____
Employer (Protected party)

_____
Employee (Noncompeting party)

_____
Date

Figure 8-5: An example of a noncompete agreement.

specify an amount of time (e.g., 3 years) and a geographic area (e.g., within a 5-mile radius of the office of the protected party). In addition, these agreements may include a clause that prevents the noncompeting party from soliciting business (e.g., contacting patients to inform them of the new practice location). It is important to understand the terms of these agreements. Failure to do so may severely impair one's ability to relocate if the job does not work out.

Mentors and Career Advancement

Finally, the APRN should be aware of the role of mentors and issues of career advancement. **Mentoring** is a relationship between a novice and an expert in any given profession in which advice is shared to further a mutual goal of career advancement. This relationship has as its most important functions[42]:

- Preparation for a leadership role
- Promotion of career success and advancement
- Enhancement of self-esteem and self-confidence
- Increased job satisfaction
- Strengthening of the profession

Building a relationship with a mentor requires a strong foundation of similar values, goals, and abilities for successful career advancement. Again, the personal mission statement, discussed earlier, can help in establishing this relationship. Knowing oneself and knowing the character of the mentor become the cornerstones for a successful match.

The characteristics of good mentors consist of a set of behaviors that include guiding, supporting, and teaching as well as good communication skills, good judgment, appropriate use of power, well-honed people skills, an ordered personal life, and a good sense of humor.[43] The novice professional who attracts a good mentor has been shown to possess six major character traits:

1. Good performance
2. Right social background
3. Striking appearance in a suit (either gender)
4. Social affiliation with the mentor
5. Flair for demonstrating the extraordinary
6. High visibility

The best age difference between mentor and protégé is said to be a half generation, or 8 to 15 years. A greater age difference may create a parent-child relationship. Prospective protégés in their late 20s and early 30s generally look for a match with mentors in their 40s.[43] The problem of the gender gap in the work environment particularly affects women's choice of mentors. The gender disparity demands that women choose strong, powerful mentors to help them advance. The alliance with a mentor may help counteract the effect of bias and gender type expectations not experienced by men.[44]

A single role model, or mentor, does not always meet the needs of every novice professional. An alternative to the traditional mentor model is proposed by Haseltine and colleagues.[45] These authors have urged young professionals to actively participate in the creation of their professional identity by choosing advisors and considering multiple role models. The process of career goal attainment can be furthered not just with a single mentor, but with a group of professionals who work at different levels of career advancement. The **patron system** is a continuum of benefactors whose roles are to guide, support, and advocate for the novice. It is composed of **peer pals, guides,** and **sponsors.** The peer pals are people with whom the novice shares information and strategies and, most importantly, who act as sounding boards for new ideas. Guides offer invaluable information about the organizational structure and suggestions for avoiding the wrong people or pathways as well as point out the right people and shortcuts toward a goal. Guides may be a coworker but also may be an administrative-support person, such as a secretary or research assistant. The sponsor is a less powerful figure than the mentor.

Often these three alternatives—peer pals, guides, and sponsors—are more accessible to the novice professional than the mentor and may be available immediately. The perfect mentor relationship may be discovered later during the networking process. The patron system functions on a more horizontal plane than the vertical, hierarchical mentor system. The advantage of the horizontal link is the wider range of contacts for information and career advancement. Always it should be remembered that career advancement and support should be built on mutual trust and a fair exchange of information.

Summary

The APRN should keep focused on his or her personal goals and stay true to a well-thought-out, carefully researched marketing plan. Having a simple philosophy of life can often work wonders in guiding professionals to their dream job. In *The Four Agreements,* Don Miguel Ruiz offers a practical guide to personal freedom. He proposes that one will succeed in life by simply following these rules:

- Be impeccable with your word.
- Don't take anything personally.
- Do not make assumptions.
- Always do your best.[46]

APRNs must abide by their individual code of ethics. They must develop a philosophy that matches their own values and beliefs. The job is an extension of who we are and therefore should reflect one's personal values. Taking the time to develop a personal mission statement may be the hardest and the most beneficial step towards marketing oneself.

The marketing strategies discussed in this chapter allow APRNs to present both themselves and their role in the most effective manner. They also clarify the major points of employment for the employer as well as for the prospective employee, allowing each to make a decision regarding the job based on a foundation of well-defined facts.

SUGGESTED LEARNING EXERCISES

1. A colleague in another discipline claims that APRNs are not particularly cost-effective and that there is no evidence for how clients perceive the quality of care provided by these professionals. Relate the findings from major studies about the cost and quality of advanced practice registered nursing, and outline indicators that have been consistently evaluated to support the quality of advanced practice nursing care.

2. A physician colleague challenges that one of the sources of resistance to APRNs is that they compete with physicians' practices. Give examples of how nurses in advanced practice can substitute or compensate to provide medical care in underserved areas of health care. Recall that "underserved" can have several interpretations, such as insufficient numbers of providers, inadequate insurance systems, poor geographic access, and so on.

3. **Résumé and cover letter:** Identify a hypothetical professional job opportunity for which you would like to apply. In response, write a cover letter and enclose your professional résumé.

4. **Professional practice statement (PPS):** Develop your individual PPS (i.e., job description) for a hypothetical job. This assignment builds on the cover letter and résumé developed in Question 3. The PPS must include clinical, administrative, research, and education

components. Although it will not be necessary to create supporting policy statements or clinical privilege lists, these considerations should help to frame the writing of the PPS.

5. Role-play an interview, including a discussion of salary and benefits. Consider how you can incorporate optimism into your preparation for the job interview and the description of your expected work.

6. What analogies can be made to the characteristics and functions of a mentor? What concerns or cautions are frequently made regarding gender? Evaluate the logic of these assumptions, identify unstated assumptions, and propose solutions or conclusions. Identify the characteristics of a mentor you would choose. How could you introduce the idea of their cooperation in the patron system?

7. Consider your present employment. Create a list of possible peer pals, guides, and sponsors. What made you choose these individuals?

8. Review Harrold's seven rules of success. Look at your résumé and interview notes to see if you have reflected these rules in those documents.

REFERENCES

1. McNeil, NO, and Mackey, TA. (1995). Unpublished material.

2. Woods, DK, and Cardin, S. (June 2002). Realizing your marketing influences. Part 2, Marketing from the inside out. *J Nurs Admin* 32:6.

3. Crandall, R. (2002). *Marketing Your Services: For People Who Hate to Sell.* McGraw-Hill, NY.

4. Covey, SR. (1989). *The Seven Habits of Highly Effective People.* Simon and Schuster, NY.

5. Tri, D. (May 1991). The relationship between primary health care and practitioners' job satisfaction and characteristics of their practice setting. *Nurse Practitioner* 16(5):46–54.

6. Fisher, R, and Brown, S. (1989). *Getting Together: Building Relationships As We Negotiate.* Penguin, NY.

7. Harrold, F. (2008). *The Seven Rules of Success.* Pegasus Books, NY.

8. Seligman, M. (2006). *Learned Optimism.* Vintage Books, NY.

9. Gallagher, SM. (1996). Promoting the nurse practitioner by using a marketing approach. *Nurse Pract* 21:36.

10. McCormack, M. (1984). *What They Don't Teach You at Harvard Business School.* Bantam Books, NY.

11. Berragin, L. (March 1998). Consultancy in nursing and opportunities. *J Clin Nurs* 7(2):139–143.

12. Schweitzer, S. (1991). The relative costs of physicians and new health practitioners. In Record, JC (ed), *Staffing Primary Care in 1990: Physician Replacement and Cost Savings.* Springer, NY.

13. Greenfield, S, et al. (1978). Efficiency and cost of primary care of nurses and physician assistants. *N Engl J Med* 298:305.

14. U.S. Congress, Office of Technology Assessment. (1986). *Nurse Practitioners, Physicians Assistants and Certified Nurse-Midwives: A Policy Analysis.* U.S. Government Printing Office, Washington, DC.

15. Crosby, F, Ventura, MR, and Feldman, MJ. (1987). Future research recommendations for establishing nurse practitioner effectiveness. *Nurse Practitioner* 12:75.

16. Gabay, M, and Wolfe, SM. (1995). *Encouraging the Use of Nurse-Midwives: A Report for Policy Makers.* Public Citizens Publication, Washington, DC.

17. Brown, D. (October 2007). Consumer perspectives on nurse practitioners and independent practice. *J Amer Acad NPs* 19(10):523–529.

18. Green, A, and Davis, S. (April 2005). Toward a predictive model of patient satisfaction with nurse practitioner care. *J Acad NPs* 17(4):139–148.

19. Morris, W, ed. (1981). *The American Heritage Dictionary of the English Language.* Houghton Mifflin, Boston.

20. APRN Joint Dialogue Group. (2008). *Consensus Model for APRN Regulation: Licensure, Accreditation, Certification and Education.* http://www.aacn.nche.edu/. Accessed February 16, 2009.

21. American College of Nurse-Midwives. (1978). *Essential Documents: Definition of a Certified Nurse-Midwife.* Washington, DC.

22. Council on Accreditation of Nurse Anesthesia Education Programs. (1994). *Standards for Accreditation of Nurse Anesthesia Education Programs.* Park Ridge, IL.

23. Boyd, NJ. (1993). The Merit and significance of clinical nurse specialists. *J Nurs Admin* 21:35.

24. Mallison, M. (1993). Nurses as house staff. *Am J Nurs* 93:7.

25. Collins-Fulea, C, ed. (1996). *An Administrative Manual for Nurse-Midwifery Services.* Kendall-Hunt Publishing, Dubuque, IA.

26. Puetz, BE. (1983). *Networking for Nurses.* Aspen Publishers, Rockville, MD.

27. Petras, K. (1989). *The Only Job Hunting Guide You'll Ever Need.* Poseidon Press, NY.

28. Kent, GE. (1991). *How to Get Hired Today!* VGM Career Horizons, Lincolnwood, IL.

29. Casey, R. (1993). *How to Find a Job: Your 30 Day Action Plan.* Thomas Nelson Publishers, Nashville, TN.

30. Crandall, R. (2002). *Marketing Your Services: For People Who Hate to Sell.* McGraw-Hill, NY.

31. Vick, J, and Furlong, J.(2008). *The Academic Job Search Handbook,* 4th ed. University of Pennsylvania Press, Philadelphia, PA.

32. Editors of VGM Horizons. (1996). *Résumés for Health and Medical Careers.* NTC Publishing Group, Lincolnwood, IL.

33. Monster.Com Resume Center. Healthcare Resume Success Story—Multiple Resumes for Multiplied Success. http://resume.monster.com/restips/healthcare/successstory/. Accessed May 12, 2003.

34. Dikel M, and Roehm, F. (2008). *Guide to Internet Job Searching, 2008–2009 Edition.* McGraw-Hill Publishers, NY.

35. Tysinger, J. (2001). *Resumes and Personal Statements for Health Professionals.* Galen Press, NY.

36. Leeds, D. (1991). *Marketing Yourself.* HarperCollins, NY.

37. Bazan, K. (2008). *The Art of Follow-Up After a Job Interview.* QuintCareers.com.

38. Monster.com Interview Center. Ten Tips to Boost Your Interview IQ by Carole Martin. http//interview.monster.com/articles/challenge/. Accessed February 16, 2009.

39. Santiago, A. (2008). The Seven Deadly Sins of Job Interviews—Top Seven Things Not To Do On An Interview. Available at http://www.About.com.

40. Buppert, C. (August 1997). Employment agreements: clauses that can change an NP's life. *Nurse Practitioner* 22(8):108–119.

41. Parsons Technology. (1995). *Quicken: Family Lawyer.* Intuit, Hiawatha, IA.

42. Vance, C. (1989). Is there a mentor in your future? *Imprint* 36(5):41.

43. Alleman, E, et al. (1984). Enriching mentor relationships. *Personal Guide Journal* 62:329.

44. Babcock,L, and Laschever, S. (2007). *Women Don't Ask.* Bantam Books, NY.

45. Haseltine, DP, Rowe, MP, and Shapiro, EC. (1978). Moving up: Role models, mentors and the patron system. *Sloan Management Review* 19:51.

46. Ruiz, Don Miguel. (1997). *The Four Agreements.* Amber-Allen Publishing Co., San Rafael, CA.

Deirdre K. Thornlow received her master's degree in cardiopulmonary nursing from the University of California-Los Angeles, and her PhD in nursing from the University of Virginia. Dr. Thornlow's experience as an advanced practice nurse includes the roles of cardiovascular clinical nurse specialist in the United States and integrated care pathway coordinator in the United Kingdom. Dr. Thornlow has held numerous quality management positions throughout her career, including Assistant Vice President, Quality Management for Carolinas Healthcare System and Director of Quality Operations at The George Washington University Hospital. She served as gerontology program director for the American Association of Colleges of Nursing (AACN) and is currently an assistant professor of nursing at Duke University where she teaches in the master's and doctoral nursing programs. Her health services research interests include acute care quality and patient safety.

CHAPTER 9

Advanced Practice Nursing: Inquiry and Evaluation

Deirdre K. Thornlow, PhD, RN, CPHQ

CHAPTER OUTLINE

PRACTICE-BASED EVIDENCE
Evaluating practice and outcomes of care to improve quality and patient safety
Leading data-driven improvement efforts

EVIDENCE-BASED PRACTICE
Ensuring practice is based on evidence
Translating evidence into practice

PRACTICE INQUIRY
Engaging in practice inquiry
Research–practice exchange
Practice-based research networks

APRN INQUIRY AND EVALUATION COMPETENCIES
Practice-based evidence competencies
Evidence-based practice competencies
Practice inquiry competencies

SUMMARY

SUGGESTED LEARNING EXERCISES

CHAPTER OBJECTIVES

After completing this chapter, the reader will be able to:

1. Delineate strategies for one's own advanced practice registered nurse (APRN) role that enhance practice inquiry and evaluation and relate these to other topics in this text, such as critical thinking, change and leadership, and excellence in practice.

2. Compare and contrast the role of the APRN in evaluating practice-based evidence and facilitating evidence-based practice.

3. Analyze the impact of the "research–practice gap" on clinical care and outline strategies APRNs can use to narrow the gap.

From the time of Hippocrates, the dictum "First, do no harm" has prodded healthcare providers to deliver safe patient care. The 1999 Institute of Medicine (IOM) report *To Err is Human: Building a Safer Health System* brought to light how far the American healthcare system had strayed from this edict.[1] More recent reports indicate that significant progress toward transformational improvement in quality and patient safety is still necessary.[2,3] Despite spending nearly $2 trillion annually on healthcare services, American adults receive just half of recommended care for the leading causes of death and disability.[4] Similar findings have been reported for children, who receive recommended care only 46% of the time,[5] and the odds are even slimmer for older adults, with approximately only one-third of recommended care delivered for a subset of geriatric conditions such as dementia, falls, and urinary incontinence.[6,7] Real progress toward superior healthcare quality requires a more rapid translation of evidence into practice and a far greater emphasis on quality outcomes.

Advanced practice registered nurses (APRNs) are well poised to lead this transformation by engaging in more robust practice inquiry and evaluation. Schooled in the principles of research at the master's and doctoral levels,[8,9] APRNs use research methods and the scientific process every day to evaluate patient outcomes and responses to treatments, to solve problems, to make clinical decisions, and to answer questions regarding clinical practice and care delivery. Knowledge of research enables APRNs to read critically, to evaluate published research, and to function as agents of change in planning, implementing, and sustaining innovation in practice. As such, APRNs are often viewed as leaders who can facilitate the implementation of evidence-based practice into the culture of an organization.[10]

Practice inquiry and evaluation comprise integral components of the advanced practice roles and not only serve to narrow the gap between research and practice but also enable continued improvement in the quality and safety of patient care. The purpose of this chapter is to describe the role of the APRN in evaluating practice-based evidence, facilitating evidence-based practice, and engaging in collaborative practice inquiry. Necessary competencies for success in these APRN roles are outlined.

Practice-Based Evidence

The scientific orientation of clinical nursing practice was formed by Florence Nightingale, who instructed nurses to use objective, sound observations, not just as information or interesting facts, but to save lives and to increase the comfort and safety of those for whom they cared. As far back as the 1860s, this mandate heralded the need to methodically relate interventions to desired improvement in outcomes. Her use of the scientific approach to practice led Nightingale to describe the profession as the "science of nursing."[11]

Evaluation of nursing care processes and patient outcomes remains an integral component of advanced practice nursing. Advanced practice nursing is the application of an expanded range of practical, theoretical, and research-based competencies to phenomena experienced by patients within a specialized clinical area of the larger discipline of nursing. It is defined by three primary criteria: graduate education, certification, and practice focused on patients and families. While direct clinical practice remains the central competency, research skills, including the use and implementation of evidence-based practice, comprise a core competency.[12] Lately, process and outcome evaluation has garnered significant national attention, with regulatory and accrediting agencies incorporating quality measurement into their expectations.

APRNs are well positioned to evaluate practice and clinical outcomes, to benchmark and identify best practices, and to lead data-driven improvement efforts designed to improve quality and patient safety. APRNs often serve as the link between the patient and care evaluation and between research and practice. Statements by the National Organization of Nurse Practitioner Faculties (NONPF) and the American Association of Colleges of Nursing (AACN) contend that nurse practitioners (NPs) should "practice continuous quality improvement based on professional practice standards and relevant statutes and regulation."[13]

The AACN master's essentials[8] require competency in evaluating practices and programs, and these competencies are further expanded in the doctorate of nursing practice (DNP) essentials.[9]

Evaluating Practice and Outcomes of Care to Improve Quality and Patient Safety

Patients, providers, insurers, regulators, and purchasers continue to demand improvements in healthcare quality and safety. This push appears justified, as research demonstrates that the majority of medical errors, or adverse events, are preventable[14,15] and hospitalized patients who experience a medical error remain hospitalized longer and accrue greater costs when compared to controls.[16,17]

Tired of reimbursing for poor-quality care for its covered patients, the Centers for Medicare and Medicaid Services (CMS) joined the Hospital Quality Alliance (HQA) in a public-private collaboration designed to improve the quality of care provided by the nation's hospitals by measuring and publicly reporting that care. The goal of the Alliance program is to identify a robust set of standardized and easy-to-understand hospital quality measures that would be used by all stakeholders in the healthcare system to improve quality of care and that would enable consumers to make informed healthcare choices. The "Hospital Compare" website provides a mechanism for publicly reporting information about the quality of care delivered in hospitals in the United States (http://www.hospitalcompare.hhs.gov). As further testimony to their desire to reward only good-quality care and safety, in October 2008 the CMS eliminated payments for hospital-acquired infections and other "never events," defined as preventable adverse events that should never occur in health care.[18] Healthcare entities other than hospitals face tough scrutiny as well in terms of regulation and quality oversight. Web sites similar to the CMS Web site house comparative data for public viewing for nursing homes (http://www.medicare.gov/NHCompare) and home healthcare agencies (http://www.medicare.gov/HHCompare/Home). Additionally, the National Committee for Quality Assurance (NCQA) has developed the Healthcare Effectiveness Data and Information Set (HEDIS), a tool used by more than 90% of America's health plans to measure performance on important dimensions of care and service.[19]

The intent of quality measurement, and most specifically public reporting of quality measures, is to increase transparency and support value-based purchasing. Value-based purchasing posits three major goals[18]:

- Cost avoidance—avoiding paying for care that does not work
- Cost reduction—reducing unnecessary variation in delivery of care
- Cost benefit—implementing care that improves outcomes and reduces morbidity and complications

The evidence regarding the effectiveness of public reporting is mixed, yet early studies indicated that states that had public reporting systems experienced more rapid declines in cardiac surgery mortality than those states without public reporting.[20,21] One dramatic example was reported by Chassin,[22] who found that deaths from cardiac surgery fell 41% over the first four years of New York's reporting program. Public reporting is here to stay and expanded reporting, including the incorporation of new measures, will continue. Public reporting of core measures promotes benchmarking, evidence-based practice, and the search for best practices. The intent is to increase transparency, recognize top performers, and reward good performance for integrating evidence-based process measures into practice. Future initiatives are on tap, including denying reimbursement for "never events" and incorporating nurse-sensitive measures into mandatory hospital reporting.

The Patient Safety and Quality Improvement Act of 2005 required the U.S. Department of Health and Human Services (DHHS) to facilitate the creation of a network of databases to collect, aggregate, and analyze submitted reports of medical errors or near errors and to adopt standard formats for reporting information to the databases. These databases were also to make public the analysis of regional and national statistics and trends via annual reports from Patient Safety Organizations (PSOs), private entities recognized by DHHS to collect and analyze patient safety events reported by healthcare providers. Administered by the Agency for Healthcare Research and Quality (AHRQ), PSOs are new and separate from all currently existing entities addressing healthcare quality.[23] PSOs makes patient safety reporting privileged and confidential and are designed to motivate providers to dedicate more resources toward the delivery of safe patient care.

Proposed regulations provide a framework for PSOs to facilitate a shared-learning approach that supports effective interventions that reduce the risk of harm to patients. Such efforts align with the central tenet of patient safety, which is conceptualized as the avoidance, prevention, and amelioration of adverse outcomes or injuries stemming from the processes of health care.[24] The National Patient Safety Foundation (NPSF) defines patient safety as "the prevention of healthcare errors, and the elimination or mitigation of patient injury caused by healthcare errors" (http://www.npsf.org/au). A goal of patient safety, therefore, is to reduce the risk of injury or harm to patients from the structures or processes of care.[25] APRNs play a critical role in evaluating the safety and quality of patient care and implementing evidence-based practices designed to prevent harm and improve care to patients.

Leading Data-Driven Improvement Efforts

Quality is defined by the IOM[26] as "the degree to which healthcare services for individuals and populations increase the probability of desired health outcomes and is consistent with current professional knowledge of best practice." The IOM aims for improvement in safety, timeliness, effectiveness, efficiency, equitableness, and patient-centeredness. APRNs can provide the expertise needed to identify and lead quality and performance improvement initiatives[27] that are centered on these aims through performance improvement (PI), which is defined as a practice in which individuals work together to improve systems and processes with the intent of improving outcomes for a specific population or in a specific setting.[28] PI is achieved through interventions that target providers, practitioners, plans, and/or patients. CMS defines a PI project as a "set of related activities designed to achieve measurable improvement in processes and outcomes of care" whose intended process must at least be as safe as routine care, thus requiring good clinical management and routine internal oversight.[29,30]

CONCEPTUAL MODELS FOR EVALUATING QUALITY AND OUTCOMES RESEARCH

Conceptual models provide an overarching framework to guide APRNs in performance improvement efforts. The Quality Health Outcomes Model (QHOM)[31] is one such framework; it builds on Donabedian's[32] landmark work in assessing care quality. In 1998, the Expert Panel on Quality Health Care of the American Academy of Nursing (AAN) published the QHOM as a conceptual framework for quality and outcomes research, most specifically as a means to test relationships among the elements of structure, process, and outcomes. The QHOM takes those elements from Donabedian's seminal work in assessing the quality of care and further realigns the constructs to capture the dynamic relationships between those three elements and the patient's own characteristics. The QHOM posits reciprocal, rather than linear, interactions among the four constructs, thus serving as a useful conceptual guide for healthcare systems researchers.[33]

Several investigators have used the QHOM model in acute and community care to organize their choice of variables among the four constructs and to build evidence regarding the quality of health care. Mayberry and Gennarro[34] applied the model to a review of second-stage labor in obstetric care and reported that interventions such as cesarean delivery and epidural analgesia differed in their quality outcomes depending on system and client characteristics. Radwin and Fawcett[35] retrospectively used the model to frame their work in identifying components of several aspects of patient characteristics, interventions, and systems of care of oncology patients. More recently, the model was used to evaluate a community-based exercise program for elderly Korean immigrants.[36] In these studies, the QHOM served as a conceptual guide for research and provided a useful method for advancing outcomes research and evidence about the quality of health care.

PRACTICAL IMPLEMENTATION OF PERFORMANCE IMPROVEMENT

While conceptual frameworks guide research development and the empirical evaluation of quality, practical implementation of performance improvement (PI) centers on the PI process. This process includes:

1. Identifying the problem
2. Selecting a team to assist with improvement efforts
3. Choosing the appropriate QI method for the improvement goal
4. Applying PI tools to clarify understanding of the problem and understand any variation in process (e.g., flow charting, histograms)
5. Implementing proposed improvement solutions
6. Evaluating and sustaining the improvement gains

Problem Identification and Prioritization

APRNs have a variety of data sources they can use to identify and prioritize opportunities for improvement. Internal data sources include organizational- and unit-level performance improvement data such as quality scorecards and risk management data, including adverse event and incident reports.

Typically, PI efforts focus on problems that are high volume, high risk, high cost, or problem-prone. Addressing high-volume procedures or high-volume patient populations ensures that efforts focus on a majority of patients. APRNs may also choose to concentrate on procedures that are high risk or that carry a high mortality or liability risk when not done properly. Problem-prone implies that repeated incidents of similar types of injuries or harm require attention. For example, an APRN may be charged with finding a better way to manage the risk of falls in older postoperative patients. Certainly, high cost and/or resource-intensive procedures may necessitate review and improvement. Regardless of whether issues are high volume, high risk, high cost, problem-prone, or some combination, APRNs should ensure that areas identified for improvement strategically align with system-wide priorities. Aligning quality and administrative strategic initiatives into one overarching strategy increases the likelihood for success.

Benchmarking

Benchmarking comprises a key component of data-driven performance improvement efforts and facilitates identification of opportunities for improvement. Xerox made "benchmarking" a household term in the 1990s when it used this method to transform its business and profit strategy. Benchmarking in health care is most commonly defined as setting, seeking, and attaining an ideal target, or gold standard, that has been achieved by a group or organization known for its quality of services.[37] Both internal and external comparisons are necessary in benchmarking, using key metrics that are measurable and relevant. Identifying best in class through outcomes comparisons with peer organizations should comprise 10% to 25% of the benchmarking effort, and 75% to 90% of the effort should go toward understanding the process that produced the best-in-the-class performance. APRNs might ask, "How did that particular hospital or clinic achieve top decile performance? What are they doing right, that we need to be doing?" Choosing organizations to be benchmarked against is a critical decision and care must be taken to avoid selection bias. APRNs must be sure that patient characteristics such as age, comorbidities, and severity of illness and organizational characteristics, such as case mix index, are risk-adjusted, increasing the likelihood that peer-to-peer comparisons are accurate.

Several sources for benchmarked data exist, including the American Nurses Association (ANA) National Database of Nursing Quality Indicators (NDNQI) (http://www.nursingquality.org/); the Hospital Quality Alliance, as outlined above; the Universal HealthSystem Consortium (http://www.uhc.edu/); and the AHRQ, whose Healthcare Cost & Utilization Project network (HCUPnet) provides access to health statistics and information on hospital inpatient and emergency department utilization via its online query system (http://hcupnet.ahrq.gov/). Specialty organizations, such as the Vermont-Oxford Network (http://www.vtoxford.org/), with databases devoted to specific populations also provide excellent benchmarking venues.

Choosing Pertinent Indicators

Indicators are valid and reliable quantitative measures of structure, process, and outcome that are related to one or more dimensions of performance.[38] Most quality improvement leaders struggle to find a balance between measures that are scientifically sound and those that are feasible to implement with limited resources.[39]

Selected indicators used to gauge performance should consist of a balance of structure, process, and outcome measures. Structural measures focus on the internal characteristics of an organization and its personnel by addressing the infrastructure needed to support quality of care and delivery of services.[38] Human, organizational, and physical resources are examples of structure standards and may include such indicators as staffing levels of registered nurses (RNs), percent of nurses certified in a specialty, and presence of intensivists in critical care units. Process measures focus on whether activities within an organization are being conducted appropriately, effectively, and efficiently; they generally focus on the behaviors, activities, interventions, and the sequence, or work flow, of caregiving events.[38] Completion of nursing assessment within 24 hours, timely administration of antibiotics to patients with pneumonia, and provision of smoking-cessation counseling are examples of process indicators.

Quality of care is a dimension of the process of care, not an outcome. Outcomes are assessed to provide an indication of the level of quality achieved during the care delivery process. Outcome measures focus on the resultant effect on patients and/or organizations[37] or a change in the current or future health status attributed to antecedent health care and client attributes of care. Basically, outcome indicators measure the effectiveness of interventions or the effectiveness of care.[38] Misusing "process as outcome indicators," such as identifying "accuracy in nursing documentation" as an outcome indicator is incorrect; documentation is a process that centers on the care provider, not the care recipient.

Although process indicators should be collected, they are not acceptable outcomes by themselves and should be related to outcomes at the patient or organizational level.[37] Outcomes evaluation, therefore, is defined as the evaluation of the observed results of some action or intervention for recipients of services. Outcome assessments provide the data needed to support or refute the perceived beneficial effect of some clinical decision, care delivery process, or targeted action. Outcomes measurement involves the identification of reliable and valid outcome measures; the selection of appropriate measurement methods; and attention to the timing of data collection, analysis, and reporting.[37]

Morbidity and mortality have historically been used as outcome measures. In selecting patient safety outcome measures, experts contend that an adverse event must be deemed "preventable" and the measures must be clinically meaningful.[40] Other outcome indicators include clinical endpoints such as physical or mental health status, functional status, and perception and satisfaction with care. Currently, these and similar evidence-based indicators are the focus of Joint Commission (JC) and CMS regulatory requirements. APRNs are well positioned to influence the performance of interdisciplinary teams to meet performance indicators.[37]

To address the need for standardized patient safety outcome measures, the AHRQ developed criteria for comparing risk-adjusted hospital rates for several types of preventable adverse events based on administrative data, especially data used in conjunction with the

Healthcare Cost and Utilization Project (HCUP). These patient safety indicators (PSIs) consist of 20 hospital-based indicators for medical conditions and surgical procedures that have been shown to have adverse event rates that vary substantially among institutions and that evidence suggests may be associated with deficiencies in the provision of care (http://www.qualityindicators.ahrq.gov/psi_overview.htm). In essence, the 20 accepted PSIs are a selective list of potential safety-related events that are deemed amenable to detection using administrative data, have been adequately coded in previous studies, and are sensitive to the quality of care.[41] Generally, these and other AHRQ Quality Indicators (QIs) are measures of healthcare quality that make use of readily available hospital inpatient administrative data to highlight potential quality concerns, identify areas that need further study and investigation, and track changes over time.

In addition to the PSIs, the AHRQ QIs consist of other modules measuring various aspects of quality:

- Prevention indicators, which identify hospital admissions that evidence suggests could have been avoided, at least in part, through high-quality outpatient care
- The inpatient QIs, which reflect quality of care inside hospitals, including inpatient mortality for medical conditions and surgical procedures
- The pediatric QIs, which reflect quality of care inside hospitals and identify potentially avoidable hospitalizations among children (http://www.qualityindicators.ahrq.gov)

An additional source for quality measures includes the National Quality Measures Clearinghouse, also sponsored by AHRQ, a public repository for evidence-based quality measures and measure sets (http://www.qualitymeasures.ahrq.gov/).

Nursing-Sensitive Indicators

APRNs should ensure that "nursing-sensitive" measures are included in unit and organizational performance improvement programs. Patients are hospitalized because they require nursing care, and evidence strongly suggests that focusing on nursing would improve patient safety.[42] Maas and colleagues[43] coined the phrase "nursing-sensitive" to reflect patient outcomes that are affected by nursing practice. The National Quality Forum (NQF), a private, not-for-profit group that was created to develop and implement a national strategy for healthcare quality measurement and reporting, established 15 nursing-sensitive performance measures that provide a framework for measuring the quality of nursing care.[44] In its own effort to develop national data on the relationship between nurse staffing and patient outcomes, the ANA also designed nursing-sensitive indicators, known as the National Database of Nursing Quality Indicators (NDNQI).[45]

At about the same time, the AHRQ developed the Patient Safety Indicators (PSI) to identify potentially preventable adverse events, such as central line infections, postoperative complications, and even death. Certain PSIs have been linked with nursing care. Examples of "nursing-sensitive" patient outcomes include pressure ulcers and failure to rescue, or failing to rescue a patient from complications such as cardiac arrest or shock. Savitz, Jones, and Bernard[46] compared and contrasted relevant AHRQ PSIs with the NQF and ANA indicators and found that only two of the indicators overlapped: failure to rescue and development of decubitus ulcer. An additional patient safety indicator, infections due to medical care, also overlaps with the NQF indicators.

As noted earlier, CMS has eliminated reimbursement for eight preventable hospital-acquired conditions, four of which are designated as nursing-sensitive: pressure ulcers; preventable injuries such as fractures, dislocations, and burns; catheter-associated urinary tract infections (UTI); and vascular catheter-associated infections. CMS has since released a proposed list of 43 new quality measures hospitals will need to report publicly in fiscal year 2009 to receive their full Medicare payment update. Once again, nurse-sensitive measures, including failure to rescue, pressure ulcer prevalence, patient falls, and patient falls with injury, are on the list.

Detecting and validating additional quality and patient safety outcomes that are sensitive to nursing care is crucial, as nurses represent the largest component of the healthcare workforce.[46] This link between performance and reimbursement enhances the focus on nurses' role in shaping patient outcomes. Although nurse staffing levels and skill mix have been associated with several preventable, hospital-acquired complications, including pressure ulcers, falls, UTIs, and catheter-related infections,[47–49] there was no mechanism for measuring nurses' economic contribution to hospitals prior to these CMS regulatory and reimbursement changes.[50] With additional incentives (reimbursement) designed to reduce preventable adverse events, hospitals will be under enormous pressure to determine the prevalence of these events and engage in initiatives to reduce and eliminate them. APRNs should harness this increased national scrutiny to heighten awareness of nurses' contributions to patient care. They should educate nursing staff regarding the ramifications of the reimbursement changes, the importance of accurate assessment and documentation of conditions present on admission,[50] and the importance of using data to identify opportunities for further improvement.

In sum, APRNs should select nursing measures that address inadequacies in the structure, process, and outcomes of care and should foster improvements and the capacity for improvements.[40] When selecting appropriate measures, APRNs should consider not only the reliability and validity of an indicator but also its relevance, clinical significance, and importance and base the selection on a review of the literature. The methods of data collection chosen should be feasible and result in both timely and accurate data retrieval. So too, analysis should be meaningful and interpretable; in other words, did any attempts at process change result in an improvement? Indictor types can range from proportion measures (e.g., mortality rates, readmission rates), to ratio measures (e.g., falls per 1000 patient days), to continuous measures (e.g., median time to initial antibiotic administration, average length of stay). Various levels of data, from the patient and provider level to the organization or system level, as well as the population level, should be included to ensure a comprehensive cross-mix. Additionally, APRNs should consider using standardized measures that allow benchmarked comparisons within, between, and among healthcare organizations. Once opportunities for improvement are identified and indicators selected to measure improvement, the next steps include selecting a team to assist with the improvement efforts and continuing the PI process.

SELECTING A TEAM TO ASSIST WITH THE IMPROVEMENT EFFORTS

A team is responsible for the development, implementation, and evaluation of efforts to improve performance. To succeed, the knowledge, skills, abilities, and perspectives of a wide range of disciplines must be brought together. The team or group may be an existing committee, such as the quality improvement committee or practice council; however, a task force may be the more common approach, in which a group is appointed to address a specific performance issue.[51] The composition of the team is directed by the problem selected and should include interested stakeholders. For example, a team working on pain management in older adults should be interdisciplinary and include pharmacists, nurses, physicians, and geriatricians. In contrast, a team working on ventilator-associated pneumonia might include nurses, a pulmonologist or critical care intensivist, and a respiratory therapist. Including persons in leadership positions, especially those who control finances, ensures that the team's objectives align with strategic priorities and are resourced appropriately.

Currently, hospitals face growing tensions and trade-offs when allocating nurses to the competing priorities of direct patient care or quality improvement activities. According to a study sponsored by the Center for Studying Health System Change (HSC), Draper, Felland, Liebhaber, and Melichar[52] found that hospital organizational cultures set the stage for quality improvement, including nurses' involvement. Hospitals with supportive leadership, a philosophy that quality is everyone's job, individual accountability, physician and nurse champions, and effective feedback spurred greater involvement by nurses. But even when hospitals are committed to including nurses in quality improvement, they often face various problems, including a shortage of nurses; growing demands to participate in more, often duplicative, QI activities; the burdensome nature of data collection and reporting; and the shortcomings of traditional nursing education in preparing nurses for their evolving role in today's contemporary hospital setting.[52]

Not surprisingly, hospital administrators want their best nurses at the bedside, yet these same nurses should be engaged in quality improvement efforts so that their keen observations of problems at the bedside can be transformed into effective improvement efforts for populations of patients. APRNs, with their institutional and organizational insight, possess the power to persuade administrative leaders that engaging nurses in quality improvement not only is ethically sensible but also economically savvy, given the increased national scrutiny of quality and patient safety in reimbursement models.

CHOOSING THE APPROPRIATE IMPROVEMENT METHOD AND APPLYING PI TOOLS

Choosing the appropriate PI method or model depends on the ultimate aim of the improvement project. Several models exist, including Plan-Do-Study-Act (PDSA), Six Sigma, and Lean methodologies. In a nutshell, PDSA emphasizes rapid process improvement by using small tests of improvements. Six Sigma methodology, which gained national attention in the 1980s when used by Motorola, emphasizes process, methodology, and data, with the goal of reducing defects to less than 3.4 per million, or achieving near "six sigma" perfection. Lean methodology focuses on speed, efficiency and removing waste or non-value-added activities and has as its central aim cost reduction.[53] Many healthcare organizations use a combination of methods to achieve their quality improvement goals. Regardless of the methodology chosen, all QI models basically incorporate the same essential steps.

Standardization is the first step in ensuring quality improvement. Reducing variation is critical in managing quality and enables processes to be linked to outcomes, with the ultimate aim of producing high-reliability care. Variation is present in all processes; the key is to identify and understand the causes of the variation, which may include personnel, equipment, procedures, and/or the environment. To begin, it is necessary to clarify current understanding of processes and to measure and trend the processes over time to determine whether control exists. Statistical Process Control (SPC) Charts are an excellent way to map data trends and are considered the core of any improvement program because they provide meaningful data with which to assess the current situation and measure the effectiveness of ongoing improvement activities. A full discussion of the variety of performance improvement tools used in efforts to improve quality and safety is beyond the scope of this chapter. Readers are directed to key sources for such information, including, but not limited to, the American Society for Quality (ASQ) (http://www.asq.org/); the Institute for Healthcare Improvement (IHI) (http://www.ihi.org/ihi); and the National Association for Healthcare Quality (NAHQ) (http://www.nahq.org/).

IMPLEMENTING A PROPOSED IMPROVEMENT SOLUTION, EVALUATING THE CHANGE, AND SUSTAINING IMPROVEMENT GAINS

PI teams should select feasible, practical, cost-effective, and measurable improvement solutions. As noted earlier, APRNs should identify best practices and exemplars from other organizations and/or healthcare providers and ensure that any proposed change represents an evidence-based intervention. In their role as agents of change, APRNs have the key role of anticipating barriers as well as facilitators to implementation. Overcoming resistance to change requires enormous fortitude, as is so well expressed in the quip "Change would be easy if it were not for all the people."

As mentioned, APRNs can use the increased national scrutiny and visibility of quality to make nurses' contribution to patient care more visible as well.[50] As leaders of quality improvement initiatives, APRNs have the unique opportunity to facilitate data analyses, provide surveillance and early diagnosis and treatment, and educate nursing staff regarding the importance of PI activities. And APRNs can use their advanced communication and leadership skills to direct quality improvement and patient safety initiatives. Data analyses and care evaluation will serve to demonstrate nurses' contribution to healthcare quality and patient safety.

Evidence-Based Practice

The literature has repeatedly confirmed that research findings with important implications for care are not widely used in clinical settings, despite clear evidence that such findings would improve patient care.[4–7] That is to say, a gap exists between research and practice. Although the fundamental reason for conducting nursing research is to develop a body of knowledge relative to practice, research has little value unless it is applied. Titler and Goode[54] suggested that "the conduct of research is essentially unfinished unless the findings are synthesized and applied in practice to improve patient outcomes" (p. xv). A key responsibility of APRNs is to help close the research gap by implementing research findings in practice settings.[55] Again, according to Titler and Goode,[54]

> Advanced practice nurses must embrace the pivotal leadership role they play in the synthesis and implementation of research findings. Staff nurses are essential in making the practice changes a reality at the bedside....Nursing administrators at all levels of the organization must create practice environments that support and reward use of research. (p. xv)

In addition to regulatory mandates and the Magnet certification of the American Nurses Credentialing Center (ANCC), which stipulates that nurses engage in research and evidence-based practice, a business case exists for evidence-based practice (EBP). Failure to follow best practices for two conditions (acute myocardial infarction [MI] and stroke) is the cause of more than $1.5 billion in preventable hospitalizations, or avoidable costs, per year. Jha and colleagues[56] demonstrated that following evidence-based practices was associated with lower risk-adjusted mortality for each of three conditions (MI, congestive heart failure, and pneumonia) in the national HQA program and that higher condition-specific performance on the HQA measures was associated with lower mortality rates.

As a result of such astonishing figures, organizations and investigators alike are searching for ways to improve the delivery and safety of patient care and striving to embed improved processes and patient safety practices into health care. The Evidence-Based Practice Center defines a *patient safety practice* as a type of process whose application reduces the probability of an adverse event. Evidence for the incorporation of various safety practices, including incident reporting, root cause analysis, and the promise of promoting a "culture of safety," comes from domains other than medicine or nursing. Although incorporating safety practices has been a long-standing success in fields such as commercial aviation, nuclear power, and aerospace, it has not been supported in the healthcare literature, which provides only a weak evidentiary base for the success of many safety practices.[57] When evidence does exist, organizations have attempted to translate it into practice. For example, in 2002, the National Quality Foundation (NQF) published a list of 30 evidence-based practices deemed ready for implementation, and the Joint Commission has since required at least 10 of these practices be implemented in its accredited hospitals.[58] APRNs possess the requisite skills to facilitate translation of these evidence-based interventions into practice.

Ensuring Practice Is Based on Evidence

Research utilization is a subset of EBP that focuses on the application of research findings, or the use of research findings, in any and all aspects of one's work as an RN.[59] Research utilization usually implies reading a primary research study, critiquing the soundness of its methods, and applying credible findings to nursing practice. Clinical nurse specialists (CNSs) have been engaged in research utilization since the 1970s and have led institutional efforts toward research-based practice.[60] The collaboration between nurse clinicians and nurse researchers in research utilization led to the development of the Conduct and Utilization of Research in Nursing (CURN) model. Developed in the late 1970s, the CURN model delineated six phases to achieve the goal of putting research knowledge into nursing practice.[60] The six phases are:

1. Creating an atmosphere for change by identifying specific patient-care problems
2. Evaluating current scientific knowledge of the clinical problem, institutional policies, and potential costs
3. Determining the fit of the nursing practice innovation
4. Carrying out clinical trials
5. Deciding to accept, reject, or change the innovation
6. Disseminating the innovation to other nursing practice units

RELATIONSHIP BETWEEN RESEARCH UTILIZATION AND EBP

While the terms "research utilization" and "evidence-based practice" are related, and sometimes used interchangeably, they are conceptualized differently.[59,61] EBP is more comprehensive, signaling a more systematic, rigorous, and precise way of translating research findings into practice.[62] EBP first appeared in the healthcare literature in the 1980s and referred to the practice of medicine by physicians. The concept was defined as the use of evidence from timely literature and research to guide physicians in making the best patient care decisions, at the best cost, to obtain the best outcomes.[63]

Adoption of EBP by nursing paralleled the evolution of the ANCC Magnet Recognition program in the early 1990s. EBP entails the integration of the best research evidence with clinical expertise and patient values.[64] In nursing, best research evidence refers to methodologically sound and clinically relevant research about the effectiveness and safety of nursing interventions. This research may involve randomized controlled trials, observational studies, or qualitative research. When there is enough research evidence available, it is recommended that the evidence for practice be based on the research. In some cases, a sufficient research base may not be available, and the healthcare provider may need to supplement research findings with other types of evidence, such as expert opinion and case reports. As more research is done in a specific area, the research evidence can be updated.[61]

Clinicians further support scientific research with their clinical expertise and the patient's input. Clinical expertise refers to a clinician's ability to use clinical skills and past experience to identify the health status of patients or populations, their risks, their preferences and actions, and the potential benefits of interventions. Patient and family preferences need to be considered in clinical decision making, and evidence-based clinical decisions should incorporate the patient's clinical state, the clinical setting, and the clinical circumstances.[64, 65] For example, a patient's age or severity of illness will influence the response to an intervention, and the availability of a caregiver may influence the feasibility of delivering a particular therapy; these should be factored into the decision-making process.

Since the 1990s, EBP has been advanced as a strategy to link best scientific findings, clinical judgments, clinical expertise, and clinical reasoning skills with the patient's unique characteristics.[65] Pravikoff and Donaldson[66] report that EBP should result in consistent, up-to-date nursing practice and the most effective patient outcomes. EBP can be undertaken from an individual and/or organizational perspective. Specifically, an NP can read and synthesize research, seek the expert opinions of others, and then use the information in practice. Similarly, an institution or healthcare system can make an organizational commitment to incorporate evidence into practice, resulting in clinical policies and procedures that are evidence-based.[54] APRNs have the educational background, clinical expertise, and critical thinking skills to lead the discovery of and incorporation of EBP into prevention and treatment settings. Doing so requires use of the EBP process, which includes[65-67]:

1. Developing and formulating a clear, precise, clinical question to answer
2. Conducting an efficient search of the literature
3. Critically appraising the evidence
4. Synthesizing the evidence
5. Determining the applicability of the evidence to practice
6. Implementing the evidence in practice
7. Evaluating outcomes and results of the implementation of EBP

Several models developed to guide the EBP process offer frameworks for understanding the process and for designing and implementing EBP projects in clinical settings.[67] Although each model offers different perspectives, the process is similar across models. For example, the Iowa Model of Research in Practice[68] takes an institution-focused perspective; other models offer a more broad-based approach, like the ACE-Star Model,[69] which includes a simple pictorial representation to organize and understand relationships between the various EBP stages. Still others, like the Ottawa Model for Research Use[70] and the PARIHS Framework,[71] emphasize more strongly the implementation components of EBP.

To clarify, EBP is not research. The conduct of research is the analysis of data collected from a homogenous group of subjects who meet study inclusion and exclusion criteria for the purpose of answering specific research questions or testing specified hypotheses.[67] Research design, methods, and statistical analyses are guided by the state of the science in the area of investigation. Traditionally, the conduct of research has included dissemination of findings via research reports in journals and at scientific conferences.[61] In essence, research is the generation of new knowledge, whereas EBP is the application of knowledge to practice.

IMPORTANCE OF EBP

The importance of moving toward EBP cannot be overstated. Clinicians engage in EBP to guide practice and facilitate clinical decision-making. EBP considers the relationships among the nature of the evidence, the context of the proposed change, and the mechanisms by which change will be facilitated.[72] With the ever-increasing and rapidly expanding availability of information on the Internet and from other sources, clinicians must be confident that the care they are providing is based on credible information and current best evidence. And, given the explosion of information, clinicians must consider and use practices based on recommended evidence. Increasing consumer awareness and access to information also lead patients and family members to expect their providers to demonstrate up-to-date knowledge and currency in best practices. As other providers move toward evidence-based care, nurses too must keep pace and owe a professional responsibility to their clients to do so. Use of EBP supports engagement of key stakeholders, including patients, in translating scientific findings into practice. A key role for healthcare leaders, including APRNs, is to facilitate changes in the workplace that continually improve the quality of care while meeting fiscal realities.[73]

Translating Evidence Into Practice

Researchers acknowledge that it takes 10 or more years to move scientific findings into practice.[4-7] The reason behind this lag is that educational detailing, decision-making algorithms, and reminders and alerts for clinicians are required before evidence can bring about change. Several barriers that contribute to the research–practice gap include, but are not limited to, a preference for research investigation rather than utilization, lack of clinically relevant studies in the research literature, and insufficient skill and/or experience in interpreting published studies.[74,75] APRNs and nurses in general have expressed concern that they do not have enough power or authority to change patient care practices even if research supports such initiatives. Inadequate time due to heavy workloads and competing priorities have also been identified as discouraging research efforts in clinical settings.[74,75]

With the renewed emphasis on the need to transform evidence into practice, the field of Translation Science has emerged as a means of addressing these barriers and limitations. Translation science refers to the applied effectiveness of moving evidence from the [research] bench to clinical trials and from research findings to patient care. Investigators describe the organizational, unit, and individual variables that affect the use of evidence in clinical and operational decision-making. They also test the effect of interventions aimed at promoting the rate and extent of adoption of evidence-based practices by nurses, physicians, and other healthcare providers.[76]

INITIATIVES FOR TRANSLATING RESEARCH EVIDENCE INTO PRACTICE

Recognizing that a great deal of evidence already exists, federal, regulatory, and accrediting agencies have instituted a coordinated push to incorporate it into practice. Prominent federal initiatives now center on addressing translational challenges, with translation a major focus of the National Institutes of Health (NIH) and the AHRQ-sponsored initiative, Translating Research into Practice (TRIP).[77] Funding for nursing research and other federally sponsored research programs is predicated on the ease of eventually transferring the findings to practice. Nurse researchers and other investigators must ensure that their results are generalizable and ready for immediate uptake by practitioners.[78]

This push for translation of evidence into practice is readily apparent in the ongoing and expanding requirements from the CMS-led Hospital Quality Alliance core measures reporting (http://www.cms.hhs.gov/HospitalQualityInits/33_HospitalQualityAlliance.asp), in the visibility of the Leapfrog initiatives (http://www.leapfroggroup.org), and in the recent Institute for Healthcare Improvement (IHI) patient safety campaigns (http://www.ihi.org/ihi). The aims of the IHI's "100,000 Lives" campaign were to "deliver reliable, evidence-based care for acute MI patients" (to prevent deaths) and to prevent central line infections and ventilator-associated pneumonia by encouraging hospitals to "implement a series of inter-dependent, scientifically grounded steps." The "5 Million Lives Saved" campaign followed suit in focusing its objectives on preventing pressure ulcers by "reliably using science-based guidelines for prevention"; on reducing methicillin-resistant *Staphylococcus aureus* (MRSA) infections by "reliably implementing scientifically proven infection control practices"; and on "delivering reliable, evidence-based care for congestive heart failure (CHF) patients to avoid readmissions" (http://www.ihi.org/IHI/Programs/Campaign/Campaign.htm ?TabId=1).

These initiatives align with priorities set forth in The Medicare Modernization Act of 2003 (MMA), which authorized the AHRQ to conduct and support research on outcomes, comparative clinical effectiveness, and appropriateness of pharmaceuticals, devices, and healthcare services. AHRQ's comparative effectiveness program[79] involves three approaches to researching comparative effectiveness:

1. Review and synthesize knowledge. AHRQ's network of Evidence-Based Practice Centers systematically review published and unpublished scientific evidence on what is known. Given the huge volume of studies and journal articles produced every year, it is next to impossible for providers, payers, and other key decision makers to keep up and even harder for them to weigh the evidence thoughtfully. AHRQ and its research partners synthesize the science and build a meaningful evidence base.

2. Promote and generate new knowledge. The Developing Evidence to Inform Decisions about Effectiveness (DEcIDE) Research Network studies new scientific evidence and analytic tools. Comprised of university research centers and think tanks, the DEcIDE Network conducts practical studies about the comparative clinical effectiveness, safety, and appropriateness of specific healthcare services, drugs, and devices.

3. Compile findings and translate and disseminate knowledge to decision makers. AHRQ's John M. Eisenberg Clinical Decisions and Communications Science Center transforms research results into actionable formats for stakeholders (e.g., providers, payers, purchasers, patients, manufacturers), producing guides for consumers, clinicians, and policy makers. The AHRQ initiative focuses on priority health conditions, such as cancer, diabetes, heart disease, and hypertension, selected because of their high impact on Medicare, Medicaid, State Children's Health Insurance Program (SCHIP), and other federal health programs.

ROLE OF APRNs IN OVERCOMING BARRIERS TO EBP

Federal and regulatory initiatives help, but ultimately, overcoming barriers to instituting EBP is accomplished by cultivating intellectual curiosity, by thinking reflectively about one's actions, by promoting and valuing innovation, and by creating an environment that supports questioning, evaluating current practice, and the seeking and testing of research-based solutions.[55,61,65,75] APRNs can prove instrumental in this cultural shift. They are the ideal facilitators of EBP because they possess the requisite clinical expertise, function as patient and family advocates, and understand the healthcare system well enough to negotiate effectively for the resultant changes in practice.[80] By engaging in an interactive model of knowledge translation, APRNs can facilitate translation of research into practice and bridge the research gap. This interactive approach posits a collaborative relationship between researchers and practitioners and consists of three basic actions[81]:

1. **Push,** meaning that researchers need to do a better job of communicating their study results to practicing clinicians

2. **Pull,** meaning that practice organizations need to become more evidence-based in their policies and procedures

3. **Exchange,** meaning that research should be designed to address the needs of practice, and clinicians should be engaged in the research process

The aim of this collaborative approach, discussed in greater detail in the following sections, is to remove traditional obstacles between researchers and clinicians to promote a more seamless translational process.

Practice Inquiry

Scientific inquiry and the continuing discovery of new knowledge are crucial and have the goal of generating knowledge for research-based clinical practice. Practice inquiry refers to clinical investigations that interface closely with everyday practice[78] and it is the type of research in which APRNs should be engaged. Through their participation, APRNs help to ensure the clinical relevance of the research questions[67] and the likelihood of eventual translation into practice.

Historically, research and continuous quality improvement (CQI) have operated independently of one another in healthcare settings. Today, healthcare organizations are merging these functions to help solve quality issues in the U.S. healthcare system.[82] This merging of functions has created angst among quality improvement specialists, researchers, and administrators because CQI and research share similar characteristics and are easily confused. Both ask clinically important questions, systematically collect and use patient data, apply complex statistical analyses, and have as their goal the improvement of patient care.[30] Primarily, they differ in the level of risk to the patient, as outlined below. The pressing need for APRNs and clinicians to translate evidence into practice more rapidly and effectively is a further complication.

Engaging in Practice Inquiry

Engaging in practice inquiry involves recognizing the similarities and differences between CQI and research, the types of research, and the roles the different types of APRNs have played and can play in research.

CONTINUOUS QUALITY IMPROVEMENT COMPARED WITH RESEARCH

Unique, yet somewhat overlapping, relationships exist between CQI and research.[83] Generally, CQI is differentiated from research based on such defining characteristics as purpose and process, generalizability, intent to publish, risks and benefits, degree of oversight, and protection of patient confidentiality.[84] Additional distinctions may occur at the institutional level and are driven by hospital-specific regulatory requirements that often go beyond the national requirements of the Health Insurance Portability and Accountability Act (HIPAA) for patient information privacy. The Hasting Report contributors stipulate that CQI is a necessary, integral activity for a healthcare institution, whereas research is not.[84]

CQI inferences are not causal and the process often tests potential solutions before the problem is well understood. Due to these limitations, the results are often not generalizable to other settings.[85] Alternatively, research entails systematic investigation, including research development, testing, and evaluation. It is designed to develop or contribute to generalizable knowledge with findings generally viewed as applicable to other patients, settings, or situations.[82] Anticipated risks are approved by an Institutional Review Board (IRB) and described directly to participants via informed consent.[85]

Within the general concept of research lie two different areas, basic research and applied research. Basic research entails experimental investigation to advance scientific knowledge. Immediate practical application is not a direct objective, whereas applied research focuses on specific practical application of the results. Applied researchers conduct systematic investigations used to improve patient care by collecting and analyzing data that are critical to clinical decisions. Such research studies may cross over into, or extend from, the realm of CQI, and vice versa.[82] The types of research discussed next may be basic or applied, depending on the intent.

Practice research entails using designs and methods needed to examine clinical questions related to the complexity of everyday clinical situations. The purpose of practice research is not to isolate the causal links between interventions and outcomes or to generalize intervention effect to service settings. Rather, the purpose of practice research is to examine variations in care and evaluate methods by which EBPs are introduced and adapted within a particular practice setting. By its nature, practice research encompasses the research areas of translational and EBP, clinical epidemiology and informatics, and quality of care.[78]

Outcomes research requires the use of scientific methods to measure the effect of some intervention or some process on outcomes.[37] It is directed toward populations of patients and is designed to establish care delivery standards or policy statements about best practices.

The intent of outcomes research is to demonstrate a causal connection between some change in practice or process and improvement in the observed outcome. With its emphasis on empirical evidence, the term should not be used interchangeably with the terms *outcomes evaluation* and *outcomes management*. Outcomes management is focused on the refinement of care delivery processes for the purposes of maximizing care delivery outcomes; its main intent is improving care for aggregate populations,[37] as discussed in the practice-based evidence section of this chapter.

Health services research is the multidisciplinary field of scientific investigation that studies how social factors, financing systems, organizational structures and processes, health technologies, and personal behaviors affect access to health care, the quality and cost of health care, and ultimately our health and well-being. Its research domains are individuals, families, organizations, institutions, communities, and populations. With its triad of access, cost, and quality, health services research examines how people get access to health care, how much care costs, and what happens to patients as a result of this care. The main goals of health services research are to identify the most effective ways to organize, manage, finance, and deliver high-quality care, reduce medical errors, and improve patient safety.[86]

APRNs' ROLES IN RESEARCH

Nursing research contributes to the validation of nursing outcomes, to the explanation and quantification of the unique nature of advanced nursing practice, and to the documentation of the quality of nursing care.[87] Research findings also provide essential information to policy makers about healthcare options. Conducting research provides a common language for communicating with other health professionals about the contributions of nursing to patient care and provides the means of disseminating information about nursing's effectiveness that is crucial to the survival of all four APRN roles.[88] The role of the APRN is critical in identifying issues that are important for clinical research as well as in providing firsthand insight into the research process. All APRNs across a variety of clinical settings possess this unique perspective and insight into care processes and care outcomes. APRNs work with interdisciplinary colleagues whose training required research using scientific methods. Thus there is a standardized vocabulary for exchanging findings and interpreting clinical information. Finally, because the advanced practice roles typically bridge nursing and medical functions, APRNs are ideally situated to share research findings and contribute to the scientific basis of care.[89]

Historically, advanced practice nursing research efforts focused on evaluating the value and effectiveness of the APRN role and the contribution of advanced nursing practice to patient outcomes. A brief description of some of these efforts is provided next, organized by APRN role: NP, CNS, certified registered nurse anesthetist (CRNA), and certified nurse-midwife (CNM). Outlined also are areas for future research.

Nurse Practitioners

Because the initial momentum for the nurse practitioner (NP) role came about due to concerns over gaps in healthcare services, early research focused on the unstated assumption that primary care services, as defined and provided by physicians, were adequate in every respect except quantity and accessibility.[90] The emphasis on "access" led researchers to study patient outcomes in terms of the extent to which access was achieved (e.g., number of visits), comparing NPs with physicians (MDs), and considering medical care to be standard and/or uniform.

The overwhelming majority of research on NPs has not dealt with a conceptual understanding of the practice; rather, the independent variable has been conceived of as the practitioner.[90] Further, because NPs were often seen as a subset of medical practice, the dependent variable—patient outcome—was also cast or defined in traditional medical terms. When other measures were included, they typically were patient satisfaction and acceptance.[90]

Most original studies[91]:

- Evaluated the roles of NPs in relation to physicians
- Assessed client acceptance
- Were descriptive in design
- Were conducted by investigators with limited research expertise
- Used retrospective analysis that suffered from incomplete data retrieval

One notable exception was the study by Lewis and Resnik[92] that employed randomized assignment of patients to control and experimental groups, follow-up, and multiple outcomes, including satisfaction with care, patients' knowledge about their illnesses, and system variables about the number of missed appointments and the utilization of hospital services.[91] After these early efforts, studies of NPs were done mostly by physicians, sociologists, and program evaluators (i.e., nonnurses). Many of these investigators primarily used questionnaires for data collection, did not use longitudinal designs, and lacked rigor in pretesting instruments for reliability and validity and in conducting appropriate statistical analyses.[90,91] However, not all studies suffered from these weaknesses. A well-known exception was the Burlington trial, which employed randomized controlled design, psychometrically tested instruments, and specification of patient outcomes.[91]

Studies conducted since then have had greater sophistication in method and have had more NPs involved in the investigations. They have addressed analysis of nursing components of practice, such as process and outcome measures, and factors that influenced NP performance, such as scope of the extended role, patient assignment, and economic issues.[91] Such sophistication continues, with more recent studies comparing effectiveness in care outcomes among disciplines[93] and evaluating cost-effectiveness and care outcomes of nurse-led programs.[94–96]

Clinical Nurse Specialists

Similar to the literature dealing with NPs, the clinical nurse specialist (CNS) literature before 1990 offered more information about the "role" of the CNS than about the "effectiveness" of these practitioners in patient care.[97] The tasks of documenting CNS practice and delineating the effects of interventions on patient outcomes are hampered by the complexity of the CNS role and wide variation in its implementation; thus, it is difficult to identify which of the activities are most effective in achieving outcomes. For example, in several early studies in which CNSs collaborated with other disciplines on patient outcomes, distinguishing the effects of the individual team providers on outcomes was difficult.[98] Later studies were more effective in capturing the role of the CNS in improving patient outcomes, including the classic study by Brooten and colleagues[99] that highlighted the function and effectiveness of the CNS in early discharge and home follow-up of very low birthweight infants. A more recent study evaluated care outcomes of a CNS's intervention in rheumatoid arthritis.[100]

Certified Nurse-Midwives

Certified nurse-midwives (CNMs) appear to have had the greatest leverage in documenting and reporting their contributions. Many clinically relevant and well-designed studies are available. Among the explanations for this success are the availability of data on effectiveness, establishment of linkages between data on effectiveness and health policy issues, and well-defined and sensitive outcome measures. From the inception of the role, CNMs were encouraged to gather statistics, and since 1972, this requirement has been formally acknowledged.[101]

Early statistics were primarily intended to evaluate program effectiveness and were linked to midwifery improvements in access to health care for women in rural areas.[101] Much data on infant and maternal mortality, as well as improvements in access, were collected from studies done by the Metropolitan Life Insurance Company for the Frontier Nursing Services between 1925 and the mid-1950s. In the mid-1950s, midwifery made a "deliberate" and "successful" attempt to provide services in hospitals, because most women were delivering in that setting.[101] While effectiveness had been documented in rural and underserved populations, hospital effectiveness studies included comparison of care given by CNMs and physicians using medical criteria, such as amount of analgesia given, duration of stages of labor, type of delivery, and complications. Even in later years, nurses[102] evaluated the nature of nurse-midwifery care and the relationship of clinical practice (e.g., administration of intravenous fluid, amniotomy, electronic fetal monitoring, pain medication, Pitocin augmentation) to outcomes (e.g., length of labor stages, time from labor until delivery, mode of delivery, incidence of episiotomy and laceration, and Apgar scores) in order to identify differences in intrapartum management between CNMs and physicians. As with the NP role, these effectiveness studies helped justify the CNMs' role not only to the public but also to other professionals, so that CNMs would be accepted and have access to childbearing women.

The effort was to demonstrate that CNM care was "as good as" physician care, "safe," "acceptable," and "cost-effective."[101] By the 1960s and 1970s, effectiveness studies focused on outcome measures, such as mortality rates, evidence of medical efficacy, quality of life, and cost-effectiveness. Nurse-midwives have had fewer problems in defining patient outcomes because of their obvious validity (e.g., neonatal mortality, birth weight) and their sensitivity to nursing practice interventions.[90,101] Numerous studies reported in the 1980s and early 1990s provided support for the positive outcomes of nurse midwives.[103,104] Such efforts continue, as evidenced by a recent study comparing national data on women with high-risk pregnancies cared for by CNMs with those cared for by obstetricians. Women who received care from CNMs experienced significantly higher rates of spontaneous delivery, were less likely to have instrument-assisted deliveries, and had fewer caesarean deliveries than women cared for by obstetricians.[105]

The practice of CNMs was developed through accreditation mechanisms, professional association positions, and legal parameters.[90] For these reasons and partly due to the quantity and quality of the effectiveness data that were required for public health record-keeping, there exists greater standardization for CNMs and CNMs have been able to influence health policy.[101] Further, CNM findings were relevant to practice problems, variables were easy to understand, outcomes were self-explanatory, and implications were easily connected to policy issues.[101] And finally, the nurse-midwifery literature has, to a great extent, avoided many of the oft-cited obstacles to policy creation, including isolated research findings, disjointed investigations, and infrequent replication. This focus resulted in several strong studies that provided support for the CNM role.

Certified Registered Nurse Anesthetists

Only a small percent of certified registered nurse anesthetists (CRNAs) have been involved in research, most likely because CRNAs have not received educational preparation for the research role. A significant relationship exists between working in a teaching hospital and conducting research.[106] Still, there are examples of CRNA-led research and program evaluation. Using the American Association of Nurse Anesthetists (AANA) Foundation's closed malpractice claims database, Kremer, Faut-Callahan, and Hicks[107] found that cognitive biases and inaccurate probability estimates were associated with adverse outcomes, and Jordan and colleagues[108] demonstrated that type of anesthesia provider (e.g., CRNA alone versus CRNA and anesthesiologist working together) did not have a statistically significant relationship with adverse anesthetic outcomes. Criste[109] conducted a national survey to determine whether nurse anesthetists demonstrated gender bias in treating pain. McAuliffe and Henry[110] studied nurse anesthetists in 94 countries and concluded that nurses were the main administrators of anesthesia in many countries, yet because most duties were performed inside operating rooms, the profession often lacked visibility. The authors concluded that nurse anesthetists must not only document their practice but also should participate in collaborative research at the local, regional, national, and international levels. As the majority of CRNAs and anesthesiologists practice in an interdisciplinary care team with variable staffing mix ratios, additional research evaluating practice models is warranted.

AREAS FOR FUTURE ADVANCED PRACTICE NURSING RESEARCH

The need to study the impact of nursing interventions on client response has been espoused since first advocated by Florence Nightingale in the 19th century, and even more than a decade ago, Lengacher and associates[111] reported a need for outcome research on the design and use of nursing practice models. Research establishing the value and effectiveness of chronic and acute care delivery models is warranted. This research should include evaluating APRNs' impact in disease management programs, such as the medical home and transitional care models, and evaluating and comparing the effectiveness of hospitalists and APRNs. To document effectiveness, clinical research must focus on both the processes and outcomes of APRN interventions. Outcomes regarding cost-effectiveness, access, and clinical outcomes must be woven into study designs.[80] Additionally, sources of data should be greatly increased and comparability and benchmarking improved by using standardized instruments. The literature includes a variety of valid and reliable instruments designed for such a purpose. When planning studies, APRNs should consider using established instruments to avoid the exacting process of instrument development and, more important, to allow comparisons among published findings. APRNs should also look to existing taxonomies for standardized nursing language, performance measures, decision making, and classification of nursing interventions. Furthermore, nurse researchers should consider answering research questions using existing data, or completing a secondary data analysis of quality outcomes using already-collected data. Various sets of publicly available quality and patient safety datasets are available from state, national, and private entities.

Despite increased funding and attention, a major obstacle to making widespread improvements in quality of care and patient safety has been the absence of a consensus on where to focus efforts, including how best to collect and report information on the quality and safety of health care.[112] Even a cursory review of the literature and of the 100 patient safety projects funded by AHRQ reveals a gamut of patient safety research, from studies identifying best practices for reporting medical errors to bar coding of medications and examining the effect of nurse staffing and fatigue on patient outcomes.[113]

Although clinical research efforts remain diverse, progress has been made toward identifying common patient safety outcome measures, including patient safety indicators and nursing-sensitive measures. However, additional research is needed to support the validity of these measures. The NQF assesses and rates emerging quality measures; such validation becomes increasingly important with the continual addition of nursing-sensitive outcomes to reimbursement and public reporting models. Likewise, more research is needed to measure nurses' contribution to quality of care and patient safety, other than nurse staffing. Research examining how experience, education, and critical thinking impact a nurse's ability to assess patients adequately and to provide timely intervention will provide additional evidence regarding the relationship between nursing care and patient outcomes. Research to determine the contribution of specialty nurses to the prevention of adverse events also warrants further study. Furthermore, exploring the relationship between nursing staff turnover and patient outcomes is also necessary. Disturbingly, turnover rate among nurses is more than double that for other professionals of comparable education and sex.[114] In the same vein, as the ANCC Magnet Recognition program becomes more popular, future research is needed to address the association of Magnet status to patient safety outcomes.

Certainly research on quality and safety in health care is not fully developed. To improve care we need well-designed studies using a variety of quantitative and qualitative research methods and designs. Appropriate funding and well-trained researchers from a variety of disciplines who know how to work at the interface of research, practice, and policy making are also needed.[3] Although research must be applied to the most relevant health problems and societal needs, such as the management of chronic diseases, the challenge remains to develop a more fundamental science of quality and safety. Developing and testing hypotheses about how to improve the performance of health professionals, patients, and health organizations is crucial for advancing this science. Research should focus on understanding why the provision of care and outcomes vary as well as on interventions to change behavior. Examples of such research include, but are not limited to, methods for engaging and understanding patients' roles in improving quality; how to achieve sustained change; how to guide clinicians toward scientifically correct and safe practice; how to provide new evidence to professionals at the point of care; and how to create a culture of change and continuous improvement in practice.[3]

In essence, the domains of quality, safety, and translation intersect to create a better understanding of the crucial determinants and effective and efficient methods for implementing change in practice so that interdisciplinary teams can implement research findings in a timely manner. Similarly, clinicians should evaluate the portability and effectiveness of the various EBP models on knowledge translation in practice. Equally important areas for inquiry include studying the influence of technology on the delivery of care, from assessing the impact of altered nursing practices as technological advances occur to evaluating how engineering and human factors might improve care processes and outcomes.[3]

Health services researchers are faced with the dual challenges of conducting not only complex methodological clinical research but also of conducting research in a real world environment—an ever-changing, multifaceted healthcare system. Who better to address these challenges than advanced practice nurse researchers? The overall field of patient safety and quality research is benefiting from the merging of nurses' clinical knowledge with their understanding of the healthcare system and their research abilities. The potential contribution of nursing research to improving patient safety is evident in the innovative approaches that have been documented in the literature.[113] As the health services research field grows, thecontributions of nursing researchers to patient safety and healthcare quality will also grow.

Research–Practice Exchange

Research ideas arise from one's own interests, observations of a recurring problem or unexplained phenomenon, suggestions from colleagues, and published results that recommend areas for further study.[65,67] A renewed orientation toward reflection and inquisitiveness ensures that clinical questions derived from the full array of preventive, acute, and chronic healthcare practice patterns, service models, and policy formulation are addressed by practicing professionals. Yet the challenge of interfacing research with practice requires creative solutions.[78] Teams comprised of professionals from different health-related disciplines who bridge the research–practice gap and who offer diverse perspectives and expertise are needed to participate in collaborative research designed to generate knowledge that enhances understanding of clinical phenomena, that defines optimal nursing or other interventions for patients or clinical problems, and that examines outcomes of care.[115]

Collaboration is advantageous when conducting clinical nursing research, as this approach pools complementary talents, research skills, and clinical experiences from among its members. Such collaboration may be interdisciplinary, intradisciplinary, or multidisciplinary. For example, in one interdisciplinary interpretation, a neonatal physician NP might consult with a clinical nurse researcher on the design of a study protocol, sources of funding, and implementation protocol. Intradisciplinary research collaboration occurs between nurse researchers and nurse clinicians and builds on the strengths of practice-based and academic-based models of clinical research.[89] Dufault[116] examined a model of reciprocity between nurse clinicians and nurse scientists that engaged nurse researchers, staff nurses, clinical managers, and nurse administrators to enhance research utilization. In Dufault's model, clinicians learned research methods and gained an appreciation of research, while scientists learned about clinically relevant problems and the challenges of conducting clinical investigations. Such collaboration is suggestive of Baumbusch and colleagues,[81] collaborative relationship between researchers and practitioners, outlined earlier. Multidisciplinary researchers and clinicians also may be included in nursing research, and many foundations and agencies specify that such cross-collaboration occur as a requirement for funding.

Collaborative arrangements can be instituted to increase the clinician–researcher interface, to ensure that practice informs research, and to foster mentoring relationships. Collaboration must be especially encouraged between academic and clinical institutions for mutual support in establishing programs for research and translation of research findings into practice.[8,9] Talented researchers from various disciplines who know how to work at the interface of research, practice, and policy making are needed.[3] Interdisciplinary research teams can involve nurse clinicians, nurse researchers, physicians, economists, psychologists, sociologists, anthropologists, nutritionists, statisticians, and other healthcare professionals. The chosen mix of disciplines depends on the clinical problem being investigated, the setting of the study, the desired talent pool of team members, and the goals of collaboration. Interdisciplinary research collaboration increases the visibility of nurse clinicians as uniquely skilled and contributing members of the healthcare team, promotes positive working relationships among health disciplines, and distributes the workload of a clinical investigation.[89] Blending research resources is critical to providing a scientific basis for advanced nursing practice and to providing answers to clinical questions that arise every day.

Practice-Based Research Networks

Methods for interfacing research with practice include action research, participatory research, and practice-based research, the latter being the most fully developed. The promise inherent in these models is that the research results are made more relevant; more actionable; more tailored; and more pertinent to patients, populations, and the circumstances of clinicians' practices and are completed with more immediate feedback to the practitioners.[117] The promise of this "pull" approach has led to the suggestion that if EBP is desirable, then continual practice-based evidence and collaborative practice inquiry are necessary.

Primary care practice-based research networks (PBRNs) exemplify the collaborative approach intended between practice and research. As part of the December 1999 legislation (Public Law 106-129) reauthorizing and renaming the AHRQ, leaders of the agency were directed to employ research strategies and mechanisms that would link research directly with clinical practice in geographically diverse locations throughout the country. The AHRQ leaders were also directed to include the use of "provider-based research networks . . . especially (in) primary care." AHRQ defines a PBRN as a group of ambulatory practices devoted principally to the primary care of patients and affiliated in their mission to investigate questions related to community-based practice and to improve the quality of primary care. This definition includes a sense of ongoing commitment to network activities and an organizational structure that transcends a single research project. Between 2000 and 2005, AHRQ funded four major competitive grant programs for PBRNs. In addition to funding, AHRQ supports PBRNs through a national resource center, an annual national conference, peer learning groups, an electronic PBRN research repository, and a dedicated community extranet. In 2000, the United States had approximately 24 primary care PBRNs. AHRQ has since provided direct funding for more than 50 PBRNs through targeted grant programs and has provided technical and networking assistance for many more. By 2004, AHRQ research identified more than 110 primary care PBRNs operating across the country.[118]

The Federation of Practice-Based Research Networks (FPBRN), established in November 1997, promotes the growth and development of clinical investigation in practice settings in primary care medicine. Practice facilitators (PFs), who are healthcare professionals, assist primary care practices in research and quality improvement activities. Their work goes beyond data collection and feedback and includes practice enhancement methods to facilitate system-level changes. PFs provide a framework for translating research into practice by building relationships, improving communication, facilitating change, and sharing resources in PBRNs. The work of PFs is funded from a variety of sources, including academic grants and renewable contracts with national, state, and local healthcare agencies. Nagykaldi and colleagues[119] provide examples of how the PF model was implemented in four PBRNs in the United States. However, limited information is available on the cost-effectiveness of PF interventions.

PBRNs often link practicing clinicians with investigators experienced in clinical and health services research, while at the same time enhancing the research skills of the network members. The best PBRN efforts link relevant clinical questions with rigorous research methods in community settings to produce scientific information that is externally valid and, in theory, assimilated more easily into everyday practice. Some PBRNs have existed in the United States for more than 20 years.[118] PBRNs are recognizing their potential to expand their purpose and are supporting quality improvement activities within primary care practices and the adoption of an evidence-based culture in primary care practice. Many PBRN leaders have begun to envision their networks as places of learning, where clinicians are engaged in reflective practice inquiries and where clinicians, their patients, and academic researchers collaborate in the search for answers that lead to the improved delivery of primary care.

The PBRN models, and especially the PF roles, yield positive prototypes for APRNs to emulate in their practice, whether primary, acute, or transitional care. Numerous authors[74,75,116,120] have documented the barriers that APRNs perceive in conducting and participating in research, including:

1. Inadequate facilities and organizational infrastructure for research
2. Lack of administrative incentives
3. Resistance and lack of cooperation in the work setting by administrators, other healthcare professionals, and nursing staff
4. Practice changes recommended from the findings that may be too costly to implement
5. Previous negative experiences with research
6. Isolation from knowledgeable colleagues

To advance the profession and make stronger, sustainable connections between research and practice, APRNs must remove such barriers to practice inquiry. The PBRN model offers a reasonable approach. Even simply engaging a PhD-prepared nurse in the research design, development, and evaluation of a study, with a master's or doctorally prepared APRN who can identify areas of inquiry and translate research evidence into practice offers a feasible application of this model. To apply this model for improved patient care consistently and successfully, APRNs must be competent in a range of domains.

APRN Inquiry and Evaluation Competencies

The research role is considered a core competency for APRNs and consists of three individual competencies:

- Evaluation of practice
- Interpretation and use of research in practice
- Participation in collaborative research[80] (p. 258)

These competencies relate to the components of practice-based evidence, evidence-based practice, and practice inquiry. For example, to demonstrate competence in "evaluation of practice," an APRN would be expected to evaluate relevant outcomes at the individual, group, and system levels. Similarly, to demonstrate competence in "interpretation and use of research in practice," an APRN would be expected to evaluate clinical practice guidelines for adoption in his or her specialty setting. And finally, to demonstrate competence in "participation in collaborative research," an APRN would be expected to function as a clinical expert or consultant in a collaborative research project and even be named as principal or co-investigator.

Most would agree that considerable overlap exists among the three components. For example, an APRN may determine that patient outcomes differ significantly between his or her home institution and peer-to-peer benchmarks (practice-based evaluation). Desiring to improve care, the APRN searches for evidence of best practices or treatments that may improve care for the patient population (evidence-based practice). Although the search may yield some evidence of interventions that had worked in other populations (e.g., adults in acute care), no studies might have been conducted on the APRN's population (e.g., children in home care), so the healthcare team would design a study to determine the effectiveness of the proposed treatment or intervention for the patient population (practice inquiry).

AACN advocates that master's programs should "prepare nurses to critique research and to implement changes in practice based on research data," and to "identify practice and systems problems that need to be studied and collaborate with other scientists to generate new studies based on their expertise"[8] (p. 2). A joint NONPF and AACN statement echoes this need.[13] Since then, AACN has called for transformational change in the education required for professional nurses who practice at the most advanced level of nursing, recommending that such nurses receive preparation for practice at the doctoral (DNP) level. The need for doctoral preparation emerged from multiple factors, including the expansion of scientific knowledge required for safe nursing practice and growing concerns regarding the quality of patient care delivery and outcomes. The intent of doctoral preparation is to equip specialized practitioners with the advanced competencies needed to engage in an increasingly complex healthcare environment, with the enhanced knowledge necessary to improve nursing practice and patient outcomes, and with enhanced leadership skills to strengthen practice and the delivery of health care.[9] These objectives align with The IOM[121] and the National Research Council of the National Academies[122] recommendations that nurses and health professionals be educated to deliver patient-centered care as members of interdisciplinary teams, emphasizing evidence-based practice, quality improvement, informatics, and patient safety expertise.

The *DNP Essentials*,[9] published by AACN, delineate the foundational competencies that are core to all advanced nursing practice roles. Among the essential activities described by the AACN and IOM are critiquing and using research in practice, evaluating outcomes and programs, and identifying clinical issues that can be investigated collaboratively, requiring specific knowledge, skills, and abilities.[80] The remainder of the chapter is devoted to outlining the competencies necessary for APRNs to apply practice-based evidence, evidence-based practice, and practice inquiry.

Practice-Based Evidence Competencies

Enhanced attention to quality and safety is driving the redesign of how care is delivered, monitored, and improved. In response, advanced nursing practice requires organizational and systems leadership that emphasizes practice and ongoing improvement of health outcomes. Ultimately, APRNs must ensure accountability for the quality of care and safety for the populations with whom they work; therefore, they must possess sophisticated expertise in assessing organizations, identifying systems issues, and facilitating organization-wide changes in practice delivery.[9] APRNs must be role models for others and encourage the identification of errors and hazards in care, the implementation of safety design principles to reduce or prevent their occurrence, and the continual assessment of quality of care using relevant structure, process, and outcome measures.[121]

Given the information paradigm shift and the emphasis on patient safety and quality in today's complex healthcare environment, APRNs must be adept at using information and technology to communicate, manage, and apply knowledge to practice. Possessing knowledge, skill, and ability in informatics enables APRNs to make sound decisions that are informed by data and that support high-quality, safe patient care. In this same vein, APRNs must understand the principles of informatics in order to inform and guide the design of databases that generate meaningful practice-based evidence. Necessary skills include database management, benchmarking, and analyzing and interpreting trends in practice using statistical process control charts, leading teams using various PI methodologies (e.g., PDSA, Six Sigma, Lean), and applying adequate PI tools to identify and reduce variation in care so that processes are standardized and simplified.

Balancing productivity with quality requires skill in analyzing cost-effectiveness as well. Not surprisingly, advanced nursing practice requires political shrewdness, innovative thinking, and business and financial acumen.[9] And finally, APRNs must be proficient not only in designing, directing, and evaluating quality improvement strategies within teams but also in creating and sustaining changes at the organizational and policy levels. Collaboration and clinical and professional leadership, including competence as an agent of change, comprise core competencies of advanced practice nursing.[12]

EBP Competencies

By the nature of their role, APRNs provide leadership for EBP to improve healthcare outcomes. This role necessitates competence in applying knowledge, including the skills needed to translate and integrate research into practice and disseminate new knowledge to clinicians.[9] APRNs must possess the ability to determine best practices through examining the type and level of evidence, evaluating the quality of the literature, and determining its applicability to practice.

APRNs should choose an EBP model to guide their efforts to incorporate evidence into practice. They should be confident in following the steps of the EBP process to frame meaningful and answerable clinical questions, and they should apply effective search strategies to uncover relevant evidence. To find the best evidence to answer clinical questions, APRNs should become familiar with basic principles of searching and acquire the skills needed to find the best resources, select useful sites, evaluate sites, and sort through the evidence they find. Commonly used databases include MEDLINE, CINAHL, and PubMed. The National Library of Medicine (NLM) provides its complete PubMed searching manual at http://www.ncbi. nlm.nih.gov/books/bv.fcgi?rid=helppubmed.chapter.pubmedhelp. Basic and advanced search strategies are described by Grandage, Slawson, and Shaughnessy.[123] Sources for preprocessed information including clinical practice guidelines, systematic reviews and meta-analyses are evidence-based nursing journals such as *Worldviews on Evidence Based Nursing,* the National Guidelines Clearinghouse, and the Cochrane Library.

Once studies and sources of evidence are located, APRNs must be skilled in using analytic methods to critically appraise existing literature. Critical appraisal is the process of systematically examining research evidence to assess its results, validity, and relevance prior to using it to inform clinical practice. Selecting and comparing published studies based on their research design and merits offers the best method for informing and changing practice.[124] APRNs need to have a clear understanding of research design, sampling, reliability, and validity as well as a keen understanding of statistical analyses, such as odds ratio, relative risk reduction, effect size, and confidence intervals, in order to critically appraise individual studies, systematic reviews, and meta-analyses. There are also formal systems and grading scales for evaluating not only individual studies but also a body of evidence. A report by AHRQ[125] identified seven systems as being especially useful for grading evidence based on a hierarchy of quality, and other sources are available to assist the APRN through this process.[65, 124, 126]

APRNs must then synthesize the relevant findings, identify gaps in evidence for practice, and determine applicability for practice.[127] With their knowledge of specialty practice, APRNs are well positioned to judge the applicability of the evidence base and to implement relevant findings to improve patient care. Understanding and using the principles of translation science will facilitate this movement of evidence into patient care.

Practice Inquiry Competencies

APRNs need to recognize the value of conducting research, understand the research process and their unique contributions to the process, and make participating in knowledge-generating and outcomes research a priority. Nurse investigators use research methods to predict and analyze quality and safety outcomes. Collaborating with advanced practice nurses, they design and test evidence-based interventions to change processes and systems of care, with the objective of improving quality. APRNs function as practice specialists or consultants in these research endeavors; thus, they need a solid understanding of research design principles, statistical analysis, and the scientific methods used to measure the effect of interventions on outcomes. Practice research further encompasses the research areas of translational and EBP, clinical epidemiology and informatics, quality of care, biostatistics, and policy.[78] Providing further training in these areas and encouraging nurses to coordinate and conduct interdisciplinary research to improve patient safety will amplify their contribution.

Doctoral nursing practice programs must prepare future leaders with the skills necessary to work in collaborative research teams so that they are prepared to ask clinical questions, appraise the evidence base, and translate research findings into practice. And finally, programs must incorporate health services research methods, including the analysis of large data sets and the analysis of multilevel data, to facilitate the ability of advanced practice nurse researchers to use advanced methodological approaches in patient safety and quality research.[113] The emphasis on learning and practicing these skills should be balanced by an equally endorsed orientation toward the use of such skills to interpret and apply findings reported in the research literature, as discussed above.

Teams comprised of interdisciplinary collaborators who bridge the research–practice gap and who offer diverse perspectives and expertise are needed to participate in collaborative research designed to generate knowledge that enhances understanding of clinical problems.[78] Through their participation, APRNs help to ensure the clinical relevance of the research questions by identifying issues that are important for patient care. Administrators can help create time for research by incorporating practice inquiry activities into APRN role responsibilities, allowing time for literature reviews and exploration of new ideas, and funding pilot projects on new practices. Additional strategies include instituting research journal clubs, forming research committees, promoting research presentations, subscribing to journals that emphasize research in practice,[75] such as *Applied Nursing Research*, and developing formal mechanisms for incorporating research findings into practice.

Summary

Real progress toward superior healthcare quality requires more rapid translation of evidence into practice and far greater emphasis on quality outcomes. APRNs are well poised to lead this transformation by engaging in robust practice inquiry and evaluation and by fostering an environment that supports new ideas, innovation, formalized research, quality improvement, and evidence-based practice changes. Practice inquiry and evaluation comprise integral components of the advanced practice role and not only serve to narrow the gap between research and practice but also enable continued improvement in the quality and safety of patient care.

SUGGESTED LEARNING EXERCISES

1. Consider your current or most recent place of employment.
   a. Determine clinical questions that might be examined using existing data.
   b. Propose measures (e.g., process, outcome) that can be used to address one or more of these clinical questions.
   c. Identify the database(s) where such data reside.
   d. Identify benchmarking sources and evaluate performance.
   e. Construct a potential sequence as to how you would go about improving performance and care related to your clinical question.
   f. Make a list of general areas or opportunities for conducting collaborative research or collaborating on evidence-based practice initiatives and the discipline(s) likely to participate.

2. Find a nursing home in your local area. Use the Web site http://www.medicare.gov/
   NHCompare to search by name, city, county, state, or ZIP code. Compare the quality of
   the nursing home to two other nursing homes within a 25-mile radius. Use the Five-Star
   Quality Ratings, health inspection results, nursing home staff data, quality measures, and
   fire safety inspection results to select your nursing home of choice. Explain why you
   chose this particular nursing home, and support your choice using data and tables. What
   factors most influenced your decision? Why?

3. Define translation science and evidence-based practice. Describe the relationship between
   the two. Describe your experiences with both evidence-based practice and research utilization. Clearly differentiate between the two.

4. Evaluate a set of clinical guidelines applicable to your clinical specialty. Use the AGREE
   evaluation framework (http://www.agreecollaboration.org). Outline strategies for implementing these guidelines in your current practice setting.

References

1. Kohn, LT, Corrigan, JM, and Donaldson, MS, eds. (1999). *To Err is Human: Building a Safer
   Health System.* National Academy Press, Washington, DC.

2. Commonwealth Fund. (2008). *Why Not the Best? Results from the National Scorecard on US
   Health System Performance, 2008.* The Commonwealth Fund, Pub. No. 1150.

3. Grol, R, Berwick, DM, and Wensing, M. (2008, January 12). On the trail of quality and safety in
   health care. *BMJ* 336:74–76.

4. McGlynn, EA, Asch, SM, and Adams, J. (2003). The quality of health care delivered to adults in the
   United States. *NEJM* 348:2635–2645.

5. Mangione-Smith, R, DeCristofaro, AH, Setodji, CM, et al. (2007, Oct 11). The quality of ambulatory
   care delivered to children in the United States. *NEJM* 357(15):1515–1523.

6. Ganz, DA, Wenger, NS, and Roth, CP. (2007). The effect of a quality improvement initiative on the
   quality of other aspects of health care: the law of unintended consequences? *Med Care* 45:8–18.

7. Higashi, T, Wenger, NS, Adams, JL, et al. (2007). Relationship between number of medical
   conditions and quality of care. *NEJM* (24):2496–2504.

8. American Association of Colleges of Nursing. (1996). *The Essentials of Master's Education for
   Advanced Nursing Practice.* AACN, Washington, DC.

9. American Association of Colleges of Nursing. (2006). *The Essentials of Doctoral Education for
   Advanced Nursing Practice.* AACN, Washington, DC.

10. Ahrens, T. (2005). Evidence-based practice: priorities and implementation strategies. *AACN Clinical
    Issues* 16(1):36–42.

11. Nightingale, F. (1969). *Notes on Nursing: What It Is and What It Is Not.* Dover Publications,
    New York.

12. Hamric, AB, Spross, JA, and Hanson, CM. (eds). (2008). *Advanced Practice Nursing: An Integrative
    Approach*, 3rd ed. Elsevier, St. Louis, MO.

13. National Organization of Nurse Practitioner Faculties (NONPF) and American Association of
    Colleges of Nursing (AACN). (2002). *Nurse Practitioner Primary Care Competencies in Specialty
    Areas: Adult, Family, Gerontological, Pediatric, and Women's Health.* U.S. Department of Health
    and Human Services, Washington, DC.

14. Lehman, L, Puopolo, A, Shaykevich, S, et al. (2005). Iatrogenic events resulting in intensive care
    admission: frequency, cause, and disclosure to patients and institutions. *The Amer J Med* 118:
    409–413.

15. Thomas, E, Studdert, D, Burstin, H, et al. (2000). Incidence and types of adverse events and
    negligent care in Utah and Colorado. *Medical Care* 38(3):261–271.

16. Nordgren, LD, Johnson, T, Kirschbaum, M, et al. (2004). Medical errors: excess hospital costs and lengths of stay. *J HealthCare Quality* 26(2):42–48.

17. Rojas, M, Silver, A, Llewellyn, C, et al. (2005). Study of adverse occurrences and major functional impairment following surgery. In *Advances in Patient Safety: From Research to Implementation*, Vols. 1–4, AHRQ Publication Nos. 050021 (1–4). Agency for Healthcare Research and Quality, Rockville, MD.

18. Centers for Medicare and Medicaid Services. (2007). *HHS Reports to Congress on Value-Based Purchasing of Hospital Services by Medicare*. Available at http://www.hhs.gov.news/press/2007/11/pr20071126a.

19. National Committee for Quality Assurance. (2008). http://www.ncqa.org. Accessed September 20, 2008.

20. Hannan, EL, Kilburn, H, Racz, M, Shields, E, and Chassin, M. (1994). Improving the outcomes of coronary artery bypass surgery in New York State. *JAMA* 271(10):761–766.

21. Peterson, E, DeLong, E, Jollis, J, et al. (1998). The effects of New York's bypass surgery provider profiling on access to care and patient outcomes in the elderly. *J Amer Col* 32:993–999.

22. Chassin, MR. (2002). Achieving and sustaining improved quality: lessons from New York State and cardiac surgery. *Health Affairs* 21(4):40–51.

23. Agency for Healthcare Research and Quality. (2008). Patient Safety Organizations. http://www.pso.ahrq.gov/. Accessed September 15, 2008.

24. Cooper JB, Gaba DM, Liang B, Woods D, and Blum LN. (2000). National Patient Safety Foundation agenda for research and development in patient safety. *Medscape General Medicine* [series online] 2(4):14. Available at http://www.medscape.com/viewarticle/408064.

25. Battles, J, and Lilford, R. (2003). Organizing patient safety research to identify risks and hazards. *Quality and Safety in Health Care, Supplement* ii(12):ii2–ii7.

26. Institute of Medicine (IOM). (2001). *Crossing the Quality Chasm: A New Health System for the Twenty-first Century*. National Academy Press, Washington DC.

27. Nevidjon, BM, and Knudtson, MD. (2008) Strengthening advanced nursing practice in organizational structures and cultures. In Hamric, AB, Spross, JA, and Hanson, CM (eds), 3rd ed. *Advanced Practice Nursing: An Integrative Approach*. Elsevier, St Louis, MO.

28. The Institute of Medicine Committee on Redesigning Health Insurance Performance Measures, Payment, and Performance Improvement Programs. (2006). *Performance Measurement: Accelerating Improvement* (Pathways to Quality Health Care Series). The National Academies Press, Washington, DC.

29. Jennings, B, Baily, M, Bottrell, M, et al. (2007). *Health Care Quality Improvement: Ethical and Regulatory Issues*. The Hastings Center, Garrison, New York.

30. Morris, PE, and Dracup, K. (2007). Quality improvement or research? The ethics of hospital project oversight. *Am J Crit Care* 16(5):424–426.

31. Mitchell, P, Ferketich, S, and Jennings, B. (1998). Quality health outcomes model: American Academy of Nursing Expert Panel on Quality Health Care. *J Nurs Schol* 30:43–46.

32. Donabedian, A. (1966). Evaluating the quality of medical care. *Milbank Memorial Fund Quarterly* 44(3 Suppl):166–206.

33. Swan, BA, and Boruch, RF. (2004). Quality of evidence: usefulness in measuring the quality of health care. *Medical Care* 42(2 Suppl II):12–20.

34. Mayberry, LJ, and Gennaro, S. (2001). A quality of health outcomes model for guiding obstetrical practice. *J Nurs Schol* 33:141–146.

35. Radwin, L, and Fawcett, J. (2002). A conceptual model-based program of nursing research: retrospective and prospective applications. *J Adv Nurs* 40:355–360.

36. Sin, M, Belza, B, LoGerfo, J, et al. (2005). Evaluation of a community-based exercise program for elderly Korean immigrants. *Public Health Nursing* 22(5):407–413.

37. Ingersoll, GL, and Mahn-DiNicola, VA. (2008). Outcome evaluation and performance improvement. In Hamric, AB, Spross, JA, and Hanson, CM (eds), 3rd ed. *Advanced Practice Nursing: An Integrative Approach*. Elsevier, St. Louis, MO.

38. Pelletier and Albright. (2006) In Huber, D (ed), *Leadership and Nursing Care Management*. Saunders, Philadelphia.

39. Pronovost, PJ, Berenholtz, CA, and Goeschel, RM. (2008, May 14) The wisdom and justice of not paying for "preventable complications." *JAMA* 299(18):2197–2199.

40. Zhan, C, Kelley, E, Yang, HP, et al. (2005). Assessing patient safety in the United States: challenges and opportunities. *Medical Care* 43(3 Suppl.):I42–II47.

41. Romano, PS, Geppert, JJ, Davies, S, et al. (2003). A national profile of patient safety in US hospitals. *Health Affairs* 22(2):154–165.

42. Aiken, L. (2005). The unfinished patient safety agenda. In *Web M&M: Case & Commentary*. Agency for Healthcare Research and Quality, Rockville, MD.

43. Maas, M, Johnson, M, and Moorehead, S. (1996). Classifying nursing-sensitive patient outcomes. *J Nurs Scholar* 28(4):295–301.

44. National Quality Forum. (2004). *National Voluntary Consensus Standards for Nursing-Sensitive Care: An Initial Performance Measure Set*. National Quality Forum, Washington, DC.

45. American Nurses Association (ANA). (2005). *Quality Indicators: Outcomes Measurement Using the ANA Safety and Quality Indicators*. American Nurses Association, Washington, DC.

46. Savitz, LA, Jones, CB, and Bernard, S. (2005, February). Quality indicators sensitive to nurse staffing in acute care settings. In *Advances in Patient Safety: From Research to Implementation*, Vols. 1–4, AHRQ Publication Nos. 050021 (1–4). Agency for Healthcare Research and Quality, Rockville, MD.

47. Blegen, M, Goode, C, and Reed, L. (1998). Nurse staffing and patient outcomes. *Nursing Research* 47(1):43–50.

48. Needleman, J, Buerhaus, P, Mattke, S, et al. (2002). Nurse-staffing levels and the quality of care in hospitals. *NEJM* 346:1715–1722.

49. Unruh, L. (2003). Licensed nurse staffing and adverse events in hospitals. *Medical Care* 41(1):142–152.

50. Kurtzman, ET, and Buerhaus, PI. (2008). New Medicare payment rules: danger or opportunity for nursing? *Am J Nurs* 108(6):30–35.

51. Titler, M, Cullen, L, and Ardery, G. (2002). Evidence-based practice: an administrative perspective. *Reflect Nurs Leadership* 28(2):26–27, 45, 46.

52. Draper, D, Felland, L, Liebhaber, A, et al. (2008, March). *The Role of Nurses in Hospital Quality Improvement*. Center for Studying Health System Change, Research Brief No. 3.

53. Varkey, P, Reller, K, and Resar, RK. (2007). Basics of quality improvement in healthcare. *Mayo Clinic Proc* 82(6):735–739.

54. Titler, MG, and Goode, CJ (guest eds). (1995). Preface. *Nurs Clin North Am* 30:xv.

55. Melnyk, B, and Fineout-Overholt, E. (2002). Putting research into practice. *Reflections on Nursing Leadership* 28:22.

56. Jha, AK, Li, Z, Orav, EJ, et al. (2005). Care in US hospitals—the Hospital Quality Alliance Program. *NEJM* 353(3):265–274.

57. Hojania, K, Duncan, B, McDonald, K, et al. (2001). *Making Health Care Safer: A Critical Analysis of Patient Safety Practices*, in Evidence Report/Technology Assessment No. 43 (No 01-E058). Agency for Healthcare Research and Quality, Rockville, MD.

58. Leape, L, Berwick, D, and Bates, D. (2002). What practices will most improve safety? *JAMA* 288(4):501–507.

59. Estabrooks, CA. (1998). The conceptual structure of research utilization. *Research in Nursing & Health* 22:203–216.

60. Stetler, CB, et al. (1995). Enhancing research utilization by clinical nurse specialists. *Nurs Clin North Am* 30:457.

61. Titler, MG. (2002). Use of research in practice. In LiBiondo-Wood, G, & Haber, J (eds), *Nursing Research*, 5th ed. Mosby-Year Book; St. Louis, MO, pp. 411–444.

62. Brown, SJ. (2008). Direct clinical practice. In Hamric, AB, Spross, JA, and Hanson, CM (eds), 3rd ed. *Advanced Practice Nursing: An Integrative Approach*. Elsevier, St. Louis, MO.

63. Dlugacz, Y, Restifo, A, and Nelson, K. (2005). Implementing evidence-based guidelines and reporting results through a quality metric. *Pat Safety & Quality in Healthcare* 40:2.

64. Sackett, DL, Straus, SE, Richardson, WS, et al. (2000). *Evidence-based Medicine: How to Practice and Teach EBM*, 2nd ed. Churchill Livingstone, Edinburgh.

65. DiCenso, A, Guyatt, G, and Ciliska, D. (2005). *Evidence-Based Nursing—A Guide to Clinical Practice*. Mosby, St. Louis, MO.

66. Pravikoff, D, and Donaldson, N. (2001). Online journals: access and support for evidence-based practice. *AACN Clinical Issues* 12:588.

67. Polit, DF, and Beck, CT. (2008). *Nursing Research: Generating and Assessing Evidence for Nursing Practice*. Lippincott Williams & Wilkins, Philadelphia, PA.

68. Titler, M, Kleiber, C, Steelman, V, Rakel, B, Budreau, G, Everett, L, et al. (2001). The Iowa model of evidence-based practice to promote quality care. *Critical Care Clinics of North America* 13(4):497–509.

69. Stevens, KR. (2004). *ACE Star Model of EBP: Knowledge Transformation*. Academic Center for Evidence-based Practice. The University of Texas Health Science Center at San Antonio.

70. Logan, J, and Graham, I. (1998). Toward a comprehensive interdisciplinary model of health care research use. *Science Communication* 20:227–246.

71. Malone, JR. (2004). The PARIHS Framework—a framework for guiding the implementation of evidence-based practice. *J Nurs Care Qual* 19(4):297–304.

72. Davies, B. (2002). Sources and models for moving research evidence into clinical practice. *JOGN* 31:558–562.

73. Cummings, G, and McLennan, M. (2005). Advanced practice nursing—leadership to effect policy change. *JONA* 35(2):61–66.

74. Pettengill, M, Gillies, D, and Clark, C. (1994). Factors encouraging and discouraging the use of nursing research findings. *Image J Nurs Sch* 26:143.

75. Funk, SG, Tornquist, EM, and Champagne, MT. (1995). Barriers and facilitators of research utilization. *Nurs Clin North Am* 30:395.

76. Titler, MG. (2008). The evidence for evidence-based practice implementation. In *Patient Safety and Quality: An Evidence-Based Handbook for Nurses*. AHRQ, Rockville, MD.

77. Agency for Healthcare Research and Quality. (2008). *Translating Research into Practice* (*TRIP*). http://www.ahrq.gov/research/trip2fac.htm. Accessed December 10, 2008.

78. Magyary, D, Whitney, J, and Brown, MA. (2006). Advancing practice inquiry: research foundations of the practice doctorate in nursing. *Nursing Outlook* 54:139–151.

79. Agency for Healthcare Research and Quality. *Effective Health Care Program*. http://www.ahrq.gov/research/oct05/1005RA33.htm. Accessed August 10, 2008.

80. DePalma, JA, and McGuire, DB. (2008). Research. In Hamric, AB, Spross, JA, and Hanson, CM. (eds), 3rd ed. *Advanced Practice Nursing: An Integrative Approach*. Elsevier, St. Louis, MO, pp. 257–300.

81. Baumbusch, JL, Kirkham, SR, Khan, KB, et al. (2008). Pursuing common agendas: a collaborative model for knowledge translation between research and practice in clinical settings. *Research in Nursing & Health* 31(2):130–140.

82. Harrington, L. (2007). Quality improvement, research, and the Institutional Review Board. *J Healthcare Quality* 29(3):4–9.

83. Newhouse, RP. (2007). Diffusing confusion among evidence-based practice, quality improvement, and research. *J Nurs Adm* 37(10):432–435.

84. Jennings, B, Baily, M, Bottrell, M, et al. (2007). *Health Care Quality Improvement: Ethical and Regulatory Issues.* The Hastings Center, Garrison, NY.

85. Newhouse, RP, Pettit, JC, Poe, S, et al. (2006). The slippery slope: differentiating between quality improvement and research. *J Nurs Adm* 36(4):211–219.

86. AcademyHealth. (2004). *Glossary of Terms Commonly Used in Healthcare.* AcademyHealth, Washington, DC. http://www.adademyhealth.org. Accessed December 1, 2008.

87. Hawkins, J, and Thibodeau, J. (1993). The role of research in advanced practice. In Hawkins, J, and Thibodeau, J, *The Advanced Practitioner: Current Practice Issues.* Tiresias Press, New York.

88. Papenhausen, J, and Beecroft, P. (1990). Communicating clinical nurse specialist effectiveness. *Clinical Nurse Specialist* 4:1.

89. Sprague-McRae, J. (1988). Nurse practitioners and collaborative interdisciplinary research roles in an HMO. *Pediatric Nurs* 14:503.

90. Diers, D, and Molde, S. (1979). Some conceptual and methodological issues in nurse practitioner research. *Res Nurs Health* 2:73.

91. Stanford, D. (1987). Nurse practitioner research: issues in practice and theory. *Nurse Pract* 12:64.

92. Lewis, CE, and Resnik, BA. (1967). Nurse clinics and progressive ambulatory patient care. *NEJM* 277:1236.

93. Andrus, MR, and Clark, DB. (2007). Provision of pharmacotherapy services in a rural nurse practitioner clinic. *American Journal of Health-System Pharmacy* 64(3):294-297.

94. Maljanian, R, Grey, N, Staff, I, et al. (2003). Improved diabetes control through a provider based disease management program. *Disease Management & Health Outcomes* 10(1):1–8.

95. Lenz ER, Mundinger MO, Kane RL, and Hopkins SC. (2004). Primary care outcomes in patients treated by nurse practitioners or physicians: two-year follow-up. *Med Care Res Rev.* 61(3): 332–351.

96. Rideout, K. (2007). Evaluation of a PNP care coordinator model for hospitalized children, adolescents, and young adults with cystic fibrosis. *Pediatric Nurse* 33(1):29–36, 48.

97. Lipetzky, P. (1990). Cost analysis and the clinical nurse specialist. *Nurs Manage* 21:25.

98. Rizzuto, C. (1995). Issues in clinical nursing research: documenting clinical nurse specialist role functions and outcomes. *West J Nurs Res* 17:448.

99. Brooten, D, Gennaro, S, Knapp, H, et al. (2002). Functions of the CNS in early discharge and home followup of very low birthweight infants. *Clinical Nurse Specialist* 16(2):85–90.

100. Tijhuis, GJ, Zwinderman, AH, Hazes, JMW, et al. (2003). Two-year follow-up of a randomized controlled trial of a clinical nurse specialist intervention, inpatient, and day patient team care in rheumatoid arthritis. *J Adv Nurs* 41(1):34–43

101. Diers, D, and Burst, HV. (1983). Effectiveness of policy related research: nurse-midwifery as case example. *Image J Nurs Sch* 15:68.

102. Beal, MW. (1984). Nurse-midwifery intrapartum management. *J Nurse Midwifery* 29:13.

103. Rooks, J, et al. (1989). Outcomes of care in birth centers. *NEJM* 321:1804.

104. Anderson, RE, and Murphy, PA. (1995). Outcomes of 11,788 planned home births attended by certified nurse-midwives: a retrospective descriptive study. *J Nurse Midwifery* 40:483.

105. Davidson, MR. (2002). Clinical practice exchange. Outcomes of high-risk women cared for by certified nurse-midwives. *J Midwifery & Women's Health* 47:46–49.

106. Cowan, C, Vinayak, K, and Jasinski, D. (2002). CRNA-conducted research: is it being done? *AANA Journal* 70:18.

107. Kremer, M, Faut-Callahan, M, and Hicks, F. (2002). A study of clinical decision-making by certified registered nurse anesthetists. *AANA Journal* 70:391.

108. Jordan, LM, Kremer M, Crawforth K, et al. (2001). Data-driven practice improvement: the AANA Foundation closed malpractice claims study. *AANA Journal* 69(4):301–311.

109. Criste, A. (2003). Do nurse anesthetists demonstrate gender bias in treating pain? In Craig, JV, and Smyth, RL (eds), *Evidence-based Practice Manual for Nurses*. Churchill-Livingstone, Edinburgh, pp. 21–44.

110. McAuliffe, M, and Henry, B. (2000). Nurse anesthesia practice and research—a worldwide need. *CRNA* 11:89.

111. Lengacher, C, et al. (1984). Effects of the partners in care practice model on nursing outcomes. *Nursing Economics* 12:300.

112. Altman, D, Clancy, C, and Blendon, R. (2004). Improving patient safety—five years after the IOM report. *NEJM* 351(20):2041–2043.

113. Merwin, E, and Thornlow, D. (2006). Methodologies used in nursing research designed to improve patient safety. *Annual Review of Nursing Research* 24:273–292.

114. Steele, R. (2002). Turnover theory at the empirical interface: problems of fit and function. *Academy of Management Review* 27:346–360.

115. Whitman, GR. (2002). Outcomes research. Getting started, defining outcomes, a framework, and data sources. *Critical Care Nursing Clinics of North America* 14:261–268.

116. Dufault, M. (1995). A collaborative model for research development and utilization: process, structure, and outcomes. *J Nursing Staff Development* 11:139.

117. Green, LW. (2008). Making research relevant: if it is an evidence-based practice, where's the practice-based evidence? *Family Practice*. First published online 15 Sept 2008.

118. Agency for Healthcare Research & Quality. (2008). Practice-Based Research Networks. http://www.ahrq.gov/research/pbrn/pbrnfact.htm. Accessed September 10, 2008.

119. Nagykaldi, Z, Mold, JW, Robinson, A, et al. (2006). Practice facilitators and practice-based research networks. *J American Board of Family Medicine* 19:506–510.

120. Jastremski, C. (2002). Using outcomes research to validate the advanced practice nursing role administratively. *Critical Care Nursing Clinics of North America* 14:275.

121. The Institute of Medicine Committee on Health Professions Education Summit. (2003). *Health Professions Education: A Bridge to Quality*. National Academies Press, Washington, DC.

122. National Research Council of the National Academies. (2005). *Advancing the Nation's Health Needs: NIH Research Training Programs*. National Academies Press, Washington. DC.

123. Grandage, KK, Slawson, DC, and Shaughnessy, AF. (2002). When less is more: a practical approach to searching for evidence-based answers. *Journal of the Medical Library Association* 90(3):298–304.

124. Shapiro, S, and Donaldson, N. (2008). Evidence-based practice for advanced practice emergency nurses, Part II—critically appraising the literature. *Advanced Emergency Nursing Journal* 30(2): 139–150.

125. *Systems to Rate the Strength of Scientific Evidence*, Structured Abstract. March 2002. Agency for Healthcare Research and Quality, Rockville, MD. Available at http://www.ahrq.gov/clinic/tp/strengthtp.htm.

126. Melynk, BM. (2003). Finding and appraising systematic reviews of clinical interventions: critical skills for evidence-based practice. *Ped Nurse* 29(2):147–149.

127. Newhouse, RP. (2008). Evidence synthesis: the good, the bad, and the ugly. *JONA* 38(3):107–111.

Marilyn W. Edmunds is the editor of the *Journal for Nurse Practitioners* and a number of pharmacology and procedures textbooks. She is co-owner of Nurse Practitioner Alternatives, Inc., a continuing education company for nurses and physicians, and co-author of Nursing View Points for the Web site http://www.Medscape.com.

Acknowledgement is made to Suzanne Hall Johnson, MN, RNC, CNS, whose original version of this chapter was published in *Advanced Practice Nursing*, editions 1 and 2. I applaud her overall design and content, which inform this update of the chapter.

CHAPTER 10

Publishing in Nursing Journals

Marilyn Winterton Edmunds, PhD, ANP-BC/GNP-BC

CHAPTER OBJECTIVES

After completing this chapter, the reader will be able to:

1. Develop a practical plan to evaluate the type of articles a journal selects for publication.
2. Compare format and style typically used in papers written to meet academic requirements and those of papers written for publication.
3. Outline contemporary issues to consider in submitting an article for publication.
4. Appropriately target and plan an article for publication.

Nurses in advanced practice roles are some of the most talented clinical leaders; they are developing new nursing strategies and knowledge through their clinical research and practice. Chapter 9 emphasized the importance of conducting research on clinical questions and on the practice outcomes of advanced practice registered nurses (APRNs). However, answers to clinical questions and successful techniques to expand the APRN role cannot be disseminated if the nurse does not publish their results.

While it is especially important to publish good research, it is also important to share information that increases the quality of clinical practice through other types of articles. The very nature of clinical practice is dynamic: New diagnoses are identified, treatment modalities are evaluated, and consensus statements and evidence-based guidelines that affect patient care are developed. Thus, any nurse who can make a worthwhile contribution to this literature should be able to find a way to publish it.

Prospective authors should consider that getting an article published is a transaction. Just as in business dealings, both parties to the transaction are seeking something and must be satisfied. APRNs often feel passionately about a topic, have a unique case study to share, or have learned some technique or knowledge that would help other nurses. However, they may be hesitant to approach editors about their desire to publish this work. On the other hand, editors want and need articles to publish in their journals. They are looking for articles on case studies and on new techniques or treatment strategies that provide up-to-date information as well as for articles that are innovative in their viewpoint or deal with an old issue in a distinctive way.

All authors have the same publishing challenge: how to develop a manuscript that will be accepted by a journal and that will meet the needs of the journal's readership. This chapter includes some information about writing for other media but focuses on the challenge of preparing and submitting a publishable article to a journal. Three steps are involved:

1. Choosing the journal to which you will submit your article
2. Considering all the factors that make an article publishable
3. Addressing contemporary issues that impact publication

CHOOSING THE JOURNAL AND PUBLISHER

Usually, authors believe that choosing a journal is the last thing to do when writing an article, not the first. If, however, you choose the journal wisely and know what types of articles that specific journal publishes and what is required for submission, you can shape the article to fit those requirements. This dramatically increases the likelihood that the article will be published.

Each journal has a clear market that it must please if it wishes to stay in business. Consider the following ideas as you contemplate the previous sentence:

- You are writing an article on genetic markers for breast cancer. How would your article be different if you were to send it to *RN Magazine*? *Journal for Oncology Nurses*? *Clinical Specialist*? Which of these three journals would most likely be interested in your article?

- You are a second-semester student in a clinical nurse specialist (CNS) program and are interested in cardiovascular disease. You have just struggled to learn how to assess heart sounds and correlate them to the physical examination. If you wrote an article on this topic, is there a journal with a readership who would be interested in it?

- You recently completed a medical mission to Haiti with some friends from your church. You had a wonderful time and took many photographs. You would like to share the details of your trip. Is there a nursing journal that would be interested in publishing this?

Prospective authors should consider three resources as they make a decision about which journal to approach about publishing an article. First, most journals publish author guidelines that may include a mission statement and identify their audience. You will find this information either in the journal itself or on the journal Web site. An Internet search for author guidelines should allow you to locate this information quickly. See, for example, http://npjournal.org/authorinfo.

Second, look through several issues of the journals that you believe might be appropriate for your article. Note the topics the journal features, how scholarly the publication appears, and the level of the discussion. What formats do they use? Consult their article index for the last few years to see if they have published any articles on your topic. Ask yourself the questions "Would the article I have in my head be a good fit for this journal?" and "Would I be happy to have my article in this journal?" See Table 10-1 for a summary of things to consider.

Third, once you have made a tentative decision about which journal to approach, write the editor a letter. In it, ask if the journal would be interested in publishing something on your

Table 10-1 Evaluating a Journal for Article Fit

QUESTION TO ANSWER	EXAMPLES
Who is the audience of the journal?	Clinical practicing nurses, researchers, academics, clinical specialists, APRNs, etc.
What is my message for this readership? Why would the journal audience read my article?	To update their knowledge; to learn about new research, guidelines, or algorithms; to read about a unique case study; to gain tips from an experienced nurse
What do I have to contribute to this readership?	Are you a novice? An expert? Be realistic about your skills in communicating the message to the journal audience.
Would I be happy to be published in this journal?	Consider the following: • Impact factor—Are the authors/articles included in the journal frequently quoted in other journals? • Publishing schedule (monthly vs. 2–6 issues a year) • Indexing—Is the journal indexed in the National Library of Medicine (PubMed)? Cinhal, Science Direct? • Readership—How large is the readership audience? • Additional outlets—Is the journal online as well as in print media? • Continuing education—Does the journal have continuing education activities? • Appearance—Is the journal printed in black and white or color? Does it use graphics, illustrations, and/or photos? Does it have an attractive layout?
Have I examined the journal index? What impression do I have after closely examining several recent issues of the journal?	Has the journal published on my topic recently? Does it publish on related topics? Have any of my colleagues published in this journal? Would my article seem to "fit" here?

topic and provide a few details about the format, such as whether it is research, a case study, a clinical feature, and so on.

If an author does not complete these three steps well, he or she risks writing a paper but finding no editor who wants to publish it. During the last several years the author of this chapter has had the opportunity to review 30 to 50 nursing and medical journals each month while making selections of articles to summarize for a Journal Scan column.[1] It is fascinating to see what you can learn about what is being published, the level of scholarship, the quality of research publications, who is publishing, and the flavor of a journal just by comparing issues of the same journal and by comparing different journals over time. This type of comprehensive evaluation gives you a distinct look at the world of nursing publications. You see how many journals publish quarterly versus monthly, how many journals are research-oriented, how many have themes, how many are aligned with a nursing organization, etc. You see some articles you feel should never have been published and some journals with lots of published errata. The gestalt you develop during this review process helps you formulate general impressions about where you might want to send your article for consideration.

When you choose a journal to approach, you must also consider if the journal will choose you. Just as prospective authors talk to different people about how to get articles published, editors also talk among themselves. The International Academy of Nurse Editors (INANE) is a group of about 250 nursing editors from around the world. They have a Web site (http://www.nursingeditors.org/) and a closed listserv.[2] Members correspond regularly about many facets of publishing nursing content. In 2008, they had a very animated discussion focused on things that editors did not like, or in other words, things that did not help in getting articles published.[3] Some of the things they noted were major errors, such as submitting a whole dissertation and suggesting that the editor compose a few articles from it, to small things, such as "sending me a form letter or not addressing me personally." Some of the most frequently cited behaviors are listed in Table 10-2 and many are discussed below. Being aware of these things should help the prospective author avoid making these mistakes.

Factors That Make an Article Publishable

APRNs interested in publishing should consider several factors, including not submitting student papers, following the general rules of professional writing, and carefully checking the completed article. APRNs should also become informed about what to expect when submitting an article and what to do if the article is accepted—or rejected.

Student Papers

Increasingly, APRN programs are instituting policies requiring students to write publishable papers as a condition of graduation. Particularly in the Doctor of Nursing Practice (DNP) programs, students are often encouraged to publish several practice-focused or clinical papers—first a review of the literature, second a conceptual framework or methodology, and finally their findings. Some nursing research journals accept these types of submissions, but many have a backlog of manuscripts to review and would not be pleased with this type of piecemeal submission. Also, remember that the graduate program requirements may be at variance with those of a professional article that would be accepted by the journal you have selected. Many APRN students receive high grades on academic papers and are eager to see these papers published. However, sending student papers to editors is probably the number-one reason INANE editors reject papers.[3] Therefore, it is essential to understand the difference between student papers and publishable papers.

The elements that made a good academic paper may actually be those that lead it to being rejected by an editor even before it is sent out for review. The style, the format, and the components of an academic paper are very different from those of a publishable paper. If the prospective author does not understand this, frustration and disappointment result.

Table 10-2 **Summary of Major Things That Discourage Editors From Accepting Articles**[3]

Behavior	Comments and Examples
Missing the point	• Not understanding the readership of the journal, so article sent is inappropriate for audience. • Sending a student paper • Sending a whole thesis or dissertation • Abstract same as the first paragraph of the article
Not following guidelines	• Sending graphics in wrong format • Expects publisher to get permission to reprint illustrations, photos, or quotations • References in wrong format • Failure to keep paper to recommended length • Excessive number of references • Inserting tables, figures, and graphics into the text rather than sending as separate files
Unethical behavior	• Allowing paper to be reviewed and revised, and then withdrawing it and sending it to another journal • Submitting to several journals at the same time • Plagiarism, self-plagiarism • Failure to identify financial conflict of interest of author
The little things	• Not taking time to address editor personally with query letter • Telling editor: "You are a fool if you pass this up." "I got an A on this paper, so I know you will want it" "I sent it to another journal but thought I'd give you first chance if you want it." "I worked really hard on this, so I cannot believe you rejected it."

The rejection notice may not give details on how to change the submission to make it acceptable. However, if faculty have experience publishing and are willing to mentor, they may help the student make the article more acceptable for publication.

To help understand the differences between these student papers and publishable papers, it is important to remember that classroom assignments serve a different purpose than professional publications. Student assignments are designed to help students demonstrate to faculty their understanding or knowledge of the professional writing of others and to provide critical analysis of that work, draw conclusions, or use the information in a creative manner—for example, to provide teaching materials or design research projects. For novices or beginners, the focus is on using the literature as they become acquainted with new content.[4] In contrast, the author published in professional publications is an expert who seeks to communicate something new. This may be an update on content in a given area, a unique case study that expands a diagnostic differential, an algorithm that helps experienced clinicians rethink how they approach a problem, or an exploration of new guidelines or research. It is the transition from novice to expert that is so difficult for many students to make.

How do you know if the manuscript was rejected because it looked like a student paper? Sometimes the editor or reviewer says directly that the article looks or reads like a school assignment. Perhaps you hear immediately from the editor and it is clear the article was rejected before it could even have been sent out for review. Or, if your article is sent for review, you might find that reviewers suggest extensive revision of the article to change the basic style.[4]

Unfortunately, when students with good writing skills and creative ideas submit articles that are rejected, some of them lose interest and never write again. Unless the journal is new and the editor is desperate for articles, the editor is rarely willing to spend time with prospective authors to help them make the article publishable. Often, authors have to learn the process of turning school papers into publishable papers through experience because editors do not specifically identify what they want in terms of professional style.[4]

A student's most important guide in making the transition from school paper to a professional publishable article is a close look at the format of the journal to which the student intends to submit the article. It seems common sense that if a student sends the editor something that is set up in the format required by the journal, has a consistent flow or argument to the content, and has headings or features similar to those commonly used in the journal, the editor is going to feel more comfortable with the submission and be more likely to consider it.

Although each journal has its distinctive style, there are some general components of professional writing that are universal. These are discussed in the following sections. Addressing these components will help you convert your student papers into more professional manuscripts.

The Audience

You might want to envision your reader coming home exhausted from a hard day's work. She or he picks up the mail on the way into the house and for a minute opens the journal that came in the mail. Think about what you can write to encourage continued reading and put that in the introduction.

Outlining

Student papers often place the main point or conclusion at the end of the paper. However, in professional papers, the reader should know the main point within the first few sentences so they are able to follow the logic of the argument or presentation throughout the article. Reinforce the same key point at the end of the article, but use different and more powerful words to make certain the meaning is clear.

Authors do not want to hear that they should write from an outline, but this is essential. All paragraphs should relate to the key point of the article in some way. If they do not, delete those paragraphs. A paper recently submitted for publication to the author's journal had no main point and wandered into five separate unrelated areas. They were all things that the writer had learned and wanted to share. They could have been related through use of a strong main point and sentences that pointed to the relationship. Even though the writer was given several chances to revise the article, she conceptually could never write an outline or pull it together. If you do not use an outline when you write the article and you cannot write an outline of your content after you finish it, then the final product does not hang together logically and will likely not be published.

Basic Definitions and Foundational Information

Do not provide lengthy definitions and basic foundational material that the readers should already know. Do not make the reader wade through content that is common knowledge or says the same thing five different ways. For example, if you are advocating a new way of doing things, you do not have to spend a lot of time discussing the old way of doing things. It is essential, then, to know the audience and to write at the audience's level.

Quotations

Never forget that people expect you as the author to be the expert. Therefore, people expect to learn what you think, not what others have concluded. It is expected that your writing will build on the work of others. Even after finding in the literature the expression of an idea just as you would like to have expressed it, avoid using long quotations. Summarize the literature in your own words and then give full citations and credit to the writers who influenced your thinking. Short quotes of words or phrases may enliven an article or enrich a clinical case study, but they should be used judiciously.

Previous Literature

Research articles will include an extensive review of the literature upon which the research is based. In most clinical articles, however, briefly summarize the relevant literature and analyze it to show how it relates to the ideas or content of the article. This is fundamental to the transformation from novice to expert. The literature summary should focus on the major points that the reader would not know. If the article is very sophisticated or complex, more foundational information may be required than for a less complex topic. Depending on the style of the journal, some articles and reports may have references to the literature interwoven throughout the entire paper rather than a separate literature review section.[4]

When summarizing the literature, avoid other common mistakes, such as evaluating each item separately or beginning a sentence with an author's name. For example, instead of writing,

> *Brown and Heartly concluded that the portion of the DNA strand that was damaged was more important than the extent of damage. Simmons and West argue that the extent of damage, when it occurs in the lower levels of the strand, is fundamental to cellular function. Bells concluded that both of these factors were important.*

It is more analytical to describe the findings of all researchers on a subject and reference them. Thus, you might write,

> *Researchers are now in agreement that both the portion of the strand and the extent of damage to the DNA are important in cellular function.*

Correct Format

Study previous issues of the journal in which you want to publish and determine what format seems best for your article. It may be a clinical feature, a case study, a research report, an update of old information, an algorithm, guidelines or consensus statement, an editorial, survey of literature, a personal opinion, or a project report. Some articles lend themselves to several different types of formats. If you are writing a research article, then standard research headings should be used. If you are writing a case study or clinical feature, note the organization and types of headings used for those types of articles in the journal. Do not attempt to write a clinical feature or case study using the headings of a research study. They just will not fit and will erroneously suggest that your manuscript is a research article.

Because APRNs are increasingly involved in publishing research, it is important to discuss some of the special challenges to publishing the results of a thesis, dissertation, or other research studies. When authors have spent a lot of time doing research, they often desire to include everything about their project in one paper. Articles that greatly exceed the recommended length, use small type to squeeze more content into the article, or provide pages and pages of references are rarely publishable and are usually rejected.[4] Thus, good research may never get published.

The publication of large projects presents special challenges. These reports often are not published because authors (1) lose interest in publication after they have met their graduation or grant deadlines; (2) do not know how to reduce the information into manageable portions; and (3) want to submit the research as they wrote it and not reorganize the content to fit the readership of the journal. Listed below are some of the formats APRNs might consider as they break down huge research projects into several smaller, more manageable articles[4]:

- Identify the most valuable or unique aspects of your research.
- Focus on identification of the problem.
- Describe the conceptual framework and theory development.
- Provide unique synthesis or analysis of past research.
- Evaluate the development of reliable and valid instruments.
- Provide descriptive cases.
- Explain the procedure for refining a research method.
- Craft a research report that is a distillation of your research.
- Share research implications and clinical applications.

Reference Guide and Key References

Remember, the audience for professional publications is different from the audience for school papers. For example, school papers frequently have long reference lists. While it may be important for graduate students to document many sources in their manuscripts, this may not be what a journal editor wants. Although the requirements for documentation differ among types of articles, editors often want authors to list only key references. Determining which references are the best reflects a higher level of thinking than just listing reference after reference. This selectivity requires evaluation and judgment of each of the references.

Remember that you are now writing for the readers, not a teacher. The readers are busy and want you to do some of the work for them; they are relying on you to refer them to the best references. Even readers of research articles want help in finding the most relevant articles on the problem, instrument, or methods. A list of 150 references after an article may not be as helpful as a selected list of the best 50, or even the best 20. One strategy for avoiding the use of too many references is to check on the average number of references used in similar articles in the journal. Some clinical journals have only a few references per article, whereas specialty, academic, and research journal articles may list 50 or more references.

Just as university educational programs require a specific reference style, so do journals. When you struggled to learn one reference style, you learned the importance of adhering precisely to the required format. That lesson will help you now. Consult the author guidelines in the journal or the journal's online Web site for the required reference format, then follow it meticulously. If you have a question and the author guidelines are not clear, consult recent publications of the journal to answer your questions.

The American Psychological Association (APA)[5] and the American Medical Association (AMA)[6] formats are commonly used in health-related publications. Publishing guidelines also provide guidance about how to cite articles published electronically. Web site links should be checked to make certain they are still active, and the most recent date of access should be included in the reference list.

Word processing programs that automatically generate footnotes should not be used, but other computer programs can help an author be consistent in following the format required by the journal. For example, Microsoft recently announced the release of publishing and research tools for academics. A free article authoring add-in for Word 2007 enables authors to structure and annotate their documents according to formats that publishers and digital archives require. The articles can then be converted easily to formats that facilitate their digital storage and preservation. Particularly for researchers, the new software products will also electronically embed details into articles about the research process and its results to help readers and other researchers who conduct searches in electronic databases find relevant articles more easily.[7] These tools should decrease the format failures that often result in articles being sent back to the author for corrections before any editor or reviewer even looks at them. Electronic formatting will also take the angst out of dealing with how to cite references that do not seem to fit the normal format.

Rechecking the Article

Once the article is written, the writer should review it for important finishing details, such as a strong conclusion, a well-written abstract, and an appropriate title. Then, the writer should have the article reviewed before submitting it.

HAVE A STRONG CONCLUSION

Review your conclusion again. You are restating your key idea. Are you hesitant? Hedging? Overly positive or negative? Did you overstate the findings? Put in too many ideas? Leave out something important? What final impression do you wish to leave with your audience? Make a special effort when composing and revising your final paragraphs.

FINALIZE THE ARTICLE TITLE AND ABSTRACT

Look again at the title of the article. It is surprising how many articles are mistitled. An abstract suggests the direction the article will take. When an article does not provide what was anticipated, that frequently indicates it was not properly titled. So, look again to make sure that your title communicates what is in your article.

The form of the abstract for research articles is dictated by the journal and by the research format itself. These abstracts may leave very little room for creativity. For most other types of articles, authors often seem surprised by the request to write an abstract and often just duplicate the introductory sentences to their article. Look at this task from the reader's point of view: The reader would not want to read the abstract and then find exactly the same words repeated at the beginning of the article. Indeed, the abstract represents an important piece of writing that should entice the reader to read the whole article. Authors should spend as much time crafting and polishing the abstract as they do the introduction and conclusion of the article. A well-written abstract is viewed positively by editors.

HAVE THE ARTICLE REVIEWED BY UNBIASED EXPERTS

No one likes to have someone point out things that are unclear or written poorly, but most articles benefit greatly from a review by people who are both content experts and style or writing experts. Each type of expert contributes different things to the polishing of the paper.

Because it is awkward for people to have their work criticized, it is essential to seek unbiased reviewers—people who have no vested interest in having the article published. A husband, wife, or boss is not an unbiased reviewer. They may be wonderful and experienced writers, but their comments will affect you more than comments from an unbiased person. You simply will care more about what people close to you say about your work and may feel hurt and/or defensive about every suggestion. So, ask your high school English teacher, a faculty member from whom you have never taken a class, or a distant colleague in another university for the review. You may even hire freelance writers to do style editing if you feel you are a poor writer. The potential for having your article published is greatly enhanced if you seek these reviews and follow the advice given.

Submitting the Article

Consult the table of contents or front matter of the journal to which you plan to submit the article. Find the editor's name and how and where to submit an article. In the past, authors were usually required to submit (by mail) up to three copies of the article to the journal headquarters or directly to the editor. The editor would then send copies out for reviews. In today's era of high technology, most submissions are now done electronically.

The author may be directed how to e-mail the article. It is increasingly common to be directed to a Web site where the article may be uploaded into an electronic editorial system, a comprehensive electronic platform that handles every component of the interaction between the prospective author and the publisher. An author entering the system is prompted to submit the article title; the article; any tables, illustrations, or graphics; an abstract; contact information; key words for the article; and conflict-of-interest forms. Materials are placed on a password-protected Web site where the editor reviews materials and sends an invitation to reviewers to critique the manuscript. The reviewers also review the article on the Web site and submit their reviews directly to the electronic system. When reviews are received, the editor evaluates them and decides whether to send the article back to the author for revision or to accept or reject the article. The electronic editorial system keeps a copy of all correspondence, publishing history, and versions of the article, so that nothing is lost. The authors are notified by e-mail about the publishing decision.

What to Expect From a Reviewer

Journal editors are not content experts in every field and so are at the mercy of busy clinicians and academicians for the review of articles. The beginning and end of semesters are difficult times to find two or three people who are both qualified and willing to take the time to review an article. The reviewers are not paid for their review and so volunteer their services rather altruistically. Finding sufficient reviewers for a busy journal is difficult and may take time. This often accounts for delays in letting authors know the fate of their articles.[8]

Reviewers are often content experts. They are knowledgeable about the subject matter and can help the editor determine if the article is accurate and up-to-date and would make a contribution to the target audience. Good reviewers look at the content, the structure of the article, the flow of the arguments, and the comprehensiveness of the presentation. They may make suggestions for additional references or dispute the author's interpretation of previous research. They may point out areas where writing is confusing, contradictory, inaccurate, or out-of-date, or where gaps in logic exist. They do not have to evaluate grammar, spelling, or writing style, although many of them do. They will also point out things they like, that they believe are helpful, and that make the article interesting. Reviewers make a recommendation that the article be accepted, revised, or rejected.

The editor will collect all the reviews. If the reviewers all agree, then the editor's action is clear. The reality is that not all reviewers may be content experts in the area about which the author is writing.[8] Sometimes the recommendations of the reviewers differ and the editor must make a decision. Sometimes the decision is to get more reviews.

Reviewers frequently make suggestions to improve the article. For many reasons, reviewers may ask the author to make changes that the author is reluctant to make. The author should be the expert in the area and must look at the suggestions for revision and make the decision about what to change. When the revised article is resubmitted, the author should also send a detailed response to indicate what the reviewers requested and how the reviewers' comments were addressed in the revision. The editor may then send the revised article out for additional reviews or, based on the revisions made, decide on whether or not to publish it. If the author failed to make essential changes that were recommended, the article is not likely to be accepted for publication.

The Fate of an Accepted Article

Depending on the publisher, an article accepted for publication is sent to a variety of editors (developmental, project, subject, and/or copy editors), managers, and members of the production staff. These people prepare the article for publication in a specific issue of the journal. Once the complete issue of the journal has been formatted and the graphics added, it is sent to the printer.

After the journal issue is printed (in a preliminary form), the authors and editors are notified that the articles are ready for proofreading. The editor than sends each article to its respective author(s) and sends the entire journal to a proofreader. Authors are faxed or e-mailed copies of the article as it will appear when published or asked to view their article on a Web site. At this point, authors have a chance to correct any errors but not to make any elective changes. After final corrections are made, the issue is returned to the printer to be published, bound, and mailed. This total production time often takes between two and three months. Meeting deadlines is extremely important to ensure that the journal meets its publication date.

What to Do If the Article Is Rejected

Because you have expended so much time and emotional energy seeking publication of your article, you will likely be very disappointed by a rejection letter. The editors should tell you clearly why your article was not accepted. It could be that you neglected to do some of the things that have been identified in this chapter as important in publishing. If so, this is a hard and discouraging way to learn a lesson. Occasionally, the author is not at fault. The author of this chapter recently received a wonderful manuscript but had already committed to publishing another article on the same topic and so had to reject the better article. So, do not be discouraged. Concentrate on what the reviewers and editor told you and resolve to do better with the next submission.

Writing for Other Forms of Media

Faculty and APRNs involved in scholarly activities may have opportunities to contribute to nursing knowledge in ways other than writing for journals. The APRN may be asked to write a journal supplement article or a chapter of a book or to be an author or co-author of a textbook, reference manual, or procedure guide. APRNs might be asked to write scripts for audiovisual productions, audiotapes, or PowerPoint presentations or to contribute to content for Web sites, pamphlets, annual reports, or grants.

Each of these tasks is a unique writing challenge. Just as prospective authors cannot convert their experiences writing student papers to writing publishable papers, many of the items that make successful journal articles would not be helpful in writing for these other media. When these other opportunities present themselves, APRNs should find a project director, editor, or professional writer who has experience in these types of publications to mentor them throughout the process. Learn to rely on the guidance of others rather than learning everything the hard way.

Contemporary Issues in Publishing

The APRN wishing to have an article published should also be aware of other issues, such as copyright, permissions to reprint, plagiarism, and conflict of interest.

Editors are particularly concerned about copyright violations and plagiarism, both increasingly common issues in publication. Unauthorized or extensive use of other people's published work is unethical. Editors and reviewers routinely check references to make sure that content is accurately quoted. Editors may also search for similar articles to see if content has been copied without attribution.

An array of new technology helps editors find authors who plagiarize. For example, SCOPUS is an online search engine that allows editors to search for related articles, references, and content by the same author. SCIRUS is an online search engine limited to scientific topics where editors may search by subject title and view similar articles. Other programs compare an article to other publications to detect identical phrases, sentences, or paragraphs. Cross-Ref.org and iParadigms (the creators of Turnitin) have designed an umbrella plagiarism detection program that will use iThenticate to verify the originality of material against a vast database of proprietary content that, to date, includes the archives of eight major scientific publishers as well as open Web sources. The software that will be used for this activity is called CrossCheck. Some search engines are more sensitive than others and may, in fact, suggest plagiarism when it does not exist. However, the likelihood that an author who uses other people's work without providing reference credit will be detected has dramatically increased.

Permissions

When an author's article includes previously published tables, illustrations, or photos, publication permission must be obtained from the copyright owner. The author should write to the journal or publisher who holds the copyright for the material and provide a copy of exactly what is to be used and where and when it will be used. The author often must provide this information on a form obtained from the publisher. The author should ask for a copy of the original graphics, illustrations, or photos in a .jpeg or .tif file, as photocopies or downloaded graphics in Word files cannot be used by the printer. It takes time to receive permission and it may require paying a fee, particularly for permission to reprint photos or illustrations. It is the responsibility of the author to seek and obtain these permissions, pay the fees, and to provide written documentation of the permission at the time the article is submitted to the journal for review.

Copyright

Once you publish an article in a journal, the copyright for that article belongs to the publisher or another designee, such as a professional association affiliated with the journal. That does not mean you cannot use the content in lectures or talks you give, but it does mean that you cannot duplicate the article and hand it out or publish it in other publications, newsletters, conference syllabi, or on a Web site without the permission of the publisher.

Self-Plagiarism

A new concept to some authors is the idea of self-plagiarism. Once you have published an article, you also are limited by the copyright laws. You should not duplicate your own writing in other articles. You might produce a number of different publications on the same topic, particularly if you have conducted research in that area, but you should write each article as an original manuscript. If an author writes multiple articles on the same topic, it is important to disclose this to the editor and to seek advice on how to handle any materials that may be viewed as duplicative. This is, understandably, a complex issue and authors might wish to read more extensively on it.[9]

Conflict of Interest

Conflict of interest is another contemporary concern. Congress, the U.S. Food and Drug Administration (FDA), universities, and pharmaceutical companies have been involved in discussions about whether content funded by business and industry can be truly unbiased. There is little agreement on this subject, but there is consensus that if authors receive financial support, either through grants, honoraria, or assistance with writing an article, this fact should be published with the article so that readers themselves might make the decision about whether they believe the content is biased. Prospective authors are now frequently asked about relationships with business and industry that might cause a conflict of interest. How conflict of interest is defined may be journal-specific, and so authors should request information about it as they submit their articles.

SUMMARY

APRNs have a lot of clinical knowledge to share with their colleagues. This chapter has reviewed some of the key steps in identifying journals in which to publish and how to write in a style appropriate for a professional paper.

SUGGESTED LEARNING EXERCISES

1. From the library or an online source, review six different issues of the same nursing journal. Compare and contrast the issues, and evaluate the format of articles, the ease of finding articles in the journal, the number of references, and the aesthetic design or appeal of the journal.

2. From the library or an online source, select three different nursing journals and compare them according to the items in question 1.

3. Select a topic for an article you would like to publish. Using the criteria in Table 10-1, rate the three journals selected in question 2 in terms of whether you feel your article would be a good fit.

4. Using an Internet search engine, find the author guidelines for at least two nursing journals. Compare and contrast the information available in the guidelines.

5. Go to a journal Web site and determine to whom a letter of inquiry should be sent, the address, and what the letter should contain.

6. Select a topic of interest to you from a thesis or dissertation available in the library. From the literature review, analyze and summarize the content in two to three double-spaced pages.

7. Identify at least two different articles that could be written based on the research, and write a brief outline of each article.

8. Using the author guidelines of the journal you prefer, outline a paper using a format you believe is most appropriate for your topic. Include all the other items, such as cover letter, abstract, or biographical sketch, that the journal would require with the submission.

References

1. See Medscape Journal Scan at http://www.medscape.com.

2. Baggs, JG. (2005). INANE. (Editorial). *Research in Nursing & Health* 28:1–2.

3. INANE closed listserve e-mail discussion among nursing editors, Spring 2008.

4. Johnson, SH. (2005). Publishing scholarly works. In Stanley, J. (ed), *Advanced Practice Nursing: Emphasizing Common Roles*, 2nd ed. FA Davis, Philadelphia.

5. American Psychological Association (APA). (2001). *Publication Manual of the American Psychological Association,* 5th ed. American Psychological Association, Washington, DC.

6. Iverson, C, et al. (2007). *American Medical Association Manual of Style,* 10th ed. Oxford University Press, New York.

7. McNaghan, P. (2008, July 31). Microsoft rolls out publishing and research tools for academics. *The Chronicle of Higher Education.* http://chronicle.com/free/2009/07/4049n.htm. Accessed September 25, 2008.

8. Fitzpatrick, JJ. (2008). Peer review: a 2008 report on the sacred academic cow. (Editorial). *Applied Nursing Research* 21:53.

9. Scanlon, PM. (2007). Song from myself, an anatomy of self-plagiarism. *Plagiary: Cross-Disciplinary Studies in Plagiarism, Fabrication, and Falsification* 2(1):1–10.

Linda Callahan received her nursing education at Rockingham Community College, Wentworth, North Carolina, and her anesthesia education at the Anesthesia Program for Nurses, North Carolina Baptist Hospital, Bowman Gray School of Medicine, in Winston Salem, North Carolina. Dr. Callahan received her bachelor of science in biology from Guilford College, Greensboro, North Carolina, and a master of arts in education and a master of science in nursing from California State University in Long Beach. She completed the doctorate in educational research and evaluation at Florida State University in Tallahassee. Dr. Callahan has a broad base of practice experience as an educator, clinician, administrator, and consultant. She has written numerous publications and is widely known as a continuing education lecturer in anesthesia and the sciences. She is past president of the American Association of Nurse Anesthetists. Dr. Callahan is a professor in the Department of Nursing, California State University, and remains active as a clinical anesthetist.

Mary Jeannette Mannino combines an independent anesthesia practice with medical-legal and business consulting. She is a graduate of George Washington University in Washington, DC, with a bachelor of science in anesthesia, and of Irvine University School of Law. Ms. Mannino's professional activities include having served as president of the American Association of Nurse Anesthetists in 1987–1988. She has been recognized for outstanding contributions to the profession, as the recipient of the Agatha Hodgins Award in 1996. She has written two books, *The Nurse Anesthetist and the Law* and *The Business of Anesthesia: Practice Options for Nurse Anesthetists*. She has also been editor of several journals and publications for nurse anesthetists. Her professional career has included work as an educator, manager, and clinical anesthetist. She currently practices anesthesia in ambulatory surgery in her own corporation, The Mannino Group.

CHAPTER 11

Legal and Ethical Aspects of Advanced Nursing Practice

Linda Callahan, PhD, CRNA; Mary Jeanette Mannino, JD, CRNA

CHAPTER OBJECTIVES

After completing this chapter, the reader will be able to:

1. Interpret components of the nurse-practice acts of his or her state, which define the legal scope of practice, need for collaboration, and prescriptive authority for a specific type of advanced practice.
2. Articulate the concepts of duty, standard of care, causation, and damage as applied to professional negligence in advanced nursing practice.
3. Demonstrate techniques for ethical decision making by application of a specific decision model as well as by analysis of the process of model application.
4. Discuss ethical issues currently of concern to APRNs.
5. Incorporate knowledge about caring as an ethical concept into the development of personal moral agency within a managed care setting.

As advanced nursing practice continues to evolve to new and exciting heights in the 21st century, legal issues have become more important to the practitioner, the state, and, of course, the patient. The expansion of nursing practice into areas once considered the exclusive domain of medical doctors and the independence of advanced practice registered nurses (APRNs) lead to questions of legality and standards of practice and the legendary "turf battles." Unfortunately, plaintiffs' attorneys have already recognized nonphysician providers as fair game. For example, even the best prepared certified nurse-midwives (CNMs) may become involved in cerebral palsy/fetal asphyxia cases, and nurse practitioners (NPs) are targets for failure to diagnose various cancers.[1] The law, including statutory, regulatory, and case law, is on a different time frame from science; therefore, it may be years before a concept becomes law and legal rulings become precedent. With that in mind, APRNs should look at rulings in other related fields to better understand the legality of their practices.

Certified registered nurse anesthetists (CRNAs) have set some legal trends for other APRNs. Although obvious differences exist between CRNAs, CNMs, NPs, and clinical nurse specialists (CNSs), most of the case law that sets precedent has been from the anesthesia portion of advanced nursing practice. The legal aspects of nurse anesthesia practice have been an area of discussion, myths, political activity, and clinical concerns for as long as the profession has existed. The legal definition of nonphysician anesthesia practitioners, the role of advanced nursing practice, state nurse-practice acts, and federal legislation continue to be debated in legal and political arenas. Likewise, medical malpractice concerns and the issue of vicarious liability accompany the nurse anesthetist to the operating room (OR) every day. Even though nurses have been administering anesthesia for more than 100 years, there have been constant legal challenges to the practice, for example, whether nurse anesthesia constitutes the illegal practice of medicine. These challenges continue in various formats and have been expanded to encompass all APRNs.

The American legal system functions at several levels, including laws enacted by the state and federal legislative branches, regulations at the executive levels, and the common-law system based on precedent. The legal authorization for all of nursing practice is found in nurse-practice acts; state health and safety codes; other professional practice acts, including those of medicine, dentistry, and podiatry; and federal medical laws and cases that interpret those laws. Judicial decisions on vicarious liability and professional negligence are important in identifying the standards of practice of the profession and set a precedent for future decisions.

It is important for the reader to understand that each state has the constitutional right to set its own laws and establish its own legal process. The cases presented in this chapter and elsewhere should be evaluated with that understanding. However, to complicate the issue, one state's courts will review similar rulings in other states when formulating their opinions.

Nurse Practice Acts

Each state has the obligation to protect the health and safety of its citizens. By various statutes, the state attempts to assure the public that a professional who is granted a license has met the qualifications and scope of practice as defined by the legislature. The nurse practice act is the prevailing state law that defines the practice for registered professional nurses. In recent years, recognition has been given to APRNs based on education, skills, and, frequently, certification. The majority of the states recognize advanced practice nursing, but there is no uniformity to their laws, with every state using different or unique language in framing its law. Generally, the advanced practice portions of the nursing statutes contain:

- A definition of advanced practice
- The legal scope of practice
- Educational requirements
- Collaboration and consultation requirements

Because laws regarding practice vary from state to state, it is imperative that practitioners be familiar with the laws and regulations in the state(s) in which they intend to practice. Most state boards of nursing have Web sites where the laws and regulations are available.

While the federal government leaves licensing issues to the states, it does get involved in certain areas of concern to NPs. One area, Medicare reimbursement, is beyond the scope of this chapter, but because practice and reimbursement can be closely related, APRNs and their professional organizations should be part of the political and legislative process on billing issues. Another area of federal authority that impacts advanced nurse practice is the Drug Enforcement Administration (DEA). This agency categorizes NPs as mid-level practitioners and as such requires DEA registration in order to dispense controlled substances (CFR § 1033.01 (b) (28)).

Historically, many states have considered advanced practice nursing to encompass nurse anesthetists, nurse-midwives, and nurse practitioners, but a recent trend in advanced practice nursing has been the formal recognition and definition of scope of practice in state laws of the CNS. The implementation of the role is subject to any number of interpretations and refinements. The traditional academic preparation of the CNS includes preparation as a clinician in a specialized area, as well as preparation as an educator, administrator, consultant, researcher, agent of change, and case manager. Although the educational level required has varied, master's-degree preparation is supported by the Federal Balanced Budget Act of 1997. This act defines a CNS as a registered nurse who is licensed to practice nursing in the state in which the services are performed and holds a master's degree in a defined clinical area of nursing from an accredited educational institution.[2] In addition to graduating from an appropriate educational program, completing the requirements for certification from a national specialty body and having recognition as an advanced practice registered nurse from a state agency, such as the Board of Nursing, are more frequently becoming a prerequisite for employment and the enjoyment of a full scope of practice. Managed care entities often use credentialing as a mechanism for establishing provider panel membership. Based upon credentialing status, CNSs may be able to seek provider status for reimbursement purposes from public and private insurers.[2]

The desire for peer review, self-regulation, and assurance of quality patient care are all part of the motivation for credentialing and privileging processes. However, other forces have also led many states and professional organizations to attempt to validate practitioner qualifications and ongoing competence. One of these external forces is the National Practitioner Data Bank (NPDB), which was established in 1986 to collect and release information related to the competence and professional conduct of physicians, dentists, and "other healthcare practitioners." The NPDB is a federal repository for data related to malpractice settlements and adverse actions against licensure or clinical privileges. The purpose is to prevent healthcare practitioners from changing locations without disclosure of previous misconduct or incompetence.

In the case of APRNs, only medical malpractice payments must be reported to the NPDB. It is optional for a state board of nursing to report any action against the license of an APRN. A practitioner may query the data bank, and although a report, if present, may not be deleted, the practitioner may request correction of any inaccuracies and submit a personal statement to be filed with the report. (The data bank helpline may be reached at 1-800-767-6732.) State licensing boards, hospitals, and other healthcare institutions have access to information in the data bank. Under certain circumstances, plaintiffs' attorneys may obtain data bank information, but members of the public, medical malpractice insurers, and defense attorneys may not do so. States vary in their requirements for submission of similar information on APRNs for storage in state data banks.[3,4]

Professional Negligence (Malpractice)

If a patient suffers harm from the actions of an APRN or any other healthcare professional, the legal theory that usually applies is the tort concept of negligence. Tort law recognizes the responsibility of an individual to act in the way an "ordinary, reasonable person" would under similar circumstances. A deviation from, or breach of, this reasonable person standard is considered actionable under the rules of negligence. The term "malpractice" has been used to encompass all liability-producing conduct by professionals.

For an action to be considered negligent, the following components must be present and established by the plaintiff:

- Duty
- Standard of care
- Causation
- Damages

Duty

To be held liable for professional negligence, it must first be established that the APRN owed a duty to the injured party. This may be established under contract theory or, most frequently, by a professional–patient relationship. The legal issue is whether or not an APRN has a legal duty to the patient, when this duty starts, and when it ends.

Ascher v. Gutierrez set the precedent for the time component of duty as it relates to anesthesia cases. There is not much direction from the courts on when the duty begins in anesthesia; however, it is generally considered to be when the anesthesia professional begins the continual care of the patient. When the legal duty ends has been addressed by the courts in the following case:

> *The facts as reported in the court decision show that the patient was an 18-year-old female admitted to Columbia Hospital for Women in Washington, DC, for dilatation and curettage. Thiopental was administered and shortly thereafter the patient developed a laryngospasm. Attempts to relax the spasm manually and by injections were unsuccessful. An endotracheal tube was inserted, but the patient was cyanotic, hypotensive, and ultimately had severe disabling brain damage.*
>
> *There was considerable dispute regarding the presence of the anesthesiologist in the operating room at the time of the incident. The anesthesiologist claimed he left the OR shortly after injecting the thiopental, but only after being relieved by another anesthesiologist. The plaintiff showed that the other anesthesiologist was administering an anesthetic in another section of the hospital when the incident occurred and could not have relieved on the case.*
>
> *The court ruled that once a physician enters into a professional relationship with a patient, he is not at liberty to terminate the relationship at will. The relationship will continue until it is ended by one of the following circumstances: (1) the patient's lack of need for further care, or (2) withdrawal of the physician upon being replaced by an equally qualified physician. The court ruled that withdrawal from the case under other circumstances constitutes a wrongful abandonment of the patient and if patient suffers any injury as a proximate result of such abandonment, physician is liable.*
>
> *The plaintiff was awarded $1,550,000.*
>
> *Ascher v. Gutierrez, 533 F2d 1235 (DC Cir), add 175 US 100 (1976)*

Standard of Care

Negligence law, in general, presupposes some uniform standards of behavior against which a defendant's conduct is to be evaluated. Members of the healthcare professions are expected to possess skill and knowledge in the practice of their profession beyond that of ordinary individuals and to act in a manner consistent with that added capability.

Formulation of the standard of care by which an APRN is evaluated is complex when one considers that an identifying characteristic of any professional group is its inherent right to direct and control its activities. The standards by which an APRN will be judged usually come from expert testimony and standards established by the profession. The judicial system recognizes that juries are composed of laypeople with limited or no knowledge of medical activities. For that reason, expert witnesses who are members of the profession are asked to testify about the standard of care. The rationale is that all professionals should be held to the same level of skill as their peers. Most professional organizations have formulated and published standards of practice for the profession. It is likely that those standards would be admitted into evidence in a negligence action and, though not conclusive of the standards of practice, would carry some authority.

While the courts look at expert testimony as indicative of the standard of care, they will also look at the regulatory requirements regarding protocols, collaboration, standardized procedures, or other types of physician oversight. For example, if a state has written protocols, like South Carolina, which requires "an approved written protocol," or Wyoming, which requires a "written plan of practice and collaboration," these protocols could be introduced as evidence in a malpractice case. If there is no written document validating the practice or if the incident that led to a malpractice suit was performed outside the guidelines of the practice, the APRN will have to defend that action. This may lead to an investigation by the nursing board.

LOCALITY RULE

Historically, the defined standards of care for the medical profession were limited to a specific geographic setting. This narrow ruling was interpreted to mean that one had to practice in terms of the standard of practice in one's community. However, the strict locality rule proved to be impractical and severely limited the pool of expert witnesses. The courts considered the fact that modern communications have expanded access to information and modified the rule to include practice in the "same or a similar locality."

In more recent years, the locality rule has undergone continued scrutiny by the courts, and in most jurisdictions, the standard has been expanded from a local level to a national level. For that reason, it is imperative that APRNs remain current in state-of-the-art practice for the entire country, because they will be held accountable for practice consistent with a national standard.

Causation

In malpractice actions, the plaintiff must establish that the alleged negligent act of the defendant caused the injury. This element of negligence, called causation, is an important factor in malpractice cases. Proof of causation may be based on direct testimony, usually by the use of expert witnesses.

The two most common tests to establish causation are classified as "but for" and "substantial factor." In the former, the plaintiff must prove that it was more probably true than not that the patient's injury would not have occurred but for the defendant's action. The substantial factor test requires that the defendant's conduct was a substantial factor in producing the injury. The standard most commonly applied to causation requires that the patient's injury has been "more likely than not" the result of the defendant's conduct.

Multiple causation can present difficulties in malpractice cases. The cause of the injury frequently is not easily determined to be due to a single factor. An example of this can be seen in anesthesia cases where a patient dies from hypovolemia. Was the cause of the death due to errors in surgical technique or failure of the anesthetist to adequately monitor and replace lost fluid? A plaintiff's attorney usually will attempt to ascertain multiple causation so that many defendants will be contributing to the damage awards.

Damages

The final element necessary for actionable negligence is damages. This term generally refers to the loss or injury suffered. Damages are usually categorized as general, special, and punitive.

The purpose of compensatory damages is to make an appropriate, and usually counterbalancing, payment to the plaintiff for an actual loss or injury sustained through the act or default of the defendant, thereby "making the plaintiff whole" as much as possible. **General damages** are those that flow from the wrong complained of and are often known as "pain and suffering." As a result of tort reform legislation seen recently in many states, a cap on general damages has been set by the legislatures. This cap is generally $150,000 to $250,000. **Special damages** are the actual monetary value of the negligent act and are reflected in such awards as additional money for hospital bills because of anticipated custodial care for life. **Punitive** or exemplary **damages** are awarded as punishment of the defendants for acts that the jury considers to be aggravated, willful, or wanton. Punitive damages are awarded or withheld at the discretion of the jury.

Wrongful Death

When a patient dies as the result of negligent acts of the provider, the survivors may collect for wrongful death. A number of states have wrongful death statutes that establish the bases for recovery and the maximum amount of damages that may be awarded. The issue of recovery for loss of life's pleasures and a wrongful death action were addressed in this Pennsylvania case involving a nurse anesthetist.

> A 5-year-old child, in excellent health, was admitted for a tonsillectomy and adenoidectomy (T & A). A nurse anesthetist supervised by an anesthesiologist administered the anesthetic. During the procedure, the anesthesiologist was called to an emergency in another OR. When he returned, he noticed the child was cyanotic with no apparent heartbeat. The nurse anesthetist was still administering a full concentration of anesthetic agent and was not using precordial monitoring. Emergency resuscitation restored the patient's heartbeat, but because of the prolonged cardiac arrest, he suffered severe damage and died several weeks later.
>
> The child's father filed suit on behalf of his son's estate for wrongful death. The jury awarded the estate $455,199 and the hospital appealed.
>
> The Pennsylvania Supreme Court ruled on the trial judge's instructions to the jury on the amount of damages. The trial court instructed the jury that it could consider pain and suffering and compensate for loss of future earnings and loss of amenities or pleasures of life. In the higher court's ruling, they said loss of life's pleasures or amenities is one of the elements of recovery for wrongful death and survival.
>
> Willinger v. Mercy Catholic Medical Center of Southern Pennsylvania, A2d 1188 (Pa 1978)

Proof of Professional Negligence

Except for certain exceptions, expert testimony is required to establish the appropriate standard of care in professional negligence cases. Both the plaintiff and the defendant rely on the testimony of expert witnesses to prove or to defend their case. Experts may also be used to determine causation and damages. To qualify as an expert witness, a person must possess qualifications and be knowledgeable in the area in question. The federal rules of evidence indicate that an expert be qualified by "knowledge, skill, experience, training, and education."

In an important case, the Illinois Supreme Court looked at whether a physician can be an expert witness in a case regarding a nurse. The court ruled that a physician could not testify as to the standard of care of a nurse. Although the case did not involve an APRN, the ruling helps to establish the professional status of nursing (*Sullivan v. Edward Hospital,*309 ILL. 2d 100.111-127, 806 N.E. 2d 645 20040).

Possible Exceptions to Expert Witness Requirement

Expert testimony is the primary method for establishing the standard of care for professionals. There are, however, exceptions to this rule that have a direct application to advanced nursing practice. Among these are manufacturer's instructions and medical literature.

PACKAGE INSERTS AND MANUFACTURER'S INSTRUCTIONS

Whether drug package inserts or manufacturer's instructions regarding use of equipment should be admissible as evidence of the standard of care is an interesting and a complex question. It is often common practice to use drugs in ways that deviate from the package inserts. The clinician is well aware that package inserts and other drug information protect the manufacturer and can be interpreted as being restrictive in practical situations.

Most courts hold that manufacturer's recommendations are at least admissible as evidence of the standard of care. However, they have seldom, if ever, been considered conclusive. A number of courts have upheld the admissibility of manufacturer's instructions where they are properly validated or refuted by an expert witness. It appears that most courts would not accept a manufacturer's recommendations and package inserts as conclusive evidence of the standard of care. Although the instructions would probably be admitted into evidence, expert witnesses would be called to reinforce the standard of practice.

MEDICAL LITERATURE

The rules of evidence clearly regard the use of textbooks, periodicals, and other literature as hearsay; thus, medical literature is not admissible as direct evidence to prove the statements it contains. The arguments against using this literature for establishing conclusive evidence of the standard of care are many and include the following:

- The author may not be present.
- There is no opportunity for cross-examination.
- The literature may be out-of-date.

One recommendation is that a more sensible view would be to hold medical literature as admissible under limited circumstances. Where a conflict exists between the medical treatise and the standards established by expert witnesses, a good approach would be to hold both sources admissible as evidence. The jury or the judge could then determine which source was most probative.

Other methods of establishing standard of care include standards and guidelines published by a professional organization, departmental policies, and statutes. In the past, most of the APRN malpractice cases involved CRNAs, but now some NP cases seem to be reaching the courts. An example is the following case:

> A patient was admitted to a Texas emergency room complaining of a migraine type headache, characterized by recurrent attacks of severe pain, usually on one side of the head. A Nurse Practitioner noted the patient's symptoms as a two-week-long episode of headache and vomiting, ejection of food and other matter from the stomach through the mouth, which was often preceded by nausea. The NP assessed the patient as having a migraine and administered medication accordingly. He released her several hours later after noting "slight improvement." A physician signed off on the NP's diagnosis. The following day, the patient was taken by ambulance to another hospital

where she died from a massive intracranial hemorrhage. In compliance with statutory requirements, the dead patient's family filed legal papers against the physician and the nurse practitioner.

In the lawsuit and subsequent appeal, the case against the nurse practitioner was dismissed because the complainant did not present testimony as to the applicable standard of care for a nurse practitioner. The court found that the experts qualified to render opinions regarding the applicable standard of care for physicians were not qualified to give expert opinion as to the applicable standard of care for nurse practitioners.

Simonson v. Keppard, No.05-06-00842-CV (06/04/2007) S.W.3d TX

In analyzing this case, several issues are relevant. The importance of expert testimony regarding the applicable standard of care cannot be underestimated. While policies and protocols are useful, expert testimony continues to be the gold standard in professional negligence cases. A cursory review of nurse practitioner lawsuits reveals a large number of cases where the issue is failure to diagnose or failure to refer. The APRN should conduct a review and analysis of these two issues on a regular basis.

Malpractice Insurance

Considering the independence of advanced nursing practice and the high level of knowledge and skill required, it follows that the responsibility and accountability of advanced practice leads to a greater risk of being sued. For that reason, APRNs should have professional negligence coverage through an insurance program.

The employment status of the APRN is important in determining whether to purchase an individual policy. Under the laws of agency, the employer is responsible for the acts of its employees and, as such, is responsible for defending and paying damages in a lawsuit occurring under the auspices of that employment. If the APRN is self-employed or uncertain of the adequacy of the employer's coverage, it may be advisable to purchase an individual policy. The cost of malpractice insurance is dependent on the type of practice and its potential for liability claims. Nurse anesthesiology and nurse-midwifery are the areas of practice with the highest malpractice insurance premiums.

Prevention of Negligence Suits

Even though it is important to have knowledge of the legal system, it is better never to have to be part of a malpractice suit, or if you are, to know how to defend yourself and your practice. Because medicine and nursing are inexact practices, no one, if honest about previous medical history, can predict how a patient will respond to treatments. Having strong practice standards, documenting care well, and having great communication skills are paramount to preventing lawsuits or defending against one. APRNs have a legal and ethical obligation to keep current on practice trends and continually evaluate the quality of their practices.

If you are served legal papers naming you in a lawsuit, it is imperative that you take them seriously and immediately notify your malpractice insurance carrier. It is also highly recommended that you take an active role in your defense. Make sure the attorney your insurance company assigns to you understands the nature of advance nursing practice and will be able to successfully defend your actions. It is worthwhile to review the literature relative to the incident that would justify your practice. Also, the legal system can be intimidating to medical and nursing professionals and your attorney should help you navigate it. Complications are not necessarily negligence and that should be a major consideration in defense of practice.

Additional Education in Law Needed

A major paradigm change in the U.S. healthcare delivery system is anticipated in the Obama administration. As a result, APRNs should see more practice opportunities. A recent study showed no difference in patient care outcomes in obstetrical anesthesia, whether the provider was an independent CRNA or an MD anesthesiologist. This study, along with numerous past studies, validates the safe practice of CRNAs as well as other APRNs.[5,6]

As nurses become more independent in their practices, additional education in areas of law not related to malpractice are needed. Business law, including contracts and negotiations, antitrust laws, and employment issues are areas that have been missing from nursing education. Also, a strong understanding of healthcare economics and the ability to apply those principles to developing new practice models will ensure a role for APRNs in the future.

The Patient and the APRN

APRNs must not lose sight of the patient in all of the discussions of nursing theory, critical learning, and legal standards. Most NPs and other APRNs select the advanced practice model of care because they enjoy caring for patients, and, in the end, concerns for patients' health and well-being and for the delivery of high-quality care are the highest priorities. For that reason, the integration of legal and ethical principles into clinical practice is paramount.

Nurses tend to view legal issues from a paternalistic rather than a practical standpoint. Frequently, they want to quote a law to justify a practice, when the law is rarely specific and is open to interpretation, modification, and reversal. It is much more practical for the individual APRN to use knowledge of applicable laws, regulations, and standards to determine how to manage a practice, to expect adequate reimbursement, and to go about doing what he or she knows and loves—providing high-quality patient care.

Professional Ethics

The branch of philosophy called ethics, or moral philosophy, deals with questions of human conduct. The word *ethics* is derived from the Greek *ethos,* meaning customs, habitual usages, conduct, and character. Ethics is concerned with defining the moral dimension of life in terms of duties, responsibilities, conscience, justice, and other societal concerns and issues. When an action is being described, the stated facts generally deal with what *is*, whereas ethical judgments require examination of the *why* of the action being described.

Ethical thinking is shaped by our worldview, which is, in turn, shaped by all the other dimensions of our existence. Today, the tendency is to separate ethics from traditional moral or religious beliefs. This is probably not entirely possible because every ethical system seems to raise questions about the worldview on which it is based.[7] Even though the world's great religions disagree in many ways, all attempt to point mankind to what lies beyond. Smart[7] stated that perhaps what is needed is "transcendental humanism," which he defined as valuing human welfare and seeing this welfare in the light of an eternal vision—that is, the sense of the beyond allowing one to see anew the sacredness of the person.

To think ethically requires defining the characteristics of an ethical problem. Rational choices are based on factual information but are always somewhat subjective; that is, they involve value judgment and, hence, the potential for value conflict. This is also a necessary characteristic of an ethical problem. Of necessity, the concept of choice involves freedom, or the ability to make a choice, and responsibility for both right and wrong actions. Choice requires reasoning and decision making. The whole unity of knowing and valuing that comprises an individual is used when human beings make choices, especially when the choices are difficult or perplexing. Though difficult, such judgments tend to establish precedent and justification for future activity. They may also serve as a model for future behavior.

Bioethics is the marriage of ethics and science. Ethical reasoning, unlike scientific reasoning, cannot be supported by definitive proof about what is the right or wrong action in a given situation. McManus[6] noted that ethics serves as a guide to the development of a "well-traveled trail" that may lead to better behavior and better actions among people. The APRN is often faced with concerns and conflicts between the practice of value-based clinical ethics, business ethics, and social ethics.[8] Different concerns, questions, and conflicts arise in each (Table 11-1). Current Web-based sources for further discussions of nursing ethics may be found in Table 11-2.

Table 11-1 Three Dimensions That Impact the Practice of Value-Based Ethics

Dimensions of the Workplace	Value-Based Questions of Concern to the Specific Dimension
1. Clinical ethics	What judgments about clinical behaviors can be made in light of the relationship of the nurse to the patient? What are the ethical demands and limits of service and staffing? How are these known and agreed upon, or established? What are the ethical obligations of the nurses or institution to meet the needs of individuals or families? When are needs ethically not met?
2. Business ethics	What is the obligation of the institution to act in ways that respect the rights, dignity, and values of both caretaker and client? What are the duties of the trustees, managers, and other workers as they interact with individuals and social groups?
3. Social ethics	How does the organization meet the needs of its community? How does the organization carry out tasks with providers, payers, regulators, and other entities in health care? How does this affect the larger society?

Adapted from Cofer, MJ. (2000). Thoughts on ethics: value-based ethics in the workplace. *VA Nurses Today* 8(1):12–13.

Table 11-2 Websites Devoted to Nursing Ethics

Source	Website
ANA Center for Ethics and Human Rights	http://www.nursingworld.org/ethics/
Boston College School of Nursing	http://www.bc.edu/bc_org/avp/son/ethics
Nurse Friendly Site	http://www.nursefriendly.com/
Center for Applied and Professional Ethics	www.csuchico.edu/cape
Nursing Ethics: An International Journal for Health Care Professionals	http://nej.sagepub.com
Technology's Dark Side	http://www.curtincalls.com
American Society for Bioethics	http://www.asbh.org/
Virtual Mentor: American Medical Association	http://www.virtualmentor.org/
Kennedy Institute of Ethics	http://www.kennedyinstitue.georgetown.edu

Adapted from Sullivan, BH. (2001). Linkages. Web sites devoted to nursing ethics. *Wash Nurse* 1(1):38.

Historical Perspectives

In 1937, C. A. Aikens[9] wrote *Studies in Ethics for Nurses* and included chapters devoted to truth in nursing reports, discretion in speech, obedience, teachability, respect for authority, discipline, and loyalty. Such early works focused on the morality of the individual and on the nurse's duties, obligations, and loyalties. The American Medical Association (AMA) adopted a Code of Ethics in 1847 when the organization was formed. This was a hallmark event, because before this time, there was no regulation of professional behavior. The AMA's initial Code of Ethics dealt with the relationships of physicians to each other, to the patient, and to the public. Revisions followed, with continual emphasis on professional conduct. Over time, this activity helped to solidify the idea that medicine was a dignified and honorable calling. Professional codes of ethics generally call for a covenant, or an agreement, between the client and the provider and are today viewed as a social contract.[6]

The contrast in ethical development between medicine and nursing has often been remarkable. This is due largely to the fact that nursing has historically been allied to the ideal of treating the person, rather than the disease. From this belief, the notion of the superiority of prevention over cure developed. Medicine, on the other hand, has historically emphasized curing as a response to the presence of disease. The APRN is often called on to combine the concerns of both perspectives. Complex technological problems, new legal issues, and new economic situations offer a challenging context for ethical thinking and behavior for today's APRN.

Ethical Principles

All ethical problems involve moral principles. Such principles are necessary to provide guidance for thought because universal solutions that can be applied by rote to another problem cannot be reached in most ethical dilemmas. Each ethical problem must be examined in the context of the particular circumstances. Five guiding principles are important to nursing:

1. Autonomy
2. Nonmalfeasance
3. Beneficence
4. Justice
5. Fidelity

AUTONOMY

Self-determination, or autonomy, is a basic social value. An autonomous act is an act of intention that is independent of coercion by others. This moral right was defined by Callahan[10] as follows:

> *The right to control one's body and one's treatment and the emphasis given to self-determination, privacy, freedom, and autonomy. The emphasis on not being deceived and being given complete and truthful information, all point to an important aspect of a rights-based view, namely the role of an individual patient's will in individual decision making*[10] (p. 19).

Those giving care must acknowledge and respect the autonomy of each client. It may be argued that the only permissible reason to remove a person's social or personal autonomy is to prevent harm to others. Respect for the client's autonomy and the opportunity for professional autonomy in medical practice involve possession of the threshold element of competence, the disclosure of information, and consent without duress. The presence of these three elements imposes an order on conflicting claims and offers finality, which is often sufficiently strong to override the law and prevailing custom.[6]

As a result of the Karen Anne Quinlan case of 1976 and the Nancy Cruzan case of 1989, the focus on the autonomous rights of the patient sharpened. These two cases also focused on the rights of families or surrogates to make choices for an incompetent patient. The Patient Self-Determination Act of 1990 obligated hospitals that accepted payment from federal reimbursement plans to offer education to all patients about advanced directives and to provide a means for the individual to execute an advanced directive. These events led to the recognition that the decision-making power once accorded only to physicians was now to be shared by the individual patient and any number of other chosen surrogate decision makers.[11]

To be able to make personal healthcare decisions, patients need to understand all options available to them, the possible consequences of acting on certain options, and the costs and benefits of the possible consequences. It is essential that the APRN assist patients in understanding how their decisions and values may be received in the general societal context in which they live and how their decisions might impinge on the rights of others. It must be remembered that disagreeing with the recommendation of the physician or APRN is not singularly grounds for determining that the patient is incapable of making a decision.[12]

NONMALFEASANCE

Nonmalfeasance is the concern for doing no harm or evil. Generally, the reference is to physical harm, pain, disability, and death, but harm can be defined both broadly and narrowly. Actions that inflict harm may be necessary for ultimate client well-being, but such actions always require moral judgment. Doing something and doing nothing are both actions determined by personal decision. As an example, withdrawal of treatment is often deemed a nonmaleficent decision. If "letting die" seems justifiable, the withdrawal of nutrition and hydration is usually seen as justified. The literature does not support the concept that cessation of artificial feeding and hydration is associated with pain or suffering, although there may be increased stress for caregivers and family. The principle of nonmaleficence requires an interpretation of values and the consideration of risks and benefits as part of a thoughtful and careful action.[6]

BENEFICENCE

Beneficence is the act of promoting or doing good. This principle is action-oriented and requires the provision of benefits and the balancing of harms and benefits. Ethical problems arise when benefits are conflicting. The principle of beneficence often appears at odds with the principle of veracity or truthfulness.

JUSTICE

Justice requires weighing issues and responding to the facts that are present. Philosophically, no consensus exists about what constitutes justice. The nurse in advanced practice is responsible for exhibiting just behavior and distributing comparable treatment to each client; therefore, justice is an active process. Retributive justice demands that if a client is harmed, reparation or a means by which to right the wrong be applied.

FIDELITY

Fidelity includes ideas such as loyalty, faithfulness, and honoring commitments. These concepts are the basis of a therapeutic relationship between the APRN and the patient that will exhibit stability and growth.[13]

Bases of Ethical Theory

Using the basic ethical principles, philosophers have constructed various theories that may form the bases for ethical analysis. Moral theories generally address compliance with rules, the consequences of action, or dispositions relative to behavior. These three variants are often classified into normative and non-normative approaches.

The **normative approach** explores ethical obligations and duties. This approach allows investigation of what is right and wrong, what we are to be, and what we may value.[6] At present, all humans live in a global village in which different cultures and worldviews interact.[11] In today's global society, it is essential that ethical decision-making models be inclusive of cultural variables. The Transcultural Integrative Model proposed by Garcia[14] includes four major steps:

- Awareness and fact finding
- Formulation of courses of action and determination of the best possible ethical decisions
- Identification of potentially competing nonmoral values that could interfere with the implementation of the selected action
- The implementation, documentation, and evaluation of the plan of action

At each step there is an emphasis on the incorporation of arbitration, negotiation, and consensus-building and on the use of relational strategies as part of decision formation. The cultural values, cultural identity, level of acculturation, and gender-role socialization of both the client and the APRN influence the view of each concerning the presence and seriousness of a defined dilemma. Garcia also stresses the virtues of attention to the situational context, tolerance, sensitivity, and openness as necessary elements for implementation within this model.

An optimal normative approach would call for tolerance and the formation of a society in which there is genuine plurality of beliefs and values in order to breed an ethic of "social personalism." Under this ethic, each person respects the social values of the other because there is genuine respect for that person. **Non-normative** theoretical variants presuppose universally applicable principles of right and wrong and seek systematically to provide justifiable answers to moral questions. One may assess the rightness or wrongness of an act by examining the interests of the actor or by assessing the consequences of the act itself.

Non-normative theoretical variants may take several approaches. **Deontology**, or the act of examining the interests of the actor in performing certain acts, is derived from the Greek word *deontais* ("duty"), which originally meant obedience to rules or binding duties. This sense of duty should consist of rational respect for fulfillment of obligations to other human beings. For example, the commanding duty for the health professional is to respect clients and colleagues and their right to autonomy (self-determination). Emmanuel Kant (1724–1804) asserted that respect for persons is the primary test of duty. He stated that all persons have equal moral worth, and no rule can be moral unless all people can apply it autonomously to all other human beings. The deontological approach is often applied by health professionals who work with individual clients.

Teleology (utilitarianism) is a consequentialist, paternalistic approach. The root, *telos,* comes from the Greek for "end of the consequences." All acts are evaluated as positive to the extent to which desirable results are achieved. The right action is that which leads to the best consequence and the greatest good. This is often the ethical foundation applied in the formation of healthcare policy decisions. A difficulty with this approach is the problem of defining and properly weighing the greatest good as well as deciding who should receive the act.[6]

Responses of APRNs to Ethical Issues

Rapid advances in technology make many demands on the character, education, and abilities of the APRN. Applying ethical responsibility in health care does not require the discovery of new moral principles on which to build a new theoretical system. Nor does it require one to evaluate new approaches to ethical reasoning. It does encourage professionals to lay down a proper foundation for the application of established moral rules. Society and the professions demand that practitioners be knowledgeable in the applied field of healthcare ethics and the process of ethical decision making.[6] Ethical issues facing APRNs in daily practice include, but are by no means limited to, informed consent, the right to refuse treatment, the level of competence of incapacitated patients, breaches in confidentiality, dealing with poor prognosis and terminal illness counseling, withholding of information and truth telling, resuscitation/end-of-life decisions, and genetic counseling and privacy concerns.

Laabs'[15] research indicated that maintaining moral integrity in the face of moral conflict was most important to NPs, who tended to act upon issues of moral conflict based on the meaning that the particular conflict had for them as a person of integrity. The process of decision making was influenced by the NP's work environment, role and relationship with the patient, previous knowledge and experience, and personal value perspective. The actual decision-making process required recognition of the conflict situation, drawing a line at what the NP was willing to do and not do, finding a way to meet the patient's needs without crossing this self-imposed line, and evaluating the resulting actions in terms of how well the NP's integrity had been maintained. Moral integrity may be defined as the ability to perceive oneself both as a person living a moral life and a professional who does both the good and right thing in practice. Threats to practicing with moral integrity in the workplace most often included time constraints, pressures to meet productivity quotas, lack of respect for the differing beliefs among healthcare providers, the right of healthcare providers to practice according to their conscience, and the constraints of the larger healthcare delivery system.

In 1984, Jameton defined three types of moral problems experienced by nurses in hospital settings:

1. Moral uncertainty or not being sure what the moral issue is or what moral principles might apply
2. A dilemma in which two or more moral principles may apply but clearly support two mutually inconsistent courses of action
3. Moral distress that is present when the nurse clearly knows what to do but institutional constraints make the appropriate action difficult, if not impossible[16]

Wilkinson[17] adds the concept of moral outrage, which is defined as the witnessing of an immoral act by another provider that the observer feels powerless to stop or correct. Research indicates that NPs may experience similar events but define them in different terms.[16,18,19] Types 1 and 2 above were not found to be expressive of the NP experience to any great extent, but moral distress and moral outrage required further exploration. A descriptive study conducted by Laabs [16] surveyed NPs in primary care family, adult, gerontological, pediatric, or women's health practices. The issue identified most frequently as distressing to NPs was refusal of appropriate treatment by the patient. The need to bend rules to ensure appropriate patient care and the need to function under policies and procedures inconsistent with their own personal values was second. Third was the pressure to see an excessive number of patients. Other distressful issues listed by NPs included the patients' lack of access to health care, restrictive insurance policies, restrictive formularies, inadequate allocation of resources, dealing with the rights of minors and parents, abortion issues, and competition between physicians and APRNs for patients. Other situations that NPs found highly distressing related to clinical decision making by other providers, the inability of patients to pay for services, patients not being adequately informed regarding needed care or options for care, and situations in which there were inadequate responses from agencies to whom patient abuse or neglect were reported.

Unfortunately, when moral distress or outrage are present for the APRN, a consistent theme—powerlessness and anger at the inability to remedy the situation—seems to appear. Such feelings often lead to either bending the rules covertly to ensure appropriate patient care, protectively covering themselves through extensive documentation, leaving the practice setting, or abandoning the APRN role completely.

AUTONOMY VS. BENEFICENCE

Many professional nursing organizations emphasize respect for patient autonomy as the central component of the nurse/patient relationship, but inherently bound with this respect is the obligation or duty to do that which is best for the patient and his or her health. This supports beneficence, rather than autonomy, as the central moral principle in medical/nursing ethics.[16,20]

Using as an example the identified distress experienced by the APRN when a patient refuses treatment or does not comply with other care recommendations, one can see how a conflict between respecting patient autonomy and acting beneficently can be present. Laabs[16] points out that the NP may have a strong relationship with the patient and may feel a strong moral responsibility for the outcomes of care in this individual, thereby experiencing a certain level of distress at the patient's decision not to follow treatment recommendations. This distress may indeed be a positive event in that it indicates the NP's strength of moral compass and understanding of what "the good" is in the situation. This level of distress under certain situations may inspire continued efforts by the NP to seek alternative ways to bring about positive outcomes for the patient.

Moral distress happens to nurses at all levels of practice, but stressors in the workplace and the perceived greater level of responsibility have been closely associated with the role of the NP. NPs in primary care have reported feelings of anger, guilt, powerlessness, and frustration so great in some practice situations that changing jobs or leaving advanced practice completely has seemed the only answer.[15] APRNs often cite experiencing distress related to external forces, such as an employer or consultant not taking an action that is morally correct. Additionally, there may be outrage at the immoral actions of others in the practice situation. Some writers have noted that when compared with the emergent, life-threatening ethical issues common in acute care nursing, the ethical issues experienced by the NP in the community may be more subtle, mundane, and difficult to define fully, although the issues remain complex.[15,21,22]

Braunack-Mayer [23] suggests at least four significantly different characteristics of general or primary care impact the perception and handling of ethical issues over other care settings. These characteristics include (1) the long-standing nature of therapeutic relationships that exist between patients and providers; (2) the family interactions and participation as both patients and concerned relatives; (3) the ability to adopt a "wait-and-see" attitude to watch for further development over time, which is rarely possible in hospital medicine; and (4) the incorporation of health maintenance and illness prevention strategies into the general and on-going care given by the clinician.

ETHICAL DILEMMAS

Providers are bombarded with reams of information each day in clinical practice. Consciously and unconsciously, they make selections from these data and draw conclusions about themselves, their clients, and their lives. All information carries equal weight until value is assigned by the individual. Valued information stimulates further exploration of potential meaning. Dilemmas often occur as problems that require ethical decisions emerge. A **dilemma** is a choice between equally undesirable alternatives. The two essential components of an ethical dilemma are:

1. The existence of a real choice between possible courses of action, and

2. The placement by decision makers of different values on each possible action or on the outcome of that action.

When surveyed nurses reported that when attempting to resolve ethical dilemmas, they sought the aid of nursing colleagues much more often (84%) than that of ethics committees, pastors, social workers, journals, or physicians. Ethics committees were chosen as an option in only 28% of responses, while other resources used included journals (33%), physicians (38%), pastors (48%), and social workers (45%).[17,19]

Ethical Decision Making in the Genomic Era

The unraveling and interpretation of the human genome by researchers of the Human Genome Project has broad implications for health care and society in the 21st century. Increased genetic knowledge and technological development have led to a new taxonomy for understanding disease that is predicated on the contribution of both environmental factors and genetics to the incidence and severity of disease. The increased knowledge has also led to a proliferation of techniques for and the availability of genetic testing and the promise of genotype-guided or individualized health care. This new era has been defined as the "third stage of medicine—molecular medicine."[24,25] Warner and colleagues[26] have described genetics as "the most powerful example yet" of how technological progression drives organizational change in health care.

The APRNs now entering the field will face new and never-before-considered major ethical problems grounded in genetics.[27] For example, given changing genetic technology in impregnation technology and increased potential for prenatal testing and modification of embryos, CNMs and other APRNs in women's health and pediatrics will face greater changes involving pregnancy—for example, how to become pregnant, who can become pregnant, and when pregnancy is possible. APRNs in primary care will be called upon to play a more significant role in the assessment and management of genetic risk for disease. Given such a scenario, enhanced genetics education is needed in nursing undergraduate and graduate curricula.[25,28,29]

Empowering Patients

The revolution in care that will be attributable to genetics has just begun but has already provided a wealth of information and an ever-increasing array of genetic tests with which APRNs need to cope. No nursing specialty will remain untouched. Genetics education programs that remain flexible in incorporating new discoveries need to be put in place, thereby allowing the immediate integration of new discoveries into advanced practice. The APRN should possess sufficient knowledge and critical skills to be able to fully participate in the discussion of controversial issues, as well as the appropriate application of new technologies that are and will continue to become available.[25]

Many of the ethical issues associated with genetics revolve around the need to protect patient privacy or confidentiality and at the same time protect societal interests. Patient advocacy, education regarding options, and support of the patient's right to informed consent will be an important part of the genetics counseling expected of all APRNs. The facilitation of ethical decision making is often best taught in real-life situations, and technological advances in genetics offer numerous issues with ethical implications for exploration.

In the genomic era, as intervention and technology increase in complexity, it will become increasingly difficult for patients or surrogate decision-makers to fully understand the mechanisms and potential consequences of recommended treatment. The inability to gain full understanding will compromise true informed consent and will be a threat to the concept of autonomy. At what point should the competency and judgment of the clinician rightly supersede the ability of the patient to understand what is in his own best interests? This issue, given its complexity, is certainly a topic meriting further discussion and research.[28]

Genetic Screening

Genetic screening provides an example of the concerns associated with ethical decision making in this new era. Genetic screening is a population-based means of identifying people with certain genetic structures associated with a disease or the predisposition to a genetic disease. Newborn screening is carried on in most states to identify infants with genetic disorders in which early treatment can prevent or ameliorate the sequelae. Although this seems to be in the best interest of all, there are factors to be considered. The validity of the test results is an ongoing concern because false-positive results cause unnecessary concerns for the parents and possible stigmatization of the child, whereas false-negative reports leave the child at significant risk. Criteria for effective newborn screening programs, and potentially all screening programs, as outlined by Nussbaum and asscoiates[29] include the following:

- Treatment for the disease being screened is available.
- Early treatment of the disease has been shown to reduce or eliminate the severity of the disease.
- Routine observation and examination of the child will not reveal the disease.
- A rapid and economical laboratory test that is highly sensitive and has reasonable specificity is available.
- The disease is frequent enough and serious enough in the population to warrant screening costs.
- Healthcare structures are in place to inform the parents of the findings, confirm the results, and institute the appropriate treatment and counseling.

Phenylketonuria (PKU) and galactosemia are two heritable diseases that clearly satisfy all the above criteria. Most parents would readily want their children tested at birth for these diseases, but the wishes of parents who dissent must be considered. The APRN, in the role of patient advocate, would, in a nondirective, unbiased way, make sure that the parents have adequate information about the nature of the screening, about any other genetic tests that might be part of the test battery, about any other information that might be obtained about the genetic makeup of the child or other family members, and about their right to agree or disagree to screening in accordance with the laws of the state in which they reside.

It is beyond the scope of this chapter to explore fully the social, ethical, and legal ramifications of the constantly increasing genetic knowledge that is now and will forever change medical and nursing practice. The APRN needs constantly to explore specialty-specific ethical ramifications of genetic discoveries and applications in order to make ethically responsible decisions about care and counseling offered to the individual and family. An excellent source of information is the Ethical, Legal, and Social Implications [of the] Human Genome Project. This source may be accessed at http://www.kumc.edu/gec/prof/geneelsi.html, which is a gateway to a number of other online ethics sources.

Need for Collaboration Among Healthcare Providers

The almost daily need for adequate ethical decision making should offer another opportunity for collaboration between APRNs, physicians, and other healthcare team members. In an editorial, Waldman, a physician, noted that 25 years ago the idea of collaborating with non-physicians was "akin to conspiring with the enemy."[1] He went on to say that physicians who were able to embrace collaborative practice at the outset were "blessed with the inner strength to not be threatened by professionals with a different approach to his specialty, women's health." Data from many studies have indicated that collaborative practice has improved access to care and improved patient satisfaction without eroding quality. In order to develop such skills there must be the recognition by physicians that the "sacred trust" of total responsibility for care has shifted from the primary care physician to a more fluid, patient-centered system involving medical specialists, APRNs, physician assistants (PAs), clinical social workers, therapists, and medical ethicists.[10]

Data from a recent descriptive study of third-year medical students conducted by Lomis, Carpenter, and Miller[30] indicated that the issues most frequently described as distressing were problems of communication, either with patients, families, or other healthcare providers. In this study, communication conflicts within the care team correlated with higher levels of distress than any other factor solicited from these medical students. The need for excellent collaborative skills between the physician and the APRN is of extreme importance when the need for ethical decision making is paramount in clinical and practice situations.[1]

In an earlier study, Blake and Guare[31] noted that when practitioners found themselves in ethical dilemmas, their interactions were bound up in adherence to policy, patient's rights, caring, and a shared balance between what they perceived as the ideal action versus the most realistic action. Ethical decisions continue to be complicated by perceived differences in experience, education, ethnicity, collegialism, authority, and feelings of powerlessness. Most clinicians perceived that the ethics of caring had limits, which were most often manifest when the application of ethical principles placed them in positions divergent from peers, families, patients, and the power structure within healthcare organizations.

Time and Levels of Decision Making

Decision-making models offer the nurse in advanced clinical practice an opportunity for self-examination and self-knowledge. Clinical decisions are most often of mixed character, containing moral dimensions but rarely being solely moral decisions. Ethical decision making is consistent with critical thinking. Situations must be processed by the identification of ethical dimensions within the context and by the application of principles of moral reasoning. This process offers the greatest assurance that final decisions or courses of action will be the "best." Use of the critical reasoning process produces less chance for mistakes based on ignorance, personal bias, or strong paternalism. Tong[32] holds that although there may be neither a right nor wrong answer in ethical decision making, the best decision will always be the result of consistent consensus-building, negotiation, and compromise between the major stakeholders in the clinical situation.

The complex process of ethical decision making leads to making a decision, acting on it, and justifying the action. In some situations, providers are participants, but at other times, they function only to share a point of view. Three levels of decision making are believed to exist:

1. The immediate level, which is characterized by no time for reflection
2. The intermediate level, in which there is some time for exploration and reflection
3. The deliberate level, in which adequate time exists to gather and examine information and to reach a rational decision after reflection[6]

An important construct in ethical decision making remains the concept of time. It is certainly most desirable to have time to gain understanding, to gather information, to consider and build consensus, and to plan and implement. Unfortunately, APRNs are frequently called upon to make swift decisions in situations in which time is of the essence. Such swift decisions are generally made based upon one's beliefs, and if these beliefs are sound, then the decisions made are usually defensible. From an Aristotelian viewpoint, good practice in ethical decision making is a matter of developing good habits when one has time to think. Having done so, one is more likely to make good decisions when under a time constraint.[33]

In clinical practice, providers must guard against a tendency to avoid making a choice when it is necessary to do so. Procrastination used to avoid responsibility should be avoided, as should hastened judgment that precludes careful reflection. There are levels of immediacy in decision making. However, the fact that decisions must be made immediately in some situations cannot be used to excuse the lack of thoughtful action in other situations. For example, it is justifiable to give treatment in an emergency situation (i.e., when a person is in immediate danger of death) without the patient's informed consent. However, it is not justifiable to do this in situations in which some time is available. Though often avoided, the deliberate level of decision making is by far the most common in clinical practice. Making difficult ethical decisions is often avoided because such decisions are personally taxing, require the acceptance of great responsibility, and cannot be accomplished successfully without sensitivity to the human rights and values of others.

Decisions, including ethical decisions, do not occur in a vacuum but are operant within a context that consists of an inner and outer environment. The sum of an individual's experiences make up the inner environment. The outer environment consists of the actions and reactions of others, time constraints, and material resources. It is improbable that the environmental events that modify the setting of a decision will be repeated, and the operational self brought to the decision-making situation cannot be repeated. In this sense, all decisions are unique, but not necessarily unrelated.

Need for Continuing Education in Ethics

Scanlon[34] proposes several models of ethical discernment that can be incorporated into clinical practice settings and may offer practitioners the opportunity to feel more adequately prepared to undertake independent ethical decision making. These include clinically based educational programs that help the practitioner explore his or her patient advocacy obligations and assume leadership roles in ethical discernment. This idea is supported by the work of Ulrich and Soeken[35] in which it was noted that general ethics education did not appear related to ethical conflict in practice; however, learning about ethics through continuing education events had a significant effect on autonomy in the APRNs in the study. It has been hypothesized by Hamric[36] that continuing education in ethics may allow nurses the opportunity for shared ethical discussion and decision making that are specific to practice, thereby helping them to develop the specific skills needed to deal with issues of moral agency in actual clinical care situations.

Nursing ethics groups also may provide a forum for the acquisition of knowledge and skill development through sample case critiquing and evaluation of ethics practices. Consultation with skilled ethicists and/or participation in multidisciplinary ethics committees can facilitate communication, mediate conflicts, and alleviate distress related to moral ambiguity. APRNs are an important asset to multidisciplinary ethics teams due to their unique perspective and expertise in direct engagement with the patient. If available, having APRNs participate in ethics rounds is to be desired, as this allows sharpening of assessment skills and recognition of seemingly nonimportant clinical issues that have the potential for developing into future ethical dilemmas.

Decision-Making Models

Since the early 1970s, a number of decision-making models have been developed for use by healthcare providers. Most of these models have focused on dilemmas as "triggers" for ethical analysis. An appropriate example is the Thompson and Thompson Decision Model for Nursing; it depicts a problem-solving process and allows critical review of the operant situation and assessment of all the variables and highlights pertinent ethical issues raised by the situation. Tables 11-3 and 11-4 provide the model and an analysis of the process of model application.

Table 11-3 **Thompson and Thompson Decision Model**

1. Review the situation and identify
   a. Health problems
   b. Decisions needed
   c. Key individuals involved

2. Gather information that is available to
   a. Clarify the situation
   b. Understand the legal implications
   c. Identify the bureaucratic or loyalty issues

Continued

Table 11-3 **Thompson and Thompson Decision Model—cont'd**

3. Identify the ethical issues or concerns in the situation and
   a. Explore the historical roots
   b. Explore current philosophical/religious positions on each
   c. Identify current societal views on each

4. Examine personal and professional values related to each issue, including
   a. Personal constraints raised by the issues
   b. Guidance from professional codes or standards
   c. Moral obligations to individuals

5. Identify the moral positions of key individuals by
   a. Direct questioning
   b. Consideration of advance directives
   c. Consideration of substituted judgments

6. Identify value conflicts, including
   a. Potential sources of each
   b. Possible strategies for the resolution of each

7. Determine who should make the final decision, considering
   a. Who owns the problem
   b. Whether the patient can participate in the decision process
   c. Who can speak on behalf of the patient (substituted on basis of best-interest judgment) when patient cannot

8. Identify the range of possible actions and
   a. Describe the anticipated outcome for each action
   b. Identify the elements of moral justification for each action
   c. Note if the hierarchy of principles or utilitarianism is to be used

9. Decide on a course of action and carry it out
   a. Knowing the reasons for the choice of action
   b. Sharing the reasons with all involved
   c. Establishing a time frame for a review of the outcomes

10. Evaluate the result of the decision/action and note
    a. Whether the expected outcomes occurred
    b. If a new decision process is complete
    c. Whether elements of the process can be used in similar situations

Table 11-4 **Analysis of the Thompson and Thompson Decision Model**

Step 1: Review the situation. The first step involves identifying significant components of the situation, as well as the individuals involved in making the decision. A clear understanding of the situation facilitates each subsequent action.

Step 2: Gather additional information. Additional information that may influence the situation is collected in this step. Demographic data, socioeconomic status, health status, prognosis, level of understanding, preferences, competence, and family members and/or significant others involved with the situation are examples of additional information that needs to be assessed.

Table 11-4 **Analysis of the Thompson and Thompson Decision Model—cont'd**
Step 3: Identify the ethical issues. Understanding ethics and ethical principles is essential to accurately identify the issues of the situation. Another key to successful identification of the ethical issues is to gain a historical perspective on the issues.
Step 4: Identify personal and professional values. When a nurse defines his or her personal and professional moral positions as they relate to ethical issues, the nurse is better prepared to understand his or her positions in a particular situation. Awareness of professional codes will help to identify professional values.
Step 5: Identify values of key individuals. The moral values of the key people involved in the situation are as important as the nurse's values and are assessed at this step.
Step 6: Identify value conflicts. Value conflicts can occur within one individual or between the persons involved in the situation. Understanding why conflicts exist and keeping track of how conflicts have been resolved in the past assist with the final decision.
Step 7: Determine who should decide. Many people are available to assist in making the final decision. The physician, nurse, social worker, patient's family are all involved in heath-care ethics. At this point, it must be decided who should be responsibler for the decision or action.
Step 8: Identify range of actions with expected outcomes. A clear list of alternatives helps the nurse recognize possible consequences of a decision and identify a course of action.
Step 9: Decide on the course of action and carry it out. The person must decide on the course of action.
Step 10: Evaluate results of the decision. The final step involves evaluating the decision made to determine if the outcome was the one anticipated. Evaluation also provides information that assists in future ethical decision making.

A second example, the Ethical Assessment Framework (EAF) as outlined by Cassells and Gaul,[37] may be found in Table 11-5.

Lutzen[27] argues for context-sensitive theoretical frameworks in ethics to try to grasp the ethical problems emerging from changing technology and genomic advances, as well as from new difficulties arising from changing financial compensation methods and the functional abnormalities and inadequacies of the overall healthcare delivery system.

Table 11-5 **Ethical Assessment Framework**	
Steps	**Activities**
ASSESSMENT	
1. Identify the problem.	Issues, conflicts, and/or uncertainties
2. Gather relevant facts.	Medical (objective data), contextual (subjective data), policies, state and federal laws, etc.
3. Identify methods of ethical justification to help resolve the dilemma.	Consequentialism (consequences), deontology (duty), principalism (principles), care (relationships), casuistry (cases), virtue (character)

Continued

Table 11-5 **Ethical Assessment Framework — cont'd**	
4. Consciously clarify values, rights, and duties of patient, self, and significant persons associated with the issue.	
5. Identify if there is an ethical problem.	
6. Identify guidelines from nursing and professional codes of ethics.	
7. Identify and use relevant interdisciplinary resources.	Ethics committees, ethics consultants, clergy, literature, administrators, lawyers, colleagues, etc.
8. Identify and prioritize alternative actions/options.	
PLAN OF ACTION 9. Select a morally justified action/ option from the alternatives identified.	
IMPLEMENTATION 10. Act upon/support the action/option selected.	
EVALUATION 11. Evaluate action/options taken.	Perform short- and long-term follow up

Adapted from Cassells, JM, & Gaul, AL (1998). An ethical assessment framework for nursing practice. *MD Nurse* 17(1):9–12.

An additional aid to decision making may be found in the Code of Ethics revised by the American Nurses Association (ANA) House of Delegates in 2001.[38] The changes in the document reflect the new challenges that are now facing all nurses as a result of technological innovations. The nine general provisions of the code are listed in Table 11-6.

The Codes of Ethics for CRNAs and CNMs are delineated in Tables 11-7 and 11-8. Table 11-9 provides an overview of a proposed code of ethics for NPs based on the AANP Standards of Practice.

Table 11-6 **ANA Code of Ethics for Nurses**[37]
Nine General Provisions
1. The nurse, in all professional relationships, practices with compassion and respect for the inherent dignity, worth, and uniqueness, of every individual, unrestricted by considerations of social or economic status, personal attributes, or the nature of the health problem.
2. The nurse's primary commitment is to the patient, whether an individual, family group, or community.
3. The nurse promotes, advocates for, and strives to protect the health, safety, and rights of the patient.
4. The nurse is responsible and accountable for individual nursing practices and determines the appropriate delegation of tasks consistent with the nurse's obligation to provide optimal patient care.

Table 11-6 **ANA Code of Ethics for Nurses[37] — cont'd**

5. The nurse owes the same duties to self as to others, including the responsibility to preserve integrity and safety, to maintain competence, and to continue personal and professional growth.

6. The nurse participates in establishing, maintaining, and improving health-care environments and conditions of employment conducive to the provision of quality health care and consistent with the values of the profession through individual and collective action.

7. The nurse participates in the advancement of the profession through contributions to practice, education, administration, and knowledge development.

8. The nurse collaborates with other health professionals and the public in promoting community, national, and international efforts to meet health needs.

9. The profession of nursing, as represented by associations and their members, is responsible for articulating nursing value, maintaining the integrity of the profession, and shaping social policy.

From http://nursingworld.org/ethics/chcode.htm.

Table 11-7 **Code of Ethics for the Certified Registered Nurse Anesthetist**

Preamble
Certified Registered Nurse Anesthetists practice nursing by providing anesthesia and anesthesia-related services. They accept the responsibility conferred upon them by the state, the profession, and society. The American Association of Nurse Anesthetists has adopted this Code of Ethics to guide its members in fulfilling their obligation as professionals. Each member of the American Association of Nurse Anesthetists has a personal responsibility to uphold and adhere to these ethical standards.

1. Responsibility to Patients
Certified Registered Nurse Anesthetists (CRNAs) preserve human dignity, respect the moral and legal rights of health consumers, and support the safety and well-being of the patient under their care.

1.1 The CRNA renders quality anesthesia care regardless of the patient's race, religion, age, sex, nationality, disability, or social or economic status.

1.2 The CRNA protects the patient from harm and is an advocate for the patient's welfare.

1.3 The CRNA verifies that a valid anesthesia informed consent has been obtained from the patient or legal guardian as required by federal or state laws or institutional policy prior to rendering a service.

1.4 The CRNA avoids conflicts between his or her personal integrity and the patient's rights. In situations where the CRNA's personal convictions prohibit participation in a particular procedure, the CRNA refuses to participate or withdraws from the case provided that such refusal or withdrawal does not harm the patient or constitute a breach of duty.

1.5 The CRNA takes appropriate action to protect patients from healthcare providers who are incompetent, impaired, or engage in illegal or unethical practice.

1.6 The CRNA maintains confidentiality of patient information except in those rare events where accepted nursing practice demands otherwise.

1.7 The CRNA does not knowingly engage in deception in any form.

1.8 The CRNA does not exploit nor abuse his or her relationship of trust and confidence with the patient or the patient's dependence on the CRNA.

Continued

Table 11-7 **Code of Ethics for the Certified Registered Nurse Anesthetist — cont'd**

2. Competence

The scope of practice engaged in by the Certified Registered Nurse Anesthetist is within the individual competence of the CRNA. Each CRNA has the responsibility to maintain competency in practice.

2.1 The CRNA engages in lifelong, professional educational activities.

2.2 The CRNA participates in continuous quality improvement activities.

2.3 The practicing CRNA maintains his or her state license as a Registered Nurse, meets advanced practice state statutory or regulatory requirements, if any, and maintains recertification as a CRNA.

3. Responsibilities as a Professional

Certified Registered Nurse Anesthetists are responsible and accountable for the services they render and the actions they take.

3.1 The CRNA, as an independently licensed professional, is responsible and accountable for judgments made and actions taken in his or her professional practice. Neither physician orders nor institutional policies relieve the CRNA of responsibility for his or her judgments made or actions taken.

3.2 The CRNA practices in accordance with the professional practice standards established by the profession.

3.3 The CRNA participates in activities that contribute to the ongoing development of the profession and its body of knowledge.

3.4 The CRNA is responsible and accountable for his or her conduct in maintaining the dignity and integrity of the profession.

3.5 The CRNA collaborates and cooperates with other healthcare providers involved in a patient's care.

3.6 The CRNA respects the expertise and responsibility of all healthcare providers involved in providing services to patients.

3.7 The CRNA is responsible and accountable for his or her actions, including self-awareness and assessment of fitness for duty.

4. Responsibility to Society

4.1 Certified Registered Nurse Anesthetists work in collaboration with the healthcare community of interest to promote highly competent, safe, quality patient care.

4.2 Certified Registered Nurse Anesthetists collaborate with members of the health professions and other citizens in promoting community and national efforts to meet the health needs of the public.

5. Endorsement of Products and Services

Certified Registered Nurse Anesthetists endorse products and services only when personally satisfied with the product's or service's safety, effectiveness and quality. CRNAs do not state that the AANA has endorsed any product or service unless the Board of Directors of the American Association of Nurse Anesthetists has done so.

5.1 Any endorsement is truthful and based on factual evidence of efficacy.

5.2 A CRNA does not exploit his or her professional title and credentials for products or services which are unrelated to his or her professional practice or expertise.

Table 11-7 **Code of Ethics for the Certified Registered Nurse Anesthetist — cont'd**

6. Research
Certified Registered Nurse Anesthetists protect the integrity of the research process and the reporting and publication of findings.

6.1 The CRNA evaluates research findings and incorporates them into practice as appropriate.

6.2 The CRNA conducts research projects according to accepted ethical research and reporting standards established by public law, institutional procedures, and the health professions.

6.3 The CRNA protects the rights and well-being of people and animals that serve as subjects in research.

6.4 The CRNA participates in research activities to improve practice, education, and public policy relative to health needs of diverse populations, the health workforce, the organization and administration of health systems, and healthcare delivery.

7. Business Practices
Certified Registered Nurse Anesthetists, regardless of practice arrangements or practice settings, maintain ethical business practices in dealing with patients, colleagues, institutions, and corporations.

7.1 The contractual obligations of a CRNA are consistent with the professional standards of practice and the laws and regulations pertaining to nurse anesthesia practice.

7.2 The CRNA will not participate in deceptive or fraudulent business practices.

©1986, 1992, 1997, 2001, 2005, American Association of Nurse Anesthetists.

Table 11-8 **ACNM Code of Ethics**

The Certified Nurse-Midwife has professional moral obligations. The purpose of this code is to identify obligations which guide the nurse-midwife in the practice of nurse-midwifery. This code further serves to clarify the expectations of the profession to consumers, the public, other professionals and to potential practitioners.

Nurse-midwifery exists for the good of women and their families. This good is safeguarded by practice in accordance with the ACNM Philosophy and ACNM Standards for the Practice of Nurse-Midwifery.

Nurse-midwives uphold the belief that childbearing and maturation are normal life processes. When intervention is indicated, it is integrated into care in a way that preserves the dignity of the woman and her family.

Decisions regarding nurse-midwifery care require client participation in an ongoing negotiation process in order to develop a safe plan of care. This process considers cultural diversity, individual autonomy, and legal responsibilities.

Nurse-midwives share professional information with their clients that leads to informed participation and consent. This sharing is done without coercion, or deception.

Nurse-midwives practice competently. They consult and refer when indicated by their professional scope of practice and/or personal limitations.

Nurse-midwives provide care without discrimination based on race, religion, life-style, sexual orientation, socio-economic status or nature of health problem.

Continued

Table 11-8 **ACNM Code of Ethics—cont'd**

Nurse-midwives maintain confidentiality except when there is a clear, serious and immediate danger or when mandated by law.

Nurse-midwives take appropriate action to protect clients from harm when endangered by incompetent or unethical practices.

Nurse-midwives interact respectfully with the people with whom they work and practice.

Nurse-midwives participate in developing and improving the care of women and families through supporting the profession of nurse-midwifery, research, and the education of nurse-midwifery students and nurse-midwives.

Nurse-midwives promote community, state, and national efforts such as public education and legislation, to ensure access to quality care and to meet the health needs of women and their families.

Source: ACNM Ad Hoc Committee on Code of Ethics. Approved by Board of Directors May 18, 1990.

Table 11-9 **AANP Standards and a Proposal for a Code of Ethics for NPs**

AANP Standards of Practice Professional education	Proposal for a Code of Ethics for NPs Professional education legal requirements
Competent care through assessment, diagnosis, planning, implementation, and evaluation	1. The NP should provide medical and nursing care with compassion, confidentiality, and respect for the individual, regardless of social, economic, or health status. 2. The NP's primary commitment and responsibility is to the patient, whether that patient is an individual, family, group, or community.
Patient evaluation, consultation, and equal access	3. The NP shall support access to care for all patients and should strive to effect public policies that will result in equal access. 4. The NP shall support the patient's efforts toward an optimal level of health through education, self-care promotion, consultation, and collaboration with other health care team members.
Consultation and collaboration	5. The NP shall support the patient's efforts toward an optimal level of health through education, self-care promotion, consultation, and collaboration with other health care team members.
Legal standards	6. The NP shall maintain and be accountable for accurate medical records for each patient. The NP shall not engage in fraud or deception and shall report any other health care provider that engages in such activities.
Advocacy for public health	7. The NP shall advocate for and strive to protect the rights, health, safety, and privacy of all patients. The NP should collaborate with other professionals and the public on local, national, and international levels to promote this effort.

Table 11-9 **AANP Standards and a Proposal for a Code of Ethics for NPs—cont'd**	
AANP Standards of Practice	Proposal for a Code of Ethics for NPs
Professional development, role interpretation for the public, research and advancement	8. The NP shall continue to advance personal and professional development through practice, education of the public, and lifelong continuous study, research, and activity in professional organizations. 9. The NP shall, in the provision of patient care, responsibly choose whom to serve, with whom to associate, and the environment in which to provide that care.

From Peterson M, and Potter RL. (2004). A proposal for a code of ethics for nurse practitioners. *J Amer Acad NP* 16(3):116–124.

Potential Ethical Concerns of the APRN

Potential ethical concerns of APRNs include concerns about the futility of treatment in some cases, the use of alternative/complementary treatments, managed care, and self-conflict.

Futility of Treatment

Ethics and the law give primacy to patient autonomy, which is defined as the right to be a fully informed participant in all aspects of medical decision making and the right to refuse unwanted, even recommended and life-saving, medical care. In spite of the power of this concept, it should be remembered that futile treatments are not obligatory. No ethical principle or law has ever required physicians to offer or accede to demands for treatments that are futile. Futility refers to an expectation of success that is either predictably or empirically so unlikely that its exact probability is often incalculable. Futility should be distinguished from hopelessness. Hopelessness is a subjective attitude, whereas futility refers to an objective quality of an action. Hope and hopelessness are related more to desire, faith, denial, and other psychological responses than to the objective probability that some contemplated action will be successful.

The futility of a treatment may be evident in either quantitative or qualitative terms. Futility may refer to the improbability of an event happening as a result of treatment or to the quality of the result that such treatment might produce. The process of determining futility resembles decision analysis, with one important distinction. In decision analysis, the decision to use a procedure is based on considerations of both the probability of success and the quality or utility of the outcome. A very low probability of success may be balanced by very high utility. However, when determining futility, the quantitative and qualitative aspects are treated as independent thresholds or minimum cutoff levels, either of which frees the physician from the obligation to offer a medical treatment.[39,40]

Martin[41] offers a cogent and reasonable discussion of the potential futility of mechanical ventilation in an intensive care unit of pediatric patients who develop respiratory or other organ failure following a hematopoietic stem cell transplant. While experience with this form of transplantation continues to grow rapidly, it is understood that patients who develop multisystem organ failure have little chance of long-term survival. Jacobe and colleagues[42] determined from their data that those with failure of three or more organs had only a 1-in-10 chance of survival. In this situation, there is no absolute, 100% accurate, predictive model because there continue to be occasional patients with multisystem organ failure who do achieve long-term survival. Therefore, following the guidelines of the American Academy of Pediatric Committee on Bioethics, such patients at Duke University Medical Center receive immediate, aggressive intensive care unit (ICU) care in a situation that may be viewed by some as futile. Multisystem organ failure and prolonged mechanical ventilation are two of several factors associated with poor outcomes and non-survival in this group of patients. Once aggressive ICU care with mechanical ventilation is begun, if no objective signs of improvement are noted in the first 48 to 72 hours, the chance of survival drops to less than 5%.[41]

In dealing with this potentially futile situation, Martin[41] recommends (1) early and frank discussion with the family, as well as the transplant and ICU teams, before transferring the child to the ICU; (2) immediate and aggressive treatment for acutely decompensating patients; (3) frequent reassessment of the patient's condition with realistic feedback to the family; and (4) discussion with the family about the discontinuation of or limiting of further therapy if no significant improvement is seen in 14 days. In Martin's experience, situations when life-sustaining therapy has been requested beyond a "reasonable" period of time, consideration or actual implementation of an ethics committee consultation has resulted in the ability to reach an agreement on limitation or withdrawal of life-sustaining treatments.

Use of Complementary/Alternative Medicine

Over the past 10 years, medical therapy that has been termed "complementary" or "alternative" has gradually shifted to "integrative-based medicine," particularly in the treatment of long-term chronic illness, autoimmune disorders, and cancer. Integrative medicine is conceptually a patient-centered, biopsychosocial, spiritual, holistic approach to care. Goals include the integration of complementary or alternative medical treatments within traditional medical settings and multidisciplinary teamwork. A final facet is the development of evidence-based research to support the use of alternative or complementary treatments in practice.[43]

Ethical conflicts may be present when an alternative/complementary treatment that lacks adequate research evidence of its efficacy, safety, and potential for either positive or negative interactions with other selected forms of treatment is considered or included in the plan of care. To reach a decision regarding this issue, a risk-benefit analysis of the complementary/alternative treatment versus conventional medical treatment can be approached using the framework suggested by Adams and colleagues.[44] The factors to be considered in application of this framework are:

1. Severity and acuteness of illness
2. Curability with conventional treatment
3. Degree of invasiveness and associated toxicities and side effects of conventional treatment
4. Degree of understanding of risk and benefits of the complementary/alternative treatment
5. Knowledge and voluntary acceptance of these risks by the patient
6. Persistence of the patient's intention to use complementary/alternative treatment

Managed Care

Managed care is not a new phenomenon. Zoloth-Dorfman and Rubin [45] noted that in the 19th and early 20th centuries, groups of marginalized individuals created prepaid, capitated, managed care plans in response to the problems that they experienced in securing adequate healthcare services. These attempts at prepaid care included immigrant aid societies, trade unions, and company insurance plans. Such plans developed as a response to a medical delivery system not designed to guarantee access to services for those unable to pay a fee at the time of need. The utility of such efforts is evidenced by the continuing success of Kaiser Permanente, Group Health of Puget Sound, and other nonprofit health maintenance organizations (HMOs).

Growing pressure has been placed on all providers to control healthcare costs by more rigorously controlling medical options. This produces a tension between the value of autonomy, exercised in the form of consent to use or omit various interventions, and the necessity of better control of medical resource expenditures. No consensus exists about what constitutes a just method of balancing the desires of individual patients against the diverse needs of society.

Managed care does generate concern about who will make actual treatment decisions, how decision-making authority will be established, and on which criteria clinical decisions will be made. Ulrich and Soeken[35] studied an analytic model of ethical conflict in practice and autonomy in a sample group of NPs, over 60% of whom worked in some type of managed care. A result of the study was the conceptualization of a framework that included individual, organizational, and societal/market variables and factors directly related to ethical conflict and autonomy of practice. The perception of the ethical environment of managed care was found to have the strongest effect on the presence of ethical conflict in practice as experienced by the NPs. It was recognized that professional autonomy is undergoing considerable negative stresses based on either real or perceived changes in legal requirements, societal expectations and values, the organizational environment of the workplace, the status of the NP within the delivery system, and, finally, the current political and economic environment within which practice must take place.

Today's APRN often maintains a relationship with both the patient and the health plan or employer. These entities may have very different ethical concerns and expectations about loyalty to their goals. In today's financial environment, the needs of the health plan's economic bottom line often are in conflict with the allocation of resources, including practitioner time required for optimal patient assessment and care. Although shown to have a relatively weak effect, the larger the percent of clients enrolled in managed care and the higher the market penetration in the practice region, the lower the NP's perception of professional practice autonomy. This is predicated perhaps on the additional rules, regulations, and guidelines promulgated for clinical care by many managed care entities. Ulrich and Soeken's findings regarding market penetration and perceived loss of professional autonomy are consistent with those of several physician studies.[35]

Unfortunately, unsuccessful efforts to resolve ethical conflict may weaken the provider's sense of autonomy because of the development of a sense of powerlessness as a professional. While being perhaps very realistic of the daily lives of many APRNs in very different specialties, Ulrich and Soeken[35] are careful to point out the limitations of their study. These limitations included a homogeneous sample from one state, primarily female participants, lack of predictive power of some variables in the model, and inability to define probable variability of policies in multiple, and very complex, managed care settings in more global settings. It should be noted that additional research is needed to assess the presence and impact of outcomes associated with ethical conflict in practice and autonomy in different healthcare systems. Study variables will certainly include APRN job satisfaction and/or longevity, patient health outcomes, and psychosocial issues of the practitioner and the client.

Conflict of Interest

Clients who are ill are in an inherently unequal power relationship with providers and health plans. As buyers of health care, they are rarely in a position to evaluate effectively the practice and standards of care promoted by managed care organizations (MCOs). APRNS should assume a role of advocate and educator in these situations. Strong individual moral agency is developed by reflection on personal goals and aspirations as well as by understanding the limits of one's personal and professional commitments. To develop true moral agency, the nurse in advanced practice needs to take risks in preventing all plans from calling for a gag order on healthcare providers or suppressing healthy debate on appropriate treatment modalities. Such risk taking requires courage because of both the threatened and real loss of position and status.

In today's healthcare delivery climate, conflict of interest has recently gained increased attention. Many pharmaceutical and medical manufacturing companies are receiving close scrutiny because of the potential effect of marketing strategies on patient care and management decisions made by physicians and APRNs. As a result, many healthcare organizations, governmental agencies, and academic medical research centers have developed conflict-of-interest policies for professionals who are their employees or receive funding from them. These policies are promulgated with the intent to assure the public of good professional conduct, thereby engendering consumer trust.

Medical and pharmaceutical companies are well aware that many APRNs have prescriptive authority and potentially can enable the use of specific drugs or devices in many practice settings. A conflict of interest can be said to be present when two competing interests clash, or in the case of the APRN, when the choice of drug or device becomes self-serving rather than in the best interest of the patient. Such a choice results in a moral compromise. The current focus of this debate is on developing transparency in the interactions between industry and the individual practitioner, thereby avoiding any sense of impropriety or bias.[46] The lack of such bias makes evidence-based clinical care possible in the truest sense and enhances the trust of the public in the provider's intent to have the patient's well-being and best interests at the center of any treatment proposal.

APRNs must learn to manage information accurately, work effectively in teams, integrate guidelines and clinical judgment, and manage outcomes. Both APRNs and consumers need to assume an activist role and seek positions on the boards of directors of large MCOs. APRNs must develop as expert reviewers of practice guidelines and encourage the release of such guidelines for consumers' review. Areas for future activism include striving to obtain open review of staffing patterns and reasonable compensation for providers and administrators and to secure the consumer's right to a cost rebate for improved health status or nonutilization of resources. This type of activism, properly carried out, becomes a defining opportunity for professional growth and personal advocacy of the client's right to ethical care.

SUGGESTED LEARNING EXERCISES

1. A major problem with access to health care exists in a remote rural area. The county commissioners are considering a clinic staffed by a family nurse practitioner (FNP) and a certified nurse-midwife (CNM). The county attorney obtained all the necessary permits and documents; however, one of the commissioners still has concern regarding the legality of the nurses practicing without the immediate presence of a physician. You, an FNP, and your spouse, a CNM, have been accepted to fill those positions, pending final approval of the county commissioners. They have asked you to prepare policies and procedures that would adhere to the national standards of such a practice. Prepare a model document that is realistic and practical. Assume that the state allows full prescriptive authority and off-site physician collaboration.

2. You are an experienced certified registered nurse anesthetist (CRNA) who has been asked to provide anesthesia services for a plastic surgeon in his office. You will be an independent practitioner and will be paid by the patient per case. In your state, CRNAs are not required to follow protocols or standardized procedures, and your standards of practice are determined by the profession. Prepare a document delineating the clinical policies of your practice, including pre-anesthesia evaluation and testing, selection of patients for elective ambulatory surgery, minimum equipment and supplies, and recovery discharge criteria and responsibility.

3. Prepare documents to conduct an annual legal audit of your practice. Include clinical policies, procedures, emergency situations, transfer of patients to another level of care,

medical record documentation, and review of state laws and regulations. Also include your plan for keeping current in the clinical components of your practice.

4. Form two groups. One group will represent the cancer care team (doctors, nurses, APRNs) of a large HMO. The other group is made up of those who have survived cancer for more than 5 years. Collaboratively seek to set down criteria for development of a process for making decisions about the integration of complementary/alternative treatments into conventional cancer care that respects the concerns of all the stakeholders.

REFERENCES

1. Waldman, R. (2002). A guest editorial: collaborative practice—balancing the future. *Obstet Gynecol Surv* 57(1):1–2.

2. Federal Support for the Preparation of the Clinical Nurse Specialist Workforce through Title VIII. (1997). *AACN Clinical Issues: Advanced Practice in Acute and Critical Care* 11(2):309–327.

3. Cady, R. (2003). *The Advanced Practice Nurse's Legal Handbook.* Lippincott Williams and Wilkins, Philadelphia, p. 173.

4. Hravnak, M. (1997). Credentialing and privileging: insight into the process for acute-care nurse practitioners. *AACN Clinical Issues: Advanced Practice in Acute and Critical Care* 8(1):1–8.

5. Minnick, AF, and Needleman, J. (2008). Methodological issues in explaining maternal outcomes: anesthesia provider characterizations in resource variation. *West S Nurs Res* 30(7):801–816.

6. McManus, R. (1994). Ethical decision making in anesthesia. In Foster, S, and Jordan, L (eds.), *Professional Aspects of Nurse Anesthesia Practice.* FA Davis, Philadelphia.

7. Smart, N. (1995). *Worldviews: Cross Cultural Explorations of Human Beliefs,* 2nd ed. Prentice-Hall, Englewood Cliffs, NJ.

8. Cofer, MJ. (2000). Thoughts on ethics. Value-based ethics in the workplace. *Nurs Manage* 18(1): 12–13.

9. Aikens, CA. (1937). *Studies in Ethics for Nurses,* 4th ed. W.B. Saunders, Philadelphia.

10. Callahan, D. (1981). Minimalist ethics. *Hastings Cent Rep* 11(5):19.

11. Chaitin, D, Stiller, R, Jacobs, S, Hershl, J, Grogen, T, and Weinberg, J. (2003). Physician-patient relationship in the intensive care unit: erosion of the sacred trust? *Crit Care Med* 31(5):S367–S372.

12. Iserson, KV. (1998). Nonstandard advance directives: a pseudoethical dilemma. *J Trauma* 44(1):139–142.

13. Forester-Miller, H. (1996). A practitioner's guide to ethical decision making. American Counseling Association. Alexandria, VA. Available at www.counseling.org/Resources/CodeofEthics/TP/Home/CT2.aspx.

14. Garcia, J, Froelich, R, McGuire-Kuletz, M, and Dave, P. (2008, July–August). Testing a transcultural model of ethical decision making with rehabilitation counselors. *J Rehab* 74(3):21.

15. Laabs, CA. (2007). Primary care nurse practitioners' integrity when faced with moral conflict. *Nurs* 14(6):795–809.

16. Laabs, CA. (2005). Moral problems and distress among nurse practitioners in primary care. *J Amer Acad Nurs Pract* 17(2):76–84.

17. Wilkinson, JM. (1997/1998). Moral distress in nursing practice: experience and effect. *Nurs Forum* 23(1):16–29.

18. Butz, AM, Redman, BK, Fry, ST, and Kilodner, K. (1998). Ethical conflicts experienced by certified pediatric nurse practitioners in ambulatory settings. *J Ped Health Care* 12(4):183–190.

19. Godfrey, NS, and Smith, KV. (2002). Moral distress and the nurse practitioner. *J Clin Ethics* 13(4): 330–336.

20. Pellegrino, ED, and Thimasma, DC. (1988). *For the Patient's Good: The Restoration of Beneficence in Health Care*. Oxford University Press, New York.

21. Downick, C, and Frith, L (eds). (1999). *General Practice and Ethics: Uncertainty and Responsibility*. Routledge, London.

22. Brody, H, and Tomlinson, T. (1986). Ethics in primary care: setting aside common misunderstandings. *Prim Care* 13:225–240.

23. Braunack-Mayer, AJ. (2001). What makes a problem an ethical problem? An empirical perspective on the nature of ethical problems in general practice. *J Med Ethics* 27:98–113.

24. Kaku, M. (1998). *Science Will Revolutionize the 21st Century*. Oxford Press, Oxford, England.

25. Kirk, M. (2000). Genetics, ethics, and education: considering the issues for nurses and midwives. *Nurs Ethics* 7(3):215–226.

26. Warner, M, Longley, M, Gould, E, and Picek, A. (1998). *Health Care Future–2010*. Welsh Institution for Health and Docial Care. Pontypnidd, Wales.

27. Lutzen, K. (1997). Nursing ethics in the next millenium: a context sensitive approach for nursing ethics. *Nurs Ethics* 4:218–226.

28. Barfield, RC, and Kodish, E. (2006). Pediatric ethics in the age of molecular medicine. *Pediatr Clin N Amer* 53:639–648.

29. Nussbaum, RL, McInnes, RR, and Willard, HF. (2007). *Thompson and Thompson Genetics in Medicine*, 6th ed. W.B. Saunders Company, Philadelphia, pp 487–490.

30. Lomis, KD, Carpenter, RO, and Miller, BM. (2009). Moral distress in the third year of medical school: a descriptive review of student case reflections. *Am J Surg* 197(1):107.

31. Blake, C, and Guare, RE. (1997). Nurses' reflections on ethical decision making: implications for leaders. *J NY State Nurses' Association* 28(4):13–16.

32. Tong, R. (2008). Practice precedes theory: doing bioethics "naturally." Is there an ethicist in the house? On the cutting edge of bioethics. *J Med Humanities* 29:133–135.

33. Allmark, P. (2005). Can the study of ethics enhance nursing practice? *J Adv Nurs* 51(6):618–624.

34. Scanlon, C. (1997). Models of discernment: developing ethical competence in nursing practice. *MD Nurse* 16(5):3.

35. Ulrich, CM, and Soeken, KL. (2005). A path analytic model of ethical conflict in practice and autonomy in a sample of nurse practitioners. *Nurs Ethics* 12(3):305–316.

36. Hamric, AB. (1996). Relationships between moral perspectives of care and justice, selected individuals, and contextual factors, and nurse activism in a sample of practicing nurses. (Dissertation). University of Maryland. Baltimore.

37. Cassells, JM, and Gaul, AL. (1998). An ethical assessment framework for nursing practice. *MD Nurse* 17(1):9–12.

38. American Nurses Association. (2001). *Code of Ethics for Nurses*. Available at http://nursingworld. org/ethics/chcode.htm.

39. Arnold, RM, and Kellum, J. (2003). Moral justifications for surrogate decision making in the intensive care unit: implications and limitations. *Crit Care Med* 31(5):S347–S353.

40. Lelie, A, and Verweij, M. (2003). Futility without a dichotomy: towards an ideal physician-patient relationship. *Bioethics* 17(1):21–31.

41. Martin, PL. (2006). To stop or not to stop: how much support should be provided to mechanically ventilated pediatric bone marrow and stem cell transplant patients? *Respir Care Clin* 12:403–419.

42. Jacobe, SJ, Hassan, A, Veys, P, et al. (2003). Outcome of children requiring admission to an intensive care unit after bone marrow transplantation. *Crit Care Med* 31(3):1299–1305.

43. Ben-Arye, B, Schiff, E, and Golan, O. (2008). Ethical issues in integrative oncology. *Hematol Oncol Clin N Amer* 22:737–753.

44. Adams, K, Cohen, MH, Eisenberg, D, et al. (2002). Ethical considerations of complementary and alternative medical therapies in conventional medical settings. *AMM Intern Med* 137(8):660–664.

45. Zoloth-Dorfman, L, and Rubin, S. (1995). The patient as commodity: managed care and the question of ethics. *J Clin Ethics* 6:339.

46. Erlen, JA. (2008). Conflict of interest. *Orthop Nurs* 27(2):2.

Anita Hunter is a professor at the University of San Diego (USD). A pediatric nurse practitioner (PNP) since 1975, from Northeastern University, she has practiced, served as health consultant, conducted research, and taught nurse practitioner (NP) and other graduate students nationally and internationally. Dr. Hunter's work has extended into Northern Ireland, Ghana, Uganda, China, Taiwan, Mexico, and the Dominican Republic. She is Director of MSN and International Nursing as USD and is currently involved in an extensive collaborative project in Uganda to build the first children's hospital in the country. Since 1994, Dr. Hunter has taken over 700 nursing students and faculty to the aforementioned countries for short-term clinical immersion experiences involving developing and implementing clinical practice, health education, lay educator health programs, community cottage industries, and health consultative services that have benefited thousands of people. She has published innumerable articles and, through her work as first chair of the Global Advancement Committee with the National Organization of Nurse Practitioner Faculties (NONPF) and the International Nurse Practitioner/ Advanced Practice Nursing Network (INP/APN) Policy and Standards Committee, was instrumental in developing the standards and scope of practice protocols for the APRN in the international arena.

Katherine Crabtree is a professor of nursing at Oregon Health & Science University (OHSU). She received her BS and MS in nursing from the University of Michigan and her doctorate in nursing science from the University of California, San Francisco. She has been an adult nurse practitioner since 1975 and has taught nurse practitioners since 1977 at Michigan State University, OHSU, the University of California at San Francisco, and Wayne State University. She is faculty teaching in Doctor of Nursing Practice program (DNP) at OHSU. She lived in Thailand for one year teaching and consulting on advanced nursing practice throughout the country. She currently teaches international students in nursing at the doctoral level. She served four years as chair of the NONPF Education Guidelines and Standards Committee and led the revision of core competencies and co-directed the federally funded *National Validation of NP Competencies for Adult, Family, Gerontological, Pediatric, and Women's' Health Nurse Practitioner*. She is currently co-director of the project to blend adult and gerontology nursing competencies for nurse practitioners at the doctoral level; this project is being conducted jointly by the American Association of Colleges of Nursing (AACN) and NONPF and funded by the Hartford Foundation. She now serves as secretary on the executive committee of NONPF.

CHAPTER 12

Global Health and International Opportunities

Anita Hunter, PhD, CPNP, FAAN
Katherine Crabtree, DNSc, APRN-BC, FAAN

CHAPTER OBJECTIVES

*At the completion of the chapter, the
reader will be able to:*

1. Discuss the interrelatedness of the
health of people around the world.
2. Describe some of the global challenges
facing advanced practice nursing in
developed and developing nations.
3. Examine how competing national
priorities influence health needs.
4. Examine how the competencies needed
by advanced practice registered nurses
(APRNs) in the United States are
translated/incorporated internationally.
5. Recognize the ethical and spiritual
aspects of developing culturally
responsive care.
6. Identify preparations needed, available
resources, and opportunities for
international nursing assignments.

Consider the following: If the world consisted of 100 people who represented the demographics present today, then 6 would have 59% of the world's wealth, 80 would live in poverty, 70 would be illiterate, 50 would suffer from hunger and malnutrition, and only 1 would have a university degree. The developing world has faced and is facing many crises not common to industrialized nations. If you have never experienced the horror of war, the solitude of prison, the pain of torture, or the slow death of starvation, then you are better off than 500 million people. In a community in Uganda, 17,000 children under age 5 die yearly from malaria and its complications. This is equivalent to a jumbo airliner filled with children crashing weekly. These statistics draw attention to global health needs beyond the borders of the United States and show how health is affected by war, famine, natural disasters, and political upheaval. Nurses need to recognize their responsibility to help improve the lives and well-being of people around the world. Thinking about health globally brings new issues into focus and invites new visions for our future.

What once were the unique health challenges of people in less developed countries—challenges related to social injustices, loss of human rights, and lack of access to food, housing, safety, and health care—are now becoming common health problems of people all over the world. Global warming, increasing global violence, the declining global economy, and the depletion of oil and food supplies all contribute to the current global health crisis. Preventable conditions like malnutrition, communicable diseases, environmental poisonings, and chronic health problems, whether physical or mental, are taxing the traditional healthcare systems of the world nations. It will take alternative healthcare models, nongovernment organizations (NGOs), APRN-led initiatives, and a commitment to social justice and human rights to improve health and well-being globally. Such actions must be culturally congruent, culturally responsive, and culturally acceptable to the people for whom interventions are planned. See Figures 12-1 and 12-2.

What the Problems Are

The health of the peoples of the world is affected by many factors, some specific to particular areas of the world, others widespread. In this section, some major concerns and factors contributing to the global health crisis are outlined.

Lack of immunization is one major factor. As people cross boundaries and enter new communities they may bring with them a host of health problems that may not be common in

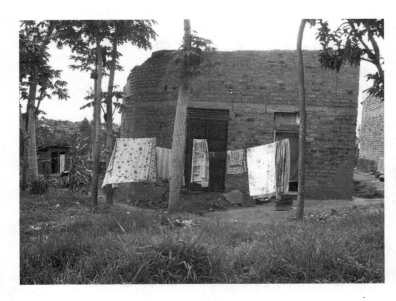

Figure 12-1: Typical village dwelling in Uganda.

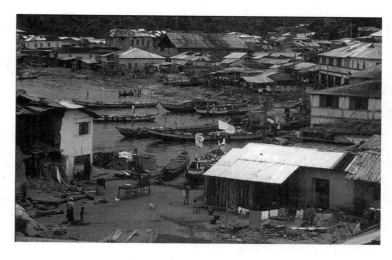

Figure 12-2: Fishing village in Ghana.

their host nations. Measles, malaria, tuberculosis, and pertussis have increased in the United States because many immigrants lack immunization against these diseases. People in the United States who now choose not to immunize themselves or their children may also increase the risk for the spread of some diseases.

Zoonotic diseases, or diseases transmitted from animals to humans, are also increasing, caused, at least in part, by the increasing encroachment of humans and domesticated animals on the land inhabited by wild animals.[1] Anthrax, tuberculosis, brucellosis, and scabies are a few examples of such cross-contamination evident in Uganda (personal communication, Dr. Gladys Kalema-Zikusoka, October 2008). Human immunodeficiency virus (HIV) is probably the greatest example of zoonotic disease transmission; once isolated to Africa, it now has become a global problem with devastating results. See Figures 12-3 and 12-4.

Increasing populations, migration within countries, and natural disasters are significant factors not only in contributing to the spread of disease but also to many social problems. The world's increasing population is wreaking havoc on depleted viable lands. Migration within countries occurs because indigenous people who are no longer able to sustain themselves in outlying communities travel to larger cities, looking for employment to feed themselves and

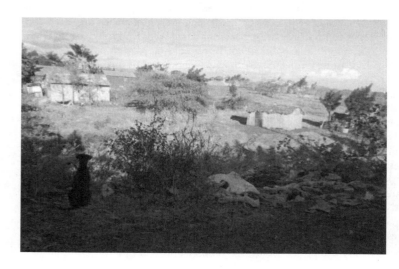

Figure 12-3: Homeless community in the Dominican Republic.

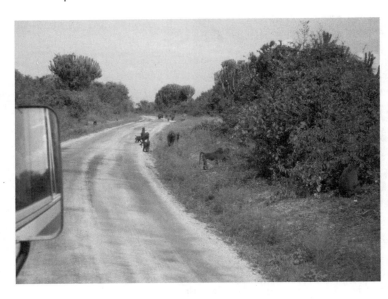

Figure 12-4: Baboons in Uganda are known to spread zoonotic diseases.

their families. However, jobs are scarce and many of these people end up living in poverty in shantytowns under unsanitary conditions that breed disease. Frustration and a sense of hopelessness often lead to the separation of families, personal or child exploitation, and substance abuse.

The shantytowns that many people are forced to live in are often located in areas subject to natural disasters, such as floods and landslides/mudslides that destroy lives, homes, food, and what little worldly goods the people have. Depletion of crops and the cost of transporting food or cultivating food affect those most in need of these goods. Foreign relief agencies try to provide food for people just to survive in the short term, but they do not change the prospects of a dim future for stability and family health. As frustrations mount, individuals become increasingly vulnerable to political and military coups that promise better conditions and a brighter future, but often fail. These conflicts bring violence, including rape, murder, and social destruction.[1]

Migration between countries also presents problems. Whether escaping from undesirable sociopolitical or physical living conditions or merely seeking a better life, waves of immigrants continue to strain global resources. Immigrants fleeing their homelands are often confronted with issues of prejudice, discrimination, unemployment, and poverty in their new lands. Nations plagued by civil war and political corruption are faced with chronic poverty, unstable leadership, and lack of economic development.[1] These conditions adversely affect not only the health of their citizens but also the health of bordering nations and potentially others around the world.

The *reallocation of government resources* to meet problems not directly related to health issues also plays a role. When peoples' health and social welfare are not prized, available resources are frequently used to meet other governmental priorities. Ignoring illiteracy, hunger, and poverty, while directing resources toward other national goals, precludes reaching an optimal level of health nationally and globally. International communications and media portrayal of conflicting lifestyles, economic discrepancies, racial prejudice, and differing religious beliefs create a climate of dissatisfaction and distrust, which can turn to hate, frustration, hostility, and sometimes war. Acts of terrorism are increasing. Nations that felt safe and insulated from political unrest and ethnic wars are now required to reallocate resources to protect themselves from these threats, leaving fewer resources to meet the healthcare mandates of society.

The *age of the population* is also a factor in global health. While the population of the world's developed nations is aging rapidly, many developing nations still report that 60% of their population is under the age of 15 years (http://en.wikipedia.org/wiki/File:Median_age.png). In these countries, the average age remains 45 years. Lives are lost or shortened because of unmanaged chronic health problems, such as diabetes, and cardiac and respiratory conditions. In some countries, the shortened life expectancy is related to immigrants seeking refuge from genocide, military coups, famine, or long-standing wars. Epidemics of disease can spread rapidly in immigration camps and, if uncontrolled, to the rest of the population. Whether health services and resources are allocated haphazardly or deliberately, the nation is, in effect, making decisions about who shall live and who shall die. Ultimately, these decisions affect the number of children who grow to be adults and the number of adults who survive to become elders.

The allocation of national resources and health standards in one nation also impacts other nations who may have to divert resources needed to provide health care for their own citizens. All of sub-Saharan Africa and many other nations lack the financial resources and trained health professionals to achieve the health goals set by the World Health Organization (WHO) (http://web.worldbank.org). With the world at our doorstep, the WHO has mandated that nurses, especially APRNs, take a leading role in correcting the disparities in healthcare delivery, filling the deficit of healthcare providers that currently exists, and addressing the unmet health needs of peoples around the world.[2] See Figure 12-5.

Where, How, and What Interventions Should Be Implemented

Too many people around the world are not receiving care or are receiving inadequate care. Interventions to address health and human rights are fundamental to achieving global health, but where, how, and what interventions should be implemented?

Interventions occur in needy countries. They typically address basic public health issues, such as improving the living environment (e.g., through improved sanitation and a safe water supply); addressing the causes of major health problems, such as malaria, tuberculosis, dysentery, malnutrition, and zoonotic diseases; and assessing the physical and mental health consequences of violence and social injustice. International involvement requires participants to make a commitment, to respond to invitations for help, to collaborate with the local

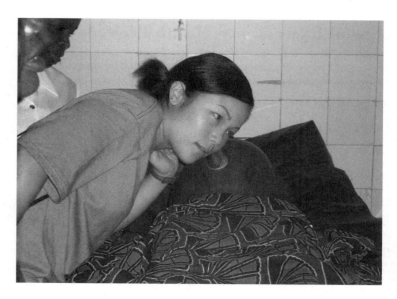

Figure 12-5: A USD student listening to fetal heartbeat with a typical Ugandan fetoscope.

population so they will be able to help themselves, and to practice from an ethical and culturally responsive perspective. Effective interventions are pertinent to the health problems being addressed and culturally sensitive.

Some interventions used in the United States are inappropriate for use in other parts of the world because people cannot afford them, the people do not support the use of life-saving technology, and/or they do not take care of the survivors. A commitment to address global health and human rights means valuing the life of every human being and their right to health care.

The needs of the underserved populations are best met on their own soil, with their own resources, and with their own people. APRNs can play a role in implementing this by traveling to other countries where they can teach the people about basic health concerns and help them use their own resources to improve their health. This process requires teaching the basic tenets of public health, the principles of accessing health care, what to expect of health interventions, the right to be valued and to value others, the right to protect themselves from abuses, and the ways and means to earn a living.

Screening for disease, providing immunizations, improving nutrition and prenatal care, and ensuring clean water and sanitation for healthy communities are often the specific priorities in developing nations. However, it should be remembered that initiating these health-related programs does not save lives via medical therapies alone; they must assist in helping people learn how to help themselves through such activities as developing cottage industries, learning new life skills, and working together to change policies to protect the most vulnerable.

For decades, nurses from the United States have been actively involved in international health missions. They have been first responders in disasters nationally and internationally and have set up medical and surgical clinics providing direct patient care and health education. They have served as health consultants to health ministers in various countries and developed schools of nursing and taught faculty and students internationally. They have also served as nurses, providing direct patient care within the established healthcare system in various areas. Some have done this through formal educational or healthcare systems, some have pursued it on their own, and others have ventured into difficult territories via faith-affiliated programs. Whatever the modality, these nurses have acted on their humanitarian values and interacted with people to bring about lasting change. These nurses have made the commitment to address global health and human rights issues. These changes cannot, for the most part, be achieved by military force or governmental rule.

Characteristics of Successful International Health Projects

Certain intervention projects have met with widespread success. Paul Farmer and other experienced international healthcare activists all concur that the most successful projects and their participants share the following characteristics[1,3]:

- The health professionals are invited by the people, not the government. Most health initiatives have been undertaken by nongovernmental faith-based organizations, which offer nondenominational health care/education to all. Interested persons can locate outreach efforts to developing communities around the globe. Other U.S.-based initiatives often operate within universities with schools of nursing and/or medicine or out of hospitals offering specialized surgical services. Many other countries also offer disaster relief, humanitarian aide, and health care/education; additional information about these programs can be located on the Internet.

- The participants have a philosophy of altruism, cultural respect and responsivity, and a desire to help those less fortunate live better lives. Participants typically pay their own way and live and work with the people. Such positioning allows participants to get to know the community—how the people live, what the health problems are, and how the people care for one another. It develops a sense of trust and of oneness and community.

■ No governmental sponsorship from political parties is involved. Federal grants may support individual research or other initiatives as extensions of the project, but the overall project is an NGO (non-governmental organization) operation. No drug company or medical company sponsors the project either. Drug and medical companies may, however, be contributors to the project, again operating through the NGO.

■ Projects that have incorporated as an NGO with advisory boards established at the community level in both the helping and assisted communities are formed. The intent of the project is that it belongs to and is managed by the people in the assisted community. The helping community (an international NGO) may provide support and make recommendations. Oversight and successful implementation require cooperation of both partners.

■ No services are given for free. Whatever is given for free is not valued by the people for whom it is intended. Even the poorest will pay in whatever way they can for better health care; such payment can be in labor, goods, or cash.

■ Short-term clinical immersion projects, usually 2 to 3 weeks in length, occurring several times a year, are most effective. Such projects accomplish specific goals, such as conducting a needs assessment or training program; allowing the assisted community to operate on its own once the base has been established, such as running a local clinic, hospital, or training program; and encouraging regular follow-up, evaluation, refinement, and movement to the next goal, such as expansion of the current project or replication of the model in another area of need.

■ Multidisciplinary teams consisting of health professionals, business experts, peace and justice experts, scientists, and others may be necessary to help a community care for itself and support itself. With these programs, communities may develop a stronger sense of self-respect through their success in improving the life of the community.

■ It is imperative to make a commitment to a community in need for at least 3 to 5 years with a timetable for withdrawal and a plan for turning the operation over to the assisted community. Projects that continue beyond that time period run the risk of making the assisted community dependent on the helping organization. Projects committed for shorter periods seldom assist a community to achieve better health or improve human rights. Those who participate are changed individuals, often improving their professional practice because of the cultural responsivity they have acquired and the respect they have gained for those whom they helped.

■ Teams that work with the local providers teach and learn together, often improving the skills of both professional and lay participants. Collaboration communicates to the local people that both parties respect and value one another's expertise, leading to improved access to local health care. The collaborative efforts of physicians from Cuba, England, Ireland, Japan, and the United States and nurses from England, Ireland, and the United States have made significant contributions to the betterment of health in many communities in Africa, South America, the Caribbean, Southeast Asia, and the Balkan countries.

Lastly, all successful projects completed a full community needs assessment that included:

■ Identifying the barriers and facilitators to health and well-being

■ Conducting focus groups with the local people, politicians, and business people

■ Examining the environment to identify the greatest risks and most vulnerable people

■ Identifying how health care could best be provided

■ Meeting with the community to discuss options and having the community choose its plan of action

A plan imposed on the community does not belong to them and is not generally accepted. Changes that grow out of interaction with the community, rather than those imposed by "outsiders," are more lasting. The community must also be willing to accept the responsibility for improved lives and saved lives and incorporate those living with disabilities.

Ethics and Spiritual and Cultural Responsivity in a Global Environment

Ethics and spiritual and cultural respect are learned behaviors that arise from values such as respect for human dignity, freedom, and equality. Practicing in an ethical, culturally, and spiritually responsive manner is essential when working in the global arena. Ethical practice means respecting the civil rights of people, treating all people equally and humanely, advocating on behalf of those in need, valuing life, and facilitating dying with dignity.

Cultural competence is a concept that refers to an ability to interact effectively with people of different cultures.[4] It may be comprised of four components: an awareness of one's own cultural worldview, one's attitudes toward cultural differences, one's knowledge of different cultural practices and worldviews, and one's cross-cultural skills. Such competence may be an idealistic goal and achieving it may be unrealistic without living in the culture, because it implies knowing all aspects of a culture and its beliefs, values, and practices. However, being culturally respectful and responsive is achievable, as demonstrated on the following Web site: http://www.intime.uni.edu.multiculure/curriculum. Because each country consists of multiple cultures, all one can hope to achieve is to understand this and value and respect the life/values/practices of each and every human being, no matter what culture, and to try hear the voice(s) of others when working to improve life, health, and well-being.

Unfortunately, cultural and spiritual tolerance are often lacking in relations among people from different backgrounds within and across national borders. Some long-standing conflicts can erupt into conflagrations that lead to genocide. Recent and current evidence of genocide continue to be reported in Darfur, Rawanda, Zambia, the Congo, Iraq, and in some countries in the Balkan area. Even in highly developed nations, civil unrest may arise as ethnic minorities compete to meet their needs and preserve their values and communities, often within a hostile society. In many countries around the world, a nurse of one color, gender, class, ethnic heritage, or religion does not provide care to a patient who is a different color, class, ethnic heritage, or religion without risk to self and family. Such social divisions make it difficult to meet the needs of people in many countries.

Chase and Hunter[4] discuss cultural and spiritual responsivity as part of the advanced practice role. Being culturally responsive means the APRN integrates the health and illness perspectives and practices of patients and families when developing healthcare interventions. Cultural and spiritual responsivity reflects a mind-set that recognizes—and avoids—ethnocentricity. Instead of viewing how the patient can fit into the nurse's world because it is assumed the nurse knows best (ethnocentrism), the nurse acquires an understanding of the patient's world and examines how to fit into that world. The culturally responsive nurse incorporates communication patterns, social organizations, heritage, spirituality, biological variations, beliefs, traditions, and practices that the patient values into the plan of care (ethnorelativism).

Ethics and cultural and spiritual responsivity are attributes critical for the APRN practicing in a country or community outside of his or her own experience. Without these competencies, efforts to address health and social disparities may be for naught.

The APRN Role Outside the United States

The role of APRNs as health consultants, health educators, and health providers is critical to the health and even survival of people. Grace Madubuko,[5] Coordinator of Nursing Affairs, West African College of Nursing in Nigeria, described the needs that can be addressed by

APRNs: screening and triaging patients, monitoring those with chronic illnesses, screening for and managing breast and cervical cancer, teaching people how to prevent the spread of HIV/AIDS and other sexually transmitted diseases (STDs), reducing maternal/child morbidity and mortality, promoting nutrition, and alleviating the health effects of poor sanitation.

Much of the focus of the advanced practice role abroad is on promoting public health and delivering services to populations at risk, especially mothers and babies. APRNs and nurses also are needed to help stem communicable diseases and promote prenatal health by providing programs that rely on laypersons trained to carry on the work locally and spread knowledge in the community. Programs, such as the Community Lay Health Educators, are designed to train lay individuals to teach the most impoverished and isolated people how to create a healthier environment in which to live. Topics commonly discussed by these lay health educators include improving sanitation, encouraging hand washing, and explaining the need to protect from mosquitoes by using netting and eradicating mosquito breeding grounds to prevent such diseases as malaria and dengue fever. Lay health educators also discuss venting enclosed cooking areas to prevent chronic respiratory problems, boiling water to free it of disease-causing microorganisms, rehydrating infants afflicted with dysentery, and wearing shoes to prevent parasitic infestation. Improving nutrition, encouraging safe sex, explaining about family planning, and encouraging breast feeding and developing healthier "formula" feedings for newborns are also important topics.[6,7] Public health is the key to survival for the people of the world, and collaborative efforts among nursing, medicine, and public health professionals, political leaders, and the lay community are needed to achieve the health goals of each developing country.

Where APRNs Have Served

Many APRNs from the United States, including the authors, have served in formative roles as consultants to ministries of health, as directors of nursing services in international hospitals such as The Holy Innocents Children's Hospital in Mbarara, Uganda, and/or have worked with schools of nursing, faith-based healthcare initiatives, and orphanages to develop nurse-led health interventions, nursing outreach services, community lay educator programs, and improved nursing educational curricula and regulation of advanced practice. They have served in countries such as Thailand, Canada, Ghana, Uganda, Mexico, the Dominican Republic, Honduras, Ecuador, Zimbabwe, Kenya, Tanzania, and Albania. Others have participated in disaster relief measures after such world tragedies as the tsunami of 2004, Hurricane Katrina, earthquakes, and the genocide in Darfur, to name a few. Still others have been instrumental in the success of international surgical teams whose goals may be providing ophthalmological surgeries or repairing cleft palates or congenital cardiac or neurological anomalies.

Learning About Opportunities

A multitude of international opportunities awaits the APRN committed to making a difference in the health and well-being of the people of the world. A search of the Internet reveals existing opportunities of proven and sustainable activities affiliated with NGOs. Many nursing schools have also developed international opportunities for students: the University of San Diego, the University of California at San Francisco; Oregon Health & Science University, Duke University, Marquette University, and the University of Michigan among them. Each school has provided varied services to people of other nations, including direct patient care, program development, cottage industry development, training of community/lay health educators, and consulting and preparing nurses to care for the people. Regardless of the affiliate organization, the APRNs interested in global health should seek opportunities that meet the aforementioned characteristics of successful global health outreach initiatives.

Those who are planning to practice as APRNs abroad after graduation need to plan sufficient lead time to accomplish their goals. Some universities are offering graduate-level certification courses to prepare health professionals to practice abroad. APRNs will need to locate policies and applications related to practice abroad and acquire the documents required by the specific host country and sponsoring agency. Many countries restrict practice to persons who are fluent in the native language.

The Web sites http://www.globalhealth.gov and http://www.usaid.gov are useful resources. The Web sites of global organizations, such as the UN Refugees Agency, Red Cross, International Rescue Committee, and International Centre for Migration and Health, which address disaster and emergency relief as well as development during the post-conflict phase, are also good resources.

Community and public health nursing skills are paramount to reversing the effects of poverty due to war, drought, flood, and famine experienced by many people in Third World nations. The skills needed by APRNs in these situations are an intimate knowledge of the community's needs and the ability to obtain and organize resources to meet these needs on a continuing basis. The APRN must earn the trust of the community, understand the beliefs and concerns of the people, and be able to communicate complex ideas and concepts simply and clearly. In addition to extensive clinical knowledge and skills, these APRNs must be politically and socially astute to remain trusted members of the community and to survive the changing political landscape. See Figure 12-6.

Globalization of Advanced Practice Registered Nursing

Some of the less developed countries sponsor advanced education for their nurses in developed countries such as the United States. These nurses historically have been sent to the United States and their education sponsored by their government so that they can return to their country and use their acquired knowledge to improve the health of the citizens. Unfortunately, not all of those nurses return to their native countries, creating a "brain drain" of intellectual resources that further depletes the potential leadership and talent available to meet the sponsoring nation's health goals.

Over the past several years, with the mandate from the WHO and the support of the International Council of Nurses (http://www.icn.ch/policy.htm), more and more countries have begun the educational preparation of their own APRNs.[11] Governments are increasingly willing to bring nurse educators from developed nations to their country to train larger groups of nurses. This often reduces costs and encourages nurses once trained to remain in their native lands. APRNs are traveling the world to share their professional knowledge and skills.

Basic problems in the systematic dissemination of food and medications to those in need further frustrate the efforts of nurses in countries where resources are scarce and the need is great. At times, nurses, because they are the only persons with professional health knowledge available, are sought after to perform medical procedures that would otherwise be performed by physicians. See Figure 12-7.

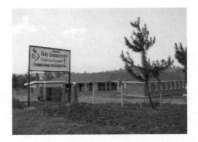

Figure 12-6: The hospital built by nursing students and faculty in Mbarara, Uganda.

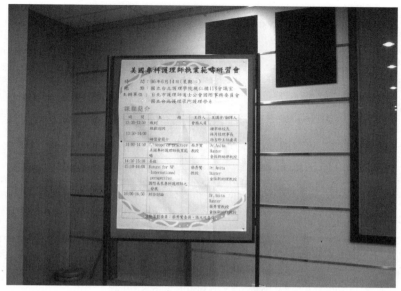

Figure 12-7: Teaching program for NPs in Taipei, Taiwan.

Similar frustrations are encountered by nurses educated abroad who return to their home countries often to find their attempts to implement new knowledge and to change the system frustrated by a lack of resources for quality nursing care, terrain and roads that limit access to health care, illiteracy, and poverty.[5–10]

In Latin America and the Caribbean, because of a lack of physicians, nurses have historically been primary care providers (personal communication with Dr. Leda McKenry, 2008). Using models of public health nursing reminiscent of Lillian Wald's and Mary Breckenridge's, these nurses have successfully cared for the people of their countries. Many have been educated as nurse-midwives and some have become family nurse practitioners. They create and manage community clinics and home healthcare agencies to bring health care to rural underserved areas. In addition, these nurses train lay community health assistants and health educators to assist in health screenings, risk identification, and health teaching.

The "village" phenomenon in Africa is similar. Here, lay professionals are often the traditional birth attendants and healers who use herbal therapies and local health practices. Few rehabilitation hospitals, eldercare complexes, or orphanages exist. Access to health care is limited primarily to acute care facilities. People care for one another at home with traditional means. Nurses in several African nations, including Ghana, South Africa, Nigeria, and Zimbabwe, as witnessed by coauthor Anita Hunter, have built on these practices by establishing traveling clinics or local clinics to reach out to those in the "bush," who cannot access healthcare services.[3,5]

Some countries also provide outreach healthcare services and aid to persons outside their geographical borders. There are many examples of nurses from one country helping people in other countries as part of a "friendly neighbor" program. Two examples illustrate the diversity of assistance that is provided. Nurses in Israel have established an education program to help Ethiopian refugees understand food labeling so they can make informed food choices to meet cultural and health needs.[12] Japan has sponsored the development of a community-based NGO, a hospital for mothers and children, a primary school, and a vocational training school for the impoverished people of the Zia Colony of Pakistan.[12]

The International Nurse Practitioner/Advanced Practice Nursing Network (INP/APN) provides a forum for advanced practice nurses in every nation to join in advocating for global health. The organization has defined advanced practice nursing for the global community and established policies related to education, standards of practice, and scope of practice for the APRN in the international arena. From the International Council of Nurses and the INP/APN network (http://icn.apnetwork.com) the following information about international NPs is available:

- In Canada, NPs are becoming more abundant. They address the needs for cost containment, increased access to care, and health promotion and disease prevention.
- In Australia, the role has been evolving, extending across the vast regions of the country into Tasmania.
- New Zealand, which is further along in its use of APRNs than Australia, has implemented the NP role to increase access to care, provide affordable care, reduce inequalities, and benefit the public, particularly the indigenous population who live in areas where there are often no other healthcare providers.
- In the Netherlands, the lack of physicians drove the need to develop the NP role. The NPs' efforts center on supporting holistic care and demonstrating positive outcomes.
- In Sweden, NPs have filled the gap in geriatric care.
- In Fiji, the NP is prepared to practice in rural and remote communities and is often the sole healthcare provider to a community.
- In Korea, Taiwan, and Thailand, the NP role is expanding exponentially. Throughout these countries, graduate programs for preparing APRNs are evident. In Japan, where the nurse-midwifery role is well established, the first NP educational programs are being launched.

Authors have worked with regulators in Canada in the development of their NP licensing exam and in Taiwan for both certification and licensing exams. The licensing exam in British Columbia, Canada, consists of both a written and a standardized patient-focused assessment exam. This type of exam is in keeping with the trend toward professional performance exams for health professionals in the United States, including such exams in dentistry and medicine and probably nursing in the future. The expense of conducting these exams is a deterrent, but protecting the safety of the public may outweigh the expense, which is passed along to the examinee.

APRN Impacts on Global Nursing Practice and Education

There have been APRNs in the United States since the early 1900s, including pioneers like Mary Breckenridge and Lillian Wald, working in both rural and city communities. These early examples of advanced nursing practice exemplified serving unmet community needs and helped prepare the way for other types of advanced practice. In 1965, the first NP, Loretta Ford, with the help of physician Henry Silver, developed the role of the pediatric nurse practitioner (PNP) in the community. The types of advanced practice nursing continue to expand to meet different needs. APRNs may move across settings to care for their patients' needs, whether they are in the home, an outpatient agency, a primary health arena, an acute care agency, or an extended care facility.

Four roles requiring special certification with the APRN licensing classification—the clinical nurse specialist (CNS), the nurse practitioner (NP), the certified registered nurse anesthetist (CRNA), and the certified nurse-midwife (CNM)—currently comprise advanced practice nursing in the United States. These APRN roles include delivery of direct care involving the assessment of health, ordering and interpreting diagnostic tests, prescribing medications, and performing common medical procedures for the designated patient population as well as consulting, educating, advocating, evaluating care, and applying research. Regardless of the population served or the setting for care, advanced practice nursing in the United States is characterized by complex decision making, independent functioning, and advanced knowledge and skills obtained through graduate nursing education, either at the master's or the doctoral level.[13] See Figure 12-8.

Changing Educational Requirements for APRNs in the United States

The education of APRNs is changing in the United States. Educational programs are offering a new degree called the Doctor of Nursing Practice (DNP) as preparation for nurses in advanced practice. This preparation is aimed at developing leaders who will improve the quality of healthcare delivery and improve patient outcomes in the complex system of health care unique to the United States. The change is a significant one for employers, patients, and other health professionals. Its impact will be evaluated as graduates assume their responsibilities and create a new vision of healthcare delivery. The dissemination of advanced knowledge may also benefit global health efforts that are on the horizon, but given that the trend toward the DNP as the entry into advanced practice is just now occurring, it may be some time before the impact is felt abroad. Some of the preparation acquired by the DNP may prove especially helpful in designing innovative models of care to improve access and quality of care while reducing cost (http://www.aacn.nche.edu/DNP).

The quality of the care APRNs strive for in the United States is compassionate, evidence-based care that meets national standards for practice. Regardless of the population (e.g., pediatric or geriatric) or setting (e.g., hospital or office-based), the APRN is expected to provide quality care that builds on an expanded knowledge base from the humanities and biopsychosocial and behavioral sciences. Such advanced clinical knowledge, critical thinking, clinical judgment, and communication skills can be used to address complex problems, including family dysfunction and chronic and life-threatening illnesses. Critical components of the APRN role are promoting healthy growth and development from birth to death and helping to resolve psychosocial issues and ethical dilemmas.

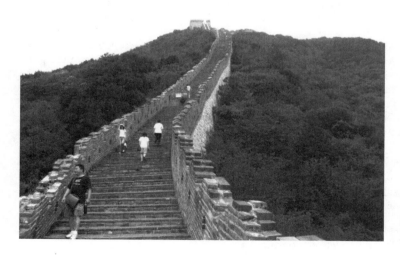

Figure 12-8: Great Wall of China.

Reimbursement Issues

Most APRN services are reimbursed by private payers and third-party payers. Federal regulations address Medicare reimbursement for APRN services. More and more NPs are recognized as primary care providers (PCPs) on managed care panels and receive reimbursement for their services from Medicare under their own provider numbers.[14] However, the problem of reimbursement and the cost of health care and health insurance create gaps in access to quality care for the uninsured and working poor. APRNs are helping to close this gap, providing care to indigent people and other underserved individuals and families. In such cases, there may be little, if any, reimbursement. When reimbursement for services rendered is lacking, people are denied access to health care and the sustainability of the practice is jeopardized.

Growing Recognition of the Contributions of APRNs

The valued contributions of the APRN over the past 40 years have brought recognition and acceptance by the public and the healthcare system in this country and abroad. The role of the APRN has been viewed by the federal government as a cost-effective means of extending care to many citizens who would otherwise go without health services. Federal support of educational programs to prepare NPs has allowed the role to expand and develop models of care emulated around the world. The following are examples of the federally funded National Health Service Corps (NHSC) practice and educational programs:

- Arizona—Combining Native Traditions and Modern Medicine
- California—Building a Healthier Community
- Colorado—Interdisciplinary Approach Is Necessity in Remote Regions of Colorado
- Washington DC—Community Spirit Alive and Well in DC
- Iowa/Illinois—Certified Nurse-Midwives Attentive to Mothers
- Maine—Improving Patient Management of Diabetes
- Minnesota—Rural Community and Good Mental Health
- New York—Improving Oral Health in a New York Community
- North Carolina—community-wide universal healthcare program
- South Carolina—providing mobile health care to underserved populations

Over the years, the NHSC has helped prepare 22,000 clinicians through such program initiatives as these and by offering educational scholarship programs, such as the National Health Service Corps or the Loan Repayment program requiring 2 years of service at a NSHC-approved site in a Health Professional Shortage Area. (See http://nhsc.bhpr.hrsa.gov for more information.)

Satisfied consumers recognize the value of APRN care, and public acceptance has allowed the role to flourish. Many physicians have recognized the value of adding NPs to their practices. However, to maintain this caliber of practice and professional respect, it is important to prepare APRNs for tomorrow's practice, not just today's. NONPF has assumed a leadership role in setting the educational standards for APRN education in the United States. The International Council of Nurses (ICN), in consort with the INP/APN Network, has assumed the leadership role in setting the standards for APRN education internationally.

NONPF Core Competencies for APRNs in the United States

Based on the work of Patricia Benner[15] and Karen Bryczynski,[16] NONPF developed core competencies for entry-level NP practice in the United States regardless of specialty.[13] Benner's original four domains of nursing practice have evolved into seven domains of practice[13]:

- Management of patient health and illness status
- Nurse practitioner–patient relationship

- Teaching-coaching function
- Professional role
- Managing and negotiating the healthcare delivery system
- Monitoring and ensuring the quality of healthcare practice
- Cultural and spiritual competence

The 2002 national project, undertaken by NONPF and the American Association of Colleges of Nursing (AACN) with funding by HRSA, further developed these competencies.[13] For a complete list of the core and advanced practice competencies, see the NONPF Web site (http://www.nonpf.com) or the AACN Web site (http://www.aacn.nche.edu).

A national panel of NP educators, along with representatives from accrediting and credentialing organizations, developed these advanced practice competencies, which have been endorsed by 19 national organizations. These competencies provide educators, employers, and federal funding agencies a guide for the educational programs preparing NPs in five primary care practice areas: adult, family, gerontological, pediatric, and women's health. Similar national validation processes were used to develop advanced practice competencies for psychiatric-mental health and acute care NPs. These competencies are currently undergoing revision and updating. National consensus-based competencies for advanced practice nurses guide curriculum development, state licensing, national board certification and accreditation of educational programs in the US.

A new initiative to blend the adult and gerontological nurse practitioner competencies for NPs serving adults and the elderly is underway as a joint project of AACN and NONPF with funding from the Hartford Foundation. These competencies address doctoral expectations for NPs serving these populations and are intended to increase the number of individuals prepared to care for the growing population of elderly (http://www.nonpf.com).

Spread of NONPF Core Competencies Internationally

To date, the NONPF core competencies that describe foundational competencies have served as a model for APRN education in 19 countries.[11] While working with NPs in Taiwan recently, coauthor Anita Hunter found evidence of their use as well as of the implementation of standardized patient exams (SPEs) in conjunction with completion of a board certification exam as a requirement for entry into the APRN role. Coauthor Katherine Crabtree working with Canadian regulators in British Columbia found that they are also implementing standardized clinical exams for advanced practice licensure. Certifying boards in the United States may soon adopt a similar process.

Preparation for APRN practice in other countries is very different from that required in the United States. APRNs mentoring nurses around the world need to be aware of the rich variety in cultures and environments and adapt both teaching methodologies and expected competencies. Most importantly, to be successful, adaptations must be culturally relevant. Individuals sensitive to the beliefs, values, and customs of the people of a particular country can assist others within that culture design and develop appropriate educational programs to prepare APRNs for practice in that culture. In addition, APRN consultants must be culturally savvy to help international colleagues achieve the fullest scope of practice possible in their countries and support their colleagues as they learn to negotiate the political and social structures.

The Influence of the ICN and INP/APN Network on APRN Practice

The ICN and INP/APN have endorsed the definition of health care put forward by the WHO:

> *Primary health care is essential evidenced-based health care practice, brought to the individual, family, and community, at the primary, secondary, and tertiary levels, and is universally accessible, affordable, and able to be a self-sustained practice in that country.*[2,17]

This definition encompasses the work of many nurses around the world, including bachelor's- and master's-prepared nurses, those who perform diagnostic or surgical procedures, midwives, those who provide health promotion, and those who provide acute and chronic illness care and public health care.

This definition has framed the work of the ICN, INP/APN Network, the American Academy of Nurse Practitioners (AANP), the Royal College of Nursing (RCN), NONPF, and a multitude of other nursing organizations around the world. It defines the practice characteristics and educational preparation needed to become an APRN. These organizations, working collaboratively through the INP/APN Network, have defined the NP/APRN as: a registered nurse who has acquired the expert knowledge base, complex decision-making skills and clinical competence for expanded practice in primary health care, the characteristics of which would be determined by the context in which s/he is licensed to practice. Given the country in which one practices, an advanced degree—for example, a master's degree—is recommended for entry-level practice in the expanded role.[12] The characteristics of nurses practicing in the expanded role should include:

- The ability to integrate research, education, practice, and management
- The opportunity to practice a high degree of professional autonomy
- The opportunity to have one's own case load and [provide] case management
- The acquisition of advanced decision-making and diagnostic reasoning skills, advanced health assessment skills, and clinical competence
- Prescribing, referral, and hospital admitting rights
- Legislation that confers and protects the titles of Nurse Practitioner/Advanced Practice Nurse/Clinical Nurse Specialist/Nurse Midwife (http://www.icn.ch/networks)

Currently, not all nations can provide the education for advanced practice nurses, endorse the scope of practice, or adopt a restricted title for advanced practice nurses. It is not uncommon for nurses prepared in many developing nations to be expected to practice as APRNs, yet not be legitimized by the political or medical establishments of those nations.[5,12] Traditional beliefs about the role of women and the traditional practices of physicians have impaired the forward movement of nursing in these countries. Unstable political systems in developing countries also impede long-term planning for health services and education of advanced practice nurses.

Differences in the etiology and treatment of diseases in developing nations also require modification in the educational preparation and scope of practice of the APRN. In the United States and other developed nations, one of the major aspects of the APRN role is to ameliorate or stabilize the conditions associated with unhealthy lifestyles and teach the adoption of health behaviors for better self-care. In developing nations, the nurse must focus on public health and other environmental factors, such as poor air and water quality, inadequate nutrition, or lack of sanitation, that give rise to disease or complicate disease responses and treatment. Thus, differences in roles and educational preparation must be recognized in defining APRN practice in developed and developing nations. While working with APRNS in Uganda, Hunter found that many practicing in an APRN capacity were prepared at the diploma level but had acquired advanced skills from experience and/or through special training by doctors so they can help those who are most removed from access to medical care.

Preparing nurses to educate others about the principles of health, nutrition, hygiene, and prevention of disease allows the dissemination of healthy practices and prevention of illness in villages lacking resources and access to more advanced technology. The valuing and recognizing of what nurses do in their world where educational and healthcare resources are limited may give credence to the legitimacy of the nurses' expanded role in these developing nations.

NP Role and Education in Other Developed Nations

In developed countries, the APRN role and educational qualifications are similar to those in the United States.

In the United Kingdom (UK), NPs are required to complete an advanced educational program beyond basic nursing training. These programs vary in length and lead to a bachelor's degree, postgraduate diploma, or master's degree. In the UK, NPs are well prepared to become autonomous and/or interdependent practitioners, with full prescribing rights. They function in community-based clinics, specialist hospital units (e.g., dermatology, cardiology, accident and emergency, minor injury units, and oncology) and in projects working with the homeless and male and female sex workers in inner-city areas. NPs lead the Minor Injury Units and are linked to physicians at nearby hospitals by telemedicine, if consultation is needed, and work as part of a professional team in both primary and secondary care. The NP/APN role in the UK is being adapted to fit the national healthcare system and to meet the unique needs of the people, including the itinerant population known as the "travelers"; new refugees; an increasing number of homeless, mentally ill, and elderly persons; and those from rural or underserved areas of the country. However, data from a national survey conducted by the University of Central England revealed many of the more than 60 different advanced practice nursing roles identified in the UK are located within hospital settings, rather than in community settings. The challenge of differentiating the NP role and defining the scope of practice and role characteristics acceptable to patients, communities, and government remains.[11]

Canada's national healthcare system is similar to that of the UK, and the NP/APN role is very similar to that in the UK system. The scope of practice varies among the Canadian provinces just as it does from state to state in the United States and Australia. The advanced practice role differs depending on whether the population the NP is working with is urban or rural. In the major cities, the CNS/APN works collaboratively with the physician within the hospital in an interdependent relationship. This model is similar to the CNS role in the United States, focusing on patient, educator, and staff development. The APRN in the rural community assumes a more autonomous position, working in a position similar to the general practitioner model, with the physician remote from the practice site.

In an effort to provide a national umbrella for advanced practice nursing in Canada, the board of directors of the Canadian Nurses Association finalized a broad framework to guide its development. The framework, which includes core competencies, provides national consistency in the key elements defining advanced nursing practice, yet allows provinces to adapt the model to their regional needs and pursue legislation to enact and enable the role. The Registered Nurses Association of British Columbia and the Ministry of Health in Ontario have developed entry-level competencies for NPs adapted from the NONPF core competencies. The number of NPs practicing in Canada has risen significantly since 2002, up at least 40% (http://www.cna-aiic.ca/CNA).[18]

In Australia, the development of the NP role is attributed to a shortage of medical practitioners, especially those willing to work in rural, aboriginal health care. The Nurse's Registration Board has been working for more than 8 years to implement the NP role, which is designed along the lines of the NP role in the United States and encompasses assessment, diagnosis, treatment, and prescriptive authority. Because of the mostly rural nature of their practice, NPs practicing in these areas may have total medical responsibility for the community. Therefore, stringent education and accreditation criteria have been established to ensure public safety and to support the autonomy of the role. Changes have been made in the Nurse's Act, the Poison and Therapeutic Goods Act, and the Pharmacy Act to pave the way for implementation of the NP role. As the NP role is adopted, issues surrounding education, titling, and licensure are at the center of the debate. The sociopolitical struggle for recognition and protection of the NP title and for full scope of practice are similar to the struggles experienced since 1965 by NPs in the United States.[12]

APRN Roles in Other Nations

In developing nations, the role of the APRN centers on those of the clinical registered nurse anesthetist (CRNA) and the certified nurse-midwife (CNM).

CRNA ROLE IN DEVELOPING NATIONS

The nurse anesthetist has become a critical component of care for people in developing countries. Many undeveloped nations have few anesthesiologists and rely mainly on nurse anesthetists. In 1989, an international organization of nurse anesthetists, the International Federation of Nurse Anesthetists (IFNA), was established. Membership has flourished and the organization has become an authoritative voice for nurse anesthetists worldwide. The IFNA has developed standards of education and practice and a code of ethics (http://www.aana.com).

The Health Volunteers Overseas (HVO) organization offers programs to prepare nurse anesthetists in developing countries. This nonprofit, volunteer organization founded in 1986 offers more than 50 training programs in 25 developing nations, promoting health care in the least developed nations of the world through training and education in 10 specialty areas (http://www.hvousa.org/fact.cfm).

CERTIFIED NURSE-MIDWIFERY (CNM) ROLE IN DEVELOPED AND DEVELOPING COUNTRIES

The role of the APRN as a certified nurse-midwife is specific to the United States. In other countries, this role is usually fulfilled by a layperson, rather than a nurse. It is a well-known and well-respected role around the world. Many midwives in developing nations are not nurse-midwives. They are midwives trained in programs offered by their governments or they are untrained local attendants; unfortunately, less favorable outcomes for both mother and infant have occurred with the less trained or untrained attendant. Though specialized training for this role is required for nurses practicing in developed countries, it often is not required in developing countries where there is no money or access to trained personnel to teach others. People in those areas are only able to access what is available or affordable. Such financial destitution afflicts over 75% of the world population.[1]

Preparing APRNs With A Global Perspective

To participate in international opportunities to contribute to the improvement of health globally, nurses must understand exactly what the needs are, learn about the country they will be working in, and provide for their own health and safety. They also need to be educated on what to do.

Twofold Need

The need for APRNs is twofold:

1. There is a need for knowledgeable public health nursing consultants who can design and implement community-wide programs. Such programs should include training laypersons to be community health educators who can serve the larger community. Training should include teaching about health priorities, maintaining health, preventing diseases, obtaining immunizations, accessing good nutrition, improving sanitation, obtaining prenatal care, and preventing sexually transmitted diseases.

2. There is a need for experienced APRNs to help nursing educators around the world develop educational programs to prepare quality APRNs who are able to provide health care for the people of their nations.

Placement Opportunities

Several private and public organizations help to place APRNs and other nurses overseas. Their Web sites describe current needs abroad, the types of opportunities available for health professionals, and potential sponsoring organizations. Some religious organizations, such as Northwest Medical Teams (http://www.northwestmc.com), recruit health professionals for foreign mission assignments. Some nurses choose short-term assignments of a few weeks or months. Long-term contracts may stipulate a two-year or longer commitment.

Doctors without Borders (http://www.doctorswithoutborders.org), Volunteers in Medical Missions (http://www.vimm.org), and Mercy Corps (http://www.mercycorps.org) dispatch teams of healthcare providers to disaster areas to provide emergency relief services. Nursing Students Without Borders (http://www.vcu.edu/so/nswb) is a national organization that was established in 2000 by student nurses who wanted to become involved in global health activities before graduation; it is based on the Doctors without Borders model. These nurses have performed health services in the United States as well as in El Salvador. Chapters are appearing at several universities. Nurses are also occasionally recruited by foreign governments to set up healthcare services, organize facilities, and train staff.

There are many incentives for engaging in international nursing practice: altruism, respect, providing assistance, and sharing knowledge and resources. Financially, salaries may not compete with those afforded health professionals in the United States, but cost of living may be substantially less, thus allowing for net savings.

Need to Respect the Local Customs

As guests of the country in which they live, nurses must honor the customs of the country regarding dress and deportment. For example, in the Middle East nurse consultants may live in a restricted community or compound with other foreign nationals. There may be restrictions on the type of clothing worn for leisure and work. Eating, sleeping, and bathing areas are often segregated by gender. Often, the role of women is more restricted abroad than the role of women in U.S. culture. Women may not be allowed to travel unescorted, and they may not be allowed to provide physical care to patients of the opposite gender.

Regardless of the country in which a nurse is working, cultural sensitivity and responsivity are critical. Respect for religious observances, social structure, parenting practices, traditional health and illness beliefs, and marital relationships are necessary for a nurse to be successful in any capacity.

Need to Know and Prepare for the New Environment

Before participating in international health efforts, health providers need to be prepared to work with the people in their environment and be knowledgeable about local health problems. Available therapies may be limited or differ from the treatments the APRN has used previously. Some countries may lack vaccines and prescription medications available in the United States. Universal precautions may not be practiced. Medical supplies may be in short supply. Shipped medical equipment and drugs may be delayed or not arrive due to lack of permits, transportation problems, or diversion. Equipment may be older and low technology may be the norm. Laboratory tests may be unavailable and treatment may be empirical. Differences in water and food supplies and lack of electricity and refrigeration require adjustment. Temperature extremes and high altitudes also may create health hazards.

Protection for the APRN includes up-to-date immunizations prior to departure. A list of required immunizations is available through the Centers for Disease Control and Prevention (CDC) for travel to any country in the world: http://www.cdc.gov/travel. The CDC also issues health alerts, designating areas where there are known health risks. Protection against disease is important when practicing and living in rural areas or when responding to natural or manmade disasters. Often, special permits are required to enter some countries. Travelers may be screened to prevent the spread of disease such as severe acute respiratory syndrome (SARS) or H1N1 (swine flu) before receiving permission to leave an area where there has been an outbreak.

Communication and transportation delays are common and expected. Persistence and detailed directions are often needed to locate specific places due to a lack of adequate signs for travelers to find their way.

Passports and work visas are often required. Obtaining these documents before departure may require additional time and planning. Work restrictions may limit the ability of the nurse to practice abroad due to differences in licensing and educational requirements. Personal safety may be an issue in countries where political unrest is the norm and sentiment against the United States is high.

Reputable organizations require and may provide preparation in the language and culture (beliefs, customs, values, and social, political, and religious structures) before departure. APRNs entering the international arena are responsible for educating themselves about the people and the culture where they will be living and working. Knowledge of priority health problems, their causes, how they are managed, and their long-term outcomes is important preparation for success. Knowledge of personal values, beliefs and prejudices is essential. The ability to help nurses from a variety of cultures work together in harmony under disaster conditions and during periods of high stress is paramount to success. Flexibility and having a sense of humor also can be a tremendous advantage in the face of the multitude of adjustments that will most likely be necessary. The ability to tolerate uncertainty, problem solve, and adapt innovative approaches is key. Patience with unfamiliar, complicated regulations is a necessity.

Need for Educational Preparation Within the APRN Curriculum

Using the NONPF core competencies[13] as a framework, the following activities could be developed within the curriculum to provide APRNs with a broad global perspective:

- Provide professional role learning activities
  - Debate the strengths and weaknesses of a global perspective on nursing policy, economics, management, and role.
  - Identify ways to improve access to care for immigrant populations.
    Contact nurses or others in an international community via the Internet or at nursing conferences.
  - Discuss cultures, populations, or communities of interest to identify the socio-economic and political barriers to furthering their health; explore the effect of these barriers on health policy development, nursing practice, and economic, social, and religious factors within that community.
- Managing and negotiating healthcare delivery systems.
  - Incorporate cultural learning activities in core or general graduate courses.
- Identify the regional, national, and global context of care for different populations. Present case studies and problem-oriented scenarios on how to negotiate the U.S. healthcare delivery system.
- Monitoring and ensuring the quality of healthcare practices
  - Identify political and professional activities needed in an international organization. One example of such an organization is the ICN and its INP/APN Network, whose goal is to facilitate the development of global standards of practice and education through the sharing of resources and information to help overcome some of the current world health problems.
- Demonstrating cultural responsivity
  - Identify different cultures, populations, or communities of interest and use the Internet and literature to plan assessment and intervention strategies.

- "Adopt" an international community within a developing nation, identifying health needs of a particular population and planning culturally appropriate interventions for that population.
- Assess and plan health-related activities to assist a new immigrant community within the United States.

■ Teaching-coaching function, APRN-client relationship, and management of client health/illness status
- Identify pathophysiological and pharmacological variations in the presentation and treatment of disease states and responses to medical treatment in given populations.
- Explore complementary and alternative health practices of a specific culture, population, or community and their compatibility with modern medical interventions.
- Identify health problems of a specific culture, population, or community using case studies and problem-focused scenarios, identify how to assess and manage these health problems, develop culturally appropriate and manageable interventions to prevent further recurrence, and assist the population in accessing culturally appropriate care. Include the newest concerns related to zoonotic disease transmission.
- Participate in short-term domestic international service-learning programs and clinical cultural-immersion experiences.
- Establish faculty practice models for community health and international health.
- These practice environments serve as learning centers for nurses, facilitate mentorship, and provide arenas for scholarship whether in research, teaching, or clinical practice.

SUMMARY

We live in a global society. As the world grows smaller, APRNs are becoming increasingly aware that people around the world are interdependent. Despite differences in skin color, language, dress, and religion, people are more similar than dissimilar. Although the causes of illnesses APRNs treat in other countries are local, some illnesses are becoming global experiences. Global health needs are rising, resources are diminishing, and emigration of future nurse leaders is occurring in the countries least able to afford such losses. WHO has called upon APRNs to correct disparities in healthcare delivery and address the health needs of peoples around the world. APRN roles and education programs are being developed around the world, particularly in other developed countries. Advanced practice nursing has a responsibility for the health of the world; APRNs are well suited to meet these needs.

SUGGESTED LEARNING EXERCISES

1. Identify where you would locate information about advanced practice opportunities abroad. Select a country and obtain information on advanced practice nursing in that country.

2. Identify the immunizations you would need if you were going to spend several months working with an international healthcare relief organization in rural areas of a South American country such as Nicaragua, or in sub-Saharan Africa, Eastern Europe, or Southeast Asia.

3. Describe personal and professional characteristics you would look for in hiring an APRN to develop a new community-based rural health clinic in a developing nation. State why these characteristics are important to the success of the program.

4. Describe the competencies you would expect an APRN to possess before seeking a position in international health. Identify and plan for the differences in role responsibility, health access, health problems, and management of identified problems.

References

1. Farmer, P. (2004). *Pathologies of Power: Health, Human Rights, and the New War on the Poor.* University of California Press, Berkeley.

2. Siddiqi, J. (1995). *World Health and World Politics: The World Health Organization and the U.N. System.* University of South Carolina Press, Columbia.

3. Hunter, A, and McKenry, L. (2001). An advanced practice international health initiative: the Ghana Health Mission. *Clinical Excellence for Nurse Practitioners: Intern J of NPACE* 5(4):240–245.

4. Chase, S, and Hunter, A. (2002). Cultural and spiritual competence: curricular guidelines. Monograph. National Organization of Nurse Practitioner Faculties, 19–28.

5. Madubuko, G. (2001). *Nurse Practitioner/Advanced Nursing Practice Development in West Africa.* White paper of the International Nurse Practitioner/Advanced Practice Nursing Network. http://www.icn.ch/networks_ap.htm#reports. Accessed May 6, 2003.

6. Fawcett-Henesy, A. (2001, Second Quarter). Disparity versus diversity: meeting the challenge of Europe's underserved populations. *Reflections on Nursing Leadership* 18–19.

7. Avotri, J, and Walters, V. (1999). You just look at our work and see if you have any freedom on earth: Ghana women's account of their work and their health. *Social Science & Medicine* 48(9):1123–1133.

8. Douglas, M. (2000). The effect of globalization on health care: a double-edged sword. *J Transcultural Nurs* 11(2):85–86.

9. Appel, AL, and Malcolm, P. (1999). The struggle for recognition: the nurse practitioner in New South Wales, Australia. *Clinical Nurse Specialist* 13(5):236–241.

10. Diamond, J. (1999). *Guns, Germs, and Steel: The Fates of Human Societies.* W.W. Norton & Co., New York.

11. Pulcini, J, Yuen-Loke, A, Gul, R, and Jelic, M. (2007). *An International Pilot Survey on Advanced Practice Nursing: Education, Practice and Regulatory Issues.* ICN-INP/APN Survey.

12. Duffy, E. (2001). *Evolving Role and Practice Issues: Nurse Practitioners in Australia.* White paper of the International Nurse Practitioner/Advanced Practice Nursing Network.

13. National Organization of Nurse Practitioner Faculties & American Association of Colleges of Nursing. (2002). *Nurse Practitioner Primary Care Competencies in Specialty Areas: Adult, Family, Gerontological, Pediatric, and Women's Health.* U.S. DHHS, HRSA, Rockville, MD.

14. Buppert, C. (2003). *Nurse Practitioner's Business Practice and Legal Guide.* Aspen, Gaithersburg, MD.

15. Benner, PE. (1984). *From Novice to Expert: Excellence and Power in Clinical Nursing Practice.* Addison-Wesley, Menlo Park, CA.

16. Bryckzynski, KA. (1989). An interpretive study describing the clinical judgment of nurse practitioners. *Scholarly Inquiry for Nursing Practice: An Interpretive Journal* 3(2):113–120.

17. World Health Organization. (1978). *Alma-Alta 1978. Primary Health Care.* "Health for All" series No 1. Geneva, Switzerland.

18. Canadian Nurses Association. (2000). *Advanced Nursing Practice: A National Framework.* Ottawa, ON. Available at www.cna-nurses.ca.

Eileen O'Grady is a certified adult nurse practitioner and wellness coach and serves as visiting professor at Pace University's Leinhard School of Nursing in New York City. Dr. O'Grady has held a number of leadership positions with professional nursing associations and as a founder of the American College of Nurse Practitioners (ACNP). She was a 1999 Policy Fellow in the U.S. Public Health Service Primary Care Policy Fellowship and in 2003 was given the ACNP's Legislative Advocacy Award for her leadership on nurse practitioner policy issues.

Dr. O'Grady serves as the policy editor for the *American Journal for Nurse Practitioners* and is a monthly columnist in *Nurse Practitioner World News*, providing commentary on health policy issues. She teaches health policy and political competency to doctoral nursing students at Pace University. She is in private practice as a wellness coach, in which she employs an evidence-based approach with patients to create wellness visions and achievable goals that reverse or entirely prevent disease.

Dr. O'Grady has authored numerous articles and book chapters on primary care, health policy, and sports medicine. She has taught nurses and physicians around the United States as well as around the world with the U.S. Peace Corps.

Dr. O'Grady holds an associate of applied science degree from Marymount University in Arlington, Virginia, a bachelor's of science degree from George Washington University, a master of public health degree from George Washington University, and a master of science in nursing and a doctorate in philosophy from George Mason University. She has dual citizenship in Ireland and the United States.

CHAPTER 13

Advanced Practice Nursing and Health Policy

Eileen T. O'Grady, PhD, RN, NP

CHAPTER OBJECTIVES

After completing this chapter, the reader will be able to:

1. Analyze the fundamentals of the health policy-making process in the United States.
2. Compare and contrast the major contextual factors and policy triggers that elevate issues to the policy agenda and influence health policy making in the United States.
3. Differentiate between the current and emerging health policy issues that impact advanced practice registered nurses (APRNs) and the populations they serve.
4. Summarize the critical elements of political competence.

"The highest patriotism is not a blind acceptance of official policy, but a love of one's country deep enough to call her to a higher plain."—George McGovern, Politician

"Most people are not for or against anything; the first object of getting people together is to make them respond somehow, to overcome inertia."—Mary Parker Follett

"Sentiment without action is the ruin of the soul."—Edward Abbey

Engaging in health policy is central to the advanced nursing practice role. It requires intervening on behalf of the public, rather than on behalf of individuals at the clinical level. APRNs witness on a daily basis the consequences of policies that harm patients and populations and violate human dignity and value. These powerful clinical experiences can become potent influencers in policy formation for the APRN who integrates these experiences with two additional skill sets: the ability to analyze the policy process and the ability to engage in politically competent action. The APRN movement has made great progress over the last four decades, practicing in every sector of health care. This chapter describes the tensions among cost, quality, and access to health care; the policy process; current APRN policy issues; the skill sets of a "politically competent" APRN; and strategies for influential organizations.

Health policy development is the process by which society makes decisions, selects goals and the best means for reaching them, handles conflicting views about what should be done, and allocates resources to address needs. *Politics* is an indirect method of influencing decision making through the human ego and power relationships, rendering some aspects of policy making nonrational. Health policy has many definitions and there is no concurrence among authors. Longest (2006)[1] defines health policy as:

> *authoritative decisions pertaining to health or the pursuit of health, made in the legislative, executive, or judicial branches of government that are intended to direct or influence the actions, behaviors or decisions of others. This includes groups or classes of individuals (e.g., the poor, physicians, or newborns) or types or categories of organizations (e.g., non-profit hospitals, pharmaceutical companies, schools of nursing).*

Florence Nightingale embodied the leadership role in shaping health policy. She spent most of her life compiling the evidence base used to powerfully sway members of Parliament to enact health policy aimed at making people whole. Her early recognition of the power of evidence to inform policy led to her induction in the Royal Society of Statisticians in Victorian-era England. Although the APRN movement has made astonishing progress, APRNs could be effectively engaging to a much larger degree in health policy formulation. This chapter may serve as an inspiration to strengthening the social covenant that APRNs have with the public, just as Florence Nightingale had with Londoners on the receiving end of Victorian health policies.

Tensions Among Healthcare Costs, Quality, and Access

There is a fundamental tension in the 21st century healthcare system in achieving an appropriate balance between access and quality without excessive increases in costs (Fig. 13-1). The emphasis on healthcare quality stems from a large body of research documenting serious quality problems due to poorly developed systems of care.[2] Access to care cyclically becomes a priority as unemployment rates increase, causing the number of uninsured to swell, or U.S. Census reports are released indicating alarming numbers of uninsured. As systematic quality measures are implemented, healthcare costs frequently increase, at least initially.[3] There is widespread consensus among all stakeholders that extensive and far-reaching systematic reform is needed in our healthcare finance and delivery systems.[4]

Costs

In 2008, total national health expenditures were expected to rise 6.9%—two times the rate of inflation. Total spending was $2.4 trillion in 2007, or $7900 per person, representing 17% of the gross domestic product (GDP), an astonishing increase from 5.2% in 1960.[5] U.S. healthcare spending in the future is expected to increase at similar levels, reaching $4.3 trillion in 2017, or 20% of GDP.

Healthcare costs have spiraled upward at an alarming rate. The average health insurance premium per year for an individual is $4,404 and $12,680 for family coverage. This constitutes a 119% increase since 1999.[3] These rising health insurance premiums are accompanied by increasing co-pays and deductibles and rising employee cost-sharing expenses that threaten access to health care. Employees must pay a larger percentage of the premiums, larger co-pays, and more out of their pockets—or choose to go without insurance. These costs also negatively impact healthcare businesses as they try to balance costs with job growth and competitiveness. In cost per hour, American manufacturers pay more than twice as much on health benefits as most of their foreign competitors.[6]

The number of underinsured adults in the United States—that is, people who have no health coverage or coverage that is so meager they often postpone care because of high medical expenses—has risen dramatically a Commonwealth Fund study finds.[7] As of 2007, there were an estimated 72 million uninsured or underinsured adults in the United States, up 60% from 2003, and 43% of people with health coverage said they were "somewhat" to "completely" unprepared to cope with a costly medical emergency over the coming year. Escalating healthcare costs create spillover effects in the larger macroeconomic realm as well. In a study of foreclosures and bankruptcy, half of all foreclosures were directly linked to medical debt; in 2008, medical crises were estimated to have put 1.5 million Americans in jeopardy of losing their homes.[8]

There is broad consensus that our healthcare system is riddled with inefficiencies, excessive administrative expenses, inflated prices, poor management, inappropriate care, waste, and fraud. These problems significantly increase the cost of health care and health insurance

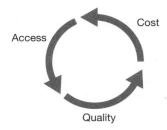

Figure 13-1: The tensions between cost, quality, and access.

for employers and workers, which, in turn, affects the security of families and the economic stability of our nation.

Quality

Currently, we are undergoing a revolution in health-care quality. Purchasers insist on knowing what value they are getting for their dollar, so more metrics are being made available. Today, many people who interact with the healthcare delivery system are deeply dissatisfied with their experiences. The Institute of Medicine (IOM) defines quality as "the degree to which health services for individuals and populations increase the likelihood of desired health outcomes and are consistent with current professional knowledge."[9] Healthcare quality is frequently described as having three dimensions: quality of input resources (certification and/or education of providers), quality of the process of service delivery (the use of appropriate procedures for a given condition), and quality of outcome of service use (actual improvement in condition or reduction of harmful effects).

Evidence of quality problems include:

- Unacceptably high rates of avoidable healthcare errors resulting in disability or premature death. Medical errors result in an estimated 100,000 deaths per year in hospitals in the United States.[10]

- Underutilization of services causing needless complications, higher costs, and lost productivity for millions of Americans. On average, American adults receive just over 55% of recommended care for the leading causes of death and disability.[10]

- Overuse of services causing unnecessary and costly procedures that impose risks on patients. One example is the U.S. caesarian section rate, which is now at 31%, an increase of 41% since 2000. The World Health Organization[11] recommends that the safe caesarian section rate for industrialized nations should not exceed 15%.

- The wide pattern of variation in healthcare practices, suggesting that health care, for the most part, is not delivered from an evidence base. This is most evident across geographic areas as well as in specific clinical areas in which racial and ethnic minorities experience serious disparities in access and outcomes.[12,13]

In addition to differential access and healthcare outcomes for the uninsured versus the insured, racial and ethnic disparities exist in all clinical areas, including heart and renal disease, pain management, asthma, and cancer. The causes are multifactorial and the federal government has made the reduction of racial and ethnic health disparities a major priority for research and intervention funding.[12,13]

Access

Access, the third source of tension in the healthcare delivery system, is an individual's ability to obtain appropriate services. Health insurers today are allowed to deny individuals coverage for any reason or condition. Insurers are also permitted to raise premiums without warning or rationale.

A lack of insurance compromises the health of the uninsured because they receive less preventive care, are diagnosed at more advanced disease stages, and, once diagnosed, tend to receive less therapeutic care and have higher mortality rates than insured individuals. Efforts to improve access often focus on providing/improving health insurance coverage. The IOM report[14] on the consequences of uninsurance notes that working-age Americans without health insurance are more likely to:

- Receive too little medical care and receive it too late;

- Experience more acute sickness and die sooner; and

- Receive poorer care when they are hospitalized, even for acute situations like injuries from motor vehicle crashes.

The uninsured are increasingly paying "up front"—before services are rendered. When they are unable to pay the full medical bill in cash at the time of service, they can be turned away, except in life-threatening circumstances. This raises disturbing questions about our society. The lack of coverage pushes the uninsured into highly inappropriate venues; for example, 20% of the uninsured say their usual source of care is the emergency room[2] as compared to 3% of those with insurance coverage. A more affordable option for the uninsured with discrete primary care problems has been the recently established retail health clinics, largely staffed by nurse practitioners (NPs); this option is, however, limited. Simply put, it is quite risky to be uninsured. Studies estimate that the number of excess deaths among uninsured adults ages 25 to 64 is in the range of 18,000 a year. This mortality figure is more than the number of deaths from diabetes (17,500) within the same age group.[15]

The most common barrier to access is insufficient financial resources. According to one study, over a third of the uninsured have problems paying medical bills. The unpaid bills were substantial enough that many had been turned over to collection agencies, and nearly a quarter of the uninsured adults said they had changed their way of life significantly to pay medical bills.[16] The degree of debt that many of the uninsured have or think they will incur creates a major barrier for them in seeking needed health care, unless they are in a life-threatening situation.

Other barriers to access also exist. Geographic barriers are created when providers are practicing at a distance from communities or when patients are unable to travel to services due to disability or lack of time or transportation. Organizational barriers occur when health systems are unable to employ an appropriate health workforce. Many rural towns are facing a shortage of nurses and need to close hospital units as a result. Sociological barriers include discrimination due to gender, race, ethnicity, sexual preference, age, and language. Cultural barriers and differing health beliefs can also create disconnects between patients accessing care and those providing it. Finally, there are educational barriers, as consumers are largely perplexed about the healthcare delivery system and the options available to them once services are required. The paternalistic framework in which health care has been delivered in the past, a framework that encouraged consumer passivity, may be partly to blame for this difficulty. High health illiteracy rates coupled with marginal cultural competency among providers are also factors contributing to the lack of access to health care experienced by many.

The benefits of having health insurance are even stronger when continuity of coverage is taken into account. Even being uninsured for a relatively short period of time—1 to 4 months—can be harmful to a person's health. Over the long term, uninsured adults are more likely to die prematurely than people with insurance coverage. Approximately 47 million Americans are uninsured at any one time and, as a result, are at higher risk for poorer health on every measure than people who have health insurance.[16]

The American Health Policy Process

Health policy making in the United States is a distinctly incremental process. Its key feature is that no decision is ever final and all policies are subject to modification. Just as health and heath care are dynamic, the phases of the policy-making process are highly interactive and interdependent. Health policy is highly political by nature, political circumstances continually change, and policy decisions are frequently revisited based on those changing circumstances. See Figure 13-2.

The distinctly cyclical nature of health policy making requires stakeholders to be strategic and politically competent, because there are many points along the way where policy is amenable to different forms of influence. Figure 13-3 shows the cyclical and incremental nature of the health policy-making process as it is depicted by Longest.[1]

Agenda Setting

In this country many problems related to health care go unaddressed, especially problems that are too costly and too complex to solve readily. If a healthcare issue is not considered both

Factors Influencing Public Policy

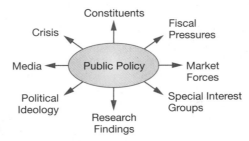

Figure 13-2: Policy triggers.

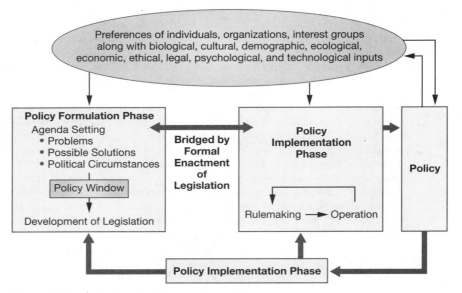

Figure 13-3: Health policy-making model. *From Longest, B. (2006). Health Policymaking in the United States, 4th ed. AUPHA/HAP, Washington, DC.*

important and urgent, it will likely never get on the agenda. Other issues, such as the large numbers of uninsured, are difficult to address because there are intense disagreements about possible solutions to expanding public and private coverage. These contentious issues often languish at the bottom of the agenda; they may receive periodic priority but are put on and taken off the agenda year after year. In order for a problem to become a priority for policy makers and to reach the top of the agenda, a confluence of three broad "streams" must occur:

1. Policy triggers (see Table 13-1)
2. Possible solutions to the policy problems
3. Political will[17]

A policy "window" opens when these three streams come together, and a policy trigger and a solution have the potential to begin the policy-making process. In most circumstances, a number of policy solutions emerge and compete with one another. This is where health services research[18]* can provide clarity. If the solutions do not have real potential to solve the policy problem, the issue will not advance in the policy-making process. The crucial third variable is political will, or creating an "open policy window"; this is the most challenging variable to predict in the policy window stream due to its high level of complexity. Political will is influenced by public opinion, the media, the strength of interest groups and their electioneering skills, executive-branch and legislative opinion leaders, and unpredictable election year pressures. Wakefield (2004)[19] identifies triggers that can propel issues to the top of the policy agenda. Table 13-1 describes policy triggers and recent examples.

Table 13-1 Factors Influencing Agenda Setting

Influencing Factor	Policy Trigger	Example of Policy Solution/Response
Crisis	H1N1 influenza pandemic	Multiple bills introduced seeking to allow states to negotiate prices with vaccine makers directly, to require health plans to withhold co-payments on influenza vaccines, and to authorize primary and secondary schools to serve as vaccination centers.
Media	Investigative reporting in the *Washington Post* exposes deplorable treatment of returning Iraqi War vets at Walter Reed Army Medical Center.	Multiple bills introduced to standardize access procedures of returning combat vets. Provisions include increasing the mental health, nursing, and outreach workforce. Advanced appropriations were authorized to enhance all aspects of veteran health care.
Political ideology	The majority party (Democrats or Republicans) will have a large impact on health policies.	The newly elected Republican leadership opposed the regulations (put into place under a Democratic leadership) that would *not* require physician supervision of CRNAs. This change in political context reversed an important decision that has large implications on the patients dependent on CRNAs for anesthesia care, mostly rural Medicare beneficiaries.
Research findings	Biomedical and health services research contributes to the policy process by clarifying problems and identifying solutions. IOM Report *To Err Is Human* estimates 98,000 people die each year as a result of healthcare errors.	A number of patient safety bills are introduced the following legislative session.

Continued

*Health services research is a multidisciplinary field of inquiry, both basic and applied, that examines the use, costs, quality, accessibility, delivery, organization, financing, and outcomes of healthcare services to increase knowledge and understanding of the structure, processes, and effects of health services for individuals and populations.

Table 13-1 **Factors Influencing Agenda Setting—cont'd**

Influencing Factor	Policy Trigger	Example of Policy Solution/Response
Special interest groups	Interest groups with strong grassroots activity and a single clear mission can have a profound impact on the public policy agenda.	The grassroots organization Mothers Against Drunk Driving (MADD) demonstrates that committed volunteer efforts can influence widespread drunken driving laws, policy, and educational campaigns.
Market forces	Medical debt becomes a major cause of bankruptcy and home foreclosures, impacting the larger macro-economic realm.	A number of bills are introduced to expand coverage and regulate the health insurance industry.
Fiscal pressures	Budget decisions are largely dependent on whether the federal government is in deficit versus surplus spending.	Downturn of the economy and deficit prompts White House Office of Management and Budget Director to slash funding for Health Services Resources and Services Administrations programs designed to enhance the primary care workforce.
Constituents	Constituents have poignant stories of loved ones with rare diseases and express concern that no private or federal research is being conducted.	The Orphan Drug bill passes into law to create incentives for companies to research drugs that do not have commercial viability. Orphan drugs are drugs for rare diseases affecting fewer than 200,000 Americans.
Litigation	Increasingly, interest groups are using litigation to challenge existing policies or obtain specificity from vague legislation.	A federal judge grants class-action status to a lawsuit that claims Wal-Mart's denial of health insurance coverage for birth control is unfair to female employees.

The Dance of Legislative Development

Of the thousands of bills introduced in each congressional session, only a small fraction will ever get to the policy formulation stage; once there, they will follow a highly prescriptive process, or "dance," in order to emerge as new public laws, statutes, or amendments to an existing law.[20] The incremental nature of making health policy and the continuous modifications to existing policies resemble dance choreography.

An important source of policy ideas is the president's State of the Union address, which outlines the laws the president feels are necessary to enact in the coming legislative session. Other proposals can come from "executive communications," often in the form of a letter from a senior member of the executive branch (an agency head, cabinet member, or the president) to members of the legislative branch. Executive communications are often a follow-up to the ideas emphasized in the State of the Union address. One of the most important executive communications is the proposed federal budget transmitted from the White House to Congress.

Once a bill is introduced by a member of Congress, it is referred to one of the 17 standing committees in the House and 16 in the Senate, each with jurisdiction over certain issues.† When more than one committee has jurisdiction over a bill, it is referred to the appropriate committees and subcommittees sequentially. The majority party controls the appointment of chairpersons to all committees and subcommittees, making political ideology a powerful predictor of both the order and pace at which legislative proposals will be considered. In addition, politically competent interest groups play a pivotal role in developing legislation pertinent to their interests to ensure their concerns and preferences are addressed. Once both legislative bodies approve the legislation, the president signs it and it becomes law.

State legislatures follow similar processes, with differences primarily of timing. Individuals should become familiar with the legislative and regulatory processes in the state(s) in which they live and practice.

Policy Implementation: Bringing Laws to Life

The policy-making process next transitions from the legislative branch to the executive branch of government, starting with the rule-making process. The pertinent federal agency is tasked with "interpreting" the law by adding highly specific rules. For example, when NPs were authorized to receive direct Medicare payment in 1998, the Center for Medicare and Medicaid (CMS) defined the education and certification criteria required of NPs in order to qualify for a Medicare provider number. Rule making is also highly procedural, and all proposed and final rules must be published in the *Federal Register*‡ to ensure that stakeholders and the public have an opportunity to participate in the process. Proposed rules are assigned a comment period, which serves as an invitation to the public and stakeholder community to negotiate, bargain, and provide evidence to support or refute the rules.

Advisory commissions, such as the Medicare Payment Advisory Commission (MedPAC),[21] are established by Congress to "help" in the rule-making process, most commonly for cases where there is widespread disagreement and conflict or a high degree of complexity. A commission is also commonly established when rules will be subject to continual revision, such as the Medicare reimbursement rates. Advisory commissions typically are comprised of members outside the implementing agency. Once the final rules are published, the actual implementation of the program begins with most of the responsibility resting on civil service employees in the federal government.

Policy Modification: No Policy Decisions are Ever Permanent

Policy decisions are often correct at the time they are made, but changes in knowledge; demographics; or technological, ethical, or legal events can cause them to become erroneous. The need for policy modification occurs when its consequences—whether intended or unintended—provide negative feedback on any phase of the policy. For example, the delinking of welfare benefits (such as food stamps) and Medicaid enrollment caused large numbers of children to become uninsured. This unintended consequence of delinking the two programs led to the creation of the Children's Health Insurance Program (CHIP) to specifically address the growing uninsurance rate among children. In fact, modern health policy is overwhelmingly derived from modifications of earlier policies. The modification phase should be understood as a continuous interrelated activity in which no decision, including public laws, rules, court decisions, or operational practices, is permanent. Whether the impact of the original policy decision is positive or negative, stakeholders will try to modify the policy to gain more

---

†Information about congressional committees can be obtained at http://thomas.loc.gov.
‡The *Federal Register* is published daily and contains presidential documents, rules and regulations, proposed rules, and notices. This document can be found on the Government Printing Office's Web site, http://www.access.gpo.gov/gpoaccess.

benefits or to retain the existing benefits. Incrementalism also allows time for compromise among diverse interests and increases the likelihood of consensus and creative solutions.

Unique Structural Characteristics of the U.S. Health Policy Arena

The Constitution of the United States is still operative after more than 2 centuries. The key to this endurance has been its flexibility: the ability of our governmental framework to accommodate tremendous change over time. The framers never imagined primary elections, the presidential cabinet, or a huge executive bureaucracy; nor could they have envisioned the growth in the nation's territory, population, and diversity; the technological advances in travel and communications; and the effects of a civil war and two world wars.[17,20,21] Yet, the constitutional framework has endured and flourished throughout these dramatic changes. The system established and fostered by the Constitution for making policy is highly procedural and formal, especially when compared to that of other nations, essentially because there is no real center of power among the three branches of government. This tends to further slow the policy-making process and contributes to incrementalism.

Since the majority of current health policies are modifications of previous policies or decisions, the modifications tend to reflect rather modest changes. Such modesty is the outcome of an intentional constitutional construct to keep power balanced among the branches of government and therefore to prevent tyranny. Incrementalism is the preferred political, economic, and social system for change in the United States.[20] Increasingly, the judicial branch is playing a more prominent role in clarifying health policies, resolving disputes, and establishing precedents, which adds another layer of formality and process. However, courtrooms are typically not an ideal venue for creating health policy, as legal proceedings define problems narrowly and the participants are not content experts.

Federalism, the construct that lies behind the separation of power between the states and the federal government, has recently shifted to devolve more power on the states. This often takes the form of block grants or program waivers given to the states to promote the concept of "states as labs." It has also become evident that each geographic area of the country may require different or varied approaches to solving health problems. Block grants with broad guidelines allow states to solve health problems unique to their region and population.

In addition to the structural, legal, and traditional bases for policy making in the United States is the factor of election-year politics. Election politics can cause policy makers to make unexpected choices in order to gain the support of an important constituent group back home. Politically charged issues can therefore often be caught in gridlock until after an election.

Table 13-2 summarizes the unique characteristics of the context surrounding the making of U.S. health policy.

The APRN Health Policy Agenda

The challenges that restrict advanced practice registered nurses (APRNs) from expressing or practicing to their full capabilities, such as payment, autonomy, and access to and acceptance in all healthcare settings, are the foci of the policy agendas of many APRN organizations. The following sections discuss some examples of policy issues that demonstrate the ongoing need for APRNs to monitor regulatory and legislative activity and the interrelationship between legislation and regulations.

Healthcare Homes

A healthcare home, or "medical" home, is, according to MedPAC,[21] a clinical setting that serves as a central resource for a patient's ongoing clinical care. The medical home is being piloted by CMS and others to see how chronic illness could be better managed at a lower cost. Qualifying medical homes currently are medical practices in, ideally, primary care or geriatrics or a multispecialty practice, such as endocrinology for diabetics. In addition to

Table 13-2 **Current Health Policy Contextual Issues Unique to the United States**

Rapidly expanding knowledge base and emphasis on evidence-based practice
Exploding chronic care needs
Revolutionary care process in antiquated systems
Web-based spirometry while the provider is still relying on clinical handwritten data
Disintermediation: Removal of the provider, consumers getting information directly from other sources
Removal of the provider, consumers getting information directly from other sources; managed care domination and backlash Workforce maldistribution
Emergence of new federalism—more autonomy to states Demographic shift: The aging of the U.S. population is the largest ever recorded in the history of the world; baby boomers are not likely to accept traditional long-term care or paternalistic illness-centered care; shrinking birth rates and growing life expectancy; changing ethnic and racial demography
Sustained interest in healthcare quality and measurement
Sustained interest and little progress in electronic health records
Continuous election-year politics make for unpredictable decision making
Minority of the electorate choosing to vote

From Institute for the Future. (2000). *Health and Health Care 2010.* Jossey-Bass, San Francisco.

receiving traditional fee-for-service payments, qualifying medical homes in the pilot studies receive monthly per-member payments for infrastructure and for comprehensive care management.

The criteria for medical homes are clearly defined to help determine if those in demonstration projects in fact improve outcomes and lower costs, especially with chronic illness. These criteria include:

- Providing the full spectrum of primary care and prevention;
- Functioning as a team to conduct care management;
- Using health information technology for interactive clinical support;
- Employing a formal quality improvement program;
- Having a 24-hour communication system and rapid access;
- Keeping up-to-date records on patients advanced directives; and
- Maintaining a contract with patients identifying the practice as their medical home.

NPs could meet these criteria and are well prepared to move into this role. However, to date, they are not included in the pilot studies. This omission renders the NP role in an enhanced primary care setting invisible. The community of NP organizations has come together to influence the concept of medical homes with the goal of expanding their scope and having them led by NPs.

The National Committee for Quality Assurance[22] is testing a more patient-centered model, the patient-centered medical home, developed by several physician groups. These groups envision a healthcare setting that facilitates partnerships between individual patients and their personal physicians and, when appropriate, the patient's family. Care is facilitated by registries, information technology, health information exchange, and other means to ensure that patients get the indicated care when and where they need and want it in a culturally and linguistically appropriate manner. These patient-centered medical homes would include lab and test tracking, referral tracking, disease registries, and an electronic, interactive healthcare record. Some of these models mention advanced practice nurses as supportive in these care delivery models, but none of them emphasizes leadership roles for APRNs, not even for those with a Doctor of Nursing Practice (DNP) degree.

The need for enhanced primary care roles is driven by a dysfunctional delivery system that has been largely unresponsive to patient needs, especially care coordination and case management. Shifting care from an organ or body-part orientation to a patient-centered model will require persistent pressure to change our healthcare culture. The core function of the healthcare home—to case manage chronic illness effectively—has historically been undervalued and invisible, but it is now proving to be the major factor in lowering cost and improving quality outcomes.[23] APRNs look at patients from their community and family context; this is fundamental to advanced practice nursing. Therefore, it seems peculiar and irrational not to have these providers assume a major leadership role in this concept.

Direct Medicare Reimbursement in Skilled Nursing Facilities

The current regulations concerning scope of practice and reimbursement for APRNS in skilled nursing facilities (SNFs) are inconsistent. Under the current Social Security Act, every SNF is required under both Medicare and Medicaid to ensure that every resident is provided health care under the supervision of a physician. In the final rules implementing the nursing facility regulations, the CMS made it clear in a preamble that regulations should allow for the effective use of NPs, clinical nurse specialists (CNSs), and physician assistants (PAs), but the statutory language prevented the rule makers from including these providers. States have the option to choose whether a Medicaid recipient's health care can be delivered under the supervision of a CNS, NP, or PA as long as these providers are collaborating with a physician and providing services within their respective scope of practice. This policy option, which allows states to opt to reimburse APRNs for services provided to Medicaid recipients, is inconsistent with policies that do not allow reimbursement to APRNs for providing services to Medicare recipients.

In addition, the Balanced Budget Act of 1997 authorized NPs to initiate care for rehabilitation services for Medicare beneficiaries, including physical therapy, occupational therapy, and speech therapy. This, too, is inconsistent with Social Security legislation. The modification needed to correct this inconsistency, which directly impacts access and the quality of care in SNFs, requires a legislative amendment to the Social Security Act to include "that the medical care of every resident be provided under the supervision of a physician *or APN or Physicians' Assistant.*"[24] Medicare reimbursement to APRNs for initiating (certifying) care for Medicare beneficiaries in SNFs will improve the quality of care because of the APRN's ability to blend the discipline boundaries of nursing and medicine, which gives them the unique cultural and language skills to communicate effectively with nurses, nurses' aides, nursing supervisors, physicians, medical directors, and medical subspecialists.

Home Health Care: A Change Is Needed

The Social Security Act stipulates that only physicians can certify and recertify Medicare home health care. However, the 1997 Balanced Budget Act authorized NPs to develop plans of care for Medicare beneficiaries receiving home health care. Rectifying the limitation in APRNs' ability to certify and recertify for home care requires a policy modification (amendment) to the Social Security Act or new legislation that would streamline the home health care certification process, which is highly burdensome to home care agencies.

Home care and long-term care are two of the fastest-growing sectors of the healthcare delivery system. If legislative changes were enacted, APRNs could play a much more important role in improving the quality of care. APRNs are well grounded in care delivery within the context of the community and the capacity of patients to care for themselves. Current restrictions on APRNs' ability to deliver services in SNFs and home care settings must be eliminated.

Professional Autonomy: Restraint of Practice

The CMS rules require certified registered nurse anesthetists (CRNAs) to practice under physician supervision in order to receive Medicare reimbursement. The rules also allow a state's governor to notify CMS of the state's desire to opt out of the supervision requirement for CRNAs. A number of states have "opted out" of the physician supervision requirement; for example, in Iowa, 91 of 118 hospitals rely exclusively on CRNAs to provide anesthesia services.[25]

CRNAs are the predominant anesthesia providers in rural and other medically underserved areas; without these APRNs, many of the facilities serving these areas would be unable to maintain surgical, obstetric, and trauma stabilization services. In addition, rural areas tend to have a high proportion of Medicare beneficiaries. Despite this, physician groups have opposed removal of the supervision requirement at both the federal and state levels, even though removal of the restriction ensures access to care for patients in rural areas and allows facilities to staff their anesthesia departments to best serve their patients. Removal of this major barrier to CRNA practice would require a rule change within CMS.

Provider-Neutral Language: Breaking the Physician Monopoly on Health Care

Use of the terms "provider or healthcare professional" rather than "physician" can have enormous impact on APRNs' scope of practice and therefore reimbursement. Legislative and regulatory recognition is needed to place APRNs on a par with providers who perform identical services. For example, language in the House and Senate versions of the Patients' Bill of Rights legislation used the term *physician,* thereby prohibiting APRNs (NPs and CNSs) from being named as primary care providers (PCPs) and certified nurse-midwives (CNMs) from being named direct OB/GYN providers. However, if *healthcare professional* were substituted, that would enable the rule makers to include providers who are licensed, accredited, or certified under state law to provide healthcare services within the scope of their practice. APRNs continue to advocate for nondiscriminatory language in all legislation and regulations proposed on the federal level. As the number of prescribers and providers who are not physicians increases, provider-neutral language would more accurately reflect the current healthcare workforce and diminish consumer confusion.

APRN Workforce: A Dearth of Data

The importance of using solid data to make a case for a policy change cannot be overemphasized. However, finding accurate, current data on the APRN workforce presents a policy challenge. Currently, there are no comprehensive databases or practice data on all APRNs across the nation, except for the most rudimentary counts. This lack of accurate workforce data is a major limitation in moving the APRN policy agenda forward. The 2010 Census will begin the gathering of federal data (to be collected by the Bureau of Labor Statistics, an important source for workforce planning data) that will distinguish among different levels of registered nurses (RNs) with advanced education. Most states do track APRNs separately from all RNs, but not all states do, so state nursing licensing data are inadequate for national APRN workforce planning needs. In addition, many APRNs hold licenses in more than one state and/or are certified in more than one practice specialty. Therefore, unless the nurse's state of residence is part of an interstate licensing compact, duplicate licenses and certifications pose another major difficulty in creating an accurate APRN database. Two groups of APRNs—CNMs and CRNAs—have robust data sets, but NPs, who constitute the largest segment of the APRN workforce, do not have a coherent national database available for research or to inform policy.

The quadrennial National Sample Survey of RNs, conducted by the Health Resources and Services Administration (HRSA),[26] is currently the best source of data about the APRN workforce supply. Since 1977, this national survey, using sampling techniques on the RN population, has estimated and characterized the size of the APRN workforce. Since the sampling technique is based on RNs and not APRNs, the sample of APRNs in many states is too small for accurate estimates.

Currently, there is no cohesive APRN data set that can address critically important policy questions that arise across the country. Policy makers frequently ask, and the APRN community must be able to answer, such questions as:

- How many APRNs work in health professional shortage areas?
- Do APRNs care for a disproportionate share of the uninsured?
- Do APRNs tend to serve in the communities in which they were educated?
- What is a typical adult NP-to-patient ratio?
- What are the work and retirement patterns for APRNs?
- How do specific practice patterns differ in relation to other providers (e.g., prescribing rates, success at behavior change, less resource usage)?
- Are the outcomes—for example, immunization rates, hospitalization rates, or chronic illness outcomes—of NP patient populations measurably improved?

Data are needed to inform these important policy questions, and APRNs must work to secure it so that it can be used to form health policies.

The lack of data also excludes the APRN workforce from large administrative and clinical data sets, including many of the important outcomes data sets designed to measure quality, such as the Agency for Health Research & Quality's (AHRQ) Healthcare Cost and Utilization Project (H-CUP), a family of healthcare databases developed through a federal-state-industry partnership, that collects longitudinal U.S. hospital care data. This data set is very powerful; it includes all payer- and encounter-level information since 1988. Databases such as H-CUP enable research on a broad range of health policy issues, including cost and quality of health services; practice patterns; access to healthcare programs; and outcomes of treatments at the national, state, and local levels. However, APRNs are currently not routinely included as a specific provider group in H-CUP. Unless and until APRNs are "mainstreamed" into large national data sets, they will remain somewhat sidelined in the policy arena.

APRN Political Competence

Political competence is the ability to understand what you can and cannot control, to know when to take action, to anticipate who is going to resist your agenda, and to determine who you need on your side to push your agenda forward. Political competence is knowing how to work through coalitions. And it is important at many levels of nursing practice and is, in fact, emphasized in the recommendations for DNP practice. Political competence involves understanding the difference between power and force; participating in civic engagement; individual skills in communication, interpersonal relationships, analysis, and conflict resolution; leadership skills; and organizational support.

APRNs and DNP: Policy Engagement in Every DNP Essential

In its *Essentials of Doctoral Education for Advanced Nursing Practice,* the American Association of Colleges of Nursing (AACN) emphasizes a high degree of mastery in political competence.[27] In fact, each DNP essential requires mastery of policy analysis and political competence in some form. For example, DNP Essential VII, which emphasizes "Clinical Prevention and Population Health for Improving the Nation's Health," requires strong skills in influencing change in healthcare financing. While this specific DNP essential emphasizes the role of APRNs in telescoping out to the population realm and back into the care of individuals, it also implies that APRNs will demonstrate political competence on behalf of populations to promote policy change.

Research, practice, and policy are sequenced links in all practice settings and are competencies expected in DNP graduates. The healthcare problems the United States is facing—our creaking, top-heavy, antiquated and inefficient system of care—need to be addressed with sensible, evidence-based reforms. There is no better provider more aptly prepared with the knowledge, scholarship, experience, and credibility to assume broad leadership in the policy arena than the DNP-prepared APRN.

Power Versus Force

There is a critical distinction between power and force in politics. Force disguises underlying motivations. Force is seductive because it resembles dominance, is divisive, and is centered in arrogance. Force exploits for the gain of an individual or organization, whereas power unifies, serves others, and attracts. Power is characterized by unassuming humility, and it accomplishes with ease what force cannot. Power is grounded on self-evident truth and requires no justification or rhetorical persuasion.[28]

Regardless of what branch of inquiry one starts from—philosophy, political theory, or theology—all avenues of investigation eventually converge on an understanding of awareness. That is, we are all connected to everyone and everything else. Invisible thoughts and attitudes are traits that can be made visible through persistence and habitual response. When we stop condemning, fearing, and hating each other (a somewhat radical departure in policy circles), we can direct our energy to our power.[28] There is an inherent dishonesty in self-serving postures and professional parochialism—for example, that "only physicians can prescribe." This belief, held by some physicians, reflects a very low level of awareness. When APRNs approach discussions in policy circles with a genuine commitment to problem solving and enhanced patient care, much needed productive energy is diffused into the conversation. By withholding counterattacks and a self-serving or parochial posture, in which the only solution comes from nurses, APRNs can elevate their capacity to bring much-needed honesty and wisdom to complex health policy problem solving. Ignorance does not yield to attack, but rather dissipates with wisdom and truth.

APRN policy representatives must be truly committed to interprofessional practice and must stop the cycle of diminishing or excluding other health professions from the healthcare marketplace in order to elevate APRNs. For example, in working on increasing immunization rates, APRNs—if truly interested in enhanced patient outcomes—must be open to vaccination by pharmacists. Immediate and outright opposition to this raises concerns about the underlying commitment to problem solving. Other concerns (e.g., injection technique) can be raised and addressed in a respectful matter, with the patient as the center of care. By clearly being on the side of the patient and improved health outcomes, APRNs can secure a place of power, rather than a position based on thinly veiled nursing parochialism. APRNs, and nursing as a whole, must ensure that the representatives they send to the policy table have a high degree of maturity (not measured by age), discipline, patience, and wisdom that reflects the power and professionalism of the APRN movement. Championing improved healthcare quality and improved access to health care are not ideals that are counter to expanded APRN practice.

Civic Engagement

American constitutional democracy is dynamic and complex. Citizens, acting individually or in groups, attempt to influence the opinions of those in positions of power. Those in power, in turn, attempt to influence public opinion. The ultimate goal of such a democracy is the widespread participation in governance by citizens who are knowledgeable, competent, and committed to the realization of the fundamental values and principles of our Constitution.[29] The Founding Fathers always envisioned that the electorate would be participatory and enlightened, committed to democratic principles, and actively engaged in the practice of democracy.

Citizens who fail to understand how government works and how to participate effectively may become alienated from the political process. To assume effective roles in our democracy at local, state, and national levels, APRNs must expand their knowledge and master the necessary skills. Having a voice in shaping health policy is a form of civic engagement. Their intellectual and participatory skills enable APRNs to apply civic knowledge as active participants capable of monitoring and influencing public policy. Because they are clinical experts who can bring important pragmatic solutions to common problems, APRNs have a responsibility to let policy makers know how policies are experienced by people in the clinical setting. APRNs who participate in health policy discourse can provide a powerful narrative about how ill-informed policy plays out and affects individuals negatively.

Individual Political Competence

Many skills are needed to be influential at the policy level. Political competence requires the creation of circumstances that can turn ideas into policies. Most of the skills needed are already strongly grounded in APRN practice. APRNs have expertise in the assessment, diagnosis, and treatment of the complex responses to human illness and problems.[30] This expertise requires depth, breadth, and synthesis of knowledge. These same skills that effectively motivate patients to make lifestyle changes can be applied to the policy arena. APRNs must continuously hone their interpersonal skills. Developing and implementing strategies requires careful listening to individuals, the collective profession, patient trends, and the political landscape in order to influence health policy decisions effectively for large numbers of patient populations.

Serving on advisory bodies is one important strategy that APRNs can use to exert influence in the health policy arena. The ability to clearly communicate, manage personal feelings, and bring evidence or a strong rationale to support one's positions makes for a highly effective advisory board member. However, also required is the ability to understand those with differing viewpoints while maintaining a focus on problem solving. In advocating for improved healthcare quality, expanded access to care, and reduced costs, APRNs engaged in the policy arena must employ the skill sets described below.

INTERPERSONAL/COMMUNICATION SKILLS

The APRN should:

- Identify and take action only on select issues about which he or she feels passionate;
- Know what outcome is desired by establishing rapport versus being right;
- Work from others' strengths and minimize weaknesses;
- Network with key stakeholders;
- Seek expertise when needed;
- Share expertise when needed;
- Communicate accurately and efficiently;
- Craft coherent arguments in written and oral form;
- Manage personal feelings and personal biases;

- Use humor, warmth, and honesty in relationships (using nonthreatening and positive intent);
- Collaborate;
- Practice persuasion skills;
- Treat patients as colleagues and trust they can think/act on their own behalf;
- Manage personal and professional boundaries;
- Create coalitions;
- Avoid the "shrill" role and respond to insults carefully and thoughtfully; and
- Interact with the media effectively.

ANALYTIC SKILLS/POLICY KNOWLEDGE

The APRN should:

- Know the policy process as well as stakeholders' views on controversial issues;
- Consider the importance of timing before intervening;
- Approach health policy issues from a genuine "solution-finding" viewpoint to increase access and quality while reducing costs;
- Develop and sustain networks within and across professions;
- Integrate an understanding of others' perspectives;
- Assess possible policy impacts, both pros and cons;
- Assess possible policy impacts on key stakeholders to strategically develop coalitions;
- Develop knowledge of individual and organizational patterns or historical positions on critical policy issues;
- Identify power/influence and develop strategies to increase one's power;
- Use data effectively to support positions;
- Engage consumer groups;
- Demonstrate a high degree of respect for other health professions and professionals;
- Stay active with the APRN professional association(s);
- Maintain a mentor *and* mentee relationship;
- Support electoral candidates interested in health care;
- Participate in the drafting of legislation during the conceptual phase of the process;
- Produce and deliver testimony in hearings to inform and refine drafted legislation;
- Help policy maker's create sensible solutions to constituent and community problems;
- Pay close attention to rulemaking; and
- Provide formal comment on proposed rules.

CONFLICT RESOLUTION SKILLS

The APRN should:

- Anticipate, assess, and respond effectively and wisely to the needs of diverse stakeholders;
- Employ systems thinking;
- Employ strategic thinking: the ability to conceptualize and articulate a vision;

- Take risks;
- Demonstrate active listening by acknowledging and clarifying verbal messages to ensure mutual understanding;
- Seek information to understand opposing viewpoints better; and
- Diffuse sensitive or difficult situations and create a climate for mutual problem solving.

Professional Leadership Skills

Using *data* effectively is a powerful tool in making the case for a policy change. Data can be critical in explaining why an issue is important. Therefore, understanding how to use and interpret data is critical to influencing policy effectively. Wherever possible, data should be incorporated into all communications—when meeting with legislators and other key stake-holders, preparing written material, talking with the media, testifying at a public meeting, or writing letters to policy makers or newspapers.

Using outside expert opinion, in the event that no data are available, is another important strategy. For example, the American Hospital Association (AHA) convened a highly diverse commission to examine the hospital and health systems workforce. This commission recommended the use of NPs as hospitalists to fulfill the care manager role in acute care settings.[31] This outside expert recommendation is a powerful tool for any APRN negotiating for hospital privileges or working to expand scope-of-practice laws.

There are two basic rules to remember when using data for policy development:

Rule 1: You will depend on data for nearly all aspects of policy development work.

Rule 2: Data alone, and especially in raw form, are seldom sufficient to change policy.

When used properly, data help persuade policy makers to think differently about an issue. Effective use of data leads people to a deeper understanding of how an issue is relevant to their lives and helps reframe issues. This reframing is one of the most powerful skills an APRN leader can have—the ability to use highly relevant data that alters the way an issue or policy is viewed by those forming the policy.

A CMS Nursing Open Door Policy Meeting provided an example of strategic use of data. The meeting began with a preview of a newsletter that was to be mailed to all 40 million Medicare beneficiaries. The newsletter described how older adults could make their care safer by asking more questions of their *physician*—a term included nine times in this one-page newsletter. The APRN leader pointed out that there were nearly 250,000 non-physician prescribing providers in the United States: more than 150,000 NPs, nearly 14,000 CNMs, 33,000 CRNAs, and more than 42,000 PAs. The APRN went on to state that using the term "physician" does not accurately reflect the current workforce that provides reimbursable care to Medicare beneficiaries and is likely to cause confusion among patients. The CMS official apologized for the oversight and revised the letter to read "healthcare professional."

APRN Organizational Design to Support Political Competencies

One of the major functions of a professional APRN association is to analyze the public environment and then to exert influence in the public policy arena. This responsibility rests with its senior executives and governing boards. Most organizations employ an administrative unit (government relations or public affairs) whose sole function is to analyze and influence public policy on behalf of members. If these units are well designed and staffed, they can provide the organization and its members the enormous advantage of lead time. The organization must have the capacity to make informed, strategic predictions about future policy so that it has the luxury of time in which to anticipate what is likely to happen. This gives the organization time to frame or influence emerging policy modifications. For example, organizations can use the lead-time advantage to talk to members, direct resources to emerging issues, engage strategic partners, and meet with policy makers when the issue is in the conceptual phase.

Achieving this level of foresight requires a high degree of political competence; it requires the organization in its environmental analysis to think strategically and long term, rather than react to each issue. APRNs who are continuously scanning the environment position themselves to find answers (or do research) concerning questions that may emerge. This activity allows organizations to fill advisory board seats with well-qualified people. The shift away from policy reactor to policy shaper could allow an APRN organization to evolve into a source of policy knowledge.

A powerful example of the use of lead time was the publication of the *APRN Consensus Model for APRN Regulation: Licensing, Accreditation, Certification and Education*,[32] in which APRN leaders anticipated more scrutiny over APRNs by policy makers and used to position themselves in the policy arena. These stakeholders came together to create a unified vision for APRNs that will significantly strengthen the APRN position in policy circles. (See the index for additional information on the Consensus Model.) Another excellent example of how the luxury of time can lead to influencing legislation and ultimately patient care occurred when Medicare regulations, which were being drafted following passage of the 1997 Balanced Budget Act, required NPs to hold a master's degree to be eligible for Medicare reimbursement. In anticipation, many NP organizations, educational programs, and certifying bodies had supported or required graduate preparation as the entry point for NP practice long before the rules were drafted. The regulations also reflected, however, concern about access to health care and included a "grandfathering provision" that allowed NPs without a master's degree to obtain a Medicare provider number (U-PIN) for a specified period following implementation of the regulations. This allowed NPs who had been practicing for many years to continue to provide care to Medicare patients. This lead time allowed the NP community to, first, create internal cohesion and, second, to provide CMSs with effective external validation.

Fragmentation of APRN Professional Organizations

Strengthening and unifying APRN organizations would go a long way toward encouraging policy makers and others to seek them out for advice and solutions to health policy issues. One of the greatest opportunities for APRNs to corral their political power has been the occasional APRN organizational collaboration on issues specific to APRNs. These loose coalitions or policy networks serve to strengthen the voice of APRNs and ensure no conflicting messages are directed at policy makers. On occasion, loose coalitions have formed to provide joint support for a policy position, but more often, the APRN movement has lacked solid structural and organizational unity. As Table 13-3 shows, the CNMs, and CRNAs, have far more unity and cohesiveness than CNSs or NPs. This organizational fragmentation leads to either competition for members, requiring APRNs to join multiple professional organizations to get the range of services they need, or APRN apathy—confusion over which organization to join leading to not joining any.

There are more than six national associations representing NPs, and until the American College of Nurse Practitioners (ACNP) was formed in 1993, there was little opportunity for the NP profession to speak with one voice. While it is important to acknowledge the uniqueness of each type of APRN, political power and influence is lost by this fragmentation. As the APRN workforce continues to grow in numbers, the APRN community will gain strength by blurring the boundaries that distinguish them from one another. As the ACNP, whose stated mission is to be fast, friendly, flexible, and funded, moves to increase unity among the NP community, additional emphasis must be placed on the unity of all APRNs to garner political resources and strength.

Important Health Policy Web Sites
Federal Government Sites

Agency for Healthcare Research and Quality: http://www.ahrq.gov

Congress: http://thomas.loc.gov

Congressional Budget Office: http://www.cbo.gov

Center for Medicare and Medicaid: http://www.cms.gov

Centers for Disease Control and Prevention: http://www.cdc.gov

FedStats (statistics from over 100 federal agencies): http://www.fedstats.gov

Food and Drug Administration: http://www.fda.gov

General Accountability Office: http://www.gao.org

Institute of Medicine: http://www.iom.edu

Medicare Payment Advisory Commission: http://www.medpac.gov

Office of Management and Budget: http://www.whitehouse.gov/omb

State/Local Health Policy

National Association of State Information Resource Executives: http://www.nascio.org

National Conference of State Legislatures: http://www.ncsl.org

National Governors Association: http://www.nga.org

Foundations

Henry J. Kaiser Foundation: http://www.kff.org

Robert Wood Johnson Foundation: http://www.rwjf.org

The Commonwealth Fund: http://www.cmwf.org

The John A. Hartford Foundation: http://www.jhartford.org

Think Tanks

Academy for Health Services Research and Health Policy: http://www.academyhealth.org

BCBS Health Issues: http://www.bcbshealthissues.com

Cato Health Institute: http://www.cato.org

Center for Studying Health System Change: http://www.hschange.com

Center on Budget and Policy Priorities: http://www.cbpp.org

Heritage Foundation: http://www.heritage.org

National Academy for State Health Policy: http://www.nashp.org

National Center for Policy Analysis-Health Issues: http://www.ncpa.org

Urban Institute: http://www.urban.org

International

Organization for Economic Co-operation and Development: http://www.oecd.org

World Health Organization: http://www.who.int

Table 13-3 **National APRN Membership Association**[s]

NP Associations	
American Academy of Nurse Practitioners (AANP)	http://www.aanp.org
*American Association of Critical Care Nurses (AACN)	http://www.aacn.org
American College of Nurse Practitioners (ACNP)[2]	http://www.nurse.org/acnp
*Association of Women's Health, Obstetric, and Neonatal Nurses (AWHONN)	http://www.awhonn.org
*National Association of NPs in Women's Health (NPWH)	http://www.npwh.org
*Gerontological Advanced Practice Nurses Association (GAPNA)	http://www.gapna.org
*National Organization of Nurse Practitioner Faculties (NONPF)	http://www.nonpf.org
*National Association of Pediatric Nurse Practitioners (NAPNAP)	http://www.napnap.org
Nurse-Midwife Associations	
American College of Nurse Midwives (ACNM)	http://www.acnm.org
Nurse Anesthetist Associations	
American Association of Nurse Anesthetists (AANA)	http://www.aana.com
Clinical Nurse Specialist Associations	
National Association of Clinical Nurse Specialists (NACNS)	http://www.nacns.org
American Association of Critical-Care Nurses (AACN)	http://www.aacn.org
Gerontological Advanced Practice Nurses Association (GAPNA)	http://www.gapna.org
Oncology Nurses Society (ONS)	http://www.ons.org
Academy of Medical Surgical Nurses (AMSN)	http://www.amsn.org

[1] Many organizations, including the American College Health Association, National Association of Neonatal Nurses, the National Association of School Nurses, and other specialty-focused organizations also have a proportion of APRN membership. This list also does not include certification entities or organizations whose primary focus is APRN education.

[2] Six national NP Associations (denoted by *) are affiliate members of ACNP. ACNP also has more than 40 state NP associations as well as individual members.

SUGGESTED LEARNING EXERCISES

1. Describe the APRN title recognition laws, prescriptive authority, and reimbursement policies in your state. Does your state appear to be restrictive in comparison to the 49 other states?

2. Create three to five pages of testimony to deliver to a legislative body (at the state or federal level) on a health problem that is important to you in your community. Clearly

identify the health policy problem and offer a legislative solution using data to inform your testimony.

3. Identify 10 ways in which you could improve your political competence.

4. Describe a current health policy issue that is important to you. Analyze where the policy issue is in the policy-making process.

5. Craft an opinion-editorial to educate the public.

Writing an Evidence-Based Opinion-Editorial (Op-Ed)

This assignment is conducted over the semester to build in numerous stages of edits and refinements in order to make the writing as strong as possible and raise the potential for publication. An op-ed is distinct from a "Letter to the Editor," which consists of readers responding to a letter previously written, a column, or a news event. You are to submit the op-ed to a news outlet in your region (e.g., the *Washington Post*, the *Boston Globe*, the *Los Angeles Times*, etc.). The purpose of this assignment is to demonstrate your political competence by educating the public about the issue, influencing public opinion, and offering policy solutions that increase quality, expand access, or reduce the costs of health care. Newspapers have policies on how to submit articles to their opinion page and most have length limits (500–700 words). Identify the media outlet you will be using and determine its op-ed policies before you begin writing. It is hoped that you will incorporate this form of patient advocacy into your professional APRN role/practice. This type of writing is not formulaic; however, the following are *suggested* components of an op-ed.

1. Establish your credibility by stating your credentials and declaring your expertise. (Do not emphasize your current role of student unless directly pertinent.)

2. Scope of the problem:
   - State how the problem impacts the public/population/disenfranchised segment of a community. Use federal or state data/statistics if available.
   - Provide a poignant, heart-wrenching personal story, if applicable.
   - Describe why the stakeholders disagree with you and inoculate their argument.
   - Identify ethical dilemmas, as appropriate.

3. Policy-based solutions:
   - Include evidence/science on why this policy solution is helpful.
   - Be *highly specific* about what sphere of government is involved and what action needs to be taken.
   - Offer policy solutions that nongovernment sectors (industry) can adapt to solve the problem (e.g., if there is a nursing shortage in a hospital, the hospital can offer scholarships to nursing aides).

4. Describe actions that readers/public can do *today* to solve this problem.

5. Predict what may happen if the problem is not fixed.

After drafting your op-ed:

Ask your peers/relatives/friends/colleagues/acquaintances who have excellent writing skills to review. Post a draft of your op-ed article for classmate peer review. Peer review at least two other students' op-ed drafts. Provide substantive feedback to each other, considering the following questions:

- Is it easy to understand?
- Does it use current federal or state data?

Grade	Global Scoring Rubric for Op-Ed
Outstanding	A thoughtful and thorough breakdown and analysis of the health policy issue; evidence-based arguments as well as a poignant narrative were included. The issue was described using a cost-quality-access framework (i.e., the policy solution will decrease costs or improve quality or access). Policy recommendations were incremental and specific to the problem. This writing excited the reader by explaining and clearly linking the policy problems to a practical solution(s). Reader feels compelled to support the policy solution actively.
Acceptable	This op-ed makes it easier for the reader to gain new understanding about the policy problem, but leaves the reader with some doubt of the linkage to the policy solution. The policy recommendation is not totally convincing, but the reader wants to know more.
Not Acceptable	This writing does not explain why anybody should care about the policy problem, so the reader is not interested in getting to the solution. Overall, the op-ed is not written in a thorough manner and leaves the reader unclear, unconvinced, and wanting more. The reader is not excited or interested in the topic.

- Does it incorporate a poignant story(ies) and/or describe what the problem means to real people?
- Does it counter or inoculate views of opposing stakeholders (with data or a sound rationale)?
- Does it describe how cost, quality, or access is impacted?
- Does it include a specific policy recommendation? Are there action steps for the public?
- Is the experience and background of the author provided?

6. Develop your health policy topic into an "action plan tool kit" that could be given to an organization for immediate use. Include the following components:

   1. Suggested evidence-based *policy recommendation(s)* and rationale
      - Sphere of government(s) or organization(s) involved
      - Action specified
      - Benefits and costs

   2. Politically competent behaviors (practice nursing with policy makers)
      - Stakeholder analysis (name of stakeholders; research or anticipate their position on policy recommendations)
      - Inoculate against opponents (use of data best)
      - Build coalitions (identify policy community: broad-based interdisciplinary strategic partners, including consumer groups; develop a grassroots campaign: identify policy community: broad-based interdisciplinary strategic partners, including consumer groups)

   3. Communication plan
      - Media plan
      - Talking points
      - 1-page summary with key points to leave with legislators

Grade	Global Scoring Rubric for Health Policy Action Plan
Outstanding	A thoughtful and thorough action plan to propel a policy into action. There was use of evidence-based arguments, using a cost-quality-access framework (i.e., the policy solution will decrease costs or improve quality or access) and a cost-benefit description, and the recommendation fits into a policy-making framework context. The policy recommendation was incremental (politically viable), specific to the problem, and aimed at the appropriate sphere of policy making. Politically competent strategies, including a stakeholder analysis, were robust and included a diverse and creative network of strategic partners. This writing excited the reader by building a compelling plan to propel the policy recommendation into action. The reader cannot identify any other action to take to move the plan forward.
Acceptable	This action plan included most of the components of a robust policy action plan. It left the reader wondering why a different sphere of policy making was not targeted, why certain data elements were not incorporated to strengthen the argument for change, or why some stakeholders were not included in the policy community. The reader was left with some doubt about the ability of the action plan to be effective. The plan is not totally convincing and the reader wants to know more.
Not Acceptable	This writing does not explain why anybody should care about the policy problem, so the reader is not interested in getting to the solution. Overall, the action plan is not written in a thorough manner and leaves the reader unclear, unconvinced, and wanting more. The reader is not excited, has doubt about the plan, or is left feeling it is more of an "Ambush Plan."

References

1. Longest, B. (2006). *Health Policymaking in the United States,* 4th ed. AUPHA/HAP, Washington, DC.

2. Corrigan, J, Kohn, L, and Donaldson, M (eds). (1999). *To Err is Human: Building a Safer Health System.* Committee on Quality of Health Care in America, Institute of Medicine, The National Academies Press, Washington DC.

3. Kaiser Family Foundation and Health Research and Educational Trust. (2008). *2008 Employer Health Benefits Survey.* Washington, DC. http://www.kff.org/content/2008. Accessed January 13, 2009.

4. Wyden, R, and Bennett, B. (2008). Finally fixing health care, what's different now? *Health Affairs* 27(3):688–692.

5. National Coalition on Health Care. (2008). http://www.nchc.org/facts/cost.shtml. Accessed January 21, 2009.

6. Nichols, L, and Axeen, S. (2008). *Policy Paper: Increasing Employer Health Costs, Lowering U.S. Competitiveness.* New American Foundation, Washington. DC. http://www.newamerica.net/publications/policy/employer_health_costs_global_economy. Accessed January 19, 2009.

7. Commonwealth Fund. (2007). *Consumer Reports. Are You Really Covered?* http://www. commonwealthfund.org/publications/publications_show.htm?doc_id=688615. Accessed January 18, 2009.

8. Robertson, CT, Egelhof, R, and Hoke, M. (2008). Get sick, get out: the medical causes of home foreclosures. *Health Matrix* 18:65–105. http://works.bepress.com/christopher_robertson/2. Accessed January 14, 2009.

9. Institute of Medicine, Committee on Health Care in America. (2001). *Crossing the Quality Chasm: A New Health System for the 21st Century.* National Academy Press, Washington DC. http://www. nap.edu/books/0309072808/html/. Accessed January 23, 2009.

10. McGlynn, EA, et al. (2003, 2006). The quality of health care delivered in the United States. *N Engl J Med* 348(26):2635–2645; updated in Asch, S, et al. (2006). Who is at greatest risk for receiving poor-quality health care? *N Engl J Med* 354(11):1147–1156.

11. World Health Organization. (1985). Appropriate technology for birth. *Lancet*; 2:436–437.

12. Institute of Medicine, Committee on the Consequences of Uninsurance. (2002). *Care Without Coverage: Too Little Too Late.* National Academy Press, Washington, DC.

13. AHRQ, DHHS. (2006). *The National Healthcare Disparities Report.* www.ahrq.gov/qual/nhdr07/-84k-2008-07-10. Accessed January 4, 2009.

14. Institute of Medicine. (2004). *Insuring America's Health—Principles and Recommendations.* The National Academies Press, Washington DC.

15. The Henry J. Kaiser Family Foundation. (2003, September). *Access to Care for the Uninsured: An Update.* http://www.kff.org/uninsured/4142.cfm. Accessed January 23, 2009.

16. U.S. Bureau of the Census. (2008, August). *Number of Americans with and without Health Insurance_Rise._Press Release.* http://www.census.gov/Press-Release/www/releases/archives/income_wealth/012528.html. Accessed January 5, 2009.

17. Kingdon, JW. (1995). *Agendas, Alternatives, and Public Policies,* 2nd ed. HarperCollins College Publishers, New York.

18. Field, MJ, Tranquada, RE, and Feasley, JF (eds). (1995). *Health Services Research: Workforce and Educational Issues.* National Academy Press, Washington, DC.

19. Wakefield, M. (2004). Government response: legislation. In Milstead, J (ed), *Health Policy and Politics: A Nurse's Guide,* 2nd ed. Aspen, Gaithersburg, MD.

20. Pfiffner, JP (ed) (1995). *Governance and American Politics: Classic and Current Perspectives.* Harcourt Brace and Company, Fort Worth, TX.

21. MedPAC. (2008, June). *Report to Congress: Reforming the Delivery System.* http://www.medpac.gov/documents/Jun08_EntireReport.pdf. Accessed January 23, 2009.

22. National Committee on Quality Assurance. *The Patient Centered Medical Home.* http://www.ncqa.org/tabid/631/Default.aspx. Accessed January 23, 2009.

23. Sidorov, J. (2008). The patient-centered medical home for chronic illness: is it ready for prime time? *Health Affairs* 27(5):1231–1233.

24. American College of Nurse Practitioners. (2002). Fact Sheet. Available at http://www.acnpweb.org.

25. American Association of Nurse Anesthetists. (2002, June 11). Press Release. http://www.aana.com/press/2002/061102.asp.

26. HRSA, DHHS. (2006). *The Registered Nurse Population: Findings from the 2004 National Sample Survey of Registered Nurses.* http://bhpr.hrsa.gov/healthworkforce/rnsurvey04. Accessed January 23, 2009.

27. American Association of Colleges of Nursing. (2006). *Essentials of Doctoral Education for Advanced Nursing Practice.* http://www.aacn.nche.edu/DNP/pdf/Essentials.pdf. Accessed January 21, 2009.

28. Hawkins, DR. (2002). *Power vs. Force: The Hidden Determinants of Human Behavior.* Hay House Inc., Carlsbad, CA.

29. Center for Civic Education. (2009). *A Framework for Civic Education.* http://www.civiced.org/index.php?page=civitas_a_framework_for_civic_education - 58k. Accessed January 23, 2009.

30. American Nurses Association. (1996). *Scope and Standards of Advanced Practice Registered Nursing.* American Nurses Association, Washington, DC.

31. American Hospital Association. (2002). *In Our Hands: How Hospital Leaders Can Build a Thriving Workforce.* American Hospital Association, Chicago.

32. APRN Joint Dialogue Group. (2008). *Consensus Model on Regulation of APRNs: Licensing, Accreditation, Certification and Education July 2008.* http://www.aacn.nche.edu/education/pdf/ APRNReport.pdf. Accessed January 21, 2009.

Margaret McAllister is a clinical associate professor and coordinator of the family nurse practitioner (FNP) program at the University of Massachusetts-Boston College of Nursing and Health Sciences and director of the post-master's nurse practitioner (NP) certificate program and co-director of the post-master's doctor of nursing practice program. She is an FNP at the University of Massachusetts-Boston University Health. Dr. McAllister received her PhD in law, policy, and society from Northeastern University and holds a clinical nurse specialist (CNS) degree in primary care nursing of adults and children from Indiana University, where she completed a Robert Wood Johnson Nurse Faculty Fellowship in Primary Care. She also has a master's degree in nursing education from New York University and bachelor's degree in nursing from Ohio State University. Dr. McAllister completed a U.S. Department of Health and Human Services Primary Health Care Policy Fellowship and has been an active mentor for the University of Massachusetts-Boston Albert Schweitzer NP Fellows. In addition, she serves as a faculty ambassador for the National Health Service Corporation (NHSC). She has served as a past member of the American Academy of Nurse Practitioners (AANP) board of directors and is a member of the Fellows of the AANP and the Society of Primary Care Policy Fellows. She serves on the executive board of the Massachusetts Coalition of Nurse Practitioners and is past president of Theta Alpha Chapter of Sigma Theta Tau.

CHAPTER 14

The Advanced Practice Registered Nurse as Educator

Margaret McAllister, PhD, RN, CNS, FNP

CHAPTER OBJECTIVES

After completing this chapter, the reader will be able to:

1. Demonstrate competencies in the teaching-coaching function of the APRN when determining the learning needs of patients, families, and colleagues.
2. Integrate the humanistic, behavioral, and social schools of learning theory when implementing the teaching-coaching competencies of the APRN.
3. Modify one's teaching-coaching actions in response to the patient's and family's needs for counseling.
4. Demonstrate the professional role of the APRN when functioning as preceptor.
5. Demonstrate the professional role of the APRN when providing continuing education for professional colleagues.

Today's healthcare system offers consumers comprehensive care beyond diagnosis, prescription, and disease management. Healthcare systems in the 21st century are cost-conscious while striving to achieve high-quality care with a focus on the identification of risk factors and on disease prevention. Advanced practice registered nurses (APRNs) are consumer advocates for health education and disease prevention. They are skilled in identifying the educational needs of consumers and colleagues in the areas of disease prevention, health promotion, chronic illness, self-care, and end-of-life care planning. Recognized leaders in healthcare services, APRNs synthesize evidence-based healthcare research to improve the quality of practices and patient care outcomes.

Healthcare consumers now receive reimbursed health education benefits in several ways. Besides providing direct one-to-one education to patients, APRNs develop community-based health education programs, apply for and receive federal and state grants for health education programs targeting at-risk populations, and provide professional continuing education (CE). The New England AIDS Education and Training Program is an example of an APRN federally funded project that targets education for at-risk populations and provides the latest education to professionals on prevention, early identification, and care of patients with HIV infection.

The APRN Role in Teaching Patients, Families, and Professional Colleagues

APRNs provide education to patients, families, and their professional colleagues as an integral part of their professional role. The teaching/coaching function of the nurse practitioner (NP) and clinical nurse specialist (CNS)[1,2] are included in national, professionally determined competencies. The competencies reflect the APRN's skill in the application of adult learning principles and learning theories. These competencies include assessing learning needs, eliciting past knowledge and experience with illness, assisting the patient to learn through the application of psychosocial principles, providing needed information, negotiating teaching goals, monitoring the patient's response to knowledge and readiness to learn, and coaching the patient in a sensitive way to reach the agreed-upon goals for health.[1(pp44–45)] APRNs impart knowledge to patients by explaining information accurately, modeling behaviors, and tutoring patients in the process of behavior change to promote and sustain health. The APRN educator also functions as patient advocate. The APRN's contribution to social movements is aligned with the health policy goals of preventing and identifying disease and improving the health of society and quality of human life.

The role of APRN as nurse educator can be direct or indirect. The direct role involves providing information to patients or groups, including families, as well as to professional health colleagues and students. The indirect role of nurse educator includes the development of patient education materials and conference proceedings, as well as comprehensive literature reviews and original research published in journals, books, policy documents, and online resources. The APRN educator role in health systems has become increasingly important as the need has grown for dissemination of evidence-based knowledge and for professionals to practice continuous quality improvement. The educator role is also important to align patient care outcomes with national chronic disease benchmarks and with state and national objectives for meeting the goals of *Healthy People 2010*. This chapter focuses on the direct role of the APRN in assessing learner needs and developing and implementing the education process.

APRNs manage patient health and illness care.[1] According to the Health Resources and Services Administration (HRSA),[1] the domains and competencies of the NP role provide a conceptual framework for the role and include health promotion, disease prevention, and teaching/coaching of the patient and family related to health and illness care. The health promotion and primary preventive education process includes responding to patient and family needs concerning immunizations, hygiene practices, balanced nutrition, exercise, and preventive healthcare practices related to one's social, environmental, and family history. Prevention education also includes teaching patients and families the importance of early identification of disease by participating in age-appropriate, evidence-based health screening practices such as skin, cervical, breast, colon, and prostate cancer screening. In the management of patient illness, the APRN provides the patient and family with the education necessary to manage chronic illness or disability (self-care). Patients with similar learning needs and health concerns can attend APRN-directed group learning experiences as part of their healthcare benefits. Social learning theory supports the utility of group learning practices as a means of achieving behavior change.

Role of the APRN in Continuing Education

In addition to providing education to patients and families, APRNs are increasingly being called upon to provide continuing education (CE) in their specialty or area of practice to their professional colleagues. Professional colleagues tend to be influenced by their own values and beliefs regarding CE and by their desire to change or improve their practice styles. A speaker who is well versed and knowledgeable in a subject and has an effective delivery style can be a strong motivator for professionals to attend an educational program and to change their practice behaviors.

CE Required by Many Boards of Nursing and Nursing Organizations

Many state boards of nursing require APRNs to complete a minimum number of CE hours to maintain licensure and/or certification. The American Academy of Nurse Practitioners Certification Program (AANPCP) requires a minimum of 75 hours of CE over a 5-year period in addition to 1000 hours of clinical practice.[4] The American Nurses Credentialing Center (ANCC) certification renewal program requires evidence of a minimum of 75 contact hours and 1000 hours of clinical practice. The ANCC provides for an additional recertification option that includes evidence of documentation of scholarship or service to the profession in one of several categories, including providing a CE program, teaching a course, publishing an article, or precepting an APRN student.[5]

Ways to Provide CE

APRNs today must learn the skills and attain the knowledge for developing and delivering CE programs. This is an important aspect of their professional role,[1,2,6,7] allowing them to emphasize quality improvement, cost controls, and evidence-based practice. One way to deliver CE programs is by speaking at the local, state, and national levels. Many APRNs voluntarily respond to the call for abstracts from nationally and internationally sponsored professional conferences. Speaking at conferences provides an opportunity for APRNs to share their clinical knowledge, expertise, and research and to build a community of clinical experts who can exchange information and join in clinically based participatory research projects. In addition to presenting at conferences, APRNs may provide CE through publishing articles and preparing online programs.

Standards for CE Credits

Professional organizations such as AANP, the ANCC, and most state nurse associations award CE credits, and standards for the credits are developed by the professional organization that has agreed to sponsor the program. The APRN must apply to the professional organization for approval of the CE program and the contact hours to be credited. This application is generally completed at the time an abstract is accepted or following a request for a CE presentation. The speaker must complete a detailed format, which is reviewed by the organization as part of the CE approval process. The application form varies among sponsoring organizations. In general, requirements include a clear description of the rationale or need for the program, the program purpose and goals, clearly written objectives as measurable behavioral outcomes, a content outline, and specific methods for evaluating the learner. Evaluation may include a hands-on return demonstration or multiple-choice questions that can be answered electronically. The applicant APRN also must submit a résumé providing evidence of his or her qualifications to speak on the subject as a CE provider. The approval process may take up to 3 months; the applicant should allow a minimum of 6 to 8 weeks to ensure that the program is approved for credits.

In general, one CE credit is given for each contact hour that the participant spends in the CE program. Methods for documenting attendance and evaluating the speaker are now generally performed electronically, thus allowing the speaker more time for delivering the content. APRNs should review feedback from the program participants as a means of improving their next speaking opportunity and learning what participants valued.

Identifying a Need for the CE Program

Prior to delivering a CE program, the APRN must identify a need for the program and be able to assure the sponsoring organization that the program will be valued by the organization's constituents. Changes in practice guidelines or changes in policies based on new evidence are some of the most prevalent reasons for CE sessions. Nationally recognized guidelines are published on the Web sites of the National Guidelines Clearing House, the Centers for Disease Control, and the National Heart, Lung, and Blood Institute. Quality improvement initiatives to decrease the rate of medical errors or healthcare disparities are other examples of reasons for CE sessions.

Outlining and Leveling Objectives of the Program

The CE program will need to have behavioral objectives appropriate to the audience and state what outcomes it intends to achieve. Many easy-to-understand Web sites explain how to write objectives and measurable outcomes and how to select objectives that are appropriate for the learner's background and level of achievement. An excellent resource for learning how to write objectives is *Gronlund's Writing Instructional Objectives,* now in the eighth edition; this simple-to-use text is an excellent reference resource.[8] Gronlund and Brookhart describe five characteristics of instructional objectives:

1. They provide a focus for instruction.
2. They provide guidelines for learning.
3. They provide targets for informative and summative assessment.
4. They convey instructional intent to others.
5. They provide for evaluation of instruction.[8(p8)]

The taxonomy, or leveling, of educational objectives[9–11] is based on three areas or domains of learning: the cognitive, the affective, and the psychomotor. Since CE provides professionals with knowledge that they can apply in practice, the instructional objectives should incorporate higher-level thinking skills and performance outcomes. Information on learning domains and related categories for the most commonly applied behavioral objectives is easily accessible on the Internet and in a number of texts. These resources can assist in developing objectives that act to organize and direct what the APRN plans for the learner to achieve as a result of the CE program.

In the cognitive domain, higher-level behavioral outcomes include application, analysis, synthesis, and evaluation. Within each of these major categories of the cognitive domain the educator can select the appropriate objective that will describe what the learner is expected to achieve at the conclusion of the educational program. The cognitive domains of knowledge and comprehension reflect lower-order cognitive skills that precede the ability to apply, analyze, or synthesize knowledge. For example, an individual who has attended a program on asthma management will be able to predict, based on knowledge and comprehension, the patient's level of asthma severity according to the guidelines set forth by the National Asthma Education Program, but the learner who can generate an action plan of care for a patient with moderate persistent asthma demonstrates the ability to synthesize information learned about asthma in the program.

In the affective domain, the APRN educator seeks to develop the learner's attitudes, motivation, and perceptions concerning health and self-care or care of others. Methods may include modeling, role-playing, case presentation, and self-reflection.

The psychomotor domain is one that includes physical movements and coordination. In nursing, we often refer to teaching students physical assessment techniques as the learning content within the psychomotor domain. Teaching students how to use an ophthalmoscope or an otoscope is a psychomotor skill; interpreting the visual findings from these instruments lies within the cognitive domain of learning.

Organizing the CE Presentation

The program should be organized in such a way that the content flows in a logical manner from general to more specific and includes case examples of how the content is applied in the clinical setting. An important skill the APRN needs to learn is how to manage delivery time so that all of the learning objectives are met. First to determine is how much time is allocated for the presentation. Second, the speaker needs to determine the nature of the audience. Is the audience made up of experienced APRNs? New APRN graduates? Or other experienced professionals such as physicians or physician assistants? The learning objectives should target the identified measurable outcomes for that specific audience, and the content should be logically aligned with the intended learner objectives. The final step is developing ways to measure the learners' achievement.

For example, in a program on electrocardiogram (EKG) interpretation, the objective for the learner would likely be mastering EKG interpretation. Thus the written objective might be: "At the end of this program, the learner will accurately identify ST segment depression as an indication of cardiac ischemia in a 12-lead EKG." The accompanying test would then provide examples of EKG strips and ask the learner to identify the one indicating cardiac ischemia. In this way, whether the objective has been met and what content has been learned is measured. Most efficient for a CE program are multiple-choice questions that flow from the content presented and that can provide feedback to the learner if reviewed at the conclusion of the program.

For example, imagine you are an APRN who specializes in asthma care and have been invited to speak to a group of experienced primary care providers, including physicians and NPs. You are asked to provide them with an update on national guidelines for the care of patients with asthma. You will have 90 minutes to deliver your message. In this case, the participants have experience and you know how much time you will have. Now you need to set priorities for achieving identified learning outcomes within the 90-minute time period.

You will want to design your teaching/learning processes not only to provide the audience with content related to the most complex aspects of the guidelines but also to allow participants time to interact and synthesize the content. The content may include new assessment criteria, changes in management guidelines, and new evidence from the research literature. You also may begin your presentation with an on-screen pretest and ask participants to answer the questions using clicker technology. By doing this, you allow participants to refresh their knowledge base and build on prior knowledge during your presentation.

Using Appropriate Learning Strategies

Appropriate learning strategies for achieving the desired outcomes should be used when organizing a talk. First, the speaker must know the subject matter, respect the audience, and determine priorities for time distribution. Strategies may also include a variety of audiovisual materials. These areas are all equally important aspects of the education process. Some practical suggestions are:

- The visual presentation should begin with the speaker's title, name, and credentials, including areas of certification and professional affiliations. An e-mail address can be included if the speaker wants participants to be able to ask additional questions.
- List the objectives and then provide the audience with an outline of the key elements of the presentation.
- Allow for sufficient contrast on the visual or slide—for example, use a bright blue font on a white background.
- Allow for only four to six lines of content per slide and use a font of 28 points or larger.
- Allow approximately 1 to 2 minutes of speaking time per slide, depending on the content emphasis.
- Pose thought-provoking questions to the audience throughout and project an attitude of approval and sensitivity regarding the subject matter.
- Allow time for and be open to questions at the end of the presentation. When speaking to a small group, the speaker may choose to respond to questions throughout the talk, if time permits.

Maintaining the Attention of the Audience

A number of principles can be applied that will benefit the audience and assist the speaker in maintaining the audience's attention:

- Encourage the learner to participate in the program. One strategy is to begin the program by asking what the learner already knows.
- Engage the learner in the problems presented. For example, ask the audience questions, allow time for comments, and listen to the participants' stories, which personalize the presentation.
- Present material in a variety of formats, including PowerPoint, video, and audio.
- Synthesize and reflect on prior information presented and summarize often.
- Use stories to demonstrate how the knowledge is applied to the clinical setting.
- Leave time for questions and attempt to meet members from the audience at the conclusion of the talk for further questions and discussion.

Early in a speaking career, it is wise to practice, practice, practice in front of a mirror or videotape or audiotape the performance. Attention should be given to hand gestures. Generally, hands should be kept at or below the waist. A speaker needs to project the voice, display enthusiasm for the subject matter, and speak at a pace that allows the audience to hear while also focusing on the content outline displayed on the visuals. Speakers should avoid reading off the screen and dropping their tone while speaking. The spoken word should embellish the material presented on the visuals and reflect knowledge of the subject matter. Another general rule is to avoid fill-in sounds, such as "um," which distract from the message as well as the speaker's creditability.

Prospective presenters are wise to seek a mentor who can help develop their presentation skills. The Fellows of the American Academy of Nurse Practitioners (http://www.aanp.org) and the Sigma Theta Tau International (http://www.nursingsociety.org.) offer professional mentorship programs, and information about these programs can be found on their Web sites. Other options include taking a course in public speaking, attending a CE program on the subject, or joining a local Toastmaster's group. The key to speaking success is in the speaker's hands.

Patient Education and Learning Theories

The science of learning theory can inform the APRN's teaching/coaching function and professional role. The main theories derive from the humanistic, behavioral, and cognitive schools of thought and are a rich resource for improving one's knowledge and application of the learning process. Learning theories help the APRN to predict the efficacy of teaching methods and serve as conceptual frameworks for organizing and directing the process of education.

Schools of Learning Theory

The three schools of learning theory discussed here—the humanistic, behaviorist, and cognitive—are philosophical perspectives that are not mutually exclusive; they share a common belief that "experience is the source of learning and that to learn is to change."[12(p66)]

THE HUMANISTIC SCHOOL

Scholars in the humanistic tradition include Carl Rogers, Abraham Maslow, and Victor Frankl. LaFrancois[13(p249)] has provided a comprehensive summary of the humanistic approach to learning and its principles, which involves paying attention to the individual's feelings, fostering self-concept, interpersonal communication, and clarifying personal. Consideration of feelings and personal values includes allowing the individual to refuse education if he or she so chooses, based on the right to self-determination. The humanistic approach focuses on inspiration through genuine communication and honest, caring, interpersonal relationships. Recognizing a patient's feelings and developing a strong interpersonal relationship with the patient and family influences their values and encourages positive beliefs.

Influencing a patient's feelings about his ability to perform self-care skills takes precedence over transferring knowledge that is retained and acted upon in a predictable way. For example, a patient's successful experience in managing diabetes under the care of the APRN, via telephone calls and support, improves the patient's feelings of self-worth and values related to diabetes self-care. Patients who feel positive about their ability to care for themselves will be inspired to participate in and follow recommendations. Their self-worth is enhanced and therefore their values and beliefs about their self-care regimen may also change.

Identifying patients' feelings and inspiring them to higher levels of self-worth through interpersonal relationships are central to success for the humanist educator. The theoretical method is particularly well suited to informing the teaching/coaching function of the APRN when teaching patients and families about chronic illness and when coaching those who need to develop lifestyle changes. Research, however, is mixed as to the efficacy of the humanistic approach. The humanistic teacher focuses on motivating the learner and believes that all humans are motivated to improve themselves. The question then becomes "Is motivation provided by the teacher the factor that drives the learning outcome or is there a basic human trait that expresses itself in response to the humanistic approach to teaching or is it that all individuals will learn under the right circumstances and conditions conducive to learning?"

THE BEHAVIORIST SCHOOL

Derived from the work by B. F. Skinner on operant conditioning,[14,15] the behaviorist, or stimulus-response, model presupposes that learning is achieved when a stimulus is applied and a desired response is achieved. The model does not consider the learner's feelings about learning, values, or beliefs. The applied stimulus can be negative or positive, depending on whether one is trying to stop a behavior such as smoking or adopt a new behavior such as weight loss. Praise from others or material items such as rewarding oneself with a new dress after losing 10 pounds are examples of positive stimuli.

Once a new behavior or goal has been reached, it must be sustained. The rewards (e.g., praise or new dress) that led to the initial behavior change may no longer be available, and unless the behavior change was accompanied by a change in the patient's feelings, values, and beliefs, the change may not be sustained. The stimulus to lose weight may have been driven by a material reward (e.g., looking good in a new dress for a daughter's wedding), but the change (losing weight) may not have been accompanied by the idea of improving health and cardiovascular risk profile. If the values and beliefs have not changed, the stimulus to control weight may be lost once the reinforcement (dress) is no longer available.

Integrating humanistic concepts into the behaviorist approach may be helpful. Using coaching skills, the APRN may ask the patient to keep a diary regarding her feelings about weight loss and to verbalize feelings about herself since she has lost weight compared to how she felt prior to losing weight. Using this technique, the APRN may help the patient discover her feelings and beliefs about health. Research has shown that multiple theoretical approaches must be considered when working with patients and families in need of behavior change.[16–18]

THE COGNITIVE SCHOOL

Learning is an internal intellectual process not open to verification by others. As people gain understanding and insight into health-related behaviors, they often store images based on these messages in the brain. Hearing the messages repeatedly over a period of time increases the potential for adopting a new behavior. Because the process of learning is longitudinal, exposure to information that builds on prior information in a variety of formats leads to some adjustments in behavior. These adjustments or changes in behavior may be subtle and the learner may not be totally aware of them. For example, patients who continue to hear the verbal message to stop smoking and are presented with a rationale or evidence to support the value of smoking cessation and then are exposed to pictures (e.g., of a lung damaged by smoking) and/or a video on the hazards of smoking (e.g., children exposed to a smoke-filled room) may change their behavior gradually. On a conscious or unconscious level, the learner may decrease the number of cigarettes smoked in a day and, with time and continued exposure to the messages, may actually set a date to stop smoking.

Albert Bandura[19] developed what is known as social learning theory (later renamed social cognitive theory), a combination of the cognitive and behaviorist theories of learning based on the supposition that the cognitive process facilitates social learning and the belief that human learning is an outcome of the interaction between one's beliefs about oneself and what one observes in the environment. Bandura emphasized the importance of learning by observing and modeling the behaviors, attitudes, and emotional reactions of others. His concept of perceived self-efficacy describes one's beliefs about achieving a future task based on experiences with the environment.

A female patient, for example, is interested in losing weight and admits to enjoying learning in social interaction with others. In the past, she has read many books on weight loss but has not been successful trying to lose weight on her own. The APRN suggests a weight-loss group meeting format for learning about adopting lifestyle changes related to diet and exercise. After listening to the testimony and stories about weight loss from others and observing the number of people attending the meetings who have lost weight, the patient self-reflects and discovers that she believes she, too, can lose weight. As weight loss begins to occur, the patient experiences an increase in her perceived self-efficacy to lose more weight.

Months later, the patient finds it difficult to keep attending the meetings and decides to monitor her weight at home. Very discouraged with her inability to sustain the weight loss after several months, she returns to the APRN. The APRN interviews the patient and asks her what she thinks helped her most to lose the weight when she attended the meetings. The patient admits that seeing others lose weight motivated her, leading her to believe she could do the same. The APRN applied the concept of self-efficacy, explaining that if she had achieved weight loss in the past, the likelihood of her achieving weight loss in the future was significant. The APRN encouraged her to attend the group weight-loss meetings and continue to pursue her goals of losing 20 pounds, or 10% of her body weight, stabilize her weight, and then identify future goals.

The process of applying social cognitive theory in practice requires knowing the learning needs of patients, recognizing how to apply adult learning principles, and assessing patients' preferred learning style. Once this has been accomplished, the APRN can assess the patient's past experience with behavior change and reinforce the patient's perceived self-efficacy.

Learning Principles and Theories of Education

Education is a process that transfers information from one human to another. The process begins when the APRN assesses the learners' motivation or readiness to learn, their ability to retain knowledge, and their values and beliefs related to acting on knowledge gained. Assessment includes attention to the developmental age, gender, and religious beliefs of the learners as well as to their individual and family values concerning health and learning. The education process transfers knowledge to the learner via a combination of verbal, written, or modeling approaches that may be incorporated into patient clinical encounters, group meetings, or computer-based interactive technologies. The reciprocal endpoint of the educative process is a change in the learner's behavior. Learning theorists argue that the process of learning is transformative; that is, the endpoint is a change in behavior or adoption of a new behavior.[20-26]

Educational theory provides the rationale and supporting constructs for the determination of learning need and the design and the implementation of the education process. Researchers have investigated the willingness to engage in learning and react to new information and the affective and behavioral responses of the learner. Rosenstock[26] identified individual factors, such as health beliefs and values concerning health, that influence a person's readiness to adopt new behaviors. In working with Hochbaurm and Kegels in the public health service, Rosenstock developed a model, the Health Belief Model, to explain the failure of individuals to obtain tuberculosis screening. Variables in the model, such as perceived susceptibility, perceived threat, perceived barriers, perceived benefits, self-efficacy, and cues to action, have been studied extensively. The APRN who assesses the patient for these variables can optimize the opportunities for success in patient adherence to a plan of preventive care. Addressing these variables through one's teaching is a useful method for the APRN educator when formulating a plan of teaching and motivating patients and families about their risk for disease.

Determinants of Learning

The "determinants of learning, adapted from Haggard, [27] are critical steps in the educator process and include:

1. Assess the needs of the learner:
   - Determine what the patient or family knows about the health condition or area of prevention.
   - Demonstrate respect for the patient and family in acknowledging their level of knowledge and skill and build a genuine interpersonal relationship.
   - Determine what new or additional information the patient needs now and in the future.
2. Assess the learner's readiness to learn:
   - Ask the patient or family if they would like to know more about the health condition or area of prevention now and in the future.
   - Determine if there are ongoing factors—physical, psychological, social, economic, or religious—that may interfere with the patient's or family's ability to learn at this time.

3. Design a teaching method that fits the learner's ability to understand and retain the information needed:

- Determine if there are any sensory deficits, such as hearing or vision loss, that may interfere with learning.

- Assess the learner's cognitive ability. Can he or she understand simple directions? Complex directions? Is there a language barrier? Is an interpreter needed?

- Assess the learner's ability to read based on knowledge of their education level or developmental stage.

- Assess their motivation to learn. What are their feelings about the subject and are they interested in learning how to care for themselves?

- Determine if the patient or family members would like to attend a group learning session or would rather read about the subject matter or be referred to a Web-based learning experience.

Adult Learning Theory

Andragogy, the theory of how adults learn, is attributed to Malcolm Knowles.[28,29] In this theory, the focus of education is on the adult learner who possesses an independent, self-directed desire to learn. A key factor in determining the learning styles of the adult and his or her motivation to learn is the developmental age of the learner. According to Milligan,[30] the teacher–adult learner relationship is linear rather than the hierarchical one seen in the teacher–student relationships of earlier developmental life-cycle stages.

The professional relationship that the APRN develops with patients, families, students, and other professionals is purposeful: The APRN provides information that is sought after by the learner. The adult learner desires health education because it meets a particular health promotion or disease management need in keeping with adult goals and objectives to be a productive member of society. Knowles[28,29] further proposes that adults build or add new knowledge onto prior life experiences, adding to their repertoire of complex skills. Adults can reflect on prior experiences and apply new knowledge to find solutions to solving problems they have experienced before. In addition, they are more likely to apply new knowledge rapidly to solve immediate problems in everyday life and less likely to seek knowledge to use at a later time. Adults' readiness to learn about health is, in part, motivated by their distinct roles in life—the demands of their work or of their family-related roles. It is important to note that Knowles's research was conducted primarily on healthy adults, so assumptions made about the application of the theory to sick individuals or older adults who may have cognitive and physical impairments may not hold true.

Several factors merit consideration when providing education for adults:[31(pp140–141)]

- Adults are self-sufficient and are more likely to seek information on healthcare subjects of immediate interest to them or their family members independently. Therefore, identifying the learner's needs or desire for information is appropriate at the time of the healthcare encounter.

- Adults bring to their relationship with the APRN previous experiences with health and illness on which they build their future understanding related to managing health and disease.

- Adults appreciate individual facts or ideas and tolerate poorly learning tedious information that is not relevant to solving an immediate need. Therefore, it is important to provide information that is relevant to the patient or family and avoid less necessary information.

- Adults are creatures of habit and respond to the need to change with considerable resistance unless it is connected to meeting the responsibilities of their job or social roles. The APRN should explore ways of integrating new health information/ recommendations into the adult's present lifestyles (e.g., how the adult might integrate an exercise program into the daily work schedule).

■ Prior negative experiences with learning in general can be a barrier to future learning. Therefore, prior to initiating learning experiences, the APRN should assess past learning experiences, readiness to learn new information, and amount of time needed to invest in the learning experience.

■ Adult learners prefer to participate actively in the learning process, rather than be passive observers. With this in mind, the APRN should seek out learning resources in the form of books or interactive tutorials, as well as online technologies that involve the learner, rather than just providing verbal information. Also, the APRN should find time at subsequent visits to follow up on questions or clarify information that the patient may have learned between visits.

■ Some adult learners, especially individuals who are extroverts by nature, may prefer to learn in a group and find social support a significant adjunct to learning. The APRN should ask patients if they would like to attend group sessions to learn how to manage their diabetes, lose weight, or recover from cancer surgery.

■ Adult learners prefer that learning be on their terms, voluntary, and self-directed, not mandatory and punitive in nature.

Patient Literacy and Readability Formulas

APRNs may provide patients with printed materials or reference online information on complex and highly technical subjects that may take longer to review than time allows in the one-to-one encounter. Providing patient education resources (PER), in both the inpatient and outpatient settings, is an appropriate way to deliver information to adults who may want to reference it in the future and/or share it with their families. When considering PER, the APRN should review the materials and ensure that they are accurate and up-to-date. Many state health departments distribute free PER, and a number of states support a health information clearinghouse where health professionals can obtain free PER, including videos on selected topics. The National Heart, Lung, and Blood Institute provides a number of excellent online resources that can be sent to a practice setting or directly to patients' homes for a low fee. One useful item is a colorful nutritional brochure on the Dietary Approaches to Stop Hypertension, known as the DASH diet. Other patient education resources can be obtained for a fee from the American Diabetes Association, the American Lung Association, the American Heart Association, and the National Osteoporosis Foundation, to name a few. A careful search of the Web will provide a list of PER related to specific diseases or conditions encountered in practice that can be ordered for free or at a nominal cost.

Assessing Literacy Levels

Adult literacy levels must be assessed whenever selecting patient education materials for distribution among a specific patient population. Literacy is defined as the ability of adults to read, write, and comprehend information at the 8th-grade level; *illiteracy* is the term used to describe adults whose reading, writing, and language comprehension range from 5th- to 8th-grade levels.

Many PER are written at a level far above the average person's reading level. The mean adult reading level in the United States is between grades 5 and 8,[5] yet most PER average above the 8th-grade level with many between the 10th- and 12th-grade levels.[7] *Healthy People 2010* reports that only 12% of adults have proficient health literacy skills; 9 out of 10 adults lack the skills needed to manage their health care adequately, and 30 million people have lower-than-basic healthcare literacy skills.[32]

Clues to illiteracy or low literacy skills include difficulty comprehending oral information, not understanding an explanation given on the prior visit, hesitancy in agreeing to read a document or leaving it behind, failure to follow directions, or asking a family member or friend to explain the information. Hearing deficits and language deficits are other factors that must be considered. Many patients will conceal their inability to read out of embarrassment. Alternative methods for delivering information, such as simple picture books and videos, as well as using the humanistic approach are considerations when teaching and coaching patients with low literacy skills.

Using Readability Measurement Tools

The APRN and nursing colleagues may choose to develop their own educational materials. In this way, the message is customized to the patient population, language, culture, and literacy level. The ease with which written or printed information can be read is termed readability.[33] The APRN should be familiar with how to apply readability measurement tools to assess the reading level of materials developed in the practice or other materials distributed to patients. These methods, however, are not foolproof and cannot assure the practitioner that the patient will comprehend what is read. Despite being able to read the text, the patient may not comprehend the message transmitted. A review of materials with patients is ideal, and family members should also be apprised of the content to be understood.

Readability formulas predict the grade reading level of text; they do not predict the comprehension of the reader. Their usefulness lies in providing a level of assurance that patients are being provided with PER that they can read based on an understanding of the literacy level of the population served. One commonly used test is the Fog Index, developed by Gunning,[34] which determines readability levels between the 4th and 11th grades. This easy method involves taking a 100-word sample from the text and determining the average sentence length and percent of words that contain more than one syllable. Another popular test is the SMOG, which is considered one of the most valid tests; rather than just the grade reading level, it assures comprehension at the reading level of the text measured. If the text measures at a 7th-grade reading level, the level of understanding is 100% for anyone reading at the 7th-grade level.[35,36] An abbreviated guide for performing the SMOG measurement is provided in Box 14-1. However, the APRN is encouraged to consult the original article for a more in-depth explanation. [35-36] A comprehensive explanation of how to use the SMOG readability formula is also provided by Bastable in his book's appendix.[31] Many readability tests, including the SMOG, can be located on the Internet and can serve as a convenient resource for the APRN.

Checking Internet Sources of Information

With maturity, adults assume responsibility for their health and welcome opportunities to reference health information on the Internet. Developing a list of recommended learning sites and having these available to patients in a printed handout is an efficient way of providing adult education on a variety of subjects.

The assessment of patient literacy levels and of readability is as important when recommending PER on the Internet as it is when considering the readability of PER distributed in the practice setting. In addition, the APRN must assess the learner's ability to access online information and their cognitive skills for understanding the written word. Therefore, the APRN should review Web sites carefully before recommending them and should stay apprised of new sites that may give updated information and/or be more interesting or readable for the learner. A committee of colleagues can be formed to review Web-based PER, which is one way of engaging colleagues in patient education, as well as gaining confidence that the PER distributed are readable, accurate, and up-to-date.

Adults with computer skills or the motivation to learn to use the computer can select learning sites that appeal to their level of education and their area of interest. In follow-up

> **BOX 14-1 | A Brief Guide to Performing the SMOG Test**
>
> 1. Count the number of words in three sets of 10 sentences each, one set near the beginning of the text, one near the middle, and one near the end. Then total all the words in the 30 sentences.
> 2. Circle all words with three or more syllables, including repetitions of the same word.
> 3. Find the nearest perfect square to your total number of three-syllable words. For example, if there are 98 three-syllable words, use 100 (10 × 10) or if the total is 51, use 49 (7 × 7).
> 4. Find the square root of the number you found in step 3; for example, if the number is 49, then the square root is 7. Then add 3 to that number (7 + 3 = 10). This latter number—10 in this case—determines the grade-level readability.
> 5. The grade level tells you that ⅔ of the students in that grade in the United States could read the sample with 100% comprehension. Or, in the example given, ⅔ of 10th-grade-level students can read the sample with 100% comprehension.
>
> The standard error of prediction is 1.5 grades in either direction.

visits, it is wise to discuss information patients have reviewed on the Internet to clarify and determine how patients may be processing or responding to information they read independently from what was recommended.

Becoming Familiar With Books on Specific Health Topics

For patients and families with higher literacy levels, selected books are often used as a way to inspire and motivate patients in the cognitive and affective learning domains, which is known as bibliotherapy. The APRN may want to learn more about books that patients are reading by visiting the local bookstore or library and reviewing the holdings in the area of health and behavior change. In addition, book reviews are often available on the Internet or published in local newspapers. Books are an excellent PER for the adult learner and may serve to motivate and help patients manage their health.

In summary, the role of the APRN in providing education to adults is more enjoyable, less challenging, and less time-consuming if adult learning principles are taken into consideration and educational processes are put in place to accommodate the needs of the adult learner. In addition, using a readability formula can assist the APRN to determine the reading level of materials developed or purchased for distribution. This process can help demonstrate a responsible approach and improve the quality of education provided to patients.

Including Family Members

Family members of patients should be approached in a similar manner and provided resources for learning about the health of their family members. Including families in patient education is important, but is often overlooked. Reeber[37] cites the role of the family as a variable critical in affecting patient outcomes. Family members contribute to the patients' emotional support, can assist with preventing patient injury, can support patients in staying on special diets, and can join with the patient in programs of exercise and rehabilitation.

Family education is critical in planning the transition of patients back into the community or to another care facility, such as long-term care. Family meetings, if appropriate, should be arranged at a time that is convenient for all members who may be playing an active role in the care of the patient. However, one key principle of family education is to identify the point person who will be responsible for supporting the patient and acting as his or her advocate. This is often easier to accomplish in the inpatient setting than in the outpatient setting, but even if more difficult in the outpatient setting, it may be useful, especially in the care of patients with chronic illness or complex health problems.

Adult learning principles should be applied to family members as well as to the patient. This includes conducting a learning needs assessment and determining the family member's readiness to learn and desire to apply knowledge to the care of the patient. In the outpatient or community setting, if patients give permission, a responsible family member who has agreed to assume responsibility for managing the patient's care may enter the room at the time of the patient encounter and be included in the education process. A family member can be a critical link to what is learned and understood by the patient. Without the family member present, the patient, due to stress, fear, or anxiety, may not hear or understand the information provided in sufficient depth to apply it safely or accurately.

Patient Counseling

Competence in providing patient and family counseling is an additional component of the teaching/coaching role of the APRN. Unlike patient education, counseling involves using skills learned in human communication and group dynamics as well as an in-depth appreciation of mental health counseling skills. Counseling principles include being open to considering the needs of the patient and family beyond the immediate management of patient health and illness care. It may involve setting aside time at the end of the encounter to ask the patient how he or she is doing in general. An empathetic, open approach to the patient or family is valued in the counseling encounter.

Establishing a trusting relationship in which one is open to hearing the patient without being judgmental is fundamental to conducting a counseling session. For example, an exchange may be:

> APRN: *"The last time we met you reported your fear about your father's drinking problem. How is that going for you now?"*

As the patient reveals feelings, the APRN should be open, listen, and avoid making judgments and giving direction too soon. The APRN should listen carefully as the patient identifies the problem, and proceed to explore the patient's and/or family's concerns about the problem, and then learn more about how the problem is affecting the family.

> APRN: *"How is your father's drinking affecting you and other members of your family?"*

The APRN should also determine if there are any economic concerns. Learn from the patient or family what has been tried previously to alleviate the problem and what were the outcomes of these attempts.

> APRN: *"Do you or any of your family members have any other ideas or solutions?"*

The goal of counseling is to have the patient and family externalize their beliefs and feelings about the situation. They may need to engage in values clarification with the APRN to determine whether their being upset and fearful about the future is rational. In so doing, the APRN can support their concerns and be empathetic.

At the conclusion of the counseling session, the APRN must be able to explore goals and have the patient or family develop recommendations they can agree to pursue. At this point, the APRN may offer a list of resources that may help them, such as the social worker at the local hospital or a recommendation that they consider talking to their minister or spiritual advisor. This phase of the counseling process provides direction, but it does not assure the family that a solution has been found.[38]

The APRN as Preceptor

For the purposes of this discussion, a preceptor is defined as a licensed healthcare professional (e.g., a nurse practitioner, a physician, a physician assistant) who role-models, teaches, consults with, assesses, and evaluates a student who formally contracts with the preceptor to learn a set of advanced nursing practice skills. Research has demonstrated that APRNs believe precepting is part of their professional role responsibility in advancing the profession and educating the next generation of NPs. The role of the NP preceptor is also defined as that of a clinical practitioner-preceptor-educator.[40] The clinical NP educator demonstrates expert patient care skills with the added dimension of teaching these expert clinical skills and knowledge to the APRN student while increasing the student's self-confidence.[41]

Models for Developing Skills and Competencies

The philosophy of educating and evaluating NP students is based on the Dreyfus model of skill acquisition adopted by Benner[42] and applied to the role development and performance of nurses. The Dreyfus model, developed by Herbert and Stuart Dreyfus in 1980, proposes that individuals apply knowledge learned to an area of practice that is either professional or technical in nature. In so doing, the apprentice progresses through a number of stages prior to reaching a competent level of performance, a process termed "skill acquisition." The process occurs over a period of time so that the apprentice's early level of competence in performing skills without supervision increases with immersion in the skill performance experience. As applied to the student APRN role, the preceptor understands that students progress along a continuum from novice to competent in achieving a safe level of competency for entry into practice.

Skill acquisition is a useful concept that guides the preceptor in assisting the learner to advance along the continuum from novice to the levels of advanced beginner, competence, expert, and proficient. Expert and proficient levels may not be reached unless learners receive intensive internship experiences in which they are immersed in clinical practice similar to that of the graduate nurse. The level of advanced beginner or competence is achieved at the master's level APRN education. The transition to the Doctor of Nursing Practice (DNP) is intended to bring graduates to a higher level of expertise; however, full expertise and proficiency may not be achieved until after a number of years of practice.[43] A guide for preceptors to consider when determining student competence is this: Competence is reached when the professional demonstrates the habitual and judicious use of communication, knowledge, technical skills, clinical reasoning, emotions, values, and reflection in daily practice for the benefit of the individual and community being served.[44]

Miller proposes a second model of developmental competency in learning.[45] This model depicts the student learner progressing from the cognitive domain of knowing to the behavioral domain of demonstrating a behavior change. The student begins with having knowledge about clinical problems, progresses to knowing how to do something with the knowledge, and then demonstrates to the preceptor what he or she can do with the knowledge. Finally, the student is able to demonstrate competence by independent actions that are based on the knowledge, thereby signifying that the behavior change demonstrates practice-based competency. This type of competency demonstrates the application of helping students achieve higher-level behavioral outcomes that require synthesis and application of knowledge rather than competency evaluated by paper-and-pencil methods.

Factors Facilitating a Preceptor's Success

A number of factors will facilitate a preceptor's success in assisting students to achieve their goals. These include:

- Knowing the overall goals and objectives for the practicum experience based on course objectives provided by the faculty
- Identifying and discussing learners' needs to meet the course objectives
- Assessing the nature of patient care encounters that will enable students to meet their learning objectives
- Utilizing appropriate teaching methods for the student and setting

- Evaluating whether the learners' objectives have been achieved
- Providing learners with feedback based on the evaluation[39]

Other factors that impact the preceptor's success include the preceptor's values, attitudes, qualities, and ethics:

- Communicating respect for the students' faculty, curriculum, and program
- Respecting the NP student as a professional nurse and adult learner
- Demonstrating the ability to cope with multiple variables in the clinical setting
- Understanding that students may not know everything they should know
- Problem-solving with students using clinical knowledge and evidence
- Addressing uncomfortable situations as they arise in a private, confidential manner
- Fostering the tenets of diversity and acceptance of difference
- Role-modeling interprofessional and collaborative communication skills
- Demonstrating sound professional ethics
- Serving as a teacher in areas where students are not knowledgeable or are outside their scope of knowledge even if they should have achieved this knowledge previously
- Recommending references and resources that students may use in obtaining information
- Holding students accountable for the application of prior knowledge
- Helping students learn through self-reflection on tasks achieved or not achieved
- Holding students accountable for evaluating their performance and learning progress during and at the end of the experience
- Encouraging students to consult and collaborate with other members of the interdisciplinary team, lead team meetings, and provide an interdisciplinary education program, if indicated
- Modeling the highest standards of quality care for patients and families[43]

Common Teaching Methods Applicable to the Preceptor Role

Teaching methods applied in the clinical setting are described in the literature and on the Web.[46–48] Prior to beginning the internship or preceptorship experience, the preceptor will have received materials from the student's school, including a course syllabus with learning objectives and a clinical evaluation tool. The preceptor should have a copy of the student's résumé and be familiar with the student's background. Ideally, the student will have also visited the preceptor for an interview and the preceptor and student have agreed to the specific days and number of hours that would be required for the experience.

Students need a specified time for orientation to the clinical learning environment. This includes becoming familiar with the physical setting, the policies and procedures that are commonly adhered to, and charting methods, as well as with electronic medical record training that may be included in orientation. Some agencies will want the student to attend a specified training program prior to beginning the experience. Students should be introduced to others in the setting and their roles and provided opportunities to observe and learn the routines related to how patients are admitted and the flow of patient care. Each agency and preceptor has its own set of clinical preferences. The student should become familiar with these preferences to facilitate a smooth learning process. The preceptor may want to have the student observe his or her practice style or may choose to allow the student to develop his or her own practice style. Part of the orientation should include a review of the clinical course evaluation with the student so that learning expectations are clear and dates for midterm and final evaluations are known by the preceptor and student in advance.

The process of educating students involves general adult learning/teaching principles. The preceptor will want to challenge the learner to act at all times in a respectful, professional manner, to be aware of patient privacy, and to develop sensitivity to differences in health values and beliefs. A preceptor should emphasize what the student can be expected to do safely based on an understanding of his or her previous level of skill and knowledge.

Each student brings to the practice setting a level of achievement somewhere from novice to competent. For each clinical experience, patients are selected based on the student's learning needs. The student should be expected to review the chart or charts and prepare for the encounter. The preceptor should strive to assist the student with critical thinking skills and application of advanced knowledge. For example, the preceptor may ask the student to think through the supporting scientific basis underlying assessment and decision making. For example, what is the drug of choice for a 45-year-old patient with community-acquired pneumonia? If this were an 85-year-old patient with pneumonia who also has chronic obstructive pulmonary disease, what antibiotics might you choose instead? And why? The attentive preceptor will provide as many opportunities as feasible for the student to learn from the clinical practice situation and apply knowledge learned in the classroom to clinical practice.

Presenting cases is an excellent learning experience that challenges the learner to organize and describe the assessment, determine differential diagnoses, and describe a plan of care with supporting rationale. This process requires discipline on the part of the student and the preceptor. Oral case presentations contribute to the student's self-confidence and the preceptor's confidence and trust in the student's development of clinical judgment. It is much easier for the preceptor to simply perform the assessment and design a management plan rather than take the time to listen to the student, challenge his or her hypothesis testing, and guide the inductive reasoning process. Preceptors may be asked to evaluate a student's performance on clinical case presentations as one method of providing feedback and evaluation to the faculty.

In many programs, students are required to submit weekly logs documenting the health problems of patients they have seen while in the clinical agency, their approach to management, the evaluation and management code for the encounter, and the level of independence or collaboration they have demonstrated in each patient encounter. No patient identifying data are included in the weekly log. Preceptors may choose to review these clinical logs with students as a way of reviewing content areas for learning, clarifying management strategies, and challenging the student to obtain evidence to support management methods. Frequently throughout the clinical day, there is not sufficient time for these exchanges, but the preceptor and student can establish time to review previous experiences at the end of the day or prior to beginning the next clinical day. This is another way for the preceptor to evaluate the student's learning needs and to plan experiences that will build on knowledge learned in prior patient encounters.

Organizing the clinical experience to meet the goals that the student has developed for clinical learning allows the student to function as an adult learner. Goal setting is a meaningful way to facilitate learning outcomes that are valued by the learner. If the student can establish learning goals on a daily basis, identify learning needs in a collaborative manner with the preceptor, and formulate objectives that can be measured, the student is more likely to be motivated and take ownership of learning outcomes.

Early in the relationship, a learning needs assessment may be difficult for the preceptor, but with time, the preceptor will come to know what the student's learning needs are and will want to take time to discuss them with the student. For example, the student may have knowledge deficits in the area of anatomy. The preceptor can guide the student to select learning methods to meet the goals and objectives. Using a feedback loop, the preceptor can build on the student's previous learning goals by providing feedback at the end of each clinical day. This methodology, referred to as the GNOME method—Goal, Needs, Methods, Objectives, and Evaluation—was developed by the University of Massachusetts-Worcester as part of the grant-funded project Teaching of Tomorrow Workshops, sponsored by the UMass-Worcester Community Faculty Development Center.[49] A helpful preceptor toolbox can be found at http://www.umassmed.edu/cfdc/toolbox/.

In summary, precepting students is a challenging but rewarding experience. Regular preceptor feedback and student self-evaluation are important to achieving learning outcomes. Reflection by both student and preceptor provides an opportunity to direct the learner to setting future learning priorities while connecting new concepts with previous clinical experiences. The student's goals, learning needs, and objectives should be assessed, prioritized, and tailored to the experience before each clinical session. The student should be assisted in selecting learning methods that will help meet these learning goals and objectives. The methods may include reading articles, observing someone else, watching a video, or developing a case study. The preceptor should challenge the learner to use critical thinking, demonstrate enthusiasm for the student's success, and provide praise as appropriate. Following graduation, and often before, many preceptors take on a mentoring role with students they have precepted.[51] Educating the next generation of APRNs is a professional responsibility and preceptor-student relationships often lead to lasting friendships and professional relationships.

SUGGESTED LEARNING EXERCISES

1. Select one of the learning theories and describe how you would apply this theory to patient education in the practice setting. Present your scenario to your colleagues for feedback and a critique.

2. Review the current *Healthy People 2010* objectives. Select a health objective that interests you and design a patient education brochure that is at the 8th-grade reading level.

3. Perform a learning needs assessment for a continuing education program for colleagues in your work setting. Discuss the learning needs with your colleagues, and seek validation for this learning need in the literature or other sources, such as a quality improvement committee. Design a 1-hour continuing education session to meet the learning need identified. Write the specific rationale and learning objectives that are measurable by demonstration or a post-test. Develop post-test questions based on the learning objectives you hope to achieve.

4. With a colleague, role-play a preceptor and student interacting after a patient encounter. Demonstrate through role-playing how you would interact with the student to develop a GNOME for the clinical day.

5. Using a simulated experience, counsel a patient who has a father who abuses alcohol. Demonstrate how you would help the patient to explore personal values and beliefs about alcohol. Demonstrate how you might help the patient discover how the problem with alcohol abuse has affected him personally. Then, advise him on what measures or resources you can recommend to help address the problem.

References

1. Health Resources and Services Administration (HRSA). (2002). Nurse Practitioner Primary Care Competencies in Specialty Areas: Adult, Gerontological, Pediatric and Women's Health. Health Resources and Services Administration, Information Center, Merrifield, VA. http://www.eric.ed.gov/ERICWebPortal/custom/portlets/recordDetails/detailmini.jsp?_nfpb=true&_&ERICExtSearch_SearchValue_0=ED471273&ERICExtSearch_SearchType_0=no&accno=ED471273. Accessed April 29, 2009.

2. National Association of Clinical Nurse Specialists. (2007, November/December). A vision for the future for clinical nurse specialist. *Clinical Nurse Specialist* 21:6:310–320.

3. Leavell HR, and Clark, EG. (1965). *Preventive Medicine for the Doctor in his Community: An Epidemiologic Approach*, 3rd ed. McGraw-Hill Book Company, New York.

4. American Academy of Nurse Practitioners (AANP). (2002). *Standards of Practice for Nurse Practitioners*. American Academy of Nurse Practitioners, Austin, TX.

5. American Nurses Credentialing Center. (2008). Certification Renewal: Professional Development Requirement. http://www.nursecredentialing.org/Certification/CertificationRenewal/ProfessionalDevelopment.aspx. Accessed April 30, 2009.

6. American Association of Acute and Critical Care Clinical Nurse Specialists. (1998). *Standards for Acute and Critical Care Clinical Nurse Specialists*. American Association of Acute and Critical Care Clinical Nurse Specialists, Harrisburg, PA.

7. National Association of Clinical Nurse Specialists. (2004). *Statement on Clinical Nurse Specialist Practice and Education*, 2nd ed. National Association of Clinical Nurse Specialists, Harrisburg, PA.

8. Gronlund, NE, and Brookhart SM. (2008). *Gronlund's Writing Instructional Objectives*, 8th ed. Pearson Merrill, Prentice Hall, Upper Saddle River, NJ.

9. Bloom, BJ, Englehart, MS, Furst, EJ, Hill, WH, and Krathwohl, DR. (1956). *Taxonomy of Educational Objectives: The Classification of Educational Goals, Handbook 1: Cognitive Domain.* David McKay, New York.

10. Mager, RF. (1997). *Preparing Instructional Objectives*, 3rd ed. Center for Effective Performance, Atlanta, GA.

11. Anderson, L, and Krathwohl, DR (eds). (2001). *A Taxonomy for Teaching, Learning, and Assessing.* Longman, New York.

12. Gleit, CJ. (1992). Theories of learning. In Boyd, MD, Graham, BA, Gleit, CJ, and Whitman, NI (eds), *Health Teaching in Nursing Practice: A Professional Model*, 3rd ed. Appleton Lange, Stamford, CT, pp 65–98.

13. LaFrancois, GR. (1994). *Psychology for Teaching*, 8th ed. Wadsworth, Belmont, CA.

14. Skinner, BF. (1974). *About Behaviorism*. Vintage Books, New York.

15. Skinner, BF. (1989). *Recent Issues in the Analysis of Behavior.* Merrill, Columbus, OH.

16. Glanz, K, Lewis, F, and Rimer, B (eds). (2002). *Health Behavior and Health Education: Theory, Research, and Practice*, 3rd ed. Jossey Bass, San Francisco, CA.

17. National Cancer Institute. (2003). Theory at a Glance: A Guide for Health Promotion Practice. http://www.cancer.gov/PDF/481f5d53-63df-41bc-bfaf-5aa48ee1da4d/TAAG3.pdf. Accessed April 29, 2009.

18. Turner, SL, Thomas, AM, Wagner, PJ, and Moseley, GC. (2008). A collaborative approach to wellness: diet, exercise, and education to impact behavior change. *J Am Acad of Nurse Practitioners* 20(6):339–344.

19. Bandura, A. (1977). *Social Learning Theory.* Prentice-Hall, Saddle Brook, NJ.

20. Combs, A. (1982). *A Personal Approach to Teaching: Beliefs That Make a Difference.* Allyn and Bacon, Boston.

21. Schon, DA. (1983). *The Reflective Practitioner*. Basic Books, New York.

22. Daloz, L. (1986). *Effective Teaching and Mentoring: Realizing the Transformational Power of Adult Learning Experiences.* Jossey-Bass, San Francisco.

23. Diekelmann, N. (1988). Curriculum revolution: a theoretical and philosophical mandate for change. In *National League for Nursing Curriculum Revolution: Mandate for Change,* National League for Nursing, New York, pp 137–158.

24. Bevis E, and Watson, J. (1989). *Toward a Caring Curriculum: A New Pedagogy for Nursing.* National League for Nursing, New York.

25. Mezirow, JD. (1991). *Transformative Dimensions of Adult Learning.* Jossey-Bass, San Francisco.

26. Rosenstock, IM. (1974). Historical origins of the Health Belief Model, *Health Education Monographs* 2:328–335.

27. Haggard, A. (1989). *Handbook of Patient Education.* Aspen Publications, Rockville, MD.

28. Knowles, M. (1990). *The Adult Learner: A Neglected Species,* 4th ed. Gulf Publishing, Houston, TX.

29. Knowles, MS, Holten, EF, and Swanson, RA. (1998). *The Adult Learner: A Definitive Classic in Adult Education and Human Resources Development,* 5th ed. Gulf Publishing, Houston, TX.

30. Milligan, F. (1997). In defense of andragogy. Part 2. An educational process consistent with modern nursing's aims. *Nurse Education Today* 17:487–493.

31. Bastable, S, and Rinwalske, MA. (2003). *The Nurse Educator: Principles of Teaching and Learning in Nursing Practice,* 2nd ed. Jones and Bartlett, Boston.

32. U.S. Department of Health and Human Services (USDHHS) (ed). (2000, January). *Healthy People 2010: Understanding and Improving Health,* 2nd ed. USDHHS, Washington, DC. http://www.healthypeople.gov. Accessed October 15, 2008.

33. Brownson, K. (1998). Education handouts: are we wasting our time? *J for Nurses in Staff Development* 14(4):176–182.

34. Gunning, R. (1968). The Fog Index after 20 years. *J Business Communications* 6:3–13.

35. Doak, LC, and Doak, CC. (1996). *Teaching Patients with Low Literacy Skills,* 2nd ed. Lippincott, Philadelphia.

36. McLaughlin, GH. (1969). SMOG-grading, a new readability formula. *J Reading* 12:639–646.

37. Reeber, BJ. (1992). Evaluating the effects of a family education intervention. *Rehabilitation Nursing* 17(6):332–336.

38. Wright, LM, and Leahy, M. (2004). *Nurses and Families: A Guide to Family Assessment and Intervention.* FA Davis, Philadelphia.

39. McAllister, M, Bergmann, M, and Nannini, A. (1997). Preceptor Role Function: An Analysis of Beliefs, Satisfaction, and Unmet Needs. Poster presentation. National Organization of Nurse Practitioner Faculties National Conference, Albuquerque, New Mexico, April 1997.

40. DeWitt, TG. (1996). Faculty development for community practitioners. Pediatric Resident Education in Community Settings: Proceedings of a Conference Held on March 23 and 24, 1996 in Chicago, IL. *Pediatrics* 98(6):1273–1277.

41. Ferguson, LM. (1996). Preceptors' enhance students self-confidence. *Nursing Connections* 9(1):49–61.

42. Benner, P. (1982). From novice to expert. *Am J Nursing* 82(3):402–407.

43. American Association of Colleges of Nursing. (2006). The Essentials of Doctoral Education for Advanced Nursing Practice. http://www.aacn.nche.edu/DNP/pdf/Essentials.pdf. Accessed April 24, 2009.

44. Epstein, RM, and Hundert, DM. (2002). Defining and assessing professional competence. *JAMA* 287:226–235.

45. Miller, GE. (1990). The assessment of clinical skills/competence/performance. *Acad Med* 65(Suppl):S63–S67.

46. Sloand, E, Feroli, K, and Beecher J. (1998). Preparing the next generation: precepting nurse practitioner students. *J Am Acad NPs* 10(2):65.

47. Heidenreich, C, Lye, P, Simpson, D, and Lourich, M. (2000). Educating child health professionals: the search for effective and efficient ambulatory teaching methods through the literature. *Pediatrics* 105(1, Suppl)231–237.

48. Dumas, MA (ed). (2000). *Partners in NP Education: A Preceptor Manual for NP Programs, Faculty, Preceptors, and Students.* National Organization of Nurse Practitioner Faculties, Washington, DC.

49. University of Massachusetts-Worcester. Teaching of Tomorrow Workshops 2004. Faculty Development Center. Available att: http://www.med.unc.edu/epic/ and http://www.umassmed.edu/cfdc/toolbox/.

50. Quirk, ME, DeWitt, T, Lasser, D, Huppert, M, and Hunniwell, E. (1998). Evaluation of primary care futures: a faculty development program for community health center preceptors. *Academic Medicine* 73(6):705–707.

51. Hayes, E. (1994). Having preceptors mentor the next generation of nurse practitioners. *Am J Prim Health Care* 19(6):62–66.

Gene Harkless is an associate professor at the University of New Hampshire where she serves as the graduate program coordinator. Dr. Harkless is also a visiting professor at Sor Trondelag University College of Nursing in Trondheim, Norway. She completed the Dartmouth Institute for Health Policy and Clinical Practice microsystem course and has served as a scholar with the National Public Health Leadership Institute. Dr. Harkless teaches clinical microsystem thinking and has presented and consulted internationally on this topic. In addition to her academic responsibilities, she continues to practice at Families First, a community health center and homeless program. She completed her bachelor of science degree in nursing (BSN) at Duke University, her master's of science degree in nursing (MSN) at Vanderbilt University, and her doctor of nursing science (DNSc) at Boston University.

CHAPTER 15

Clinical Microsystem Thinking and Resources for Advanced Practice Nursing

Gene Harkless, DNSc, FNP-C, CNL

CHAPTER OUTLINE

CLINICAL MICROSYSTEM THINKING

METHODS AND MEASUREMENTS IN IMPROVING THE WORK
  OF CLINICAL MICROSYSTEMS
    Assessment
    Establishing goals
    Implementing a change
    Measuring outcomes

CLINICAL MICRO-, MESO-, AND MACROSYSTEMS:
  IMPLICATIONS FOR APRN PRACTICE AND EDUCATION

SUMMARY

SUGGESTED LEARNING EXERCISES

CHAPTER OBJECTIVES

*After completing this chapter, the reader
will be able to:*

1. Summarize the characteristics of a
   clinical microsystem, mesosystem, and
   macrosystem.
2. Appraise the methods and
   measurements used to describe clinical
   microsystems for their usefulness in
   understanding clinical practice settings.
3. Analyze the reasons for using clinical
   microsystem thinking as an
   improvement process.
4. Apply basic principles of clinical
   microsystem thinking to a beginning
   analysis of quality improvement
   processes within one's practice setting.

In 1925, an article on the goal of nursing education stated that nursing needed to meet the challenge of rapid social and healthcare change:

> *There is a need . . . of a continual inflow of intelligent and broadly educated minds in order that . . . the new conditions, which a changing society is continually introducing, may be met with new courage and new methods.*[1]

Now, in the second decade of the 21st century, nursing continues to face the same challenges of rapid change. Much is already known about what can make health care better, including the use of best evidence, clinical knowledge, and knowledge of the design and delivery of quality service. However, as leaders, advanced practice registered nurses (APRNs) are often at a loss about how to achieve these best practices. We are uncertain whether a care team will successfully adapt a known, successful innovation and, more specifically, how each of us can get our teams to take a useful innovation and make it their own.[2]

Reconceptualizing our care teams as clinical microsystems may offer a path to achieving sustainable, tailored improvements aimed at providing the best care possible to those we serve. A healthcare clinical microsystem is defined as a small group of people who work together to provide care and the individuals who receive that care. This small team may interact regularly or on an as-needed basis, but, most importantly, their linked processes require shared information, are rooted in mutual clinical and professional aims, and are expected to achieve measurable outcomes for care and service. In this small system of care—a clinical microsystem—patients and providers meet, care outcomes are or are not achieved, risk occurs, and quality is created.[3]

Clinical microsystems are often embedded in larger systems, including both mesosystems and macrosystems. The macrosystem is easily understood as the larger organization in which the microsystem resides. The macrosystem is comprised of the organization's reimbursement, legal, policy, and regulatory environments. Leaders at the macrosystem level set the environment of the organization as one that makes possible, or diminishes, the work of the mesosystems and microsystems.[4] Leadership at the macrosystem level needs to focus on developing and supporting effective connections between and across microsystems. If macrosystems are to sustain this effort, strong mesosystems are essential. The mesosystem is the middle layer of the organization; it links macrosystem leadership with the frontline microsystems. The mesosystem can also be conceptualized as interrelated sets of "peer microsystems" that provide care to certain groups or support the care these groups receive. Clinical microsystems need to be connected, especially now as expanded interdisciplinary services, such as comprehensive diabetes care and integrated geriatric programs, are being redesigned and initiated. Interconnected and interacting microsystems become a mediating midlevel system—the mesosystem.[4]

The quality of care or care outcomes across all levels of the system can be no better than those achieved in the individual clinical microsystem. Small changes in a clinical microsystem can have large downstream effects and, most importantly, nurses and other healthcare workers can be the agents of change at the point of care. Clinical microsystem thinking and methods offer a practical and structured approach to improving quality, adding value, and reducing variation by enabling frontline caregivers to lead the process of change.[5]

Clinical Microsystem Thinking

The concept of the clinical microsystem captures a much richer description of the work and care environment than does the concept of the healthcare team. The healthcare team, viewed as individuals who work together to provide health care, is a necessary, but not sufficient, component of the clinical microsystem. The clinical microsystem includes clinical and business aims, linked processes, and a shared information environment. Its procedures, services, and care can be measured as performance outcomes. These systems evolve over time and are embedded in larger systems and organizations. Like other living and adaptive systems, the microsystem must do the work, meet staff needs, and maintain itself as a clinical unit.[5]

Clinical microsystem members include the patients and the providers, each of whom over time may have different roles, including that of patient, provider, learner, and teacher. Most importantly, the patient and patient population remain consistently at the center. In addition to the members of the clinical microsystem, the microsystem also includes the information and technology necessary to serve the common purposes of the clinical unit—improving outcomes for patients and populations, bettering the operating performance of the healthcare organization, and ensuring that the most competent and caring workforce continues to serve.[6] Functional and environmental attributes, such as offering hospitality, making good promises, seeking forgiveness, truth telling, and transparency, either support or discourage the work of the clinical microsystem. As the site of professional formation and development and the locus of client and employee satisfaction,[7] the clinical microsystem is both the agent of change and the target for improvement.

Batalden and Nelson attribute their initial idea of the clinical microsystem to Brian Quinn's book *Intelligent Enterprise*. Quinn studied outstanding service organizations and discovered that these organizations were focused on what happens to create value for the customer beginning from the first contact. This frontline interface was described by Quinn as the "smallest replicable unit."[5,7] From this first idea, the clinical microsystem approach has developed and matured.

Essential to any quality improvement effort is an understanding of how patients, clinicians, and other staff members interact and how the frontline processes of care work.[7] To better understand the way best-performing clinical microsystems work, Nelson, Batalden, and others[5] studied 20 organizations in North America, including inpatient units, ambulatory units, home health agencies, and nursing homes. The findings were published in a nine-part series in the *Joint Commission Journal on Quality Improvement* in 2003. (See complete series at http://dms.dartmouth.edu/cms/materials/publications/.) These high-quality clinical microsystems focused first and foremost on the patient and emphasized the importance of each worker in the microsystem. Excellent leadership was their hallmark, and the leaders, consistently working in nurse-physician or physician-administrator pairs, reinforced the importance of patient-centered care and the value of each staff member's contribution to care. The emphasis was on providing good care by studying the processes that determined the outcomes and then improving the outcomes. Lastly, each organization enabled innovation, the sharing of usable information, and effective communication among staff, patients, and families.[5,7]

The application of clinical microsystem thinking to clinical care began in the neonatal intensive care unit (NICU) at Dartmouth and has spread worldwide so that clinical microsystem thinking and methods are now used throughout the world. Jonkoping Health Care District in Sweden has embraced this work and has held microsystem festivals to spread the use of clinical microsystem methods in the region. In Britain, Williams and colleagues[8] evaluated the healthcare improvement claims made for clinical microsystems in the British healthcare system. They found that clinical microsystems resulted in higher staff morale, empowerment, commitment, and clarity of purpose but that they enhanced improvement and innovation only to a lesser degree. The authors conclude that more work needs to focus on patient involvement and process-outcome monitoring in order to cement the broader legitimacy of the clinical microsystem approach.

Methods and Measurements in Improving the Work of Clinical Microsystems

Based on their early work in the NICU and other settings, the Dartmouth clinical microsystem team developed, tested, and refined resource materials to help improve the work of clinical microsystems. Improvement processes account for and engage the mesosystem and macrosystem in which the microsystem is embedded. The Web site http://dms.dartmouth.edu/cms/ is the primary source for the resource materials described next. Also, an excellent textbook, *Quality by Design: A Clinical Microsystem Approach*,[9] provides a comprehensive guide to improvement work.

The improvement of clinical microsystems requires the team to focus on basics—to add value, to seek and use good science, to enable continual change, and to build community.[10,11] How to do this is based on a series of steps and processes mapped out in a series of resources available at http://dms.dartmouth.edu/cms/. The Dartmouth Microsystem Improvement Ramp is a visual representation of a systematic improvement process (Fig. 15-1). The journey begins with assessment.

Assessment

In the first step, members of a microsystem are asked to draw a picture of how the microsystem works from the patient's and/or the staff member's perspective. After doing this, the staff may recognize the foolishness of some of their work and take actions to reduce this foolishness. By doing this, they begin to see that microsystem change is possible and does not require permission. With this realization comes the question: Why are things the way they are? Thinking about this activates self-awareness and awareness of the system. Early investment in developing the microsystem team's understanding of themselves as a system uncovers more questions, which must be answered during the change process. This process, in turn, increases the team's curiosity about how to uncover hidden improvement measures.[12]

The next step in the improvement process is the assessment of the five essentials ("5Ps") of the microsystem (Box 15-1). Determining the *purpose* of the microsystem and its fit within the overall vision is the first essential. Next, the team identifies the *patients* or *people* served by the microsystem and the *professionals* who work together in the microsystem. Then, in a more challenging part of this assessment process, the caregiving and support *processes* the microsystem uses to provide care and services are mapped, and the *patterns* that characterize the microsystem functioning are recognized and described.

A detailed guide on completing this work, *Assessing Your Practice Workbook: "The Green Book,"* is found at http://dms.dartmouth.edu/cms/. From this assessment, a 5P Wall Model

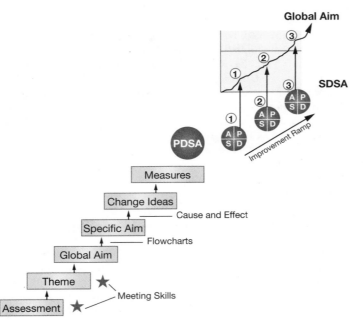

Figure 15-1: The Dartmouth Microsystem Improvement Ramp. *Reprinted with permission from Godfrey, M. (ed). (2009). Microsystem Cliff Notes. The Dartmouth Institute for Health Policy and Clinical Practice, p 7. Available at: http://dms.dartmouth.edu/cms/materials/workbooks/.*

BOX 15-1 | The 5P Wall Model Definitions and Template[16]

Purpose: To achieve the best possible outcomes for patients

Patients: Form different subpopulations such as postpartum patients, newborns, and antepartum patients

Patients interact with professionals.

Professionals: Advanced practice registered nurses (APRNs), registered nurses (RNs), licensed vocational nurses (LVNs) or licensed practical nurses (LPNs), physical therapists (PTs), occupational therapists (OTs), physicians, social workers, translators, lab technicians, etc.

Staff and patients work together to meet patients' needs by engaging in direct patient care processes.

Processes: Accessing systems and needs, diagnosing problems, creating treatment plans, and following up

The results of these interactions (patient to staff to clinical and support processes) produce patterns.

Patterns: Patterns measure safety, functional status, risk, patient satisfaction, and cost outcomes. Patterns of leadership, meetings to discuss care delivery, cultural and traditional patterns and symbols.

---

can be developed. (A blank, customizable 5P Wall Model is available at http://dms.dartmouth.edu/cms/materials/worksheets/.) See Figure 15-2.

From the 5Ps—purpose, patients, professionals, processes, and patterns—data flow charts representing different levels of detail can be constructed to map core processes and services. These flow charts can provide a rich, visual description of the work of the microsystem (Fig. 15-3).

For further study of the team's perceptions of the functioning of their microsystem, the Clinical Microsystem Assessment Tool is also available at http://dms.dartmouth.edu/cms/. This tool describes the characteristics of success found in the study of the 20 high-performing microsystems mentioned earlier and provides a definition of each success characteristic, with three descriptors covering low-functioning, mid-level-functioning, to high-performing behaviors. This tool can be used to identify the microsystem's areas of strength and weakness and present developmental opportunities that are critical for improvement.

Models developed through this process can be useful, but, as has been said, "all models are flawed, some are useful"[13] and "things should be made as simple as possible, but not any simpler."[14] Workbooks developed to structure the microsystem evaluation of inpatient units, emergency departments, outpatient primary care clinics, specialty clinics, and neonatal intensive care units are available at http://dms.dartmouth.edu/cms/materials/workbooks/.

Establishing Goals

At the next stage of clinical microsystem improvement work, assessment data are used to develop the microsystem's theme and aims or goals, both global and specific. The staff members need to gain a deeper understanding of their core processes. To effectively analyze and improve any core processes, the clinical microsystem method depends on engaging all staff members in creating and reviewing the steps at this stage. Current processes mapped out from the 5P assessment data are studied, subjected to brainstorming, and compared to benchmarks in order to develop ideas for change. Some ideas may be implemented immediately, while other ideas may require testing of the planned or proposed change. The exercise of developing fishbone diagrams, which graphically represent the factors that act as cause-and-effect

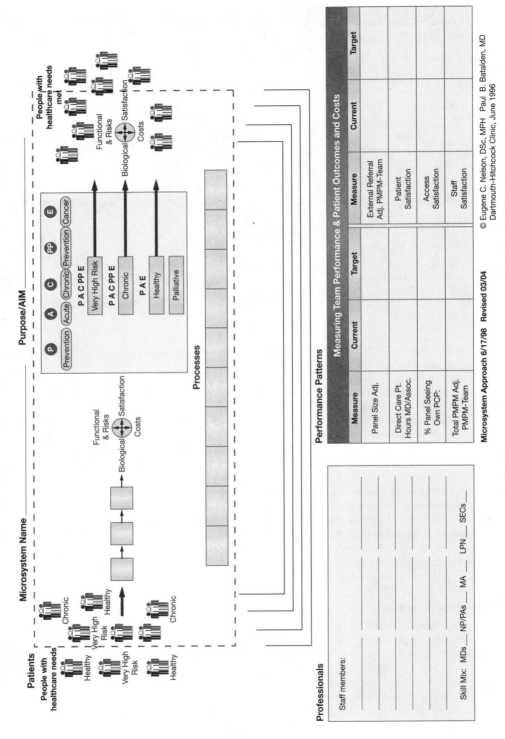

Figure 15-2: 5P Wall model. *Reprinted with permission from http://dms.dartmouth.edu/cms/materials/worksheets/*

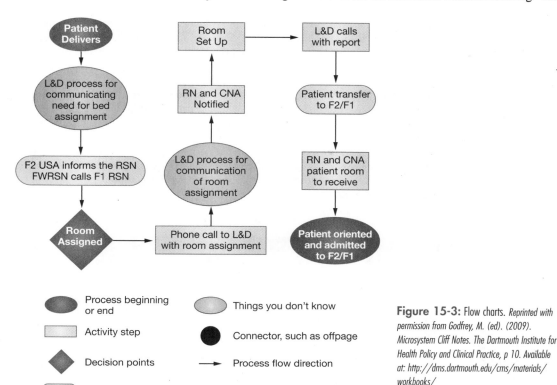

Figure 15-3: Flow charts. *Reprinted with permission from Godfrey, M. (ed). (2009). Microsystem Cliff Notes. The Dartmouth Institute for Health Policy and Clinical Practice, p 10. Available at: http://dms.dartmouth.edu/cms/materials/ workbooks/*

drivers influencing the desired result, can help identify the issue for a plan-do-study-act–standardize-do-study-act cycle (PDSA–SDSA). Next, the team members select one change to test by initiating the PDSA–SDSA process.

Implementing a Change

After the change is selected, a rapid test is conducted and, depending on the results, the process is revised or a new process is implemented. These efforts should be captured in a playbook, which is a collection of tested "best practices," or "plays," that are useful for sustaining improvement efforts, including finalized flow charts, audit tools, and a schedule of ongoing review. Useful survey tools and satisfaction measures for this effort are available at http://dms.dartmouth.edu/cms/materials/workbooks/ with helpful tutorials on interpreting these measures.

Measuring Outcomes

Integral to gaining important knowledge from the PDSA–SDSA is the ability to measure what is being done. And, it is important to know whether a change in a measure is an actual improvement. Visual displays, using a variety of charts, can help with this process by graphically representing data.[15] Specifically, run and control charts can help differentiate between common-cause variation and special-cause variation. Knowing if variation is due to a large number of small sources of variation or to special circumstances is important when directing efforts to improve on the improvement.[16]

The summary of these efforts may be a balanced scorecard depiction of the microsystem's current state of performance. Developed by Kaplan and Norton,[17] the balanced scorecard provides a graphical representation of strategic growth, core processes, customer viewpoint, and financial results. For measures, strategy, vision, and improvement initiatives can be linked with objectives and target values. Balanced scorecards provide a succinct method to communicate results and demonstrate accountability.[18] Figure 15-4 is an example of a balanced scorecard describing a neonatal intensive care unit. The scorecard describes the aim, measures, and action plans of key clinical processes balanced against the aim, measures, and action plans for financial performance; it also balances the aim, measures, and action plans for learning and growth against the aim, measures, and action plans for customer satisfaction.[19]

To reiterate, data are essential to any improvement process, and an important rule is to always measure what you value and value what you measure.[3] When beginning the outcome measurement process, keep measurements simple, be clear, and have consensus on the operational definitions. Both qualitative and quantitative data are useful. Perfection is not necessary, but the measures must be useful. To sustain the improvement work, measurement should be built into the team's daily work and job descriptions. If sampling is necessary, small, representative samples can be used. Overall, having a balance of measures is necessary. The data should capture input, process, outcomes, and cost.

Key Processes		
Aim:	**Culture of Safety: Safe/Timely/Effective/Efficient/Equitable/Patient and Family Centered**	
Measure:	1. Establish Quality & Safety Council w/regular meetings	1. Established January 2007; meeting weekly
	2. Culture of Safety Survey—share results and develop action plan	2. In process
	3. Review UOR's monthly; follow-up with actions	3. Monthly reviews; forwarding issues and concerns to appropriate persons or groups to follow-up
	4. Reviewing "Suggestion Box" concerns	4. Create a template for feedback to those who submit suggestions/concerns
	5. Review JCAHO preparedness	5. Establish report for JCAHO readiness
	6. Review Emergency Preparedness plans	6. Review/revise and update current plan
Action Plan:	See #4, #5, #6	

Learning and Growth		
Aim:	**Implement/Continue Best Practices Measure**	
Measure:	1. Establish Kangaroo Mother Care Program	
	2. Transition Feeding Protocol	
	3. O_2 Sat monitoring feedback to staff	
	4. Staffing	
	• Nurses from system partner in Oregon	
	• Tracking Chg RN w/o assignment	
	• Tracking surgery days/off unit procedures	
	• Participation in LIC	
	5. Nurse Extern/Intern/Fellowship Programs	
	6. Developed Foundation/Funding for staff to attend education/conferences	
Action Plan:		

Customer Satisfaction	
Aim:	**Patient/Employee/Physician Satisfaction: Likelihood of Recommending Providence to Others:**
Measure:	HYB.com for NICU specific results Kenexa Employee Opinion Survey
	Would you recommend this hospital to other patients – % answering "Yes"
	100 90 97 94 98 98 93 98 98 98 97 97 99 95 96 94 80 70 60 50
	Q1 Q2 Q3 Q4 Q1 Q2 Q3 Q4 Q1 Q2 Q3 Q4 Q1 Q2 Q3 03 03 03 03 04 04 04 04 05 05 05 05 06 06 06
Action Plan:	Improve scores/develop follow-up D/C phone calls

Financial Performance		
Aim:	**Achievement of NICU Net Operating Income as budgeted for 2007—roll up to PAMC**	
Measure:	1. Patient days/volumes	4. Labor costs
	2. Revenue	5. Transfers
	3. Costs/stat (UOS)	6. LOS
Action Plan:	1. Review of financial performance monthly with NICU Finance Management meeting (4th Wed). Includes supervisors, lead RT, educator, and ACNE for the Children's Hospital.	
	2. Inventory and accounting review (supervisors/manager)	
	3. Labor cost /productivity review bi-weekly with ACNE (Monthly with supervisors)	

Figure 15-4: Balanced Scorecard from a Neonatal Intensive Care Unit.[19] *Reprinted with permission. Available at:* http://dms.dartmouth.edu/cms/materials/worksheets/. See Balanced Scorecard.

Most importantly, key measures should be displayed so that staff can be aware of trends over time. This visual display, otherwise known as a data wall, or dashboard, is a mix of microsystem performance measures, along with mesosystem and macrosystem measures. Progress toward improvement goals is highlighted through this display, and improvement ideas and actions can be reinforced as well as generated. Figure 15-5 is a template that can be used to develop a data wall poster.[19]

Clinical Micro-, Meso-, and Macrosystems: Implications for APRN Practice and Education

Moving throughout the microsystem, mesosystem, and macrosystem, advanced practice registered nurses (APRNs) participate in the broader organization of healthcare institutions. Wider system responsibility, beyond the direct care level of the clinical microsystem, is expected, particularly at the Doctor of Nursing Practice (DNP) level. DNP graduates must assume organizational and systems leadership in order to improve patient and healthcare outcomes. Leading requires effective communication, and communication among and within the organization's systems is essential to any quality improvement efforts. This was one of the findings of studies of two different hospitals that shared their experiences with their quality improvement journey.[20] One hospital was a small rural facility, the other a large tertiary

SAMPLE POSTER: Microsystem Path Forward		
Names of Team Members:	**Practice Name Here** **Improvement Theme: Access and Efficiency** **Time Frame: April – November 2007**	**PICTURE OF TEAM** or other practice photo optional
Insert Fishbone(s):	**Global Aim:** Reduce handoffs, waits and delays in core processes. Starts when patient calls for appointment and ends when patient leaves office visit. We expect to improve access to appointment, reduce cycle time, optimize roles, and improve patient and team satisfaction **Specific Aims:** • Reduce 3rd available appointment for physical exam or long appointment type from 23 days to 0 days in 6 months	4 PDSA Ramps annotated with specific change ideas of identify change ideas tested for each PDSA
Insert Flowcharts: before and after changes	• Reduce cycle time from 60 min to 25 min for a 15 min appointment in 2 months. • Reduce # of phone calls for prescription refills and internal processing time by 50% in 3 months • Reduce # of no shows by 50% in one month	Key Lessons from PDSAs and Data Sample • Patient reminder calls result in significant rebooking • Morning huddles take too long using EHR for today's data needs • Reducing backlog for diabetics by lengthening revisit requires a follow-up phone call
	Measures and Results:	• Significant number of patients choose not to complete previsit card • Patients do not know that their appointment time is 15 minutes with physician
Bullet Summary of opportunities for achieving aims based on microsystem data, fishbones, current state flow charts Sample • Revisit interval for diabetes can be lengthened - no clinical bias for current standard	**Annotated Run Charts:**	**3 SDSAs** List standards in Play Book

Figure 15-5: Poster Template for Data Wall *Reprinted with permission. Available at: http://dms.dartmouth.edu/cms/materials/worksheets/. See Poster/Storyboard Template.*

organization. These hospitals described in detail the actions and activities that need to happen at the various levels and intersections of the microsystem, mesosystem, and macrosystem for transformational change to occur. These intersections of the micro-, meso-, and macrosystems are the locations of advanced practice nursing work.

APRNs need to know not only what must be accomplished but also how to accomplish it and how to coach others to do the same.[21] Developing human capability and capacity to meet these challenges may require redesigning human resource systems to integrate new values into recruitment and retention. Essential values include system-wide support for protected time to reflect and learn. Table 15-1 provides a framework for thinking about the work of leaders across the microsystem, mesosystem, and macrosystems of health care and may provide direction for nursing education and professional development.

Table 15-1 **Some Questions to Consider for Leaders at All Levels**

Macrosystem Leader	Mesosystem Leader	Microsystem Leader
• How does this work bring help/value to the patients? What stories illustrate that?	• How do the "organization's messages" move?	• How does this microsystem work? Who does what to whom? What technology is part of what you regularly do?
• What are the values that are part of the everyday work?	• How does the "macro" strategy connect to the microsystems? What helps adapt, respond to it?	• What is the main or core process of the way work gets done here? How does it vary?
• What helps people grow, develop, and become better professionals here?	• What are the microsystems doing about	• What are some of the limitations you encounter as you try to do what you do for patients?
• What helps people personally engage the never-ending safeguarding and improving of patient care?	• Muda—wasted activity • Mura—irregular work flow • Muri—stress, overwork	• When you want to change the clinical care because of some new knowledge, how does that work?
• What connects this whole place—from the patient and those working directly with the patient down to the leaders of the organization?	• How do the microsystems link strategy, operations, and people needed for successful execution?	• What are the helpful measures you regularly use here? How are those measures analyzed and displayed?
• What helps the processes of inquiry, learning, and change within, between, and across microsystems and mesosystems?	• What are the helpful cultural supports for measurably improving the quality, reliability, and value of care in the microsystem(s)?	• What are the things people honor as "traditions" around here? If you had to single out a few things that really contribute to and "mark" the identity of this clinical microsystem, what might you point to?
• What helps people do their own work and improve patient outcomes—year after year?	• What are the cultural changes required to measurably improve the quality, reliability, and value of care at the frontlines?	

Table 15-1 **Some Questions to Consider for Leaders at All Levels — cont'd**

Macrosystem Leader	Mesosystem Leader	Microsystem Leader
• What might be possible? What are some of the current limits we face?	• What is the process for identifying, orienting the microsystem leaders . . . for helping set their expectations . . . for reviewing their performance and for holding the clinical microsystem accountable for its performance?	• What do people ask questions about around here? Who asks? Who gets asked?
• What are some of the most relevant external forces for this micro-, meso-, macrosystem?		• What does it take to make things happen around here? When did it work well? Who did what?
• Do you have the measurements and feedback necessary to make it easy for you to monitor and improve the quality of your performance?	• What about my own style of work speaks more convincingly than my words about the desired "way" of work?	• How does information and information technology get integrated into the daily work and new initiatives around here?
• Are you treated with dignity and respect every day by everyone you encounter, without any regard for hierarchy?	• What helps maintain a steadfast focus on improved patient care outcomes by more reliable and more efficient systems that are regularly reflected on and redesigned?	• When you add new people here, how do you go about it?
• Are you given the opportunity and tools that you need to make a contribution that gives meaning to your life?		• How are things "noticed" around here?
• Does someone notice when you've done the job you do?		• If you to point to an example of "respect" among yourselves here, what might you point to?
• As you think about what you do and your ability to change it, what gains have been made, as you think about now in comparison with the past?		• How do the leaders get involved in change here?
• How do you actually do what you do? What changes have you been able to make? What changes are you working on now?		• How are patients brought into the daily workings and improvement of the clinical microsystem?
• What changes that you've tried haven't worked?		• Do people have a good idea of each others' work? How is that brought about?
• Do people feel compelled to regularly justify or rationalize things that happen around here?		• Do you discuss the common patterns of the way you work? And the ways you test changes in them?

Reprinted with permission. Available at: dms.dartmouth.edu/cms/materials/curriculum/

Addressing the increasingly complex nature of health care, the second generation of work on clinical microsystems focuses on the efforts or interactions between and among microsystems.[6,22] These interactions include hand-offs and transitions between microsystems and require mesosystems that support and protect patients and families throughout their healthcare experience. Microsystems working in synchrony can create a positive care experience, but the converse can also be true. Therefore, the mesosystem should be the place of safety and reliability where effective collaboration has generated clear goals. However, Godfrey[22] believes that current organizational infrastructures lack effective alignment between multiple microsystems and the mesosystem, have not optimized the microsystems, and have not identified outcome measures that link the macro-, meso-, and microsystems. Leaders who work together and value patient-centeredness over competition are needed for this new model of care delivery.[22]

To be more effective, nurse leaders can attend to commonly occurring needs within and across systems (Table 15-2). These needs determine the knowledge and skills important to APRNs as leaders within and among systems. Although the list of helpful knowledge and skills in Table 15-2 is short, the learning challenges are formidable. As nurses, APRNs can draw on their historic social mandate and disciplinary focus to attend to the illness experience and cooperate across professional boundaries to meet patient needs. In addition, APRNs need to develop expertise in the Nightingale tradition of measuring and analyzing variation in the daily healthcare process. In addition, APRNs need to master the process of change and lead in the design, implementation, and evaluation of change. Finally, practice evidence needs to inform, as well as be informed by, local processes and systems outcomes.

Learning how to do the work of healthcare systems improvement is believed to be optimal when health professionals, support staff, patients, and families share learning experiences that challenge them to design high-quality and high-value health care. The studio course method is used by the Dartmouth team to engage this learning.[23] A studio course sets up a

---

Table 15-2 Needs and Skills for Successful Microsystems[4]

Needs of Micro-, Meso-, and Macrosystems	Helpful Knowledge and Skills
Develop a vision for the desired microsystem and mesosystem future.	Develop knowledge of health care as a system and process.
Identify resource allocation strategies that address the functioning of the clinical microsystem and the optimal functioning of the whole mesosystem and macrosystem.	Attract cooperation across health professional disciplinary traditions.
Connect the desired future to current reality.	Understand patient needs and illness burdens.
Advocate for the microsystem within the macrosystem.	Plan and work in a socially accountable way.
Clarify implications of change(s).	Measure, display, and analyze variation in the daily process of health care.
Develop measures of clinical microsystem performance.	Design and test change.
Generate ideas and options.	
Identify microsystem staffing and professional development needs.	
Design and conduct pilot tests of change.	
Integrate the professional education function with daily patient care realities.	
Balance local innovation, creativity, and the needs of the whole organization.	
Receive and process complaints.	
Standardize the work and work flow appropriately.	
Execute plans.	
Respond to signals that "all is not well."	

situational challenge that engages the learner's creativity, provides an informal place of learning where participants interact with other students and faculty, and encourages open and honest critique of one's work by peers and faculty. Blueprints and models that graphically illustrate ideas are used to stimulate and represent the learner's efforts to design and innovate. These activities draw on the learner's insights, reflections, past and present learning, creativity, and intelligence.[24]

The studio course format engages the participants in the process of improving microsystems as a learning experience, with an emphasis on reflection and critique. Advanced nursing education can integrate clinical microsystem work into the curriculum by using teaching/learning strategies like the studio course format. Students would then be expected to do real improvement work, openly communicate in the teaching/learning experience, provide honest critiques, and develop skill in graphical representation of design and innovation ideas. This type of learning experience is essential in preparing the next generation of APRNs to be effective leaders and participants in real healthcare improvement and innovation.

Summary

Clinical microsystem thinking and methods offer an opportunity to engage in critical improvement work effectively through a reasoned and insightful process. This chapter provided a brief overview of clinical microsystem thinking; introduced key methods, measurements, and resources for clinical microsystem assessment; and examined implications of clinical microsystem thinking on the clinical practice and education of APRNs. Overall, a clinical microsystem approach can help APRNs learn to identify the needs of the frontline practice and the people they serve and enable frontline staff to improve their work continually and to leverage all the systems of the organization—microsystems, mesosystems, and macrosystems—to provide the best care possible.

SUGGESTED LEARNING EXERCISES

1. Consider the organization in which you work, and describe three characteristics of your clinical microsystem, mesosystem, and macrosystem. Analyze how these characteristics either enhance or hinder the interactions of these systems and either improve or constrain the work outcomes of the organization.

2. Go to http://dms.dartmouth.edu/cms/materials/workbooks/ and select a Greenbook of interest to you. Compare what you and your organization already understand and share openly about your clinical microsystem with what is suggested in the 5Ps assessment process. Analyze why this is so.

3. Reflect on past improvement processes you have experienced professionally or personally. Compare and contrast those processes with the clinical microsystem approach to improvement.

References

1. Logan, LR. (1925). The goal of nursing education. *Am J Nurs* 25(7):539–544.

2. Schlosser, J. (2003). Commentary on primary health care teams: opportunities and challenges in evaluation of service delivery innovations. *J Ambulat Care Manage* 26(1):3p.

3. Godfrey, M. (2004). *Clinical Microsystem Action Guide: Improving Health Care By Improving Your Microsystem*. Trustees of Dartmouth College.

4. Batalden, P, Nelson, E, Gardent, P, and Godfrey, M. (2007). Leading macrosystems and mesosystems for microsystem peak performance. In Nelson, E, Batalden, P, and Godfrey, M (eds), *Quality by Design: A Clinical Microsystem Approach*. Jossey-Bass, San Francisco, pp 69–105.

5. Nelson, EC, et al. (2002). Microsystems in health care: Part 1. Learning from high-performing front-line clinical units. *Jt Comm J Qual Improv* 28(9):472–493.

6. Nelson, EC, et al. (2008). Clinical microsystems, Part 1. The building blocks of health systems. *Jt Comm J Qual Patient Saf* 34(7):367–378.

7. McInnis, D. (2006, summer). What system? *Dartmouth Medicine* 28–35.

8. Williams, L, Dickinson, H, Robinson, S, and Allen, C. (2009). Clinical microsystems and the NHS: a sustainable method for improvement? *J Health Organiz and Manage* 23(1):119–132.

9. Nelson, EC, Batalden, PB, and Godfrey, MM. (2007). *Quality by Design: A Clinical Microsystems Approach*. Jossey-Bass, San Francisco, pp xliv, 459.

10. Nelson, E, Batalden, P, Huber, T, Johnson, J, Godfrey, M, Headrick, L, and Wasson, J. (2007). Success characteristics of high-performing microsystems: learning from the best. In Nelson, E, Batalden, P, & Godfrey, P. (eds), *Quailty by Design: A Clinical Microsystem Approach*. Jossey-Bass, San Francisco, pp 3–33.

11. Batalden, P. Knowing, recognizing, and acting as a health care leader at a time like this . . . (2009). dms.dartmouth.edu.

12. Batalden, PB, and Stoltz, PK. (1993). A framework for the continual improvement of health care: building and applying professional and improvement knowledge to test changes in daily work. *Jt Comm J Qual Improv* 19(10):424–447; discussion 448–452.

13. Box, G. (n.d.). Collected Wisdom. http://campus.udayton.edu/~physics/blb/wisdom.htm. Accessed May 18, 2009.

14. Einstein, A. (n.d.). Albert Einstein Quotes. Available at: http://www.brainyquote.com/quotes/authors/a/albert_einstein.html.

15. Godfrey, M (ed). (2009). *Microsystem Cliff Notes*. The Dartmouth Institute for Health Policy and Clinical Practice, Lebanon, NH.

16. Godfrey, M (ed). (2009). *Clinical Microsystem Action Guide. Improving Health Care by Improving Your Microsystem*. Version 2: Rev 4/13/2004, 2004 ed. Trustees of Dartmouth College.

17. Kaplan, R, and Norton, R. (1996). *The Balanced Scorecard: Translating Strategy Into Action*. Harvard Business Press, Boston.

18. Nelson, C, Batalden, P, Homa, K, Godfrey, M, Campbell, C, Headrick, L, Huber, T, Johnson, J, and Wasson, J. (2007). Creating a rich information environment. In Nelson, C, Batalden, P, and Godrey, M (eds), *Quality by Design: A Clinical Microsystem Approach*. Jossey-Bass, San Francisco, pp 178–196.

19. The Dartmouth Institute of Health Policy and Clinical Practice. (n.d.). *Clinical Microsystems Worksheets*. Available at: http://dms.dartmouth.edu/cms/materials/worksheets/.

20. Godfrey, M, et al. (2008). Clinical microsystems. Part 3. Transformation of two hospitals using microsystem, mesosystem, and macrosystem strategies. *Jt Comm J Qual Patient Saf* 34:591–603.

21. McKinley, KE, et al. (2008). Clinical microsystems. Part 4. Building innovative population-specific mesosystems. *Jt Comm J Qual Patient Saf* 34:655–663.

22. Nordin, A. (2009). *4 quick questions to . . . Marjorie Godfrey, adjunct instructor at the Center for the Evaluative Clinical Sciences at Dartmouth and Director for the Clinical Microsystem Resource Group.*

23. Nelson E, Batalden, P, and Godfrey, M (eds). (2007). Overview of path forward and introduction to part two. In Nelson, C, Batalden, P, and Godfrey, P (eds), *Quality By Design: A Clinical Microsystem Approach*. Jossey-Bass, San Francisco, pp 199–229.

24. Nelson, E, Batalden, P, Edwards, W, Godfrey, M, and Johson, J. (2007). Developing high-performing microsystems. In Neslon, E, Batalden, P, and Godfrey, M (eds), *Quality by Design: A Clinical Microsystem Approach*. Jossey-Bass, San Francisco, pp 34–50.

Jean Johnson is the senior associate dean for health sciences and a professor in the Department of Nursing at The George Washington University in Washington, DC. She has represented the perspective of an advanced practice registered nurse (APRN) on many national committees, including the Pew Health Professions Commission, the Institute of Medicine Future of Primary Care, and Public Advisory Board for the American Academy of Family Physicians. She has served as president of the National Organization of Nurse Practitioner Faculties (NONPF) and the American College of Nurse Practitioners (ACNP). She was the national program director of the Robert Wood Johnson Foundation's Partnership for Training Program to develop interdisciplinary education in primary care for people living in underserved areas. In addition, she facilitated the national work to develop the Consensus Model for Advanced Practice Registered Nurse Regulation. In 2009, she received the Lifetime Achievement Award from NONPF and the Associate Lifetime Membership award from the American Association of Colleges of Nursing (AACN).

Joan Stanley has served as director of education policy at the American Association of Colleges of Nursing (AACN) since 1994. In that position, she has been a member of many of the association's task forces and committees, including the Task Forces on the Essentials of Master's Education, the Doctor of Nursing Practice, the Future of the Research-Focused Doctorate, Essentials of Baccalaureate Education for Professional Nursing Practice, and the Clinical Nurse Leader (CNL) Steering Committee. She recently led the national project to develop consensus-based competencies for the adult-gerontology nurse practitioner and clinical nurse specialist. In addition, she has served as the association's representative to the national APRN Consensus Process Work and Joint Dialogue Groups, which crafted the *Consensus Model for APRN Regulation: Licensure, Accreditation, Certification and Education*. In addition, she has participated in numerous advanced practice nursing projects, including the American Nurses Association's Task Force on the Scope and Standards for Advanced Practice Nursing, The National Council of State Boards of Nursing' Advisory Committee for the Family Nurse Practitioner Pharmacology Curriculum Project, and the first, second, and third National Task Forces that developed the Criteria for Evaluation of Nurse Practitioner Programs. She also maintains a practice as an adult nurse practitioner at the University of Maryland Health System Faculty Practice Office. Before joining the AACN, Dr. Stanley was assistant professor at the School of Nursing at the University of Maryland and associate director of primary care nursing services at the University of Maryland Hospital. Dr. Stanley received her bachelor's of science degree in nursing from Duke University and her master's of science in nursing and her doctorate in higher education organization and policy from the University of Maryland.

CHAPTER 16

The Future of APRN Practice and the Impact of Current Healthcare Trends

Jean Johnson, PhD, RN, FAAN; Joan Stanley, PhD, RN, CRNP, FAAN

CHAPTER OBJECTIVES

After completing this chapter, the reader will be able to:

1. Analyze the influence of current healthcare trends on APRN practice and their possible impact on future APRN practice.
2. Analyze the potential impact of the Advanced Practice Registered Nurse Regulatory Model on APRN practice, education, certification, and licensure.

Trying to predict the future is a risky business. The healthcare environment has been in a dynamic state of change for decades amid growing concerns about the ever-rising costs of health care, the need for a strengthened primary care system, and growing numbers of uninsured. Each of these issues presents opportunities and responsibilities to APRNs. How APRN practice will be influenced by these factors will largely depend on the balance of forces that seek to limit the practice of APRNs with those that support the full scope of APRN practice. This chapter looks at the trends noted and explores their impact on APRN practice. In addition, it explores the impact of the Consensus Model for Advanced Practice Registered Nurse Regulation on APRN practice.

Emphasis on Cost Containment

All sectors of society are concerned about the cost of health care. These costs have risen faster than the general inflation of the overall economy. Health care in the United States is excellent in many ways, but its high cost has not translated into the best health outcomes.[1,2,3] Although healthcare cost inflation decreased from 9.6% in 2006 to 7.4% in 2009, it remains generally two to three times higher than the inflation rate for the overall economy.[4,5] The United States spent $2.3 trillion on health care in 2008; spending projections are $3.1 trillion in 2012 and $4.3 trillion by 2016.[6] It is anticipated that health care will consume 20% of the gross domestic product (GDP), a measure of the size of our economy, by 2020. This compares to health care being 5.2% of GDP in 1960, 9.1% in 1980, and 13.8% in 2000.[7]

An outcome or benefit of the current concerns over rising healthcare costs should be the perception that APRNs provide an option as cost-effective providers. Yet nurse practitioners (NPs) and other APRNs must continue to position themselves for and be prepared to accept this opportunity. Although APRNs as a group will not fix the problem of rising healthcare costs, they can provide a significant contribution to cost savings. NPs can address the majority of primary care health problems and provide the same or better quality of care while generally earning a lower salary than a physician. The data supporting this notion have been consistent over several decades.[8-13] The average salary of a family physician in 2008 was approximately $161,000 before taxes.[14] The average base salary for full-time NPs was $81,060 in their main practice setting, with an average total income of $87,400.[15]

Expanded APRN Practice Opportunities

A cost-effective approach to health care is a collaborative or team approach in which physicians and APRNs organize the practice in a way that each provider's skills are used to their full extent and match the needs of the patients served. Establishing practices in which physicians see more complicated or diagnostically challenging patients and APRNs manage the less complicated patients in addition to providing health promotion and clinical prevention services for all patients is one strategy that addresses cost issues. However, this approach will require states to recognize the full scope of practice for NPs and other APRNs and to recognize autonomous APRN practice.

A second way APRNs can make a significant impact on healthcare costs is to focus on chronic disease management and end-of-life care. Heart disease, stroke, diabetes, and cancer account for the majority of chronic illness in this country. Chronic diseases contribute to 75% of current healthcare costs and many of these illnesses are preventable. As the population ages, there will be an even greater need to address problems of chronic illness. The Centers for Disease Control and Prevention (CDC) has noted the following statistics related to disease prevention:

- Implementing proven clinical smoking-cessation interventions would cost an estimated $2587 for each year of life saved, the most cost-effective of all clinical preventative services.
- For each $1 spent on the Safer Choice Program, a school-based program focused on preventing HIV and other sexually transmitted diseases (STDs) and on preventing pregnancy, about $2.65 is saved on medical and social costs.

- Every $1 spent on preconception care programs for women with diabetes can reduce health costs by up to $5.19 by preventing costly complications in both mothers and babies.
- Implementing the Arthritis Self-Help Course for 10,000 individuals with arthritis will yield a net savings of more than $2.5 million while simultaneously reducing pain by 18% among the participants.[7]

These are only a few of the many examples of cost savings and improved outcomes that could be realized if APRNs and other registered nurses (RNs) took a greater role in disease prevention and chronic illness management. If APRNs position themselves to do this, as well as to take on a major role in the delivery of primary care services, the contribution to cost savings and the increased utilization of APRNs within the healthcare system could be significant. But achieving this status will require unified and continued political and policy activity by all APRNs, particularly in light of the ongoing efforts by some organized medicine groups to limit and control NP and other APRN practice.

Implementation of Electronic Health Records

Two other factors that will impact APRN practice are the widespread implementation of electronic health records (EHRs) and the emphasis on quality improvement and patient safety. These two factors are inextricably linked.

EHRs are essential to improving care because they facilitate the continued development and monitoring of quality measures. The EHR also provides practitioners and patients with alerts and reminders designed to improve continuity of care and decrease errors. The use of point-of-care technology and the EHR also provides access to references and evidence-based guidelines that provide on-the-spot information for patient care decisions. It is estimated that a 90% EHR implementation rate would save $77 billion a year in healthcare costs.[16,17] In 2005, 17.1% of medical practices used an EHR system, but by 2008, this had increased to 40% to 50% of family physician practices.[18,19] In addition, the Obama administration has made it a priority to implement EHR in 100% of all healthcare practices by 2014.[20]

APRNs will need to integrate EHRs into their practices whether they are in a group practice or solo practice. Funding through the American Recovery and Reinvestment Act (ARRA) provides financial incentives to providers who are "meaningful users." The Centers for Medicare and Medicaid (CMS) defines meaningful use as use of a certified EHR, the electronic exchange of health information to improve the quality of health care, and reporting on clinical quality and other measures using certified EHR technology.[21] The push for EHR use will be bolstered by significant federal funding through the ARRA. Payment is scheduled to begin in 2011 and the target is to have the EHR fully implemented nationally by 2014. Efforts to move this agenda forward will be overseen by the Office of the National Coordinator for Health Information Technology (HIT).

Increased Emphasis on Quality Improvement

APRNs have been involved in quality improvement at the point of care or direct care level for decades. However, now more than ever, APRNs need to take a proactive stance in the quality arena and become knowledgeable about the development of quality measures and the monitoring and analysis of outcomes. APRNs should be on EHR implementation committees as well as quality improvement committees in all practice settings. They should push their professional organizations to participate in the newly developing Nursing Quality and Safety Alliance, which will represent nursing in the formulation of policy related to quality.

Payment, particularly Medicare and Medicaid payments, has been linked to performance on quality measures in hospitals and outpatient practices. This trend will continue to grow. The CMS has considered expanding the number of "never pay" inpatient events—those for which it will not fully reimburse hospitals—from the current 11 occurrences, implemented in 2008, to as many as 73 events, many of which are directly attributable to or preventable by the level of nursing care. APRNs need to be well versed and participate in the decisions that are being made by CMS and other payers.

Increased Need for Primary Care Services

Combining with the APRN's ability to contribute to healthcare cost savings is the need for an increased number of primary care providers, specifically NPs and certified nurse-midwives (CNMs). A strong primary care system has been a hallmark of nations that have lower healthcare costs and better health outcomes. In the current payment system, physicians in specialties other than primary care have a higher financial reward; therefore, physicians have gravitated toward medical specialties other than primary care.[22] Recently U.S. medical school graduates have been filling only about one-half of family medicine residencies in the United States; the rest of the residencies are going to international medical graduates (IMGs).[23] As a result, approximately 25% of primary care physicians are IMGs. This continued decline in interest in primary care in this country is occurring at the same time that the American Academy of Family Medicine (AAFM) has estimated an increase in the need for family physicians at 39% to meet the primary care needs of the country.

The roots of the NP role in primary care go back to the 1960s and 1970s when there was a shortage of primary care providers and NPs were seen as a means of expanding and enhancing primary care services. Although some physician groups have worked to contain the practice of NPs, the American College of Physicians (ACP) has now recognized that they can play a major role in providing primary care. The ACP 2009 report states, "The College recognizes the important role that nurse practitioners play in meeting the current and growing demand for primary care" (p. 1).[24] But even though the report supports NP practice and is a major step for the ACP, the support is qualified by its statement that NPs should be supervised by physicians.

The declining interest in primary care among medical school graduates and the increased need for primary care has created a crucial gap that NPs and CNMs can fill. As with healthcare costs, the ability of this country's healthcare system to fully realize the benefit of APRNs to primary care will depend on states, institutions, and payers recognizing the full scope of APRN practice.

The alignment of the increasing need for primary care services, the skills that NPs and CNMs bring to primary care, and the recognition by key physician groups will likely support the continued growth of APRNs in primary care. In addition, the doctor of nursing practice (DNP) degree is becoming the entry-level education requirement for all advanced nursing practice. The degree provides the additional knowledge and skills that NPs and other APRNs need to assume leadership roles in many aspects of primary care, including quality improvement, policy development, outcome evaluation, and chronic care management. This additional educational preparation will be important to the success of NPs and others in responding to the call for increased numbers of primary care providers and in developing innovative strategies for improved quality and safety within a complex healthcare system.

Growing Numbers of Uninsured and Underinsured

The percentage of the population that is uninsured or underinsured has grown during the most recent economic crisis. However, for a developed country, the United States has had a relatively high percentage of uninsured even in good economic times. Even those with health insurance have postponed care because of high deductibles and co-payments. Middle-class Americans have primarily received health insurance through their jobs, but they have experienced significant erosion of healthcare benefits accompanied by increased out-of-pocket costs for premiums and deductibles.[25,26] The recent financial crisis has created the "perfect storm" in that more people are uninsured or underinsured, and the agencies that have traditionally provided services to vulnerable populations have less government support because of decreased tax revenues.

NPs, since their early beginnings in 1965, have played a critical role in caring for vulnerable populations and in improving access to care, particularly in rural communities,[27] a tradition that has remained strong across the entire APRN community. With growing numbers of uninsured and underinsured, the demand for basic primary care services and other healthcare services in which the costs are reasonable and predictable will increase. The expansion of retail clinics provides such an option to consumers; they can see an NP or physician assistant (PA) and know up front the cost of the services, many of which often do not meet the insurance requirements for deductibles. Although some primary care physicians have expressed concern that the retail clinic model will discourage people from seeing their primary care providers,[28] recent findings suggest that consumers go to retail clinics for problems that they do not generally take to a primary care physician or emergency department.[29] The retail clinic is one example of a cost-effective, accessible care model that will likely continue to evolve, with APRNs being the primary providers of care. The expectation is that the number of clinics and therefore opportunities for NPs will continue to grow.

Implementation of the APRN Regulatory Model

By 2015, the target date for full implementation of the Consensus Model for APRN Regulation, the major elements of the regulatory system—licensing, accreditation, certification, and education—will be aligned.[30] The model is intended to create a better interface among these four regulatory entities; it will also have important impacts on clinical practice. One of the most significant will be the specification that all APRNs will be licensed as *independent* practitioners for practice in one of four APRN roles—certified nurse practitioner (CNP), CNM, clinical nurse specialist (CNS), or certified registered nurse anesthetist (CRNA)—within at least one of six identified population foci: family/individual across the life span, adult-gerontology, pediatrics, neonatal, women's health/gender-related, or psychiatric/mental health.

A second significant impact of the model will be to increase the number of NPs and CNSs with the knowledge and skills to care for our growing aging population. Although combining the adult and gerontology population foci initially created concern among gerontology NPs and CNSs, it was agreed that there simply would not be enough gerontology NPs or CNSs (or physicians). Existing adult and gerontology programs will be merged to encompass an adult-gerontology population focus. Education comparable to that in the current gerontology programs will need to be incorporated into all adult NP and CNS programs, and adult content and clinical experiences will need to be incorporated into gerontology programs. The adult-gerontology NP and CNS certification examinations will transition accordingly. Transitions are always challenging, but these changes will provide a needed workforce and more flexibility in practice opportunities for the adult-gerontology NP and CNS.

Another potential effect of the APRN Consensus Regulatory Model is an increase in the number of psychiatric/mental health NPs and CNSs. The mental health needs in this country and globally remain extraordinary and there are not a sufficient number of providers prepared to meet those needs. The Consensus Model clarifies and focuses the educational requirements necessary to qualify as a psychiatric APRN. Required courses include the APRN generalist or core courses—advanced physical assessment, pathophysiology, and pharmacology— and specialized psychiatric/mental health-focused coursework, omitting much of the adult or family-focused NP or CNS program coursework.

The Consensus Model requires broad educational preparation and certification to ensure that APRNs are prepared to practice in a variety of settings and meet the needs of the designated population (across-the-life-span, pediatric, adult-gerontology, women's health, neonatal, or psych/mental health). However, the model also provides important flexibility for APRNs to be prepared in specialty areas that currently exist or will be needed in the future. Licensure will occur at the role and population level—for example, as a family NP or as an across-the-lifespan CRNA. The model will not require licensure for narrowly defined areas of practice (such as diabetes care), but will rely instead on professional organizations to establish requirements and standards of practice for specialty areas. APRNs will thus have the flexibility to specialize to meet current or emerging needs of distinct populations, such as those with diabetes or cancer. Specialization will also provide APRNs with the opportunity to evolve in their professional development and to have flexibility in employment.

The Consensus Model does require graduate preparation but does not specify a particular degree requirement. However, the model is complementary to and will remain relevant as APRN education and certification programs transition to the DNP and will have the same impact on the clinical practice of DNP graduates as for the current master's-prepared APRNs.

Summary

APRN practice is influenced by the political and policy environments at all levels, including institutional, local, state, and federal. Governmental policies impact healthcare access, cost, and quality. The current efforts to implement healthcare reform—perhaps even more intense than in the Clinton era of the 1990s—provide opportunities for APRNs, if they are prepared with the knowledge, skills, and political will to take on these challenges and opportunities to address the issues and policy concerns involved in this debate. How APRNs address the cost, quality, and access issues will depend on the vibrancy not only of APRN organizations but also of individual APRNs. The Consensus Model will strongly support and position APRNs for the growing opportunities of the future. But the significant role that APRNs can and should play in improving quality of care in the United States can only be achieved through active and continued efforts of the APRN community as a whole.

SUGGESTED LEARNING EXERCISES

1. Identify an area of dissatisfaction or concern in today's healthcare system. Detail strategies that could be used to create change or improvement in this area.

2. Identify a cohort or population in your own or someone else's practice and access and analyze outcome data for one or more measures. Compare outcomes over time. Develop strategies to improve these outcomes.

3. Obtain the nurse-practice act in your state and determine whether it is compatible with the *Consensus Model for APRN Regulation: Licensure, Accreditation, Certification & Education* (2008). If not, identify the changes that would have to be made to make it compatible. Develop a strategic plan that includes stakeholders and processes for implementing the Consensus Model within your state.

4. Access workforce data in your state and compare the number of primary care physicians per capita, the percentage of IMGs, and the number of APRNs to national data. How easy was it to access data on APRNs in your state? What sources did you use? How accurate do you believe these data are? Identify a strategy for developing a comprehensive database for all APRNs in your state.

References

1. Hussey, P, Anderson, G, Berthelot, JM, Feek, C, Kelley, E, Osborn, R, et al. (2008). Trends in socioeconomic disparities in health care quality in four countries. *International J Quality in Health Care: J of the International Society for Quality in Health Care/ISQua* 20(1):53–61.

2. Hussey, PS, Anderson, GF, Osborn, R, Feek, C, McLaughlin, V, Millar, J, et al. (2004). How does the quality of care compare in five countries? *Health Affairs (Project Hope)* 23(3):89–99.

3. Iglehart, JK. (1999). The American health care system—expenditures. *N Engl J Med* 340(1):70–76.

4. Inflationdata.com. (2009). *Current inflation: inflation rate in percent for Jan 2000–present.* http://inflationdata.com/inflation/Inflation_Rate/CurrentInflation.asp. Accessed August 17, 2009.

5. Smerd, J. (2009). *Health care cost inflation appears to slow, but statistics can be misleading.* http://www.workforce.com/section/00/article/26/43/62.php. Accessed August 17, 2009.

6. Keehan, S, Sisko, A, Truffer, C, Smith, S, Cowan, C, Poisal, J, et al. (2008). Health spending projections through 2017: the baby-boom generation is coming to Medicare. *Health Affairs (Project Hope)* 27(2):145–155.

7. Centers for Disease Control and Prevention. (2008). *Chronic disease overview.* http://www.cdc.gov/NCCdphp/overview.htm#2. Accessed August, 17, 2009.

8. Brown, SA, and Grimes, DE. (1995). A meta-analysis of nurse practitioners and nurse-midwives in primary care. *Nurs Res* 44(6):332–339.

9. Kane, RL, Garrard, J, Skay, CL, Radosevich, DM, Buchanan, JL, McDermott, SM, et al. (1989). Effects of a geriatric nurse practitioner on process and outcome of nursing home care. *Am J Public Health* 79(9):1271–1277.

10. Mullinix, C, and Bucholtz, DP. (2009). Role and quality of nurse practitioner practice: a policy issue. *Nurs Outlook* 57(2):93–98.

11. Mundinger, MO, Kane, RL, Lenz, ER, Totten, AM, Tsai, WY, Cleary, PD, et al. (2000). Primary care outcomes in patients treated by nurse practitioners or physicians: a randomized trial. *JAMA* 283(1):59–68.

12. Sox, HC, Jr. (1979). Quality of patient care by nurse practitioners and physician's assistants: a ten-year perspective. *Ann Intern Med* 91(3):459–468.

13. Spitzer, WO, Sackett, DL, Sibley, JC, Roberts, RS, Gent, M, Kergin, DJ, et al. (1990). 1965–1990: 25th anniversary of nurse practitioners. A classic manuscript reprinted in celebration of 25 years of progress. The Burlington randomized trial of the nurse practitioner, 1971–2. *J Am Acad NPs* 2(3):93–99.

14. American Academy of Family Physicians. (2009). *Median and mean 2007 individual income before taxes (in thousands of dollars) of family physicians, July 2008.* http://www.aafp.org/online/en/home/aboutus/specialty/facts/15.htm. Accessed December 22, 2009.

15. American Academy of Nurse Practitioners. (2007). *2007 AANP National NP Compensation Survey.* http://aanp.org/NR/rdonlyres/AD41DD8D-FD16-4F84-968C-F7192A0E79D6/0/NPCompensation2007.pdf 2. Accessed August 17, 2009.

16. Hillstead, R, Bigelow, J, Bower, A, Girosi, F, Meili, R, Scoville, R, et al. (2005). Can electronic medical record systems transform health care? Potential health benefits, savings, and costs. *Health Affairs (Project Hope)* 24(5):1103–1117.

17. Taylor, R, Bower, A, Girosi, F, Bigelow, J, Fonkych, K, and Hillestad, R. (2005). Promoting health information technology: is there a case for more aggressive government action?*Health Affairs (Project Hope)* 24(5):1234–1245.

18. Burt, CW, and Sisk, JE. (2005). Which physicians and practices are using electronic medical records? *Health Affairs (Project Hope)* 24(5):1334–1343.

19. DesRoches, CM, Campbell, EG, Rao, SR, Donelan, K, Ferris, TG, Jha, A, et al. (2008). Electronic health records in ambulatory care—a national survey of physicians. *N Engl J Med* 359(1):50–60.

20. Obama: All medical records computerized by 2014. *The Industry Standard.* Available at http://www.thestandard.com/new/2009/01/12/obama-says-all-medical-records-computerized-2014.

21. Centers for Medicare and Medicaid. (2009). *Medicare and Medicaid health information technology: Title IV of the American recovery and reinvestment act.* http://www.cms.hhs.gov/apps/media/press/factsheet.asp?Counter=3466&intNumPerPage=10&checkDate=&checkKey=&srchType=1&numDays=3500&srchOpt=0&srchData=&keywordType=All&chkNewsType=6&intPage=&showAll=&pYear=&year=&desc=&cboOrder=date. Accessed August 17, 2009.

22. Hu HT, and O'Malley, AS. (2007). *Exodus of male physicians from primary care drives shift to specialty practice.* Tracking Report No.17. Center for Studying Health System Change, Washington, DC.

23. National Residency Matching Program. (2009). *Results and data: 2009 main residency match.* National Residency Matching Program, Washington, DC.

24. American College of Physicians. (2009). Nurse practitioners in primary care. *American College of Physicians Policy Monograph.* American College of Physicians, Philadelphia.

25. Rowland, D, Hoffman, C, and McGinn-Shapiro, M. (2009). *Focus on health reform: health care for the middle class: more costs and less coverage.* No. #7951. Kaiser Family Foundation, Menlo Park, CA.

26. Reed, M, Fung, V, Price, M, Brand, R, Benedetti, N, Derose, SF, et al. (2009). High-deductible health insurance plans: efforts to sharpen a blunt instrument. *Health Affairs (Project Hope)* 28(4): 1145–1154.

27. Grumbach, K, Hart, LG, Mertz, E, Coffman, J, and Palazzo, L. (2003). Who is caring for the underserved? A comparison of primary care physicians and nonphysician clinicians in California and Washington. *Ann Fam Med* 1(2):97–104.

28. Bohmer, R. (2007). The rise of in-store clinics—threat or opportunity? *N Engl J Med* 356(8): 765–768.

29. Mehrotra, A, Wang, MC, Lave, JR, Adams, JL, and McGlynn, EA. (2008). Retail clinics, primary care physicians, and emergency departments: a comparison of patients' visits. *Health Affairs (Project Hope)* 27(5):1272–1282.

30. APRN Consensus Work Group and the National Council of State Boards of Nursing APRN Advisory Committee. *Consensus Model for APRN Regulation: Licensure, Accreditation, Certification and Education.* http://www.aacn.nche.edu/education/pdf/APRNReport.pdf. Accessed November 26, 2009.

Index

Note: Page numbers followed by "b," "f," and "t" indicate boxes, figures, and tables, respectively.